Pharmacology essentials for Technicians

Jennifer Danielson, PharmD, MBA, CDE

University of Washington School of Pharmacy

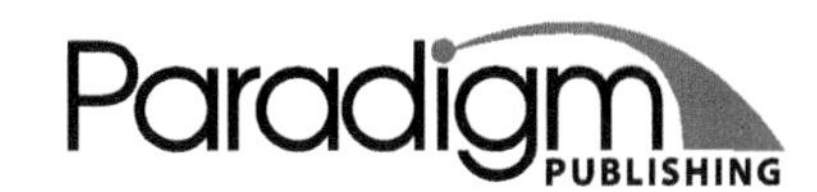

St. Paul • Los Angeles • Indianapolis

Developmental Editor Brenda Palo
Production Director Deanna Quinn
Supplements Editor Nancy Papsin
Cover and Text Designer Leslie Anderson
Sr. Production Specialist Jaana Bykonich
Copy Editor Laura Poole
Proofreader Melanie Hagge
Indexer Sandi Schroeder
Cover Images Royalty free (upper); Getty Images (lower)

Photo Credits: **2** © Paradigm Publishing, Inc.; **14** (Top) Courtesy of Tova Wiegand Green; **14** (Bottom) Courtesy of Mylan, Inc.; **15** © Paradigm Publishing, Inc.; **20** Shutterstock; **34** Shutterstock; **46** © Paradigm Publishing, Inc.; **58** Shutterstock; **63** Centers for Disease Control and Prevention; **74** Shutterstock; **79** Custom Medical Stock Photo, Inc.; **80** Custom Medical Stock Photo, Inc.; **83** (Top) Custom Medical Stock Photo, Inc.; **83** (Middle) Custom Medical Stock Photo, Inc.; **83** (Bottom) Custom Medical Stock Photo, Inc.; **89** © Allen W. Mathies, MD; **94** Shutterstock; **103** Reproduced with permission by Pfizer Inc.; **110** Shutterstock; **123** Reprinted with permission by Novartis; **127** © 2010 Rod Brouhard (http://firstaid.about.com/) Used with permission of About Inc., which can be found online at www.about.com. All rights reserved; **131** Shutterstock; **147** Shutterstock; **152** © Abbott Laboratories, used by permission; **153** (Left) Reproduced with permission by Purdue Pharma L.P.; **153** (Right) Reproduced with permission by Purdue Pharma L.P.; **164** Shutterstock; **175** Shutterstock; **176** © RP Fighting Blindness; **181** Public Domain; **196** Shutterstock; **200** James Gathany; **208** © George Brainard; **210** © Paradigm Publishing, Inc.; **217** © Paradigm Publishing, Inc.; **221** © Paradigm Publishing, Inc.; **226** Reproduced with permission by Bristol-Myers Squibb; **232** istockphoto.com; **235** Custom Medical Stock Photo, Inc.; **236** (Top Left) Shutterstock; **236** (Top Right) Shutterstock; **236** (Bottom Left) istockphoto.com; **236** (Bottom Right) © Paradigm Publishing, Inc.; **250** Shutterstock; **254** Reproduced with permission by Pfizer Inc.; **256** © Paradigm Publishing, Inc.; **258** © Paradigm Publishing, Inc.; **262** Public Domain; **265** Reproduced with permission of Shannon Hopson; **269** © Paradigm Publishing, Inc.; **273** Shutterstock; **275** © Bart's Medical Library/Phototake; **282** © Barry Slaven, MD, PhD/Phototake; **284** (Top) © Abbott Laboratories, used by permission; **284** (Bottom) © Paradigm Publishing, Inc.; **288** Shutterstock; **299** © Eli Lilly and Company, used by permission; **302** (Top) Barbara Mikula/AcclaimImages.com; **302** (Bottom) © Eli Lilly and Company, used by permission; **304** © Paradigm Publishing, Inc.; **310** Shutterstock; **322** (Top) © Paradigm Publishing, Inc.; **322** (Middle) Reproduced with permission by Merck & Co., Inc.; **322** (Bottom) Used by permission from Mayer Laboratories, Inc.; **323** © Pulse Picture Library/CMP Images/Phototake; **327** Public Domain; **332** Shutterstock; **337** © Paradigm Publishing, Inc.; **350** Shutterstock; **364** Shutterstock; **369** © Paradigm Publishing, Inc.; **373** © Paradigm Publishing, Inc.; **377** Reproduced with permission by Safety-Med Products, Inc.; **378** Reproduced with permission by Baker, Inc.; **379** © Paradigm Publishing, Inc.; **380** (Left) © Paradigm Publishing, Inc.; **380** (Right) © Paradigm Publishing, Inc.

ISBN 978-0-76383-867-6 (textbook)
ISBN 978-0-76383-870-6 (textbook + CD)

875 Montreal Way
St. Paul, MN 55102
Email: educate@emcp.com
Website: www.emcp.com

Printed in the United States of America

19 18 17 16 15 14 4 5 6 7 8 9 10

Dedicated to my daughters,
Ellen and Addison,
my little book writers.

A special thanks to my husband, Dan, for his patience as I spent many late-night hours working on this book by the glow of the computer screen. And, thanks to Connie Francis, my high school English teacher, the person who really taught me to write.

Brief Contents

Contents

Preface

Pharmacology Essentials for Technicians covers the full range of pharmacology concepts at the need-to-know level in a combined visual- and text-based approach. The emphasis is on presenting the common conditions and drug therapies that pharmacy technicians will encounter on a daily basis in both outpatient and inpatient work. Chapters are short, but comprehensive. No words are wasted, tables and photos are abundant, and reading is kept to a minimum.

Written on the foundation of the ASHP model curriculum, the textbook teaches students the competencies required in a retail, community, or institutional pharmacy setting. Aspiring technicians who complete a pharmacology course using this text will be able to

- Employ the methods for learning that are best suited to their individual learning styles
- Distinguish the normal and abnormal physiology of the body's major organ systems
- Define and correctly use the terms related to commonly used drugs and drug therapies
- Describe what happens when drugs enter the body and how they produce their effects
- List the major classifications of the drugs that affect each body system
- State the most common drugs in each classification and describe their main actions and indications
- Describe the common side effects or adverse reactions in each class of drugs

In addition to its focus on the essentials of pharmacology, the book offers a unique emphasis on addressing students' differing learning styles as identified in the Pharmacists' Inventory of Learning Styles (PILS), developed by Zubin Austin, PhD, University of Toronto. Chapter 1 introduces the concept of learning styles and the range of such styles (including auditory, visual, kinesthetic, musical, abstract, concrete, creative, and analytical). Students are encouraged to take the PILS assessment to identify their own preferred styles (dominant and secondary) and then watch for the *YourPILS* Study Tips throughout the book that relate to their particular learning style(s).

Organization of the Text

The 21 chapters of *Pharmacology Essentials for Technicians* are grouped into units based (after the introductory chapters) on the standard classification of body systems:

Unit 1: Introduction, Chapters 1–2

Unit 2: Drugs for the Immune System, Chapters 3–4

Unit 3: Drugs for the Integumentary and Skeletal Systems, Chapters 5–6

Unit 4: Drugs for the Nervous, Muscular, and Sensory Systems, Chapters 7–11

Unit 5: Drugs for the Cardiovascular and Respiratory Systems, Chapters 12–14

Unit 6: Drugs for the Digestive and Endocrine Systems, Chapters 15–17

Unit 7: Drugs for the Genitourinary System, Chapters 18–19

Unit 8: Drugs for Specialized Therapies, Chapters 20–21

For each body system, students review basic anatomy and physiology concepts as well as common diseases. Then they study the drug classes developed to treat those diseases. This structure allows readers to gain an understanding of how the disease or disorder occurs and how the commonly used drug classes work on the problem.

Appendix A titled *The Pharmacists' Inventory of Learning Styles,* offers the assessment students complete to identify their dominant learning styles, as discussed in Chapter 1. Appendix B presents recommendations for preventing dispensing errors with products that have look-alike or sound-alike drug names. The book's first index highlights the drug names and the second index highlights the key topics discussed in the chapters.

Chapter Features

Each body system chapter opens with learning objectives and an overview of the chapter content. The first major section of the chapter deals with key aspects of the anatomy and physiology for the particular body system, illustrated with colorful drawings that help students visualize the concepts. Figure captions guide students to connect anatomy and physiology with drug therapy and pharmacy practice notes.

Following this material is a section on the major diseases and illnesses that originate in or affect the body system. Photos and tables help capture and summarize the information visually for quick learning and retention. Drug therapies used by medical professionals to address the major diseases form the next content section, supplemented by numerous tables that identify drugs by generic/brand name, dosage form, route of administration, and common dose. Drug warning sticker icons in the page margins highlight important drug information that technicians (as well as patients) must be aware of, such as avoiding alcohol while taking the medication, shaking the drug solution before using it, refrigerating the medication, and taking the drug with food. Additional photos of drug therapies and drug labels supplement students' awareness of dosing and use issues, as well as look-alike and sound-alike drug names concerns.

YourPILS boxes provide tips for learning the material based on students' pharmacy-based learning styles. *Professional Focus* margin features alert students to important on-the-job considerations that aid success as a pharmacy technician.

End-of-the-chapter activities launch with a *Chapter Summary. Chapter Review* activities include a set of multiple-choice questions (*Review the Basics*), a set of matching items (*Know the Drugs*), short-answer questions (*Put It Together*), and critical thinking challenges (*Think It Through*), the final challenge involving researching on the Internet.

Additional Student Resources

In addition to in-chapter content and resources, several print and electronic resources are provided for student practice and mastery of pharmacology essentials.

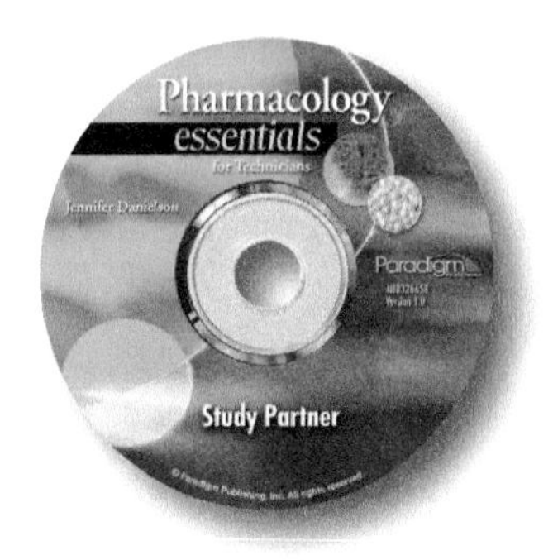

Study Partner CD

The Study Partner CD included with each textbook contains the following tools to support student learning:

- Audio drug names in MP3 format
- Games for thorough and engaging chapter content review
- Quizzes in Practice or Reported modes
- Glossary content at both chapter and book level

Student Internet Resource Center

The Internet Resource Center for this title, located at www.emcp.net/pharmessentials, provides additional resources, such as Spanish for Pharmacy Technicians, guidelines for dispensing medications, links to professional resources, and much more. Access to the site is free.

eBook

For students who prefer studying with an eBook, this text is available in an electronic form. The Web-based, password-protected eBook features dynamic navigation tools, including bookmarking, a linked table of contents, and the ability to jump to a specific page. The eBook format also supports helpful study tools, such as highlighting and note taking.

Resources for the Instructor

A printed *Instructor's Guide*, an Instructor Resources CD, and an Instructor's Internet Resource Center are provided with *Pharmacology Essentials for Technicians* to help instructors plan their courses and assess student learning.

Instructor's Guide and CD with EXAMView

The print *Instructor's Guide* offers course planning tools, suggested syllabi, chapter-specific teaching hints, and answers for all end-of-chapter exercises.

All of the resources from the print *Instructor's Guide* are also provided on the Instructor Resources CD. In addition, the CD includes the EXAMView Assessment Suite, a full-featured computerized test generator offering instructors a wide variety of options for generating both print and online tests. The test bank provides 35 questions for each chapter. Instructors can create custom tests using the chapter item banks and edit questions or add new items of their own design.

Distance-learning files, a set of content files for course management systems, are provided to instructors. Content includes chapter outlines, PowerPoint presentations, and quizzes.

Instructor's Internet Resource Center

All of the resources from the print *Instructor's Guide* and Instructor Resources CD are available in electronic format on the password-protected Instructor's section of the Internet Resource Center for this title at www.emcp.net/pharmessentials.

Additional Pharmacy Technician Textbooks from Paradigm

In addition to *Pharmacology Essentials for Technicians*, Paradigm Publishing, Inc. offers other titles designed specifically for the pharmacy technician curriculum:

Pharmacy Calculations for Technicians, Fourth Edition
Pharmacy Practice, Fourth Edition
Pharmacology for Technicians, Fourth Edition
Pharmacology for Technicians Workbook, Fourth Edition
Pharmacy Labs for Technicians

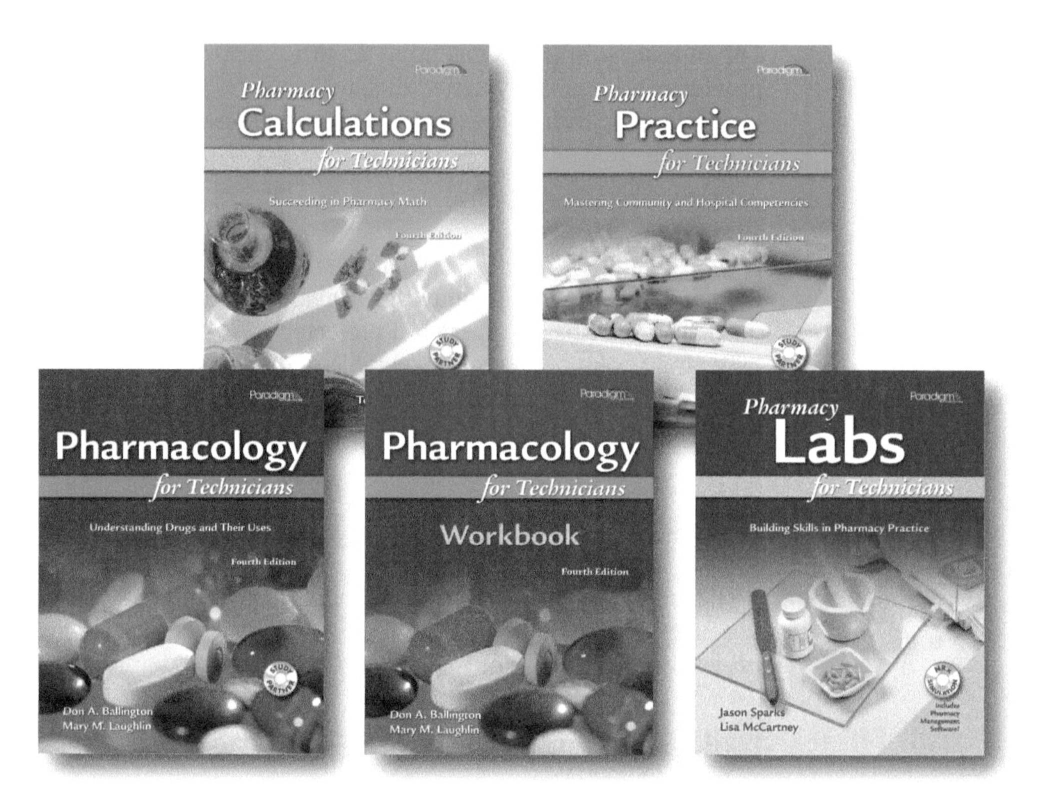

About the Author

Jennifer Danielson, PharmD, MBA, CDE, received her BS in pharmacy in 1993 from Drake University in Iowa and her PharmD from the University of Colorado in 2009. She also earned an MBA from Drake University. She is currently Associate Director of Experiential Education and Clinical Assistant Professor at the University of Washington School of Pharmacy. After a few years in publishing at the American Society of Health-System Pharmacists (ASHP), Ms. Danielson entered pharmacy academia as Director of Experiential Programs for Oregon State University, followed by a similar position at Campbell University in North Carolina. While at Campbell she taught in the introductory practice lab, communications, and drug information courses and lectured for selected topics in pharmacotherapeutics. In 2004, she became Lead Instructor and Department Chair for the Pharmacy Technician Program at Pikes Peak Community College in Colorado Springs where she taught pharmacology, calculations, pharmacy law, and community pharmacy practice. Before moving in 2007 to her current home in Seattle, she coordinated experiential education for the Nontraditional PharmD Program at the University of Colorado. Her practice interests are in diabetes care, for which she has been certified as a diabetes educator since 2000.

Acknowledgments

The author and editors would like to say a special thank you to the following contributing writers of Chapter 21 for sharing their oncology expertise:

Andrea Iannucci, PharmD, BCOP
Oncology Pharmacy Specialist
Clinical Professor, University of California San Francisco School of Pharmacy
University of California Davis Medical Center
Sacramento, California

Jeanne M. Reed, PharmD, BCOP
Oncology Pharmacy Specialist
Clinical Assistant Professor, University of California San Francisco School of Pharmacy
University of California Davis Medical Center
Sacramento, California

Tanja Bell
Oncology Clinical Technician
University of California Davis Medical Center, Inpatient Pharmacy
Sacramento, California

We would also like to thank the many reviewers who participated in the development of *Pharmacology Essentials for Technicians*.

Robert Aanonsen, CPhT
Platt College
Tulsa, Oklahoma

Catherine Ballard, PharmD
Cape Fear Community College
Wilmington, North Carolina

Danika Braaten, RPhT, CPhT
Northland Community and Technical College
East Grand Forks, Minnesota

Cheryl Buckholz
Chemeketa Community College
Salem, Oregon

Andrea Curry, BS, CPhT
Concorde Career College
Memphis, Tennessee

George Fakhoury, MD, DORCP, CMA (AAMA)
Heald College
San Francisco, California

Kristie Fitzgerald, BS
Salt Lake Community College
Salt Lake City, Utah

Steve Forshier, MEd, RT
Pima Medical Institute
Mesa, Arizona

Donna Guisado, RDA, BSOM
North-West College
West Covina, California

Paula Lambert, BS, MEd, CPhT
North Idaho College
Coeur d'Alene, Idaho

Nancy Lim, RPh, PhD
Lone Star College—North Harris
Houston, Texas

Michelle McCranie, CPhT
Ogeechee Technical College
Statesboro, Georgia

Nicole Motes, CPhT
Pikes Peak Community College
Colorado Springs, Colorado

Rebecca Schonscheck, CPhT
High-Tech Institute
Phoenix, Arizona

Sandi Tschritter, BA, CPhT
Spokane Community College
Spokane, Washington

Judy Weisbard, MPA, BS, CPhT
CuraScript Specialty Pharmacy
Orlando, Florida

In addition, we would like to offer a particular thank you to Leonard Lichtblau, PhD, and Shawn McPartland, MD, JD, CPhT, for their careful and helpful review of early pages of the textbook content and the end-of-chapter materials. Thanks also go to Andrew J. Berry, PharmD Graduate (2010) and Pharmacy Resident UC Davis, for his content contributions.

Finally, Cheryl Aiken, PharmD, RPh, of Vermont Technical College in Brattleboro, prepared the test bank materials for the Instructor's Guide CD. For the Study Partner CD, Andrew S. Bzowyckyj, PharmD, of Minneapolis, Minnesota, consulted on the drug names audio; Jeff Johnson of Minneapolis, Minnesota, created the games content; and Judy Peterson of Two Harbors, Minnesota, prepared the quiz materials. Ms. Peterson also prepared the PowerPoint slides. We thank them for their contributions.

The author and editorial staff invite your feedback on the text and its supplements. Please reach us by clicking the "Contact Us" link at www.emcp.net/pharmessentials.

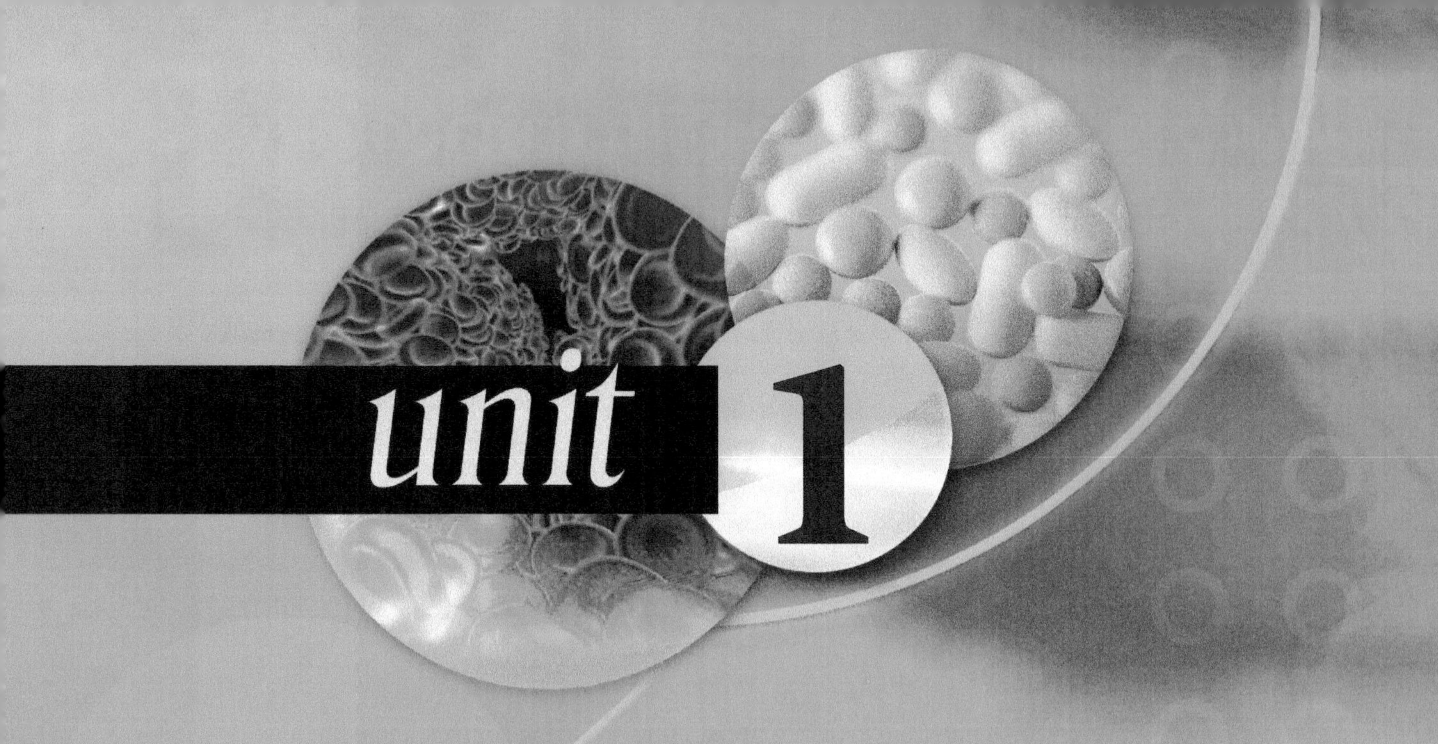

Introduction

Chapter 1 Studying Pharmacology

LEARNING OBJECTIVES

- Define the phases of pharmacology and drug therapy.
- Perform a learning styles inventory to reveal your preferred learning style(s).
- Determine which methods for learning pharmacology are compatible with your learning style(s).
- Describe major drug classes, controlled substances schedules, pregnancy categories, prescription versus over-the-counter regulations, and how drugs are classified by brand/generic names.
- Distinguish routes of administration and common dosage forms.

Interactive self-quizzes, games, audio files, and glossaries help you to learn drug names and facts.

Drugs come from a variety of naturally occurring sources, including plants, animals, and minerals. Drugs also can be produced via synthetic processes and bioengineering methods. Ultimately, drugs are used for preventing, treating, and curing illness. **Pharmacology**, simply put, is the study of how drugs from these various sources work inside the body for their intended purposes.

Pharmacology seeks to define the mechanism by which a drug works. Such definitions describe drug mechanisms of action on the molecular level, involving drug receptors and physiologic processes. Therefore, you will probably find it useful to understand a few common terms and concepts that describe how drugs exert their effects. This chapter introduces you to drug classifications and suggests methods for learning about the ways drugs work within these classes, or categories.

Understanding basic **physiology** (the study of normal body function) is useful for learning how drugs affect body processes. Therefore, most chapters begin with practical information about the way each body system works under typical conditions. When it is relevant, the corresponding **pathophysiology** (the study of abnormal body processes or disease) is then described, followed by a presentation of the drugs used to treat the pathophysiology. When you understand what goes wrong in the body, you will be better prepared to learn how a particular drug therapy works to correct or treat specific problems.

Phases of Pharmacology

Pharmacology is the study of a drug's action in the body. You may find it useful to think of pharmacology in phases (see Figure 1.1). Each phase focuses on a different part of the way drugs work, from how drugs are introduced into the body to how they behave in it. These phases dramatically affect a drug's ability to exert its desired effects.

Pharmaceutics is the study of how drugs are introduced to the body. For instance, medications are available in many oral dosage forms, such as capsules, tablets, and liquids. They are also spread on the skin, inhaled into the lungs, injected, and inserted. Pharmaceutics studies how these forms deliver drug to the body and achieve appropriate, desired drug absorption into the bloodstream. This chapter presents common drug dosage forms and routes of administration.

Pharmacokinetics is the study of how drugs are absorbed into the bloodstream (absorption), circulated to tissues throughout the body (distribution), inactivated (metabolized), and eliminated from the bloodstream over time (metabolism and excretion). Chapter 2 covers pharmacokinetic concepts in greater detail. Pharmacokinetic processes affect a drug's effectiveness, dosing schedule, and use.

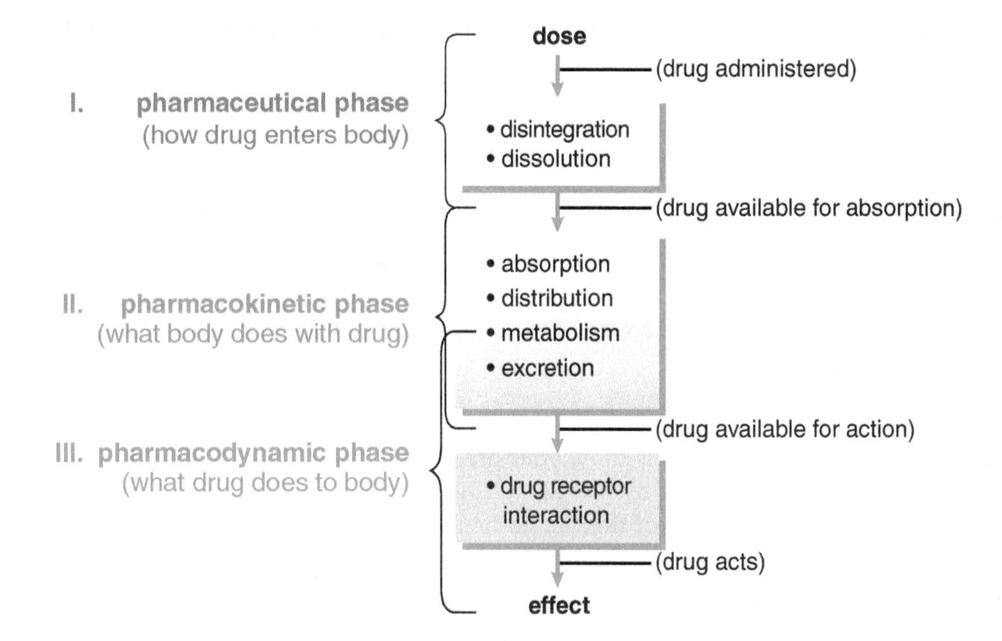

Figure 1.1
Phases of Pharmacology Therapy
For a drug to work, it must enter the bloodstream (I.), reach the site of action in a sufficient concentration (II.), and interact with appropriate receptors to cause a beneficial effect (III.).

Pharmacodynamics is the study of drugs and their receptors on the molecular level. It translates principles of chemistry to drug activity within the entire body. Pharmacodynamics is discussed in greater detail in Chapter 2. **Pharmacotherapeutics** (not pictured) is the study of how drugs are used in clinical practice for individual patients. To determine the most appropriate and beneficial drug to use for an individual patient, an understanding of pathophysiology, pharmacology, pharmaceutics, pharmacokinetics, and pharmacodynamics is necessary. Although pharmaceutics and pharmacokinetics can be considered laboratory sciences, pharmacotherapeutics is a clinical science because drugs are used and studied in real people.

Strategies for Learning Pharmacology

You may have heard that pharmacology is a challenging and demanding subject in pharmacy technician programs. In fact, many students would probably admit that the volume of information and new terminology to remember is daunting. You are being asked to learn hundreds of drug names and understand how the drugs work. Although this task can be formidable, we hope that this textbook will allow you to adopt some systematic and logical strategies for learning the material.

If you begin with an understanding of the human body's systems and then consider how each drug works on the body system(s), you can learn pharmacology *and* how to apply it. If you have not had many science courses in which anatomy or biological processes were covered, you may find this topic much like learning a new language. In a way, it *is* a new language. Medical terminology is based largely on Latin and is used extensively in the study of physiology. This text does *not* attempt to teach you medical terminology because there are many other quality texts and programs with that purpose. This text will define many key terms. We encourage you to keep a dictionary of medical terms handy so you can look up what you need as you study the basic physiology required to learn pharmacology essentials.

To best learn pharmacology, first break up the material into categories. For instance, pharmacology tends to be discussed in terms of drug classes—categories of drugs having similar characteristics. The drugs in each class work by a particular mechanism of action, behave in similar ways, and present many of the same side effects. Fortunately, drugs within a specific class are often given similar generic names, which can help your learning process. Once you learn a mechanism of action and common similarities for a drug class, you can then focus on learning the drug names associated with that class. (Admittedly, you must memorize the brand names that go with the generic drug names.)

In effect, you will learn a set of rules for each drug class and then connect the individual drugs to that set of rules. When you approach learning drug classes in this way, you will instantly know what a particular drug does and how it works by simply seeing or hearing its name. Of course, there are exceptions to these rules, particularly when it comes to side effects. First learning the commonalities that apply to all drugs in a class is easier than memorizing the individual characteristics of each drug one by one. Once you are aware of the drug class rules, you only have to remember the few exceptions.

Taking a Learning Styles Inventory

Once you know your preferred ways to receive, interpret, process, and demonstrate mastery of new knowledge, you can more efficiently and enjoyably learn any new subject or skill. In particular, learning pharmacology requires you to process a large volume of information. Many pharmacology students simply memorize facts without gaining a greater understanding. While some memorization—such as knowing generic versus brand drug names—is usually necessary at some point, relying on simple memorization often fails because there are simply too many details to remember. You will benefit by developing methods that work best for you so that you can understand and remember all you need to know from pharmacology.

Even after you complete your formal studies, you will find that lifelong learning is essential in pharmacy. The field is always changing and expanding, with new drugs coming to market regularly. Appreciating how you learn will help you to both find ways to retain large amounts of information as a student and develop new skills for learning and adapting in the workplace.

Everyone learns in different ways. For instance, some prefer to learn independently by reading alone (learning intrapersonally), whereas others prefer group interaction and discussion (learning interpersonally). Perhaps you are a concrete learner and like to deal with facts and details rather than abstract concepts. Maybe your study partner is an auditory learner who needs to hear new material out loud to remember it. Still other types of learners grasp new concepts best through:

- hands-on manipulation
- kinesthetic methods (pacing or dancing around the room while reviewing)
- logical reasoning and math
- music (studying with music playing or putting new information into a catchy tune or rhythmic phrase)
- practical approaches (boiling complex things down or arranging new concepts in your own words)
- speaking and writing
- visual presentations (needing to see words on a page to process them)
- visual-spatial methods (drawing pictures or diagrams)

Given the many ways that people learn, how can you find out your preferred methods, your own **learning styles**? You can perform a **learning styles inventory** and gain insight into how your brain works, how you prefer to receive information, understand it, and commit it to memory. Numerous learning styles inventory tools are published and available. Most are easy to use, and each has its unique take on learning styles.

David Kolb first described four learning styles (accommodators, assimilators, convergers, and divergers) in his well-known learning styles inventory in the 1980s and 1990s. His theory is based on two constructs. How you approach performing a skill (reflecting versus doing) is compared to how you process performing that new skill (experiencing versus thinking). The **Pharmacists' Inventory of Learning Styles (PILS)** is a learning styles tool that Zubin Austin adapted in 2003 from Kolb's theory. This tool works well for professionals in the pharmacy field because it is short and easy to administer, is less costly than other commercially published tools, and was developed specifically for pharmacists and individuals studying pharmacy. It is quite appropriate for your pharmacy technician studies because it uses pharmacy-specific descriptions and was validated for individuals with at least a high school education who have had some college-level coursework.

Figure 1.2 illustrates the four styles that Austin described and named: Enactors, Creators, Directors, and Producers. In only a few minutes' time, you can complete the questions and read the descriptions to learn your primary and secondary preferred learning styles. Go to Appendix A now and complete the PILS. Once you determine your preferred styles, you can use the "Your PILS" feature(s) in each chapter to find suggested exercises and activities that may help you learn the material in ways that make sense to you. Realize that everyone can learn using a variety of methods when necessary. But using methods compatible with your preferred styles makes learning easier and more stimulating.

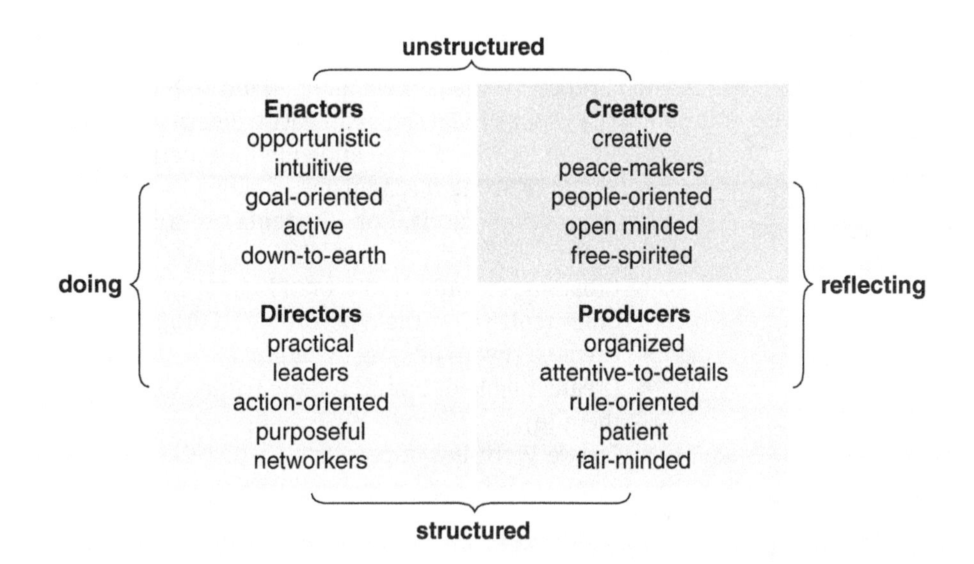

Figure 1.2
Core Constructs for PILS
Austin's PILS uses structured and unstructured learning as the vertical continuum in his learning styles adaptation, whereas Kolb used experiencing versus thinking in his original theory.

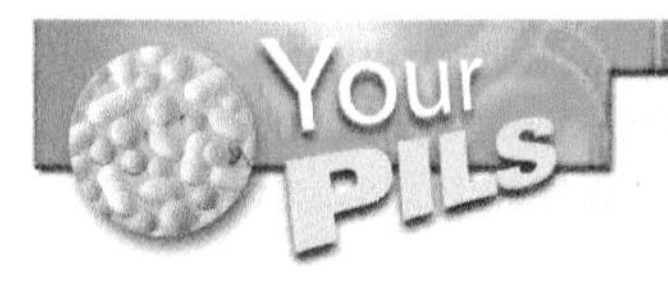

Take a few minutes now to go to Appendix A and complete the PILS assessment. Once you determine your preferred styles, you can refer to the "Your PILS" features (like this one) in each chapter for suggested exercises and activities that may help you learn the material in ways that make sense to you, based on your learning styles.

Drug Classifications

Drugs are categorized in a variety of ways, some based on legal divisions and others on mechanism of action. You will come to a thorough understanding of pharmacology and its application once you know the various ways drug categories are determined.

Brand versus Generic Drug Names

When a molecule is first discovered for its medicinal properties, its name is based on molecular structure and traditional chemical nomenclature. As the drug enters **Phase I clinical trials**, during which it is first tried in healthy human subjects, a **generic drug**

name is assigned by a government agency. If other drugs within the same family exert similar activity, the new drug's name is often somehow similar to the others in that class. During **Phase II and III clinical trials**, experimental drugs are tested in humans having the condition or disease the drug is supposed to treat.

As a drug nears the end of Phase III clinical trials and U.S. Food and Drug Administration (FDA) approval is sought, a proprietary or **brand name** is assigned by the company that will manufacture and sell it. Once a drug is approved by the FDA, it enters **Phase IV clinical trials**, called postmarketing study. The brand name can be trademarked and used for marketing purposes. It is usually easier to pronounce than the generic name, which makes marketing materials and advertising easier for the lay public to recognize and recall. During the first few years after a drug is approved, it is under patent and cannot be manufactured by any other company. Prescribers become familiar with trade names and often continue to use them even after the patent has expired.

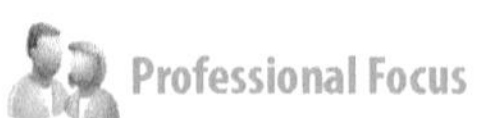

Professional Focus

When filling each prescription in the pharmacy, pause for a moment to state out loud the corresponding brand or generic name, write it out, and then recall one unique drug fact. Maybe it has a particular color or shape or is known for a particular side effect. Name its drug class or mechanism of action as you touch each tablet. As you work, quiz yourself with this hands-on strategy to learn drug names and keep on your toes!

Knowing both the brand and generic names of a drug is necessary because **generic substitution** is a regular practice. Physicians' prescriptions are often written in brand names, whereas in the pharmacy, prescriptions are often filled with generic product. Many pharmacies organize their drug inventory alphabetically by generic name. Thus, when a prescription for a brand product is received, the technician must make a mental switch or look up the generic name to locate the product on the shelf. Because generic names are often similar, you can easily determine a drug's class, mechanism of action, and common uses by simply knowing its generic name.

Although learning mechanisms of action is conceptual, learning brand and generic names involves memorization. Students use a variety of methods to memorize drug names:

- Create flash cards with a brand name on one side and its generic name on the other (color-code them according to drug class)
- Create a rhyme or song including all brand/generic names in a drug class
- Create a table of brand/generic names (leave some blanks and practice filling them in)
- Locate Web sites of products for pictures, graphics, and phonetic pronunciations

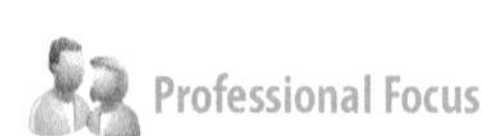

Professional Focus

One way to avoid mistakes is to bring with you both the hard-copy prescription form (the brand name is usually written on it) and the pharmacy-generated label (the generic name is usually on it) when you retrieve the product from the shelf. Compare the brand and generic names on the prescription, label, and product bottle before removing it from the shelf for counting and measuring.

Major Drug Classes

Medications are grouped into **major drug classes** according to their mechanism of action. All drugs that work in the same way are put into a particular class and usually given similar names with a common stem (see Table 1.1). Individual drug classes are then lumped into **therapeutic classes** according to their use on a particular body system. Drug classes in this text are discussed in relation to their therapeutic class. For instance, cardiovascular medications are discussed together in Chapter 12. Drug classes used to treat cardiovascular conditions include beta blockers, angiotensin-converting enzyme (ACE) inhibitors, calcium-channel blockers, and HMG-CoA reductase inhibitors (statins).

Because generic drug names within a class are often similar, learning drug actions and therapeutic uses can be relatively easy. However, you must be aware that these **"look-alike"** and **"sound-alike" drug names** are often a source of errors (see Appendix B for recommended precautions). You can also go to the Web site for the **Institute for Safe Medication Practices (ISMP)** and search for the confused drug names list. Anyone could inadvertently get two drugs within a drug class mixed up and dispense something incorrectly.

Prescription versus OTC Medications

Medications available only by prescription are considered **legend** or **prescription drugs**. These products are dispensed from the pharmacy on receipt of a prescription from a prescriber. Medications that can be bought without a prescription are called

Table 1.1 Common Drug Name Stems

Drug Class	Stem	Examples
ACE inhibitors	-pril	Lisinopril, enalapril
Angiotensin II-receptor inhibitors	-sartan	Losartan, valsartan
Antifungals	-azole	Fluconazole, miconazole
Antivirals	-vir	Acyclovir, ganciclovir
Benzodiazepines	-pam or -lam	Alprazolam, lorazepam
Beta blockers	-olol	Propranolol, atenolol
Cephalosporins	ceph- or cef-	Cephalexin, cefuroxime
Corticosteroids	-sone or -lone	Prednisone, triamcinolone
HMG CoA reductase inhibitors	-statin	Lovastatin, simvastatin
Macrolides	-thromycin	Erythromycin
Penicillins	-cillin	Amoxicillin, ampicillin
Proton-pump inhibitors	-prazole	Omeprazole
Quinolones	-floxacin	Ciprofloxacin, levofloxacin
Selective serotonin agonists	-triptan	Sumatriptan
Tetracyclines	-cycline	Doxycycline
Thiazolidinediones	-glitazones	Rosiglitazone
Tricyclic antidepressants	-triptyline	Amitriptyline, nortriptyline

over-the-counter (OTC) medications. In most cases, new drugs enter the market as prescription medications and then move to OTC status if they are safe enough to be used by patients without medical supervision. Knowing whether a drug is available via prescription or OTC helps you easily locate a requested medication. Prescription medications also have legal limitations to dispensing.

Spending time in a pharmacy is probably the most useful way to learn which drugs are available by prescription versus over the counter. Learning where each product is located—whether it is in drug stock behind the counter or on the shelves in the aisles—helps you keep legend separate from OTC medications. If that is not possible, take a look through your own medicine cabinet. As you pull out each bottle or package, you can see whether or not it is in a prescription vial. Stop at each brand name and recall from memory its associated generic name and drug class. Often, instructors teach OTC drugs as a separate group from prescription medications because learning them separately is helpful.

Controlled versus Noncontrolled Substances

Medications that have potential for abuse and dependence are categorized by the U.S. Drug Enforcement Agency (DEA) as **controlled substances**. These drugs are placed in one of five schedules, based on their degree of potential for abuse. **Schedule I** substances are illegal or only available for research or experimental purposes, whereas **Schedule II–V** drugs can be legally dispensed with restrictions on numbers of refills and quantities. Dispensing procedures and inventory control measures for controlled substances are strictly regulated at both the federal and state levels. Schedule II has the most stringent restrictions. It is crucial that all pharmacy staff be familiar with these rules and laws so as to protect patients as well as the pharmacy and its personnel. See Table 1.2 for a description of these controlled substances schedules.

Table 1.2 Controlled Substances Schedules

Schedule	Description	Examples	Restrictions
I	Drugs with no accepted medical use having highest potential for abuse. Illegal to possess, except for a few substances that can be used for research purposes (special registration and restrictions apply).	Crack, marijuana (cannabis), opium derivatives such as heroin, LSD, PCP, peyote	**Greatest**
II	Drugs with current accepted medical use having high potential for abuse. May lead to high physiological and psychological dependence.	Stimulants (amphetamines such as Ritalin), fentanyl, hydromorphone, morphine, methadone, meperidine, oxycodone, depressants (pentobarbital, secobarbital)	
III	Drugs with accepted medical use having some potential for abuse. May lead to moderate physiological but high psychological dependence.	Anabolic steroids, barbiturates, dronabinol, codeine in moderate amounts	
IV	Drugs with accepted medical use having lower potential for abuse. May lead to low physiological but moderate psychological dependence.	Appetite suppressants (sibutramine, phentermine), benzodiazepines, phenobarbital, propoxyphene, sleep aids (zolpidem, zaleplon)	
V	Drugs with accepted medical use with low potential for abuse. May lead to limited physiological or psychological dependence.	Codeine in small amounts (mostly cough syrups)	**Least**

In addition to the restrictions the DEA puts on these controlled substances, the sale of drugs considered **precursors** for making crystal methamphetamine is also limited in pharmacies. Pseudoephedrine and phenylpropanolamine are included in these restrictions. These medications have legitimate medical uses and when used properly do not cause dependence or abuse. They can be used, however, in making methamphetamine (a highly addictive and abused drug). Therefore, the sale of these drugs is limited, and they can be purchased only by patients over eighteen years old in most states. They must be stored behind the counter in the pharmacy.

Pregnancy Categories

To assess safety during pregnancy, a categorization system has been developed to help prescribers and patients determine the potential benefits and risks involved when a woman takes a medication while pregnant. All drugs marketed in the United States receive a **pregnancy categorization** (see Table 1.3). No drug is completely without side effects and 100% safe during pregnancy. However, some drugs are considered safe during pregnancy because they do not significantly cross through the placenta and enter the bloodstream of a developing fetus. Usually, the patient and her prescriber must weigh the urgency of and need for treating a particular condition with the potential adverse effects the medication may cause for the fetus.

Drugs that can cause birth defects or malformations in a developing fetus are called **teratogenic**. The degree of teratogenicity may be dependent on the stage of development of the fetus. For instance, some drugs can cause severe defects and even spontaneous abortion early in a pregnancy (first trimester) but have little to no effect late in the pregnancy (third trimester). Still other drugs are considered dangerous at all times during pregnancy.

Because it is difficult to conduct studies in pregnant subjects, categorization of risk is often based on data from animal studies. Consequently, definitive facts about risk to a mother or her developing fetus are not known. These pregnancy categories were developed with this limitation in mind.

Related to pregnancy and a drug's ability to cross the placenta is a drug's ability to enter breast milk and thus be ingested by an infant who is breast-feeding. Although no special categorization system is available for breast-feeding characteristics, such information is available through reputable sources and drug manufacturers. Pharmacy technicians should refer patients inquiring about drug safety during breast-feeding to the pharmacist, who can consult with proper sources and discuss options.

Table 1.3 Pregnancy Categories

Category	Definition
A	Controlled studies show no risk. Adequate, well-controlled studies in pregnant women have failed to demonstrate risk to the fetus.
B	No evidence of risk to humans. Animal findings show risk, but human findings do not. *Or* If no adequate human studies have been done, animal findings are negative.
C	Risk cannot be ruled out. Human studies are lacking, and animal studies are either positive for fetal risk or lacking. *Or* No animal studies have been conducted, and there are no adequate and well-controlled studies in pregnant women to determine risk. However, potential benefits may justify potential risks.
D	Positive evidence of risk. Investigational or postmarketing data show risk to the fetus. Nevertheless, potential benefits may outweigh potential risks. If needed in a life-threatening situation or a serious disease, the drug may be acceptable if safer drugs cannot be used or are ineffective.
X	Contraindicated in pregnancy. Studies in animals or humans, or investigational or postmarketing reports have shown fetal risk that clearly outweighs any possible benefit to the patient.

Alternative and Complementary Treatments

Patients use many forms of treatment besides those generally accepted and recognized by **Western medicine** (often called traditional medicine). In the United States, we tend to think of drug therapy primarily in terms of prescription and OTC products. We forget sometimes about herbal products, vitamins, and dietary supplements. Because Western medicine relies on the scientific method, whereby truth is determined only through observation and controlled experimentation, we tend to discount therapies that do not have large volumes of published studies and research data to support them.

Many alternative therapies come from **Eastern medicine**, an older type of medicine that uses many herbs and alternative therapies and recognizes a person's spiritual being and balance. Eastern medicine looks at the whole person, along with spiritual beliefs, and uses natural ingredients to promote and achieve health. Western medicine is highly influenced by objective evidence and its treatment modalities tend to be summoned only when something is wrong. Increasingly, practitioners of Western medicine are recognizing that natural, holistic, and alternative strategies for treatment can complement traditional methods to achieve greater health and overall well-being.

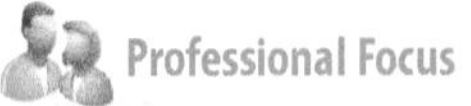

Professional Focus

If the pharmacy where you work sells vitamins and herbal products, take some time to learn about them and why patients use them. Supporting patients' choices for overall health and well-being requires more than just filling prescriptions accurately. Recognizing the whole person—not just a patient's medical condition and corresponding drugs—improves patient care and customer service. Alternative treatments can augment traditional drug therapy to improve ultimate outcomes.

The FDA considers vitamins and herbal products to be **dietary and nutritional supplements** and regulates them as food, not as drugs. They are not regulated for safety and efficacy as are prescription or OTC products. Many have legitimate uses, and others have yet to be proven to have beneficial drug activity. Dietary supplements are permitted to claim that they can support the structure, function, or health of the body, but they may not be marketed for the treatment of, prevention of, or cure for a specific disease or condition. Some of these products interact with prescription or OTC drugs, so patients must realize that even natural products can be harmful. Pharmacists can help patients weigh the potential benefits with the risks (including financial outlay) of these products before choosing to buy them. This text includes discussion of the most commonly used herbal and natural products as they relate to each body system, but it is not a comprehensive guide.

Knowledge of a few alternative medicine terms is useful. **Homeopathy** involves treating an ailment with a substance, usually an herb, that causes an effect similar to the ailment itself. However, multiple dilutions are made of the herb so that only the "essence" of its activity remains in the final product. **Chinese medicine** uses Eastern medical philosophies of holistic health. It employs the balance of yin and yang and often uses **acupuncture** and herbs. Acupuncture inserts needles at specific points on the body to unblock energy channels, whereas **acupressure** applies pressure to those points to enhance energy flow. Acupuncture and acupressure started out in Eastern and Chinese medicine practices, and they are widely used in the United States today to augment other therapies.

Chiropractic therapy may not be considered Eastern medicine, but it uses similar approaches. Chiropractic therapy uses nondrug modalities such as manipulation to achieve better body alignment and health. It can also employ natural and herbal products. **Ayurveda** is a form of East Indian medicine that involves spiritual and whole-body well-being and employs changes in diet and lifestyle in its treatment modalities. **Biofeedback** is another method used to control body function. Patients are taught to use mental exercise and relaxation to slow their heartbeat, lower blood pressure, and reduce stomach problems. Biofeedback has also been useful against lower back problems and tension headaches.

Common Pharmacy Abbreviations and Terms

Although there is a movement to limit using too many abbreviations, they are still used extensively for ordering, preparing, and administering drug therapy. Most prescribers write prescriptions and medical orders by using abbreviations. Familiarity with these **prescribing terms** and **pharmacy abbreviations** is essential for interpreting orders quickly and dispensing them accurately.

Many abbreviations used in medicine and prescribing are based on Latin or Greek terms. Thus, knowing the Latin terms can sometimes help you remember the abbreviation. Others are simply shortened versions of English terms. Learning these terms and abbreviations may feel like learning a different language, but you must commit them to memory to work efficiently in the pharmacy.

Medication Errors

Proper familiarity with common pharmacy terms and abbreviations also requires that you be aware of their propensity for causing medication errors. A **medication error** is an event in which a patient is harmed by a medication in some way that could have been prevented. The mistake could be made on the part of the prescriber writing an order, the pharmacy personnel dispensing a medication, a nurse or caregiver administering a drug, or the patient taking the medication. Thousands of patients are hospitalized every year as a result of medication errors and misuse. Working with medications and patients on the front line makes the job pharmacists and technicians do crucial to ensuring good patient care. Poor handwriting, bad communication, and unfamiliarity with proper meaning and use of abbreviations create opportunities for mix-ups and mistakes. Technicians must remain diligent in their use and interpretation of abbreviations to avoid harm to patients.

Correct drug administration involves giving the right drug to the right patient at the right time in the appropriate strength and route (see Figure 1.3). Technicians should stop to ask, "Is this right?" or "Does it make sense?" for each of these components of a prescription or medication order. Questions to ask yourself are:

- Is the correct patient listed on the drug order?
- Does the dose ordered seem to make sense for this drug?
- Does the strength ordered make sense for the drug and its dosage form?
- Is the frequency or timing of doses appropriate for this drug?
- Does the route of administration match up to the drug, its intended use, and the dosage form ordered?

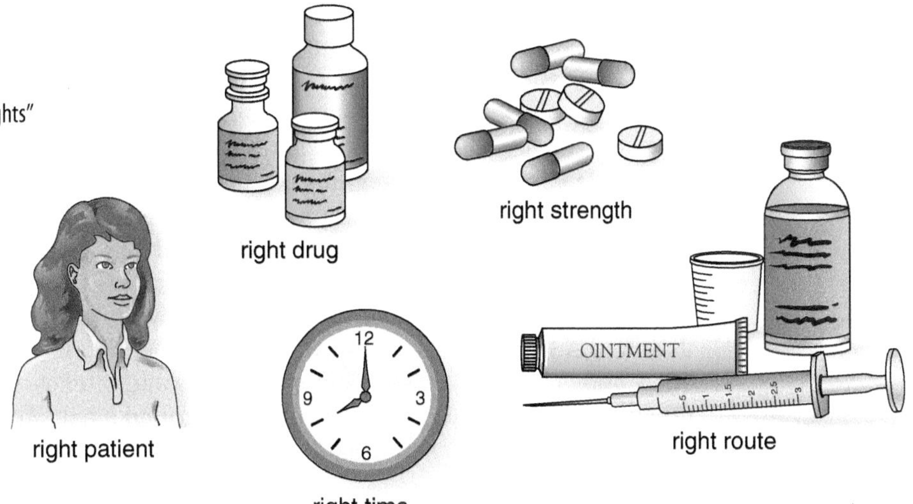

Figure 1.3
"Rights" for Correct Drug Administration
A problem with any one of the "five rights" can result in a medication error.

right drug
right strength
right patient
right time
right route
OINTMENT

Several efforts are under way in a variety of practice settings to address medication errors. Patient safety groups as well as regulatory and monitoring agencies within healthcare are concerned with this issue. The ISMP publishes a list of abbreviations that most pharmacies and institutions are trying to eliminate from use. Because the list is long and changes periodically, it is best to view the updated ISMP Table of Error-Prone Abbreviations on the ISMP Web site. A glance through the table will show you that these abbreviations can easily be misread for a variety of reasons. Technicians must follow procedures to promote accuracy and patient safety, including curbing use of these **dangerous abbreviations**.

Dosage Forms and Routes of Administration

For a drug to be effective, it must be administered in a way that allows it to reach the appropriate site of action in a sufficient amount to produce the desired effect. Drug delivery is, therefore, dependent on the **dosage form** (how it is delivered) and the route by which it is administered. If the drug must enter the bloodstream to reach its site of action, then a **systemic effect** is desired. The drug must be absorbed or administered directly into the bloodstream. If the site of action is a specific area or tissue where the drug can be administered directly without first traveling through the bloodstream, then a topical or **local effect** is needed.

Systemic Routes of Administration

Systemic **routes of administration** are used when a drug is intended to enter the bloodstream and travel to its site of action. A variety of dosage forms is available for each systemic route. Having a variety of forms enhances drug delivery because the most effective form for an individual patient can be used. Form variety also provides options for patients with difficulties taking or using any one route (see Table 1.4).

Table 1.4 Systemic Routes and Corresponding Dosage Forms

Route of Administration	Most Common Dosage Forms
Buccal or sublingual	Tablet, spray, lozenge, troche
Oral	Tablet, capsule, liquid, suspension
Parenteral	Injectable, solution, some suspensions
Rectal	Suppository, solution
Transdermal	Patch, paste, cream, ointment
Implant	Drug encasement carrier

Oral The **oral** route (**peroral** or **PO**, meaning giving a drug by mouth) is the most convenient and cost-effective means of delivering a drug systemically. The majority of medications dispensed today is given as pills (tablets or capsules) by the oral route. Usually, oral dosage forms are swallowed and then absorbed into the bloodstream through the gastrointestinal system.

A wide variety of dosage forms is administered by the oral route. Dosage forms given orally include solid dosage forms such as **tablets** and **capsules** and **liquid forms** such as **syrups**. Tablets can be coated or uncoated. Coatings can affect absorption rates or may simply improve taste or appearance. Most tablets are swallowed whole, but some are intended to be chewed before swallowing. Many oral liquids are **solutions** (liquids with dissolved substances), and some are **suspensions** (liquids with particulate matter). Suspensions must be shaken before each dose and often refrigerated as well. With most oral dosage forms, onset of effect occurs at around a half an hour after swallowing.

A few tablets dissolve quickly on the tongue and are absorbed directly in the mouth. These tablets are called **orally disintegrating tablets (ODTs)**. Other dosage forms that dissolve and absorb within the mouth itself include **sublingual** (under the tongue) and **buccal** (in the cheek) tablets. Those forms that dissolve and absorb in the mouth start acting within a few minutes.

Figure 1.4
Intramuscular Injection
Typically, a 1-inch needle is used and is injected at a 90-degree angle to ensure that the drug is administered within the muscle tissue.

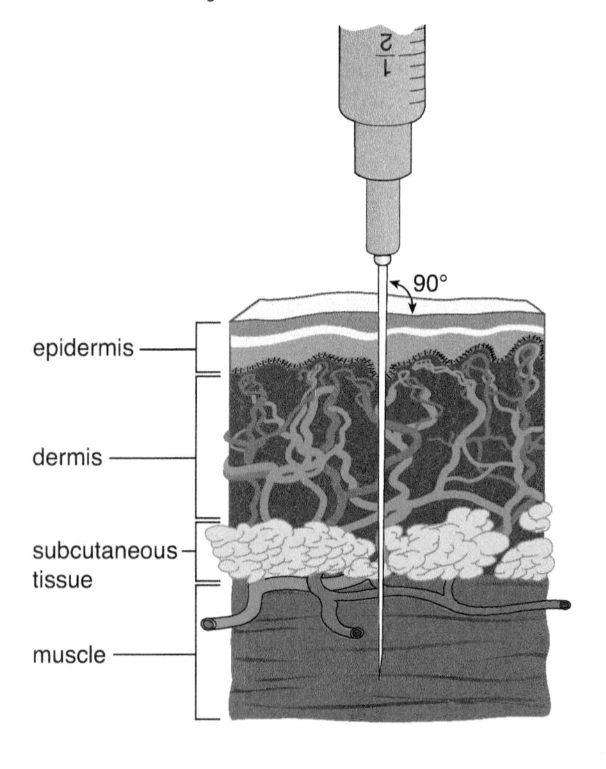

Parenteral Routes Drugs delivered via the **parenteral** route are administered by injection. Usually, the intention is to deliver the drug systemically. These routes are useful for patients who are unconscious or otherwise unable to swallow when rapid action is needed, or for those drugs that have a large first-pass effect (see Chapter 2).

Intramuscular (IM) IM injections are given directly into a muscle (see Figure 1.4). The most common muscles used for IM injection are the **deltoid** in the upper arm and the **gluteus medius** in the buttocks. The drug is absorbed into the blood supply within the muscle and distributed throughout the body. The most common dosage form used via the IM route is solution.

Intravenous (IV) IV injections are given directly into a vein (see Figure 1.5). When repeated or **continuous infusion** of a drug into a vein is needed, a small catheter (plastic tube) is inserted into a vein and left in place while IV fluid containing the drug runs through it into the blood. IV solutions are the dosage form of choice for this route. A **peripheral IV line** is most often inserted into a vein in the arm, wrist, or hand. A peripheral line is used when small amounts of fluid need to be given or the time over which the fluid will infuse is a few days or less. A **central IV line** is inserted into one of the larger veins in the upper chest area near the clavicle (collarbone). This type of line must be inserted surgically and is used when large volumes of fluid must be given, many repeated infusions will be needed, or the time over which the infusion is needed is longer than a few days.

Figure 1.5
Intravenous Injection
The size and angle of the needle used for IV injections depend on the area of the body and the vein into which the drug is delivered.

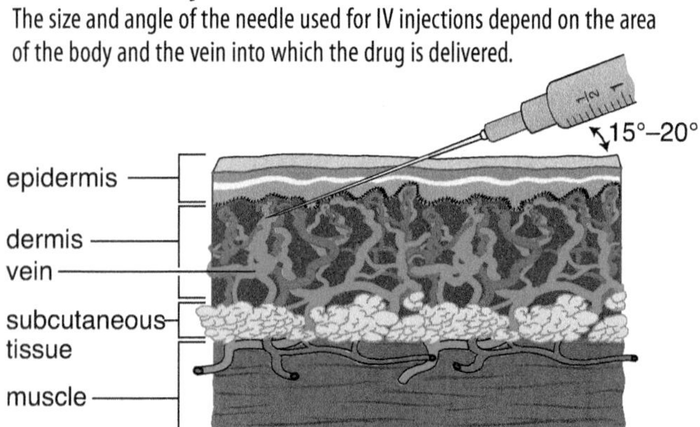

Subcutaneous (SQ or SC) Injections given into the fatty tissue under the dermal layer of the skin and above the muscular tissue are called **subcutaneous** (see Figure 1.6). Common subcutaneous injection sites are the abdomen, upper thigh, and back of the upper arm. The drug is absorbed through the blood supply to the area of the injection over the next few minutes to hours, depending on the drug. Dosage forms used via this route are solutions and some suspensions.

Intrathecal (IT) and Epidural Injections that are given into the spinal column between vertebrae in the back are **intrathecal (IT)** injections. **Epidural** injections use a small catheter to deliver a drug directly into the spinal column over time. These types of injections are used most often for regional anesthesia, such as in childbirth and delivery. These types of injections must be mixed and administered under strict aseptic technique so as not to introduce pathogens into the central nervous system. These injections are administered exclusively by anesthesiologists or anesthetists, but pharmacy technicians may be involved in preparing the products if their institution supports surgical or birth and delivery services.

Intradermal (ID) Injections that are given just underneath the top layer of skin (epidermis) are **intradermal (ID)** injections (see Figure 1.7). This type of injection is used for **tuberculosis (TB) skin tests (PPD)**, local anesthesia, and allergy skin testing. Because these types of injections are given most often in a physician's office or clinic setting, a pharmacy does not usually prepare these products. However, as a healthcare worker, you will become familiar with them because you may be required to get an annual PPD test for TB exposure. Many employers now require this test.

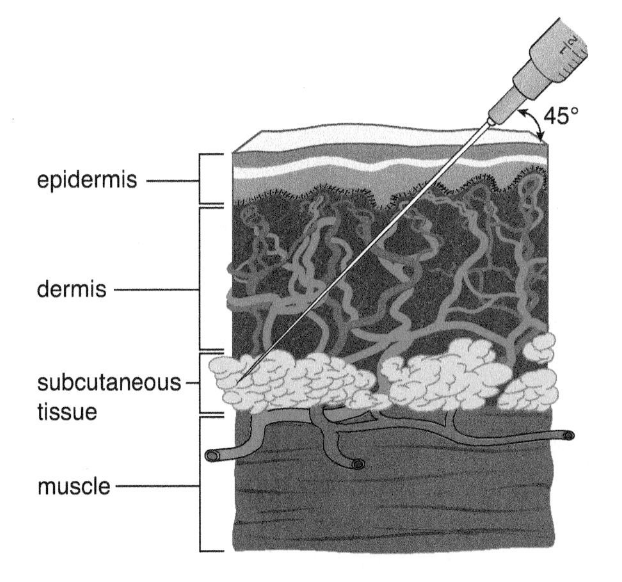

Figure 1.6
Subcutaneous Injection
Some subcutaneous injections, such as those for insulin, use a very fine, short needle and are injected at a 90-degree angle. For others, a 1-inch needle injected at a 45-degree angle ensures that the drug is delivered into subcutaneous tissue, not the underlying muscle.

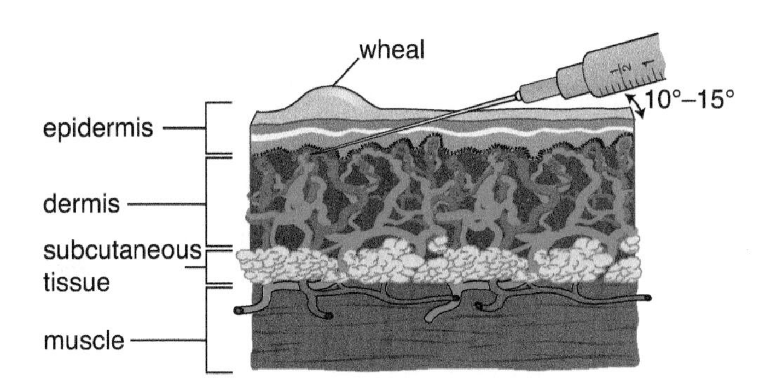

Figure 1.7
Intradermal Injection
After an intradermal TB injection, the patient must return within two to three days to have an appropriate healthcare professional examine the injection area. Redness and swelling at the site indicate possible previous exposure to TB.

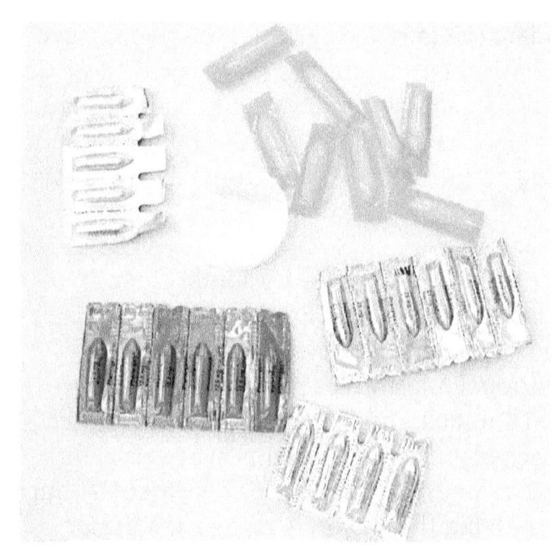

Suppositories use wax or another semi-soft medium that liquefies when warmed to body temperature. In contrast, enemas are liquid solutions inserted into the rectum and held in place for a period of time before defecation.

Rectal Drugs delivered via the **rectal** route are inserted into the rectum and allowed to melt or dissolve in place. Systemic absorption usually occurs through the mucosal lining, and thus many dosage forms given this way are intended for systemic effect. However, a few are intended for local activity, such as when treating hemorrhoids. Dosage forms include suppositories and enemas.

Transdermal Systemic effect is not usually the goal of dermal preparations, including most lotions, creams, and gels that are spread and rubbed on the skin. The **transdermal** route, however, involves applying a drug delivery system, such as a patch with adhesive backing, to the skin so that the drug is slowly absorbed through the skin over time (see Figure 1.8). Transdermal patches can be applied and left in place for a period of time (hours to days) to allow a gradual and even absorption of a drug. Occasionally, a cream or paste is used for transdermal delivery.

Implant Various forms of **implants** are available for drug delivery. In most cases, such implants are inserted just below the skin to release a drug slowly over time (months to years). Long-term treatments (such as birth control) work best for this route.

Figure 1.8
Transdermal Drug Delivery

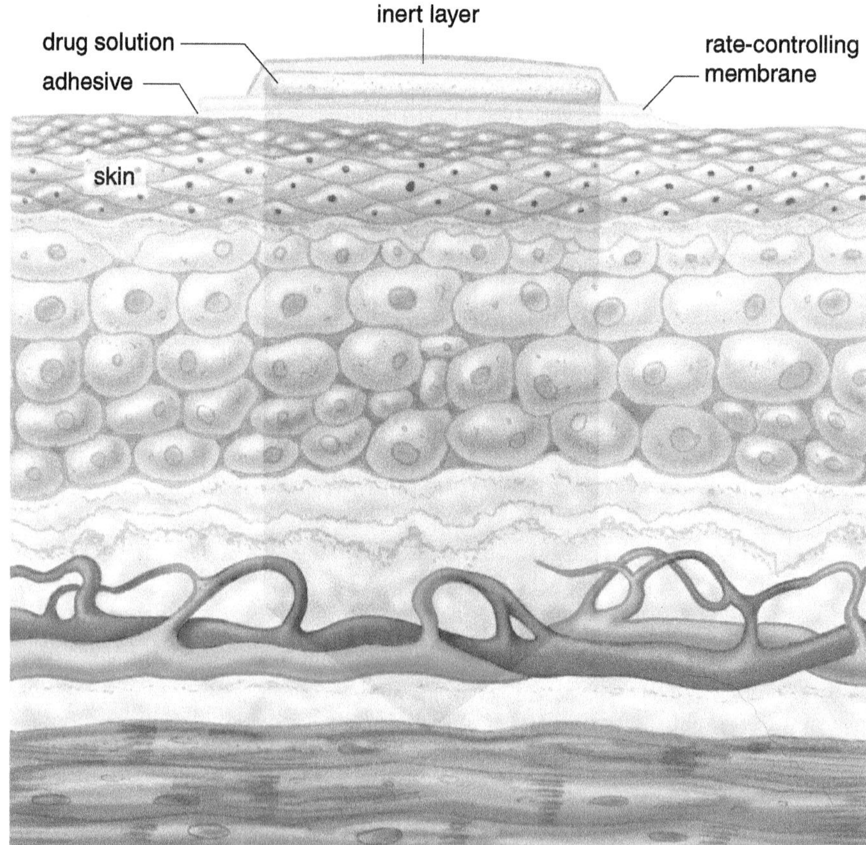

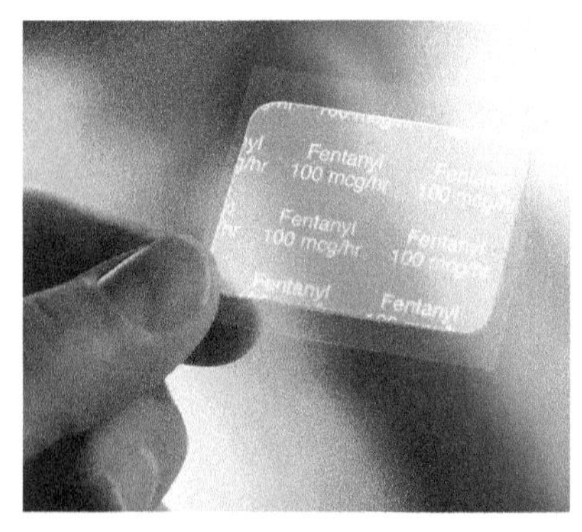

Transdermal drug delivery has become popular among patients who find it difficult to remember to take a pill every day. The convenience enhances their ability to adhere to therapy.

Topical Routes of Administration

Topical routes of administration are used with the intention that the drug will not be systemically absorbed. In many cases, the potential for systemic absorption exists with these routes but normally occurs to such a small extent that for all intents and purposes the effect is strictly local. The topical route is not limited to application on the skin. Drugs can be delivered topically to lung tissue, eyes, and the vagina without significant systemic absorption (see Table 1.5).

Table 1.5 Local Routes and Corresponding Dosage Forms

Route of Administration	Most Common Dosage Forms
Dermal	Cream, lotion, ointment, powder, solution
Inhalation	Metered dose inhaler, dry powder inhaler, nebulizer solution
Intranasal	Spray, solution
Ophthalmic	Solution, ointment
Otic	Solution, suspension
Vaginal	Cream, gel, suppository, solution, ointment, tablet

Dermal Preparations applied topically to the skin are known as **dermal**. Various creams, lotions, gels, ointments, powders, solutions, and pastes are spread or sprayed on the skin to treat local infections, wounds, sunburns, and rashes. If applied over a large enough area in a large quantity, systemic absorption is possible. Therefore, patients must follow instructions closely.

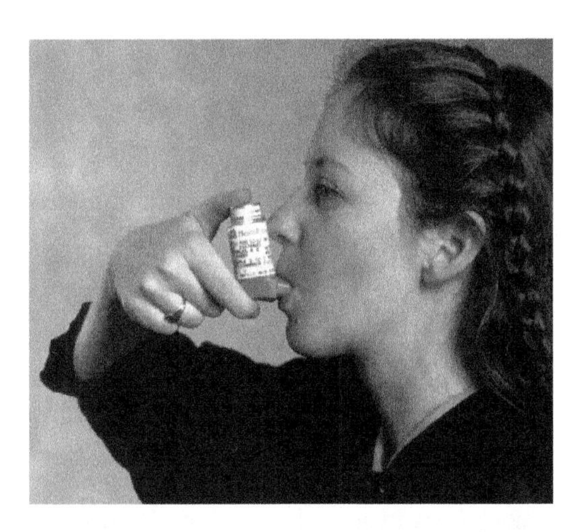

Inhalers are devices in which a canister containing medication delivers a consistent dose, spraying it into the air. Patients place the inhaler in their mouth and inhale the spray into their lungs as they actuate (depress) the inhaler canister. Sometimes inhalers are used along with a spacer, a tube in which the drug is suspended while the patient inhales, which greatly enhances the drug's ability to travel deep into the lungs. Refer to Chapter 14 for a photo of an inhaler with a spacer.

Inhalation Some devices deliver a drug into the lungs by **inhalation**, where a patient breathes it in through the mouth. Metered dose inhalers, dry powder inhalers, and nebulizers all deliver drug by inhalation. Although systemic absorption is possible, inhalation allows for direct treatment to lung tissue without significant systemic side effects in most cases. Patients must learn proper inhalation technique for adequate drug delivery and activity.

Intranasal Drug products that are sprayed into the nose are called **intranasal**. In most cases, a liquid dosage form, such as a solution, delivers the drug to the nasal mucosa. Most intranasal products are intended for local activity, but a few are formulated to achieve systemic absorption. Patients should not sniff forcefully to assist the spray to enter the nose. Doing so pulls the drug too far back into the sinus and down the back of the throat, missing the intended site of administration.

Ophthalmic Eyedrops and eye ointments are examples of **ophthalmic** dosage forms that deliver a drug topically to the eye (see Figure 1.9). Systemic absorption is possible but usually limited with ophthalmic dosage forms, which include solutions and ointments.

Figure 1.9
Ophthalmic Administration
Mastering the application technique for eyedrops may not always be easy, but the benefits of administering a medication without systemic side effects are appealing and often necessary.

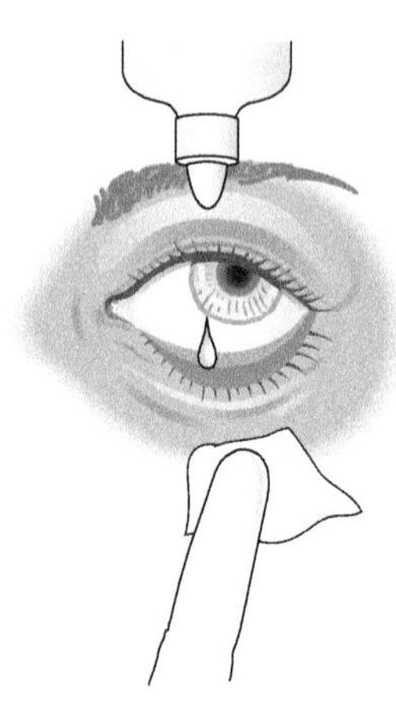

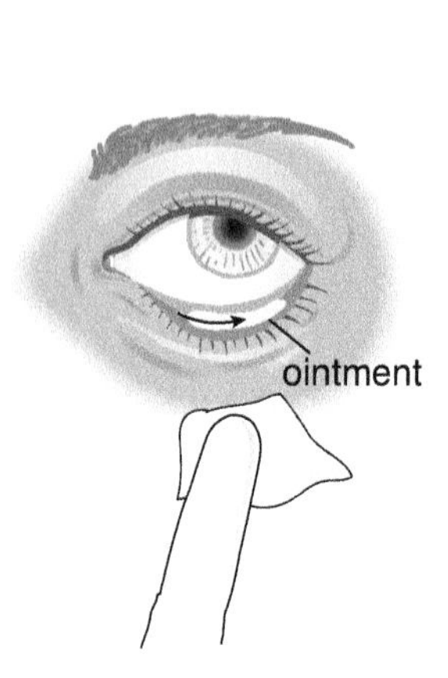

Otic Preparations delivered into the external ear canal are called **otic** (see Figure 1.10). Otic preparations, usually eardrops, are instilled into the ear canal, but the eardrum prevents systemic absorption. Dosage forms include both solutions and suspensions.

Figure 1.10
Otic Administration
It is best for patients to turn their head horizontally and pull on the earlobe while squeezing the bottle to allow drops to fall into the ear canal. For adults, pull upward, but for children under 3 years old, pull downward.

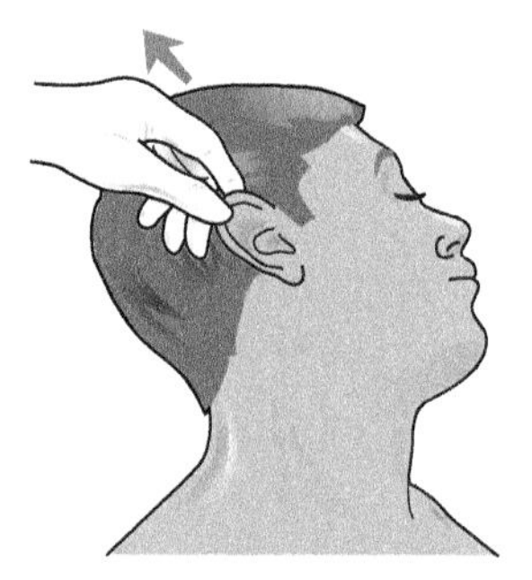

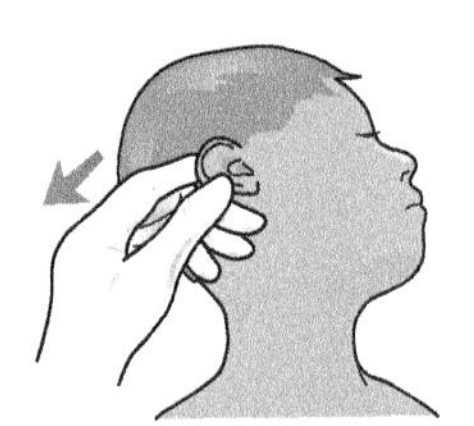

Vaginal Another method of drug delivery is **vaginal**, which is achieved by inserting and applying medication into the vagina. Typically, systemic absorption is not intended but is certainly possible. Only a few products delivered vaginally are intended for systemic absorption. Dosage forms given via the vaginal route include creams, gels, solutions, suppositories, ointments, and tablets. In most cases, patients use a vaginal applicator to aid delivery.

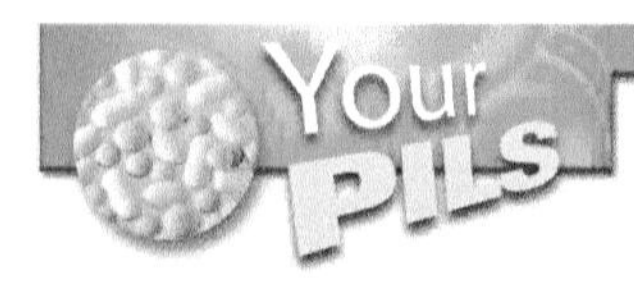

To learn routes of administration and corresponding dosage forms, try one of these methods. If you are an Enactor, pull everything out of your medicine cabinet and categorize each product into its route of administration and dosage form. If you are a Producer, make a chart of all routes of administration on one axis and dosage forms on the other, and then place a check mark in each column and row where the dosage form makes sense to give by the corresponding route. If you are a Director, take a trip to your local pharmacy and make a note of all routes and dosage forms available for OTC items familiar to you. And if you are a Creator, watch the national evening news hour and make note of all drug product advertisements, and then look up the routes and dosage forms available for each.

Chapter Summary

Pharmacology is the study of how drugs work in the body. Learning mechanisms of action for various drugs requires some familiarity with the physiological processes of the body and how those are altered in disease and illness. When learning pharmacology, you must commit many drug names to memory, in addition to gaining a conceptual understanding of each mechanism of action. Therefore, it helps if you can employ ways of learning that fit best with your preferred style(s) of learning. Taking a learning styles inventory is a useful step toward conquering the large volume of material to be learned in this topic area.

Drugs are categorized in several ways. First, drugs are put into classes that have similar mechanisms of action. Drugs are also divided into prescription (legend) and OTC products. Some prescription medications are controlled substances due to their potential for dependence and abuse. These controlled drugs are categorized into five categories, based on their degree of potential for abuse. Last, medications are ranked into pregnancy risk categories that help prescribers and patients determine the safety and risks of taking various drugs during pregnancy.

Another category of drugs, dietary supplements and natural products, are not regulated by the FDA as prescription and OTC medications are. These items include vitamins and herbal therapies that can be purchased by patients. Familiarity with these products and a general awareness of alternative and complementary treatments are useful for pharmacists and technicians because many patients use them.

Familiarity with the common terms and abbreviations used in healthcare is essential to operating with competence and efficiency in the pharmacy. You should be aware that many of these abbreviations can be easily confused and contribute to medication errors.

Finally, this chapter reviews routes of administration and common dosage forms used for each route. As you learn how various drugs work, you should also learn how they are delivered to the body to exert their activity. For instance, technicians working primarily in the inpatient setting should be familiar with injectable drugs. Those working in the outpatient or retail setting should become familiar with oral drugs.

Chapter Review

For the following sets of exercises, write the exercise heading, exercise numbers, and your answers on a separate sheet of paper. Your instructor may direct you to turn in the sheet of paper or discuss your answers as a class.

REVIEW THE BASICS

Choose a, b, c, d, or e as the correct answer to each multiple-choice question.

1. Which of the following is the study of abnormal physiological processes within the body?
   a. pharmacology
   b. physiology
   c. pathophysiology
   d. pharmacokinetics

2. Which of the following is the name given to a drug when it enters Phase I clinical trials?
   a. chemical
   b. generic
   c. brand
   d. proprietary

3. Which of the following are drugs that can be sold directly to patients without an order from a prescriber?
   a. legend
   b. prescription
   c. over-the-counter
   d. controlled substances

4. Which of the following controlled substance Schedules includes illegal substances?
   a. I
   b. II
   c. III
   d. IV
   e. V

5. A drug in which of the following pregnancy categories would be considered the safest to use during pregnancy?
   a. A
   b. B
   c. C
   d. D
   e. X

6. Which of the following dosage forms would be least likely to produce a systemic effect?
   a. antibiotic ointment applied to a small area on the skin
   b. anti-inflammatory tablet taken by mouth
   c. antibiotic solution given intravenously
   d. a and b only
   e. b and c only

7. Which of the following best describes drug administration that would result in a local drug effect?
   a. injecting a medication intravenously via a peripheral catheter
   b. applying a transdermal patch to the skin
   c. applying a lotion to a rash on the skin
   d. swallowing a tablet that gets absorbed in the gastrointestinal tract

8. Which of the following is most often considered a topical route of administration?
   a. intradermal
   b. buccal
   c. inhalation
   d. all of the above

9. Into which of the following muscles are intramuscular injections given most often in the pharmacy?
   a. abdominal oblique
   b. deltoid
   c. gluteus maximus
   d. gluteus medius

10. Which of the following publishes lists of easily confused drug names and error prone abbreviations so that medication errors can be avoided?
    a. DEA
    b. FDA
    c. ISMP
    d. all of the above

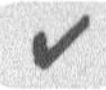

KNOW THE DRUGS

Match each category with its corresponding drug classification system.

Drug Classification System	Category
1. Category X	a. Alternative and complementary treatments
2. Schedule II	b. Prescription medications
3. Legend	c. Major drug class
4. "Statins"	d. Controlled substances
5. Eastern medicine	e. Pregnancy categories

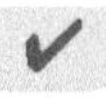

PUT IT TOGETHER

For each item, write down either a single term to complete the sentence or a short answer.

1. _______________ is the proprietary name given to a drug when it is marketed (enters Phase IV clinical trials).
2. Drugs with a legitimate medical use in the United States and having the highest risk potential for dependence and abuse are Schedule _______________.
3. Liquid codeine cough syrup is usually Schedule _______________.
4. Drugs that pose risk to a developing fetus, when evidence shows that harm to the fetus outweighs the potential benefits of taking the drug, are put in pregnancy category _______________.
5. _______________ is not a controlled substance but is limited in sale because it is considered a precursor to methamphetamine.
6. List three dosage forms that could be given by each listed route of administration.

   oral

   vaginal

   dermal

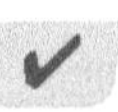

THINK IT THROUGH

Read and think through each numbered scenario carefully, and then write several sentences in reply to the question(s) presented. Question 4 requires you to do some Internet research before completing your answer(s).

1. Mr. McDonald is given Protonix (a drug used to reduce stomach acidity and prevent gastroesophageal reflux) and told to take one tablet each morning, preferably on an empty stomach. He returns to the pharmacy complaining that this new medication is not helping his heartburn at night much at all. When asked how he is taking it, he states he is taking one tablet by mouth as instructed on an empty stomach at bedtime. Which of the "five rights" of drug therapy is wrong?
2. Describe differences between Eastern and Western medicine.
3. Name four parenteral routes of administration and describe how they differ.

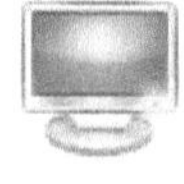

4. **On the Internet**, find a few Web sites about learning styles and take an inventory of your own preferences. What style(s) do you seem to prefer? What did you learn about yourself in doing this exercise? Do you think the tools and Web site you chose are reputable and reliable for their content and assessment of your learning style(s)? Think of three ways you could use your preferred style(s) to approach learning pharmacology.

Chapter 2 Drugs in the Body

LEARNING OBJECTIVES

- Identify the main principles of organic chemistry, pharmacodynamics, and pharmacokinetics.
- Describe how those principles influence the behavior of drugs in the body.
- Describe how atoms combine to form different kinds of molecules.
- Distinguish how pH affects behavior of acidic and basic drug molecules.
- Identify the key components of the dose-response curve that represent therapeutic range, efficacy, potency, and steady state.
- Describe factors that influence absorption, distribution, metabolism, and excretion of drugs from the body.

Interactive self-quizzes, games, audio files, and glossaries help you to learn drug names and facts.

The ways that drugs behave in the body depend on the principles of organic chemistry. Organic chemistry is the study of the structure, properties, and reactions of carbon-based compounds. Learning basic concepts and principles of organic chemistry will add great depth to your understanding of how drugs behave in the body and how they are chosen for individual patients. This chapter introduces the general concepts that govern the chemical makeup of drugs and discusses principles that affect how they get into, move around in, and exit from the body. Last, this chapter covers differences in patient populations that change the chemical characteristics and behavior of drug therapy. Pharmacy technicians with an understanding of these concepts and how they apply to specific patients will better grasp how drug dosing and therapy decisions are made in the practice setting.

Atoms and Molecules

All matter can be broken down to its most basic unit, the **atom**. All matter—including the human body—is made up of atoms. Ninety-two different types of atoms, or **elements**, exist naturally on Earth. Chemists have chosen to organize and display the elements in a particular arrangement (see Figure 2.1).

The **periodic table of the elements** arranges the naturally occurring elements, along with those synthesized in the laboratory setting, into rows and columns that group atoms by their chemical properties. Elements in the same column have similar properties and reactivity, affecting the way they combine with other molecules. Elements in each row increase in size and mass (from left to right), which also helps predict behavior.

Atomic Structure

Atoms are made up of a nuclear center and an outer shell. The nucleus is a small core of solid matter, including protons and neutrons, and the outer shell is an orbital space where electrons circulate. Each element has a unique number of electrons and protons (see Figure 2.2).

Protons have a positive electrical charge and determine an element's atomic number, as shown in the periodic table of the elements. Protons have measurable mass and are found in the nucleus. **Neutrons** are also in the nucleus and are neutral, neither positively nor negatively charged. However, they have mass and add to an atom's atomic weight. **Electrons** have a negative charge and seek to balance the electrical

Figure 2.1

Periodic Table of the Elements

Elements in the same group tend to behave in similar ways when combining with other elements.

Periodic Table of the Elements

	I A	II A	III B	IV B	V B	VI B	VII B	VIII	VIII	VIII	I B	II B	III A	IV A	V A	VI A	VII A	0
1	1 H 1.008																	2 He 4.003
2	3 Li 6.939	4 Be 9.0122											5 B 10.811	6 C 12.011	7 N 14.007	8 O 15.999	9 F 18.998	10 Ne 20.183
3	11 Na 22.99	12 Mg 24.312											13 Al 26.982	14 Si 28.086	15 P 30.974	16 S 32.064	17 Cl 35.453	18 Ar 39.948
4	19 K 39.102	20 Ca 40.08	21 Sc 44.956	22 Ti 47.9	23 V 50.942	24 Cr 51.996	25 Mn 54.938	26 Fe 55.847	27 Co 58.933	28 Ni 58.71	29 Cu 63.546	30 Zn 65.37	31 Ga 69.72	32 Ge 72.59	33 As 74.922	34 Se 78.96	35 Br 79.904	36 Kr 83.8
5	37 Rb 85.47	38 Sr 87.62	39 Y 88.905	40 Zr 91.22	41 Nb 92.906	42 Mo 95.94	43 Tc (97)	44 Ru 101.07	45 Rh 102.91	46 Pd 106.4	47 Ag 107.87	48 Cd 112.4	49 In 114.82	50 Sn 118.69	51 Sb 121.75	52 Te 127.6	53 I 126.9	54 Xe 131.3
6	55 Cs 132.91	56 Ba 137.34	57 •La 138.91	72 Hf 178.49	73 Ta 180.95	74 W 183.85	75 Re 186.2	76 Os 190.2	77 Ir 192.2	78 Pt 195.09	79 Au 196.97	80 Hg 200.59	81 Tl 204.37	82 Pb 207.19	83 Bi 208.98	84 Po 210	85 At 210	86 Rn 222
7	87 Fr 215	88 Ra 226.03	89 +Ac 227.03	104 Rf (261)	105 Db (262)	106 Sg (266)	107 Bh (264)	108 Hs (269)	109 Mt (268)	110 Ds (271)	111 Rg (272)							

• Lanthanide series	58 Ce 140.12	59 Pr 140.91	60 Nd 144.24	61 Pm 145	62 Sm 150.35	63 Eu 151.96	64 Gd 157.25	65 Tb 158.92	66 Dy 162.5	67 Ho 164.93	68 Er 167.26	69 Tm 168.93	70 Yb 173.04	71 Lu 174.97
+ Actinide series	90 Th 232.04	91 Pa 231	92 U 238.03	93 Np 237.05	94 Pu 239.05	95 Am 241.06	96 Cm 244.06	97 Bk 249.08	98 Cf 252.08	99 Es 252.08	100 Fm 257.1	101 Md 258.1	102 No 259.1	103 Lr 262.11

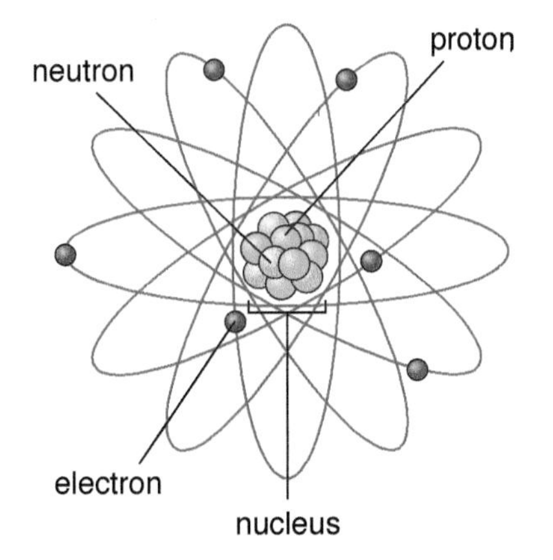

Figure 2.2

Atomic Structure

Electromagnetic forces keep an atom together but do not allow electrons and protons to touch.

charge of an atom; thus the number of electrons normally equals the number of protons. Electrons weigh so little that they do not contribute significantly to the mass of an atom. The interplay of electrons and their effect on electrical charge determine the chemical activity of an element and its ability to combine with other atoms.

Ions are atoms or molecules with an electrical charge. When electrons are separated from an atom, energy is released and a positively charged ion is formed. When an extra electron is added to an atom's orbital, a negatively charged ion is formed. When neutrons are added to an atom, the charge does not change, but the atom becomes heavier. This type of atom is called an **isotope** and is often radioactive. Isotopes are used in nuclear medicine to perform imaging on the body, such as in cardiac catheterization.

Professional Focus

Nuclear pharmacy is a specialty practice in which radioactive isotope material (usually called dye) is prepared for imaging procedures. Technicians and pharmacists working in this field must receive specialized training to handle radioactive materials.

Chemical Bonds

Atoms combine by exchanging electrons in their outer shells. This exchange occurs in two ways. Atoms can share electrons, or they can transfer them completely to another atom. Sharing electrons is called a **covalent bond**, a strong bond that creates a neutrally charged molecule (see Figure 2.3).

Ionic bonds occur when one element has entirely lost and another has gained electrons, but the two atoms remain connected by electromagnetic attraction (see Figure 2.4). One atom becomes positively charged, and the other is negative. Each

Figure 2.3
Covalent Bond
In a covalent bond, electrons share orbitals around the nucleus.

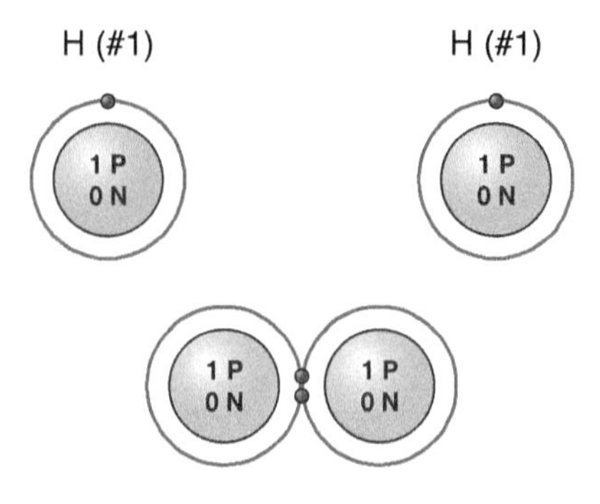

Figure 2.4
Ionic Bond
Sodium (+) and chloride (–) combine via ionic bonds to make table salt.

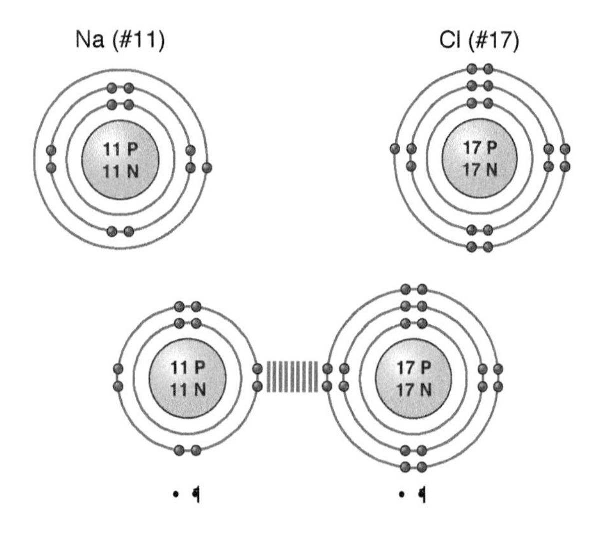

Figure 2.5
Ampicillin Molecule
The amino functional group in ampicillin is shown as NH_2, and the carboxyl functional group is shown as COOH.

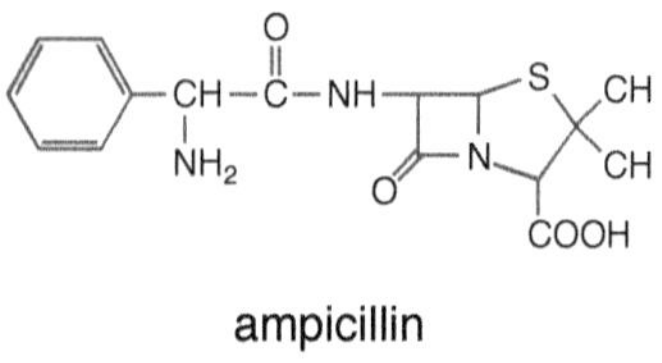

ampicillin

atom is individually referred to as an ion, because it has a charge. Ionic bonds are considered to be polar. They are weaker and more easily broken than covalent bonds.

In the body, most substances are made up of molecules using covalent bonds. In fact, all organic material contains carbon, an element that combines with other atoms or elements primarily by covalent bonds. Some molecules, such as minerals and electrolytes, exist in the body as ions. Examples of ions in the body are sodium (Na^+), potassium (K^+), and chloride (Cl^-).

Molecules and Functional Groups

When two or more atoms combine via covalent or ionic bonds, a **molecule** is formed. Some molecules form the structure of the body itself, and others, called biochemicals, react with each other to conduct various physiological processes.

Organic molecules have a **carbon backbone** that occurs in chains of atoms strung together or in ring-like structures. Forming rings is a unique property of carbon that allows it to behave in ways conducive to organic life. On each backbone you find **functional groups**, which are the side portions of a molecule that give it the chemical properties that allow it to react with others in specific ways. Each functional group has a specific shape and particular tendency to react according to its chemical properties. Molecules react only with those receptors in the body that are shaped similarly, much like a lock and key. A drug's activity can be predicted by examining its molecular shape and functional groups (see Figure 2.5).

Isomers are compounds (i.e., molecules with differing types of atoms) with the exact same chemical makeup (the same number and types of atoms), but they are not arranged the same way within space. Many times, isomers of the same molecule are mirror images of each other (called **stereoisomers**). A drug product may contain a mixture of stereoisomers, one having more drug activity, and the other causing more side effects.

The most common molecules in the body are carbohydrates, peptides, lipids, and nucleic acids. **Carbohydrates** are an essential part of nutrition. Breaking bonds in carbohydrate molecules, such as glucose and fructose, produces energy that the body can use to sustain life. Large carbohydrate molecules, such as starches, are used in building cell membranes or stored for energy. **Peptides** are composed of amino acids and are the building blocks of protein molecules. Proteins are most often used to build tissue but can also be used for energy. **Lipids** are molecules that form long chains of covalently bonded carbon and hydrogen atoms. Lipids are soluble in fat or oil and are used to create hormones and other active biochemicals. **Nucleic acids** are part of deoxyribonucleic acid (DNA), which forms the genetic material contained in the nucleus of each cell. DNA serves as the road map for the body's processes and growth cycle.

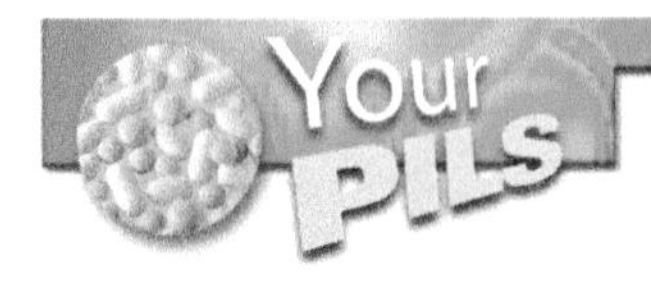

No matter what learning styles you prefer, using hands-on manipulation reinforces concepts involving spatial relationships of molecules. Whether you work in a group, as Creators prefer, or alone, as Producers prefer, you might find building molecules using a toy building-set (such as Tinkertoys®) useful to understanding how bonds are formed and why functional groups affect molecular behavior. Using such a toy, try building two molecules that are stereoisomers (mirror images) of each other.

Acids and Bases

Understanding acidic and basic properties of molecules is useful because most drugs are either weak acids or weak bases. These properties affect how drug molecules enter and behave in the body. The **pH scale** is a way to measure acidic and basic properties of substances. Substances with a low pH (below 7) are **acids**, and those with a high pH (over 7) are **bases** (see Figure 2.6).

The pH scale measures the propensity of a molecule to shed or take on hydrogen ions. **Hydrogen ions** are created when an electron orbiting a hydrogen atom is lost, leaving a lone proton with a positive charge (H^+). In a sense, acidic molecules donate protons to other molecules. Basic molecules easily accept protons. Those molecules that have the ability to donate multiple hydrogen ions are considered strong acids, and those that donate few are weak acids. The opposite is true for bases.

When acids and bases come together and an exchange of protons occurs, the remaining molecules become ionized (positively or negatively charged). Ionization affects drug activity, because ionic molecules cannot easily cross membranes and enter the bloodstream. For example, putting a basic drug with a high pH into the acidic stomach facilitates the exchange of many protons, creating ionic molecules that are difficult to absorb into the bloodstream. Conversely, if an acidic drug enters the acidic environment of the stomach, more of it will get absorbed because few molecules will shed protons and most will remain neutrally charged.

Figure 2.6

pH Scale for Acids and Bases

Gastric acid in the stomach has a pH around 2 to 3.

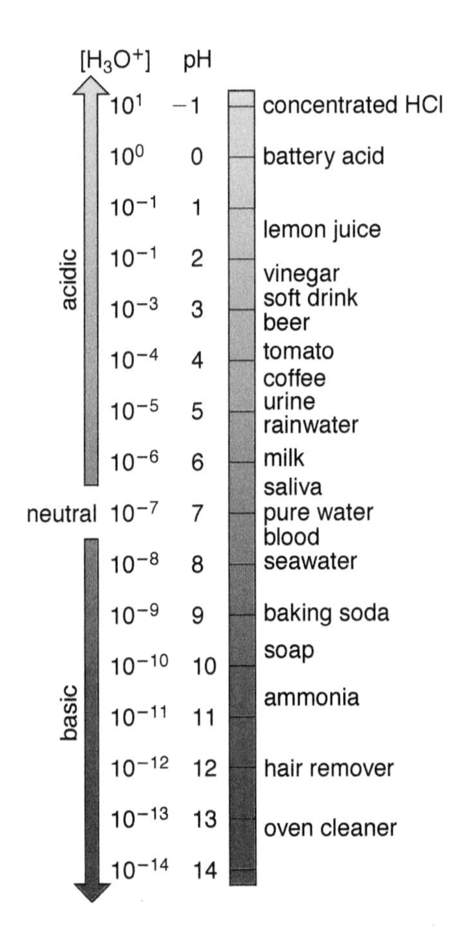

Pharmacodynamics

Generally, drugs work by mimicking, enhancing, or blocking the activity of substances that are usually already present in the body. In most cases, drug molecules interact with **receptors** on the surface or inside of specific cells. This interactive process is explained by **drug receptor theory,** which is based on a **lock and key mechanism** (see Figure 2.7). Cells of the body have many different receptor molecules (or locks) on their surface and various substances (or keys) fit exactly into them. Usually, these "key" substances are produced or processed within the body. That is, they are endogenous chemicals that act as messengers for communication and for regulating physiological processes. When a messenger molecule connects with a receptor, it triggers a series of reactions within the cell.

Pharmacodynamics is the study of drug receptor theory at this molecular level and how that interaction translates to drug activity on the entire body. Through pharmacodynamics, you can determine a drug's **mechanism of action** and, therefore, its effect on the body. Drug molecules mimic the molecular shape of the body's endogenous

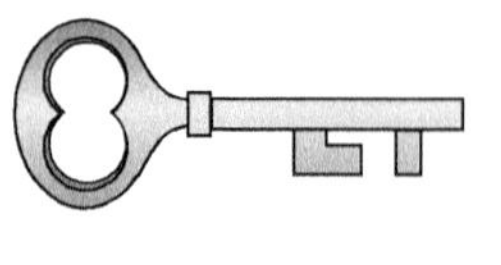

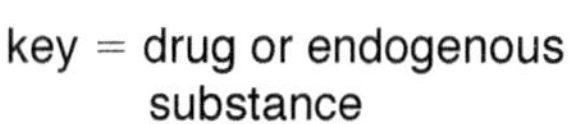

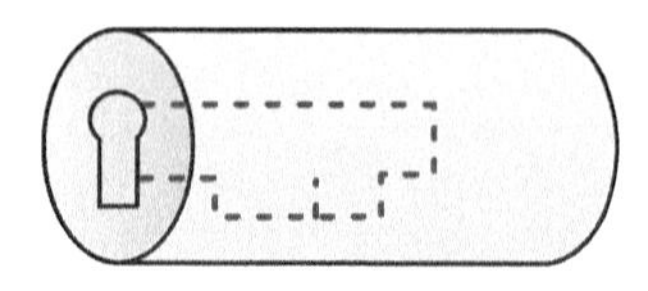

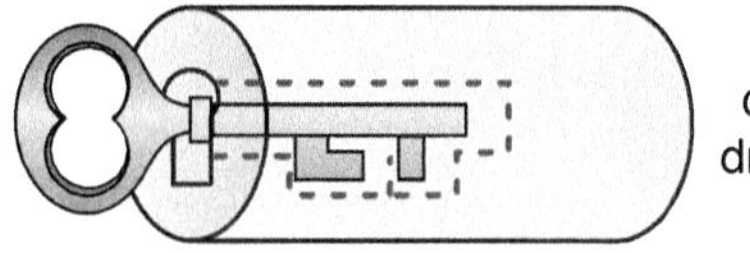

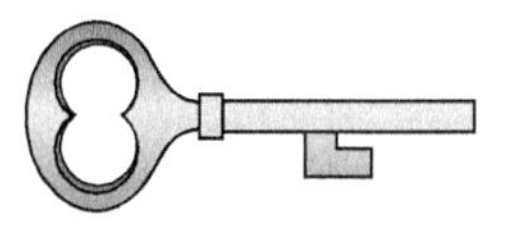

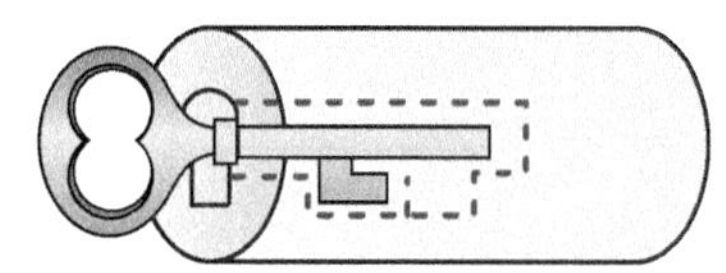

Figure 2.7
Drugs and Receptors
Drug molecules are similar to but not exactly the same as endogenous molecules. Their slight differences can be the reason why side effects occur.

chemicals and then either produce similar effects or block the activity. Logically, you can see why drugs with similar molecular shape are categorized together, because they interact with the same receptors and thus have similar activity.

Drugs whose activity is to stimulate a specific response when binding to receptors are **agonists**, and those drugs that block a response when binding to receptors are **antagonists**. Antagonists block a response in one of two ways. They can either directly inactivate the receptor, blocking its ability to trigger a response. Or they can bind to the receptor in a competitive fashion, keeping other agonist molecules from binding and then triggering a response. When a drug binds with high affinity to a receptor, it sticks to the receptor longer—perhaps even permanently. Those drugs with low affinity for a receptor may bind quickly and then fall off easily, which can lead to a short duration of action.

Dose-Response Relationship

For a drug to be effective, it must reach its site of action in a large enough concentration to produce a measurable effect. In other words, enough of the drug molecules must reach the site of action to elicit a significant response. A drug's safety for use depends on its ability to reach desired concentrations without producing too many toxic effects. Therefore, proper dosing hinges on achieving the desired effect without producing unwanted effects.

This relationship between dose and effect is depicted graphically as a **dose-response curve** (see Figure 2.8). This graph displays concentration of drug in the bloodstream over time. The curve shows that increases in dose result in increased response. Eventually, a **ceiling effect** is reached in which no further increase in dose produces additional response.

Proper drug dosing aims for blood concentrations in the middle of this curve, the **therapeutic range** (see Figure 2.9). The lower threshold of this range is the **minimum therapeutic concentration**. Drug dosing must achieve at least this concentration to gain any measurable effect. The upper edge of this range is the **toxic concentration**; above this concentration the incidence of toxic effects may outweigh any benefit of the drug and thus pose too great a risk.

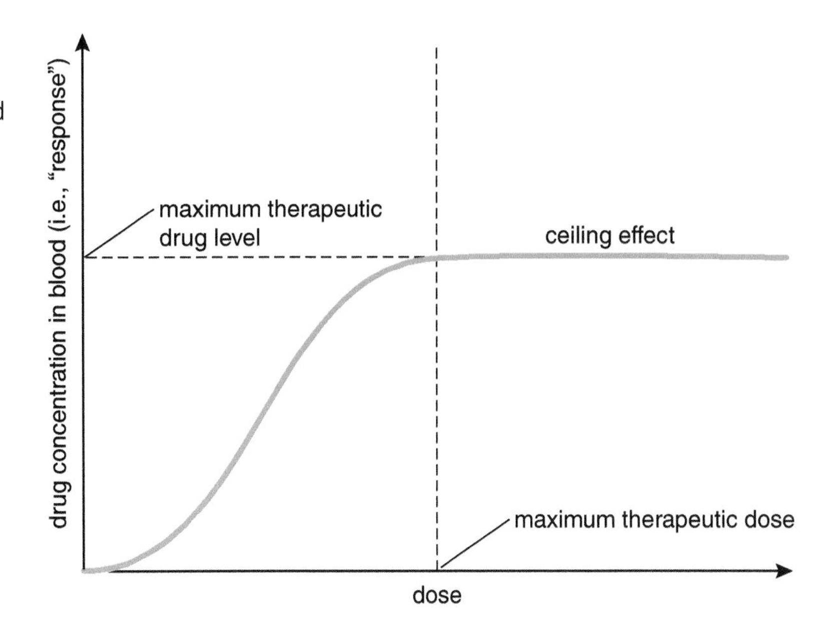

Figure 2.8
Dose-Response Curve
The ceiling effect is usually dangerously high and associated with many toxic effects and even death.

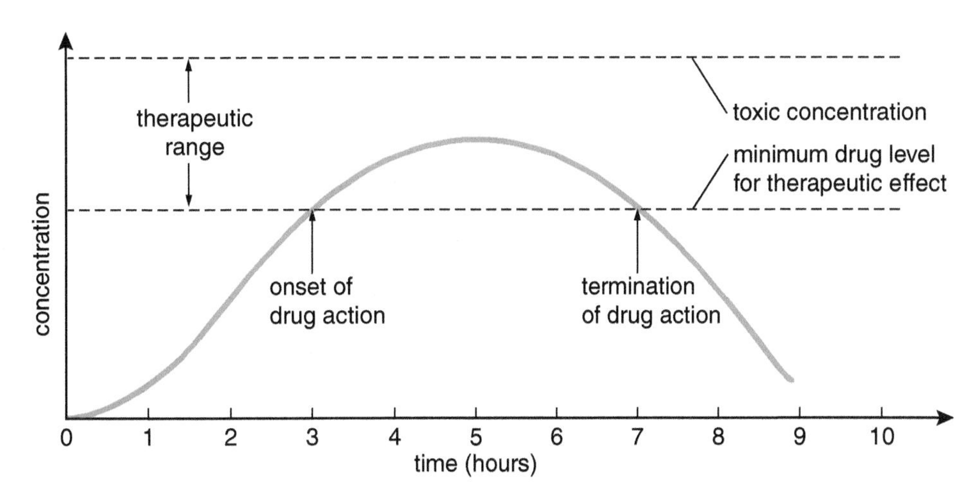

Figure 2.9
Time-Response Curve
Some drugs have a narrow therapeutic range whose minimum therapeutic and toxic levels are close to each other. In these cases, drug dosing must be monitored closely to ensure the appropriate amount of drug is given to produce desired effects without overshooting and causing toxic effects.

The dose-response curve can be used to determine drug **efficacy** and **potency**. When a dose-response curve is lower in vertical height for one drug compared with another, the first drug is considered less effective. When the curve is shifted horizontally left or right as compared with another drug, the potency differs. For instance, a drug that achieves the same response as another drug but at a lower dose (left shift) is more potent.

For drugs with which a constant concentration in the therapeutic range is desired, timing of doses is important. Figure 2.10 shows how repeated doses are timed to produce an average drug concentration that remains in the therapeutic range. When this constant concentration is maintained, **steady state** is achieved. Up to five doses, if timed appropriately, may be required before blood concentrations reach steady state. When time is of the essence, a **loading dose** is given. A loading dose is a dose that is large enough to bring blood concentrations up to the therapeutic range immediately. Subsequent doses keep levels at the steady state.

The point at which a drug is at the lowest concentration between doses is called the **trough**. The **peak** is when the concentration is at its highest. For some drugs, peaks and troughs are measured to be sure they are high and low enough. Drug levels aid prescribers in making certain that patients get maximum benefit but avoid toxicity. Pharmacy technicians are sometimes asked to assist pharmacists in retrieving drug concentration levels from laboratory data. Once steady state has been reached and the prescriber is sure that peaks and troughs are appropriate, monitoring may become less frequent.

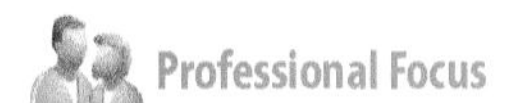

Professional Focus

In hospitals, pharmacists often assist prescribers in dosing medications with narrow therapeutic ranges or drugs that have severe side effects associated with elevated peaks and troughs. When helping gather laboratory results for drug dosing, you should be sure to record the time doses are given in relation to when blood draws are performed. Blood draws taken at the wrong time can render lab results useless for drug dosing.

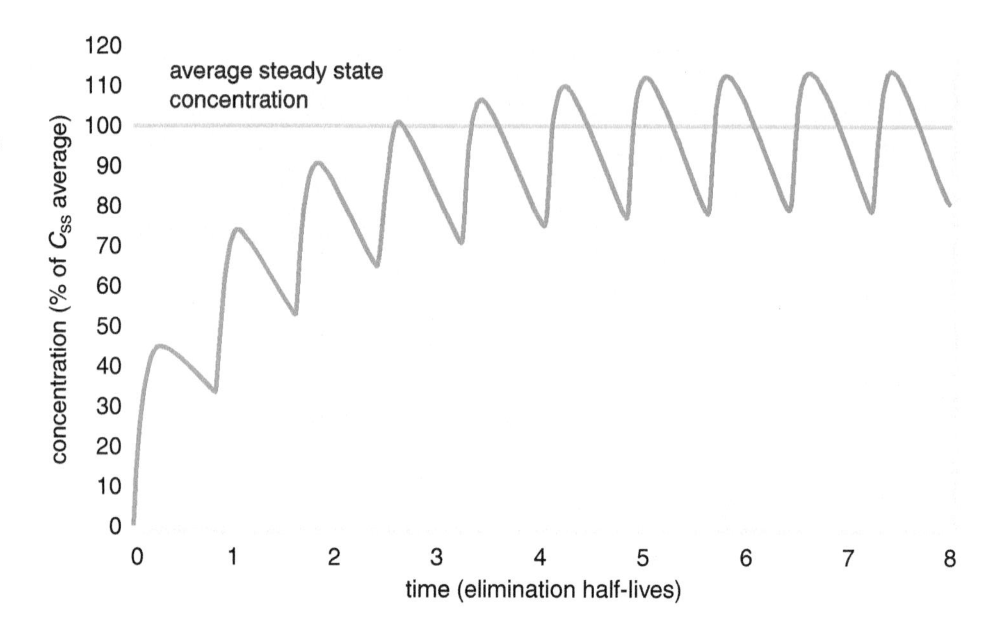

Figure 2.10
Steady State
Another way to maintain a steady concentration in the therapeutic range is to give a continuous infusion.

Pharmacokinetics

The study of **pharmacokinetics** uses mathematical modeling to observe and predict how a drug enters, moves around, and leaves the body. In other words, pharmacokinetics studies how drugs are absorbed, distributed, and eliminated from the bloodstream (see Figure 2.11). This entire process can be described in terms of four phases: absorption, distribution, metabolism, and excretion.

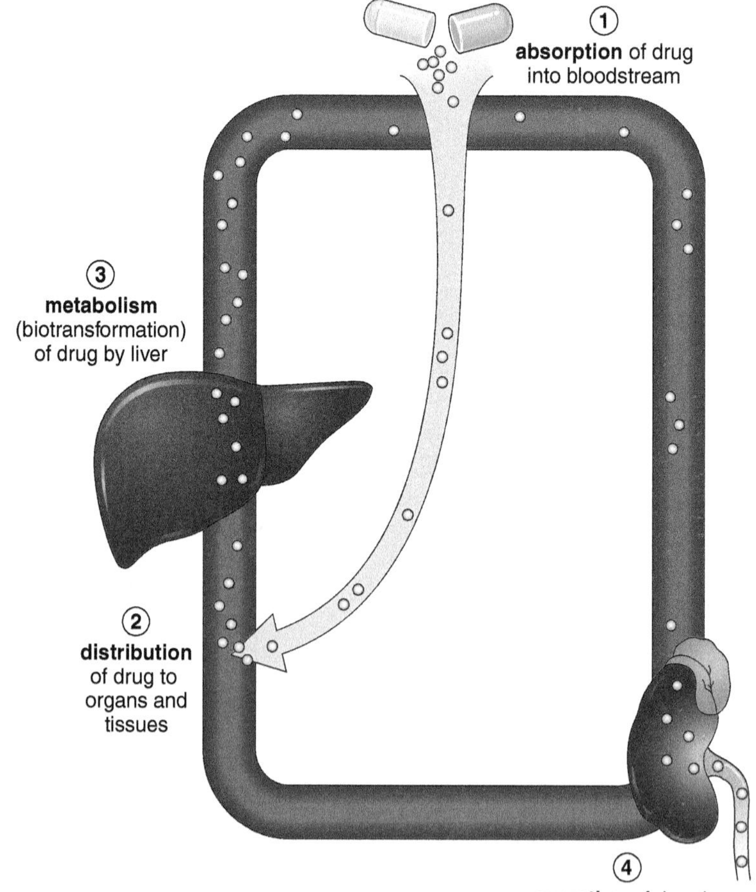

Figure 2.11
Pharmacokinetic Process
Most oral drugs enter the bloodstream through the lining of the intestines, where all blood flow goes through the liver before entering the rest of the body.

Absorption

Absorption is the process by which drugs enter the bloodstream. It is measured as the rate and extent to which a drug moves from the site of administration to the circulating blood. On the time-response curve (see Figure 2.9), absorption is the upward-sloping part of the curve. Absorption affects the onset of drug action as well as the extent of action. For instance, if a drug is quickly and easily absorbed, the onset of action is fast and the effect is noticeable and great. If the absorption is slow and incomplete, only a small amount of drug reaches the bloodstream and gets to the intended site of action.

The route of administration affects absorption by enhancing or limiting systemic effect. For example, oral administration is used frequently because it usually results in good systemic absorption through the small intestines. Intravenous administration skips the absorption step entirely by administering drugs directly into the bloodstream. Topical routes do not always produce a measurable systemic effect because absorption is usually limited.

Dosage form affects absorption by taking advantage of solubility properties to regulate the release of drug molecules. Before a drug can enter circulation, it must dissolve. Therefore, solid dosage forms usually result in slower absorption rates than do liquids. Transdermal patches release drug slowly, so that absorption through the skin is steady and incremental. Some tablets and capsules are specially manufactured or coated for specific solubility properties. Orally disintegrating tablets (ODTs), also referred to as rapidly-dissolving tablets, are quickly absorbed when placed on the tongue because they instantly dissolve in saliva. Coated tablets take longer to dissolve and absorb.

Acidic and basic properties of drugs and their environment affect drug solubility and ultimately drug absorption. When a basic drug is in an acidic environment, it dissociates into ionic particles, which cannot cross membranes easily. Acidic drugs placed in an acidic environment do not easily dissociate, and thus more drug will be absorbed.

The transport mechanisms that drugs use to cross membranes also affect absorption. Molecules cross membranes by active and passive transport mechanisms (see Figure 2.12). Crossing membranes between the site of administration and the circulatory system is necessary for drug activity. **Active transport** mechanisms use energy to bring drug molecules across a membrane, whereas in **passive transport** mechanisms molecules move across on their own. An example of an active transport mechanism is the sodium/potassium exchange pump, which requires ATP for energy (Na-K-ATPase, aka, sodium pump). These proteins, which traverse the cell membrane, use energy to pump potassium into, and sodium out of, cells. Because active transport mechanisms are limited by the availability of energy sources, they can become saturated, or maxed out, which limits overall absorption.

Figure 2.12
Transport Mechanisms
In simple diffusion, molecules move either directly through the membrane itself or through an open channel.

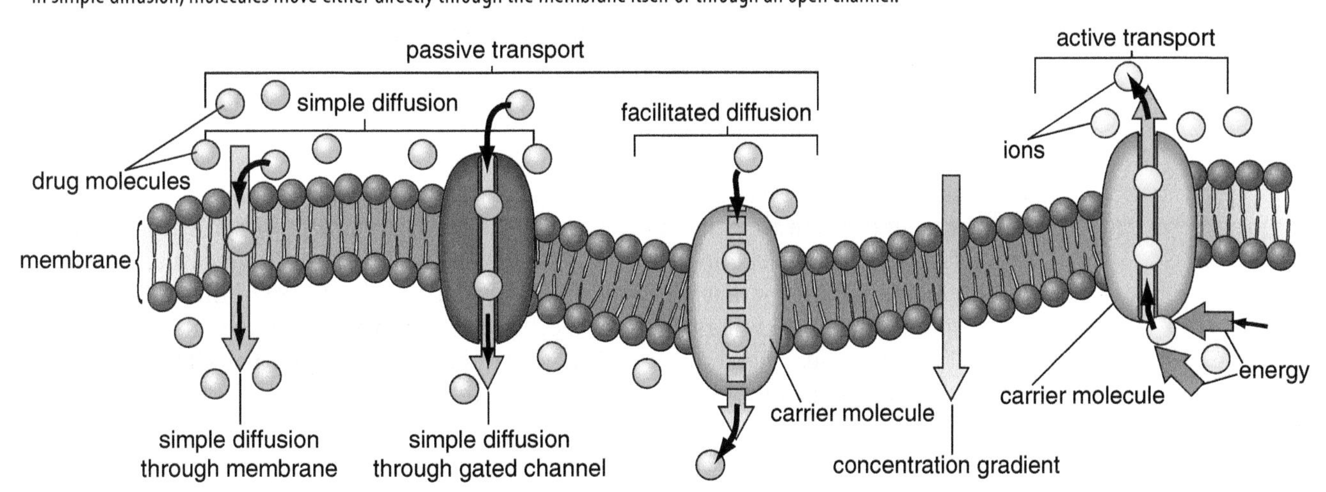

Passive mechanisms, on the other hand, are usually driven by **concentration gradients**. Drugs absorbed via passive transport move from an area of high concentration (the site of administration) to an area of low concentration (the bloodstream). Thus, higher doses typically produce greater absorption. Diffusion is a passive transport mechanism by which many drugs are absorbed because molecules simply move along a concentration gradient.

Last, blood flow and surface area affect absorption. For instance, the gastrointestinal tract may not have a conducive pH for a drug to be absorbed. But the great amount of surface area and good blood flow to the small intestine overcome this limitation to absorption. Surface areas that are large, thin, and have good blood supply, like those of the small intestine and lungs, can easily affect systemic absorption.

Distribution

Distribution is the process by which drugs move around in the bloodstream and reach other tissues of the body. Consequently, distribution is highly affected by blood flow. If blood flow is poor in a particular tissue or area of the body, few drug molecules are able to reach it. On the other hand, organs with high blood flow (for example, the heart, kidneys, liver, and lungs) are exposed to drugs easily.

A measurement known as **volume of distribution (Vd)** indicates how a drug is distributed within the compartments of the body. For example, a highly water-soluble drug stays in the bloodstream—the primary compartment for water-soluble drug distribution. However, if a drug is highly fat- or lipid-soluble, it can accumulate in fatty tissue and then slowly be released back into the bloodstream over time. This second example is referred to as a **two-compartment model**. Drugs are usually distributed to one- or two-compartment models. Drugs that have more than one compartment for distribution must be dosed accordingly in order to avoid accumulation over time and increased potential for toxicity.

Two other factors greatly affect distribution: **protein binding** and the blood-brain barrier. Some drug molecules have a high affinity for protein molecules and thus bind to proteins, such as albumin, that circulate in the blood. When drug molecules are bound to proteins in the blood, they are not free to reach the intended site of action. If a drug binds to a large extent (90% or better), distribution is affected. If two highly protein-bound drugs are given together, they compete with each other for binding sites, leaving more of both drugs to roam freely in the blood. Therefore, they are more easily distributed. If dosing is not adjusted accordingly, both drugs can cause toxic effects.

The **blood-brain barrier (BBB)** is a physical layer of cells that affects distribution of drugs to the central nervous system. Although oxygen and carbon dioxide molecules easily pass across the BBB to reach brain cells, most larger drug molecules do not. This barrier is structured to allow only select molecules through. It serves as a good defense mechanism for preventing harmful substances from reaching delicate brain tissue, but may also limit access for desired drug therapy.

Elimination

Elimination is the process by which drugs leave the body. Elimination can be measured as the rate and extent to which a drug leaves the bloodstream. On the time-response curve (see Figure 2.9), elimination is the downward sloping part of the curve. **Half-life** **($t_{1/2}$)** refers to the time it takes for half (50%) of a drug to be cleared from the blood. It takes approximately eight half-lives for a drug to be completely eliminated from the body. Two processes, metabolism and excretion, affect elimination half-life. Drugs can be deactivated via metabolism first and then excreted from the body, or they may be excreted unchanged.

Metabolism The liver contains enzymes that metabolize drugs and other substances in the body. Its purpose is to detoxify the blood. The liver is considered the primary site of drug metabolism. Drug **metabolism** is, therefore, highly dependent on blood flow to the liver as well as the efficiency and function of enzymes located there. In some cases, drugs rely on metabolism to activate them. These are called **prodrugs**.

First-Pass Effect Because blood coming from most of the gastrointestinal system goes through the liver before entering the rest of the body's circulation, many drugs undergo the **first-pass effect**. This effect refers to the liver metabolizing drugs as they "pass," or travel through it. As a result, the full drug dose does not reach the body, and its systemic effect is lessened or effectively eliminated. For those drugs that are quickly and easily metabolized by liver enzymes, this first-pass effect is especially problematic, and alternative routes of administration that bypass the liver must be used.

Drug Interactions Many liver enzymes are involved in metabolism; the **cytochrome P450 enzyme system** most frequently deactivates drugs. Cytochrome P450 enzymes that metabolize drugs are numbered. Common ones include 1A2, 2A6, 2C9, 2D6, and 3A4. Drugs that interfere with these enzymes can affect other drugs that need these enzymes for proper elimination. Two drugs that use the same enzyme system, when given together, can compete for elimination and increase potential for toxicity. It's easy to see how the cytochrome P450 system is a common source of drug interactions.

Excretion The process by which drug molecules are removed from the bloodstream, **excretion** primarily occurs in the kidneys, the organs responsible for filtering substances from the blood and making urine. Excretion can also occur via bile, feces, sweat, and exhalation. Usually, excretion is highly dependent on blood flow through the kidney as well as kidney function itself. Like transport mechanisms that control entry into the bloodstream, excretion can occur by active or passive mechanisms. Ionization also affects excretion, because highly ionized drugs cannot easily cross membranes to exit the bloodstream. The pH of urine can therefore affect ionization and elimination rates.

Special Populations

The specific characteristics of individual patients affect the pharmacokinetic properties of the drugs they take. Although some population generalizations can be made, no two patients are exactly alike. Awareness of these differences is important when choosing the best drug for each patient, as well as for dosing and delivering it in a way that will be both safe and effective.

Differences in age and function of the liver and kidneys create the most problems, but other factors also influence pharmacokinetic parameters. In regard to gender, females have higher body fat content (compared to males), which affects drug distribution. Metabolism rates are often higher in men than in women, again affecting drug elimination. In pregnancy, gastrointestinal motility slows, allowing more time for absorption. Blood volume also increases, effectively lowering the concentration of blood proteins and distribution. Urination also increases, affecting elimination. In severe cardiovascular disease, blood flow decreases, altering blood supply to vital organs such as the liver and kidneys. In hyperthyroidism, the metabolism rate increases in the liver, enhancing elimination.

Age Very young and very old patients pose the greatest risks to safe drug therapy because the pharmacokinetic behavior of drugs varies widely in these populations. In **pediatric practice** (infants and children), infants are of greatest concern, because their body makeup and liver function are different from those in adults. Babies have higher body water content, so drugs that are highly water-soluble will distribute well, making toxicity an issue. Blood circulation is also very good in pediatric patients. However, liver function is not fully mature at birth. It takes months to years for all liver enzyme systems to become fully functional. Therefore, absorption, distribution, and metabolism are all affected in infants and children.

In **geriatric practice** (elderly patients), you must consider several different effects on pharmacokinetic parameters. First, acidity in the stomach is usually decreased in older adults, which translates to a higher pH. Drugs that need a highly acidic (low pH) environment for absorption are affected. Older patients tend to have higher body fat content, so drugs that are highly fat-soluble may distribute well and accumulate. As people age, both kidney and liver function decrease, so elimination drops dramatically. Blood flow to these vital organs also decreases with age. Doses are usually decreased and dosing intervals increased to accommodate altered absorption, distribution, and elimination in older patients.

Liver Disease Because metabolism occurs primarily in the liver, problems in **liver function** can greatly affect drugs eliminated via metabolism. Cirrhosis, hepatitis, and other liver diseases can severely affect liver function. In these cases, doses must usually be adjusted downward.

Kidney Disease Because excretion happens most often through the kidneys, problems with **kidney function** greatly affect drug elimination. Both acute and chronic kidney failure make a difference in a drug's ability to leave the body. If doses are not adjusted accordingly, drugs accumulate and cause toxicity.

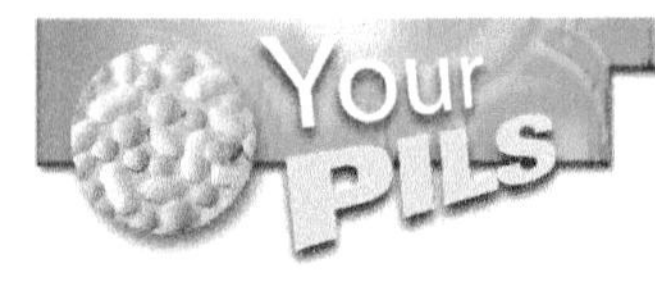

Grasping concepts related to pharmacokinetics can be difficult. Producers and Directors may find it useful to redraw the dose-response curve to represent the influence of various factors on absorption and elimination. Enactors and Creators may find group discussion valuable for reasoning out the effects that changes in absorption, distribution, and elimination have on the dose-response curve and drug behavior.

Chapter Summary

The atom is the smallest unit of matter. Atoms are made up of positively charged protons, uncharged neutrons, and negatively charged electrons. The periodic table of the elements categorizes elements, or types of atoms, into groups with similar chemical properties. When atoms bond together, they combine via covalent or ionic bonds to form molecules. Common molecules found in the body are carbohydrates, lipids, proteins, and nucleic acids. Each of these molecules contains various functional groups that give them particular qualities that predict how they behave in the body. The same may be said about drug molecules. Their functional groups and behavior in acidic and basic environments determine how drugs are absorbed, distributed, and eliminated from the body.

Pharmacodynamics studies how drugs act on the body at the molecular level. Drug receptor theory helps explain drug activity. Receptor agonists stimulate a response, whereas antagonists block a response.

Pharmacokinetics is the study of how drugs move around in the body. The four phases of pharmacokinetics are absorption, distribution, metabolism, and excretion. Mathematical models describe these phases, and graphical representation describes how drugs enter and exit the bloodstream. Drug dosing depends on these concepts.

Various factors affect individual patient pharmacokinetic parameters for drug therapy. Factors such as age, gender, liver/kidney function, and certain disease states affect how drugs are absorbed, distributed, and eliminated. Such characteristics are taken into account when choosing appropriate drug therapy and dosing.

Chapter Review

For the following sets of exercises, write the exercise heading, exercise numbers, and your answers on a separate sheet of paper. Your instructor may direct you to turn in the sheet of paper or discuss your answers as a class.

REVIEW THE BASICS

Choose a, b, c, or d as the correct answer to each multiple-choice question.

1. Which of the following is the part of an atom that is negatively charged and orbits around the nucleus?
   a. proton
   b. neutron
   c. electron
   d. isotope

2. Which of the following is a chemical bond between atoms wherein electrons are shared?
   a. covalent
   b. ionic
   c. polar
   d. stereoisomer

3. Which of the following is true of acidic substances?
   a. Acids easily accept hydrogen ions (H^+).
   b. Acids easily donate hydrogen ions (H^+).
   c. Acids exist in their ionic form when put in an acidic environment.
   d. Acids exist in their nonionic form when put in a basic environment.

4. Which of the following is the membrane transport process that moves drug molecules from the site of administration into the bloodstream according to a concentration gradient (high to low)?
   a. diffusion
   b. active transport
   c. sodium/potassium ion pump
   d. none of the above

5. Which of the following factors could affect the absorption of an oral drug?
   a. poor blood flow to gastrointestinal tract
   b. changing the pH of the stomach (such as taking an antacid)
   c. dissolving the drug in water before swallowing
   d. all of the above

6. In which of the following routes of administration would you most likely encounter problems with the first-pass effect?
   a. oral
   b. intravenous
   c. transdermal
   d. inhalation

7. If someone had alcoholic liver cirrhosis, which pharmacokinetic phase would most likely be affected?
   a. absorption
   b. distribution
   c. metabolism
   d. excretion

8. Which of the following is the term for the time it takes for the concentration of drug in the blood to drop to half?
   a. onset of action
   b. duration of action
   c. half-life
   d. volume of distribution

9. The hepatic cytochrome P450 enzyme system affects drugs in which phase of pharmacokinetics?
   a. absorption
   b. distribution
   c. metabolism
   d. excretion

10. Which of the following phases is represented in the upward-sloping portion of the dose-response curve?
    a. absorption
    b. distribution
    c. metabolism
    d. excretion

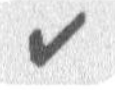

KNOW THE DRUGS

Match each major types of body molecule with its corresponding description.

Body Molecule	Body Molecule Description
1. Carbohydrates	a. Molecules that form the building blocks of protein and tissue
2. Peptides	b. Molecules that form hormones and biochemicals
3. Lipids	c. Molecules that form sugars and are used for energy
4. Nucleic Acids	d. Molecules that form genetic material (DNA) inside cells

PUT IT TOGETHER

For each item, write down a single term to complete the sentence, the correct letter in response to the multiple-choice question, true or false, or a short answer.

1. Protein binding within the bloodstream primarily affects ____________ of a drug.
2. Water molecules move across membranes by diffusion like drug molecules do. If a cell were placed in a solution of pure water, which of the following would happen? Explain why you chose your answer.
   a. Water would enter the cell, which may burst.
   b. Water would leave the cell, which may shrivel.
   c. Nothing, the concentration gradient is equal.
3. True or False: A leftward shift in the dose-response curve for one drug compared with another means the drug is less effective.
4. For the following organs of the body, describe how the phases of pharmacokinetics are different in an infant as compared with a normal adult.

   Body fat

   Liver

   Kidney
5. Describe the difference between an agonist and an antagonist drug.

THINK IT THROUGH

Read and think through each numbered scenario carefully and then write several sentences in reply to the question(s) presented. Question 4 requires you to do some Internet research before completing your answer(s).

1. Describe two ways that the pharmacokinetics of drugs are altered in the elderly patient population and explain what happens to that phase.
2. If a patient had severe diarrhea that drastically increased gastrointestinal motility, what pharmacokinetic phase would be affected? Why?
3. Someone has end-stage renal disease from diabetic nephropathy. What pharmacokinetic phase would be affected and in what way? Describe how the dose-response curve would change for such a patient. How would this affect drug dosing?

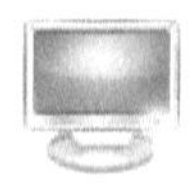

4. **On the Internet**, locate information about renal dosing for metformin (commonly prescribed in the outpatient setting) and cefuroxime (commonly ordered in the inpatient setting). What changes in dose are necessary for these drugs in patients with kidney dysfunction or failure? *Hint:* Manufacturers' Web sites often have FDA-approved labeling that includes guidelines for renal dosing. If you work for a hospital or retail pharmacy, look in the professional references and resources (such as *Micromedex* or *Drug Facts and Comparisons*) provided to you online through your employer.

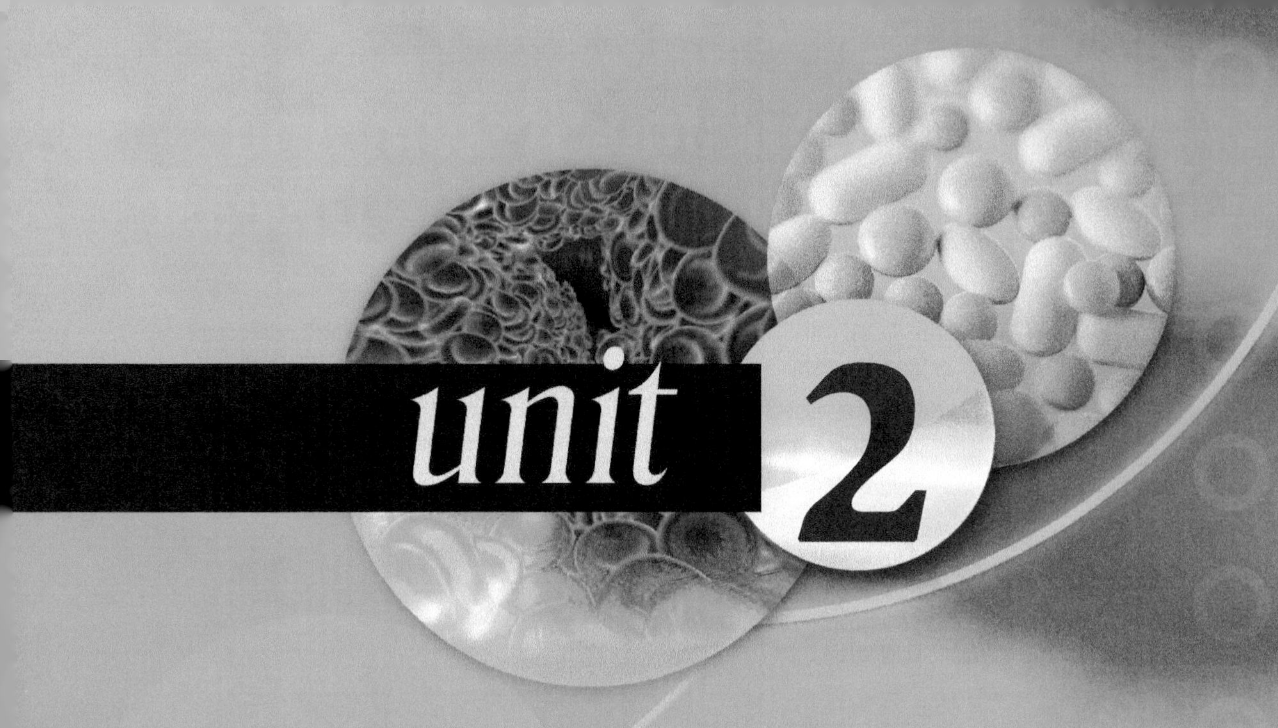

Drugs for the Immune System

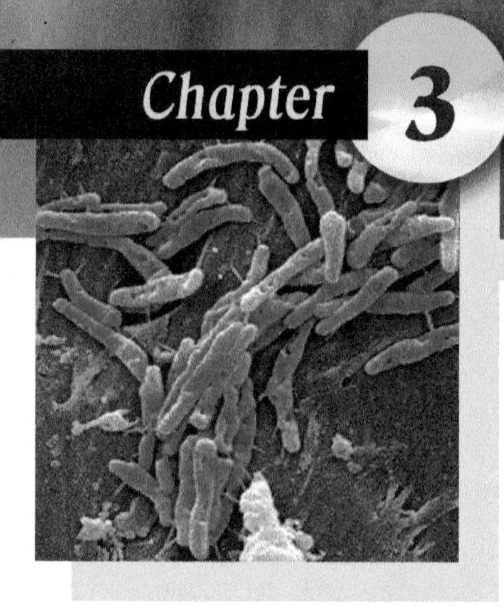

Chapter 3 The Immune System and Drugs for Infectious Diseases

LEARNING OBJECTIVES

- Describe the basic anatomy and physiology of the immune system.
- Explain the therapeutic effects of the prescription medications, nonprescription medications, and alternative therapies used to treat common infections.
- Describe the adverse effects of the prescription medications, nonprescription medications, and alternative therapies used to treat common infections.
- Identify the brand and generic names of the prescription and nonprescription medications used to treat common infections.
- State the common doses, dosage forms, and routes of administration for prescription and nonprescription medications used to treat common infections.

Interactive self-quizzes, games, audio files, and glossaries help you to learn drug names and facts.

Before discovery and development of the first antibiotics and vaccines in the early twentieth century, infections were the most frequent cause of death. Through the "Age of Antibiotics," great strides in treating infectious diseases changed the nature of healthcare, at least in industrialized countries. These days, infections are usually fully cured using drug therapy, and long-term complications are relatively few, compared to other chronic conditions, such as cardiovascular disease and diabetes.

The purpose of this chapter is to describe the immune system and explain the use of antimicrobial agents in treating infections that commonly afflict this system. The most frequently encountered pathogens (bacteria, viruses, and fungi) are described along with the typical infections they cause. The number of antimicrobial drugs is large and varied, making this a long chapter. However, knowing these drugs will be useful because technicians work with such medications on a daily basis in all patient care settings. Other disorders of the immune system, including autoimmune diseases and immunization against future infection, are covered in Chapter 4.

Anatomy and Physiology of the Immune System

The **immune system** is the body's built-in defense mechanism against invading **pathogens**, the foreign organisms that cause infection. The immune system works on two levels—a local level, right at the site of a cut or wound, and a systemic level. The localized process is called **nonspecific immunity**, the **innate response**, or **inflammation** (see Figure 3.1). Inflammation involves mast cells, complement, and mediator chemicals such as histamine, leukotrienes, and prostaglandins.

When pathogens get into the bloodstream, a systemic immune response ensues. This process is called **acquired immunity** and involves a whole different set of cells. **Leukocytes** (**white blood cells**, or **WBCs**) mount this systemic response. Neutrophils, eosinophils, basophils, and monocytes are all types of WBCs that directly attack foreign cells such as bacteria. **Lymphocytes** (T and B cells) are WBCs that detect specific pathogens such as viruses (see Figure 3.2). **T cells** are responsible for **cellular immunity**, the process of detecting cells that are infected with viruses and initiating the immune response. **Killer T cells** attack cells of the body that have already been infected with a virus, and **helper T cells** release lymphokines that stimulate B cells to go into action. **B cells** provide **humoral immunity**, the process of making antibodies to prevent further infection. B cells mature into plasma cells that release antibodies, which fight off viruses before the viruses infect cells.

Figure 3.1
Inflammation: Nonspecific Immunity
Increased numbers of WBCs, improved blood flow, and fluid accumulation from increased vascular permeability combine at the site of an infection to cause redness and swelling.

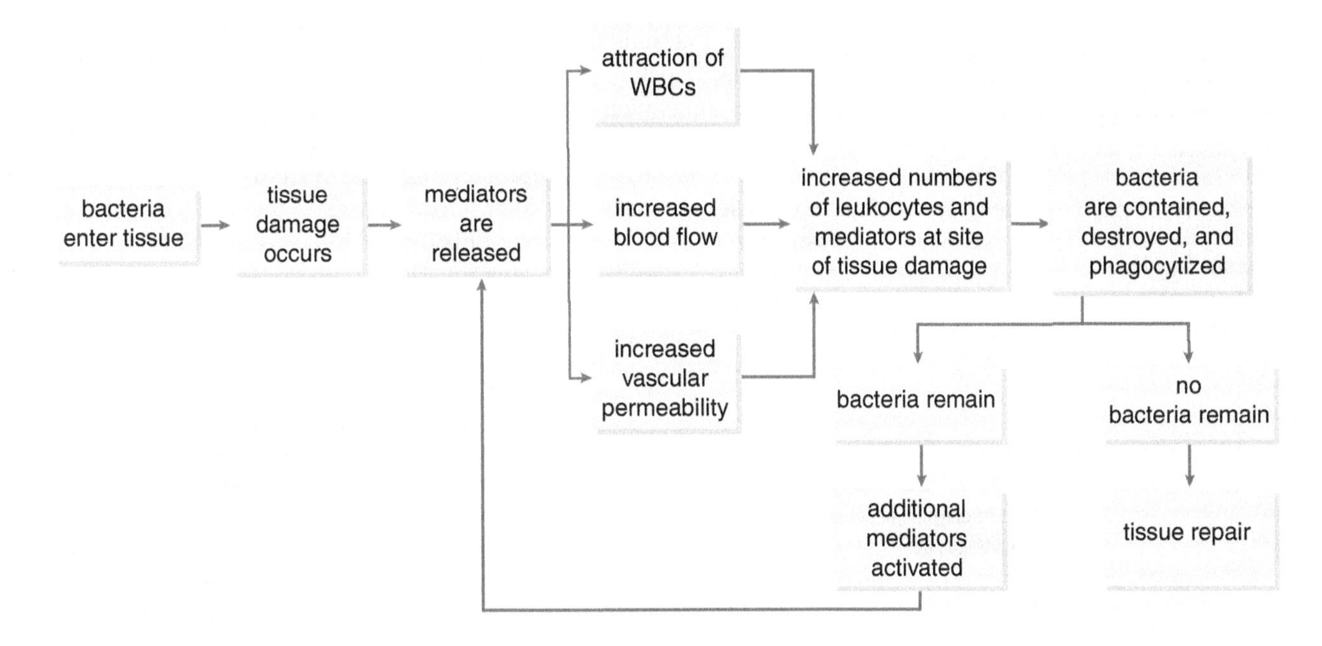

Figure 3.2
Acquired Immunity
Killer T cells directly attack cells infected with viruses, whereas helper T cells release substances that stimulate B cells to produce antibodies.

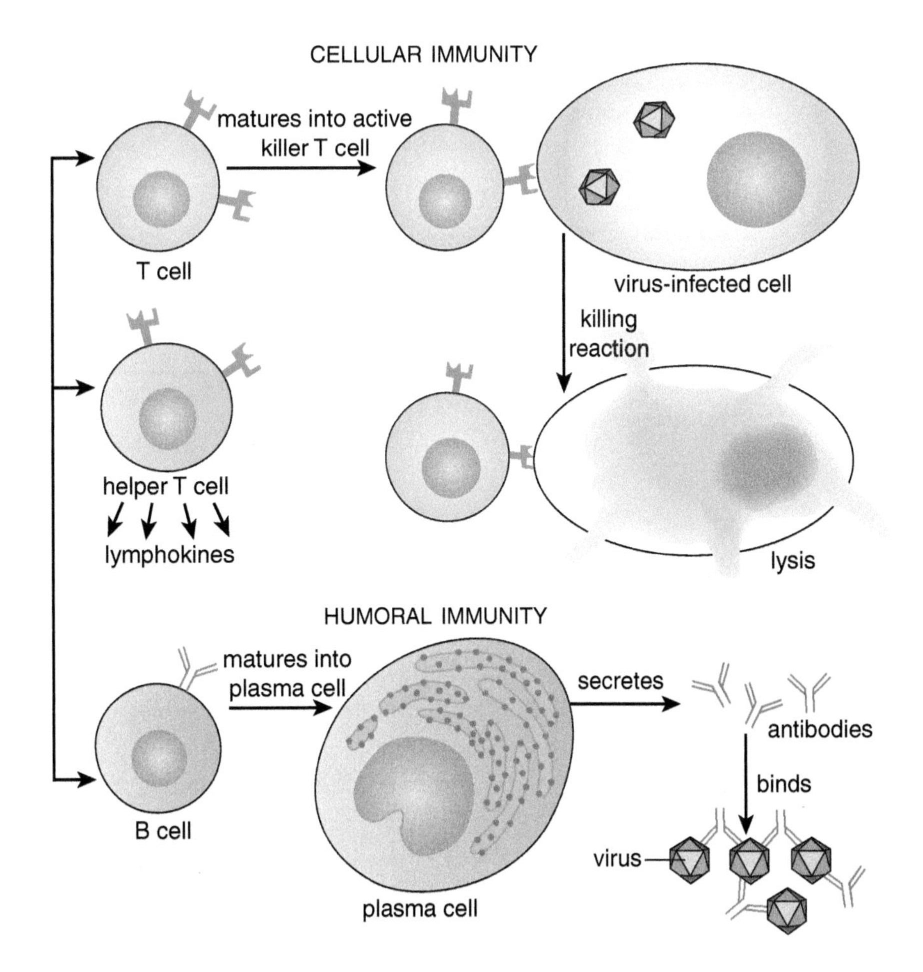

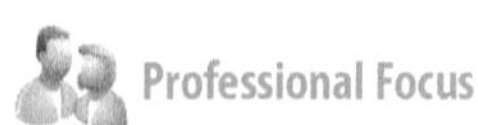

Professional Focus

During an active infection, the **WBC count** elevates (> 10,000 cells/mcL). When the body cannot fight off an infection on its own, antibiotics are used. In some institutions, pharmacy technicians assist pharmacists in determining whether an antibiotic is working by gathering laboratory results such as **complete blood count (CBC)**, which includes WBC count.

Antibodies help our bodies to remember specific pathogens in case we encounter them again. They allow the body to detect an infection early and mount a quick response before the infection causes symptoms or illness.

Laboratory tests to detect antibodies for specific viruses, such as **human immunodeficiency virus (HIV)**, can be used to check for exposure. If antibodies to a particular virus are found in a blood sample, that individual has been exposed either through natural contact or through a vaccine. Depending on the type and amount of antibodies measured, you can determine whether someone has been infected through exposure or is immune due to vaccination.

The immune system operates largely within the **lymphatic system** (see Figure 3.3). The lymphatic system is a set of vessels that filter **lymph**, the fluid that leaks out of the bloodstream into tissue spaces around the body. This fluid is filtered through **lymph nodes** before it is dumped back into the bloodstream. The lymph nodes are where foreign pathogens are often detected and destroyed by WBCs. During an active infection, these lymph nodes can become swollen and sore. For example, swollen tonsils and neck glands are signs of this process when someone has an upper respiratory tract infection (RTI).

Figure 3.3
Lymphatic System
Clusters of lymph nodes are located in the neck, armpits, and groin.

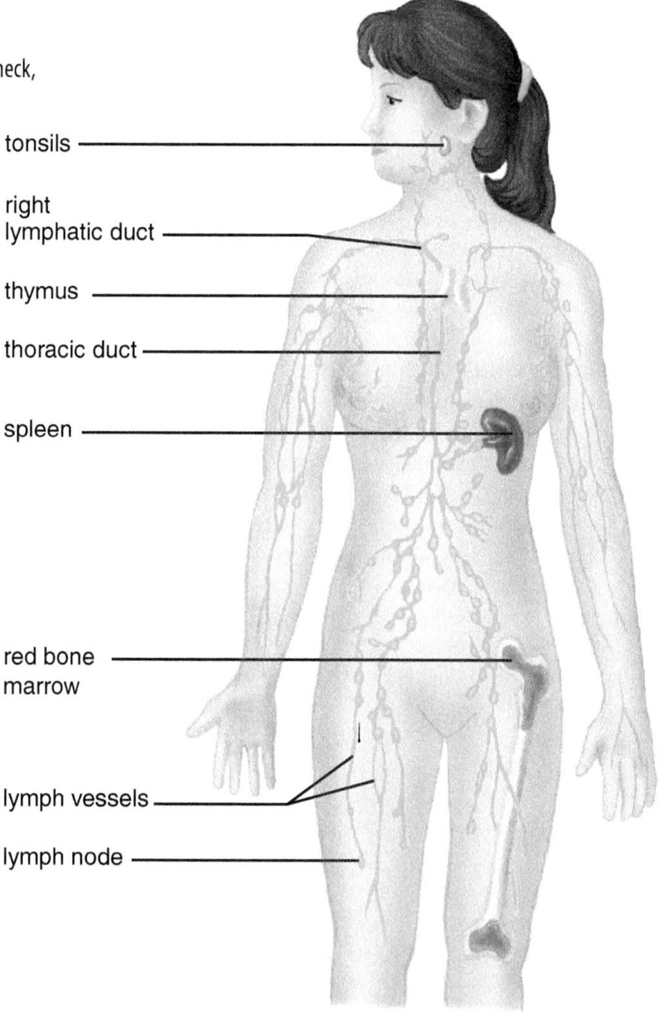

Bacterial Infections

Bacteria are single-celled microorganisms that live practically everywhere. For example, many bacteria can be found on the skin and in the bowels at all times. These skin and bowel organisms only cause disease when they either grow out of control or gain entry to the blood. Other bacteria are harmful (pathogenic) whenever they invade.

Figure 3.4
Characteristic Bacteria Shapes
Spherical bacteria (a) are called cocci. Rod-shaped bacteria (b) are called bacilli. And spiral-shaped bacteria (c) are spirochetes. *Streptococcus pyogenes*, the bacteria that cause strep throat, is round and grows in chains.

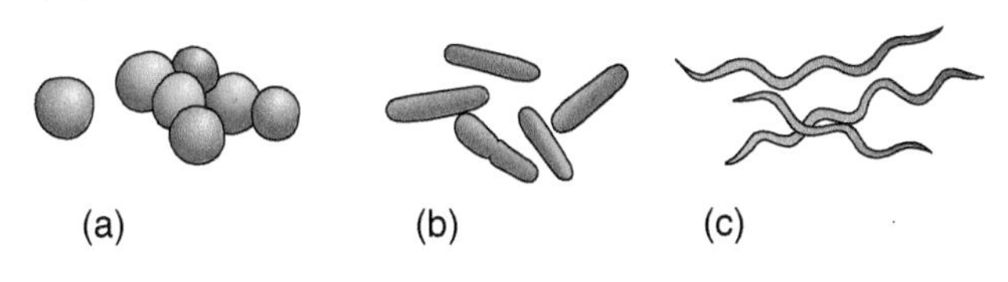

Sometimes, pathogenic bacteria produce toxins that cause many of the signs and symptoms experienced when infection is present.

Bacteria are either **aerobic**, needing oxygen to live, or **anaerobic**, meaning they can survive in an environment void of oxygen. Bacteria are classified by their shape and arrangement of growth (see Figure 3.4). If bacterial cells grow in chains or lines, their name begins with "strep." If they grow in clusters, their name begins with "staph." If they grow in pairs, their name begins with "diplo." For instance, *Staphylococcus aureus*, a common bacterium found on the skin, is round and grows in clusters like grapes. See Table 3.1 for more information.

Finally, bacteria are said to be either **gram-positive** or **gram-negative**. This classification comes from a staining technique named after its developer, Hans Christian Joachim Gram. In this technique, a purple stain called crystal violet is applied to the bacteria, and then they are viewed under a microscope. Gram-positive bacteria have a thick cell wall that absorbs this stain and appears purple. Gram-negative bacteria have a thin cell wall that does not absorb this stain.

Drugs for Bacterial Infections

Antibiotics are used to treat bacterial infections. They are not effective against viral infections. Antibiotics are either **bacteriostatic** or **bacteriocidal**. *Bacteriostatic* means the drug does not necessarily kill the pathogen but hinders its growth and progression, allowing the body's immune system to fight it off. *Bacteriocidal* means that the drug kills the pathogen. Bacteriocidal drugs are used on the most difficult infections to treat, especially for patients whose immune systems are not functioning well.

Antibiotics are chosen based on their **spectrum of activity** on pathogens suspected to cause an infection. For example, penicillin covers gram-negative, aerobic bacteria, so it could be used for infections such as *Streptococcus pyogenes* (strep throat). To facilitate diagnosis and choice of drug treatment, a sample or swab of the bacteria is taken from the patient and grown in culture in the laboratory. Then, various antibiotics are tested on the culture to determine which drug has the best activity on the pathogen. This laboratory test is called a **culture and sensitivity (C&S)** test. The amount of drug needed to inhibit growth of the bacteria is called the **minimum inhibitory concentration (MIC)**, a result often reported along with the C&S results.

When choosing appropriate drug therapy, the pharmacist must also take into account **antibiotic resistance**. Some bacteria have developed defense mechanisms that resist or inactivate antibiotics used on them. For instance, many bacteria that cause common respiratory tract infections (RTIs) are now resistant to the most frequently used drugs, like amoxicillin. **Nosocomial infections**, those that are acquired while in the hospital or nursing home, are often drug resistant and difficult to treat. In these cases, the common first choice of therapy cannot be used, because the bacteria are already resistant. More powerful (and expensive) drugs must be used.

Antibiotic resistance is a growing problem as we use more and more of these common drugs. Therefore, prescribers must be mindful of using antibiotics when they are not really needed and should be diligent in ordering antibiotics with a limited spectrum of activity first before advancing to more powerful drugs. If a patient were to develop an infection that was resistant to the most powerful antibiotics, no therapy would exist to treat the infection—a dire situation that could cause death. Patients can help reduce resistance by taking the entire course of therapy to prevent reemergence of resistant organisms. As a pharmacy technician, you should apply an auxiliary label for all antibiotics, warning patients to take the medication until it is gone.

TAKE UNTIL GONE

Table 3.1 Common Bacteria and Infections

Gram Stain	Shape	Bacteria	Associated Infection(s)
Aerobic			
Positive	Cocci	*Streptococcus pneumoniae* *Streptococcus pyogenes (Group A)*	Respiratory tract infection (RTI) and/or pneumonia Strep throat
Positive	Cocci	*Staphylococcus aureus* and other *Staphylococcus* spp.	Skin infection Endocarditis
Positive	Cocci	*Enterococcus faecalis, faecium*	Intestinal infection, urinary tract infection (UTI)
Positive	Bacilli	*Bacillus anthracis*	Anthrax
Positive	Bacilli	*Gardnerella vaginalis* *Lactobacillus* spp.	Vaginal infections
Positive	Bacilli	*Listeria monocytogenes*	Meningitis
Positive	Bacilli	*Clostridium tetani* *Clostridium perfringens* *Clostridium botulinum* *Clostridium difficile*	Tetanus Gangrene Botulism Intestinal infection
Positive	Bacilli	*Corynebacteria diphtheriae*	Diphtheria
Negative	Cocci	*Neisseria meningitidis* *Neisseria gonorrhea*	Meningitis Gonorrhea
Negative	Bacilli	*Escherichia coli* *Klebsiella* spp. *Proteus* spp. *Enterobacter* spp. *Shigella* spp.	Intestinal infection
Negative	Bacilli	*Salmonella typhi*	Typhoid fever
Negative	Bacilli	*Yersinia pestis*	Plague
Negative	Bacilli	*Pseudomonas aeruginosa*	Various difficult-to-treat infections
Negative	Bacilli	*Haemophilus influenzae*	RTI
Negative	Bacilli	*Vibrio cholerae*	Cholera
Negative	Coccobacilli	*Bordetella pertussis*	Pertussis
Negative	Coccobacilli	*Helicobacter pylori*	Stomach ulcers
Anaerobic			
	Cocci	*Peptococcus, Streptopeptococcus*	Dental infection
	Bacilli	*Bacteroides fragilis*	Abdominal infection Sepsis
Miscellaneous			
Spirochetes		*Treponema pallidum* *Borrelia burgdorferi*	Syphilis Lyme disease
Atypical		*Mycoplasma pneumonia* *Legionella* spp.	RTI and/or pneumonia
Atypical		*Mycobacterium tuberculosis*	Tuberculosis (TB)
Gram-negative		*Chlamydia trachomatis*	Chlamydia and pelvic inflammatory disease (PID)

The choice of oral versus intravenous (IV) antibiotic therapy depends on the site and severity of the infection as well as the organism suspected to be causing it. In most cases, antibiotics are best given at even intervals throughout the day. In children, antibiotics are dosed for an entire day, based on the child's weight, but are given in divided doses. Doses provided in this text are presented as general guides for recognizing when a prescribed dose is out of the ordinary. You should refer to the package insert or other reliable sources to verify proper dosing and double-check dose calculations for children so as not to accidentally overdose them.

Penicillins This class of drugs kills bacteria by inhibiting the formation of their cell wall, without which the cell cannot survive. All penicillins have a **beta-lactam ring** as part of their molecular structure. Unfortunately, some bacteria are resistant to penicillins because the bacteria produce an enzyme called **beta-lactamase** that breaks apart this ring structure, rendering the drug inactive. For this reason, some penicillin products are available as a combination of penicillin with a **beta-lactamase inhibitor**.

Penicillins are used for a variety of infections and are most frequently prescribed for RTIs, strep throat, syphilis, gonorrhea, tooth/gum infections, ear infections, and endocarditis. Certain penicillins are used for some skin infections, meningitis, and even bacteremia (bacterial infection in the blood). They are most effective on gram-positive bacteria.

Penicillins work best when taken on an empty stomach, but if stomach upset occurs, they can be taken with food. They should not be taken with fruit juice or cola because the acid in these drinks can deactivate the drug. See Table 3.2 for dosage and routes of administration for common penicillins.

Side Effects Common side effects of penicillins include stomach upset and diarrhea. Taking them with food can help with these side effects. Other rare but more severe side effects include mental disturbances, seizure, kidney damage, and bleeding abnormalities. These particular side effects tend to occur more often at higher doses and with the IV route.

Cautions and Considerations Allergy to penicillins is common, affecting as many as 10% of patients. Approximately 10% of those patients who are allergic to penicillin will also be allergic to cephalosporins, another class of antibiotics that inhibits cell wall formation. Therefore, technicians should always inquire about all drug allergies when dispensing either one of these antibiotics.

Some bacteria have become resistant to methicillin, an old penicillin used for difficult staphylococcal infections. The antistaphylococcal penicillins (also called penicillinase-resistant) have largely replaced it in practice. **Methicillin-resistant *Staphylococcus aureus* (MRSA)** infections are resistant to all antistaphylococcal penicillins and thus few drugs can treat them. Special precautions are used to protect against the spread of this bacteria to other patients. For instance, access to the affected patient's hospital room will be restricted, and anyone who enters will have to wear protective gear such as a gown, mask, and gloves.

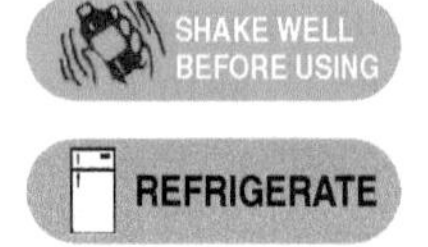

Oral penicillins in liquid form are suspensions, so they should be shaken well before every dose. Most of these suspensions must also be refrigerated. Pharmacy technicians should take care to apply warning labels about shaking and refrigeration when dispensing these products. Suspensions prepared with water are good for only fourteen days from the mixing date. Any medication left over after treatment should be thrown away.

Although IV preparations are often used in conjunction with other antibiotics, such as aminoglycosides, for difficult infections, they should not be mixed into the same IV bag.

Cephalosporins Like penicillins, **cephalosporins** are drugs that kill bacteria by inhibiting the formation of their cell wall. Cephalosporins are divided into four groups, called

Table 3.2 Common Penicillins

Generic (Brand)	Dosage Form	Route of Administration	Common Dose
Amoxicillin (Amoxil, Trimox)	Tablet, chewable tablet, capsule, suspension	Oral	Pediatric: 20–45 mg/kg/day in divided doses Adult: 250–875 mg taken 2–3 times a day
Ampicillin	Capsule, suspension, injection	Oral, IM, IV	PO: 250–500 mg QID IM/IV: Varies by age of patient, typical doses range in hundreds of milligrams a day in divided doses
Penicillin G	Injection, powder for injection	IM, IV	Varies by age of patient Typical doses range in thousands to millions of units a day in divided doses
Penicillin V (Pen VK)	Tablet, solution	Oral	Pediatric: 25–50 mg/kg/day in divided doses Adult: 125–250 mg every 6–8 hours
Antistaphylococcal Penicillins			
Dicloxacillin	Capsule	Oral	Pediatric: 12.5 mg/kg/day in divided doses Adult: 125–250 mg every 6 hours
Nafcillin	Injection	IV	500–1,000 mg every 4 hours
Oxacillin	Solution, injection	Oral, IV	PO: Pediatric: 50–100 mg/kg/day in divided doses Adult: 500–1,000 mg every 4–6 hours IV: varies by age of patient, typical doses range in hundreds of milligrams a day in divided doses
Extended-Spectrum Penicillins			
Piperacillin	Injection	IM, IV	Varies depending on route and type of infection treated Usually given multiple times a day
Ticarcillin	Injection	IM, IV	Varies depending on route, patient age, and type of infection treated Usually given multiple times a day
Combination Penicillins			
Amoxicillin + clavulanate (Augmentin)	Tablet, chewable tablet, oral suspension	Oral	Pediatric: 20–45 mg/kg/day in divided doses Adult: 250–500 mg every 8–12 hours
Ampicillin + sulbactam (Unasyn)	Injection	IM, IV	Pediatric: 300 mg/kg/day in divided doses Adult: 1.5–3 g every 6 hours
Piperacillin + tazobactam (Zosyn)	Injection	IV	Pediatric: varies by age and weight of patient, usually given multiple times a day Adult: 3.375 g every 6 hours
Ticarcillin + clavulanate (Timentin)	Injection	IV	Varies by age of patient Typical doses range in hundreds of milligrams a day in divided doses

generations. In general, first-generation cephalosporins work best on gram-positive bacteria, and as you move up through the generations, activity against gram-negative bacteria increases. Overall, cephalosporins are used for upper and lower RTIs, skin infections, some urinary tract infections (UTIs), infection prophylaxis during surgical procedures, and some deep-seated infections. The second-generation cephalosporins are used for respiratory infections caused by *Haemophilus influenzae* and for otitis media (ear infections). The third-generation cephalosporins are used for severe gram-negative infections. The fourth-generation cephalosporin, cefepime, is used for *Pseudomonas* infections that are difficult to treat.

Some cephalosporins should be taken with food, and others should be taken on an empty stomach. For example, cefditoren should be taken with food but not with antacids. Refer to the package insert to verify proper instructions with regard to food. Common cephalosporins and their dosing information are found in Table 3.3.

Side Effects Common side effects of cephalosporins include nausea, vomiting, diarrhea, headache, and dizziness. Most of the time, these effects are tolerable. Other rare but more severe side effects include mental disturbances, seizures, heart palpitations, and bleeding abnormalities. These particular side effects tend to occur more frequently at

Table 3.3 Common Cephalosporins

Generic (Brand)	Dosage Form	Route of Administration	Common Dose
First Generation			
Cefazolin (Ancef)	Injection	IM, IV	250 mg–1 g taken every 6, 8, or 12 hours (dosing depends on type of infection being treated) Also given prior to/during surgical procedures
Cephalexin (Keflex)	Tablet, capsule, oral suspension	Oral	Pediatric: 25–50 mg/kg/day in divided doses Adult: 250–750 mg every 6 hours
Second Generation			
Cefaclor (Ceclor)	Tablet, chewable tablet, capsule, oral suspension	Oral	Pediatric: 20–40 mg/kg/day in divided doses every 8 hours Adult: 250 mg every 8 hours or 375–500 mg every 12 hours
Cefdinir (Omnicef)	Capsule, oral suspension	Oral	Pediatric: 7 mg/kg every 12 hours or 14 mg/kg every 24 hours Adult: 300–600 mg every 12–24 hours
Cefixime (Suprax)	Oral suspension	Oral	Pediatric: 8 mg/kg/day Adult: 400 mg a day
Cefotetan (Cefotan)	Injection	IM, IV	500 mg–3 g every 12 hours
Cefoxitin (Mefoxin)	Injection	IV	1–2 g every 6–8 hours Also given prior to/during surgical procedures
Cefuroxime (Zinacef)	Tablet, oral suspension, injection	Oral, IM, IV	PO: Pediatric: 20–30 mg/kg/day divided twice a day Adult: 250–1,000 mg twice a day IV: 750 mg–1.5 g every 8 hours Also given prior to/during surgical procedures
Third Generation			
Cefditoren (Spectracef)	Tablet	Oral	200–400 mg twice a day
Cefotaxime (Claforan)	Injection	IM, IV	IM: 0.5 g–1 g single dose (for gonorrhea) IM/IV: 1–2 g every 4–12 hours depending on severity of infection
Ceftazidime (Fortex, Tazidime)	Injection	IM, IV	Pediatric: 30–50 mg/kg every 8–12 hours Adult: 1–2 g every 8–12 hours
Ceftibuten (Cedax)	Capsule, oral suspension	Oral	400 mg once a day
Ceftriaxone (Rocephin)	Injection	IM, IV	Pediatric: 50–76 mg/kg once or twice a day Adult: 1–2 g once or twice a day
Fourth Generation			
Cefepime (Maxipime)	Injection	IV	1–2 g every 8–12 hours

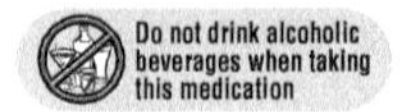

higher doses and with the IV route. Some of these serious effects can be worsened by alcohol intake, so patients should avoid alcohol while taking a cephalosporin.

Cautions and Considerations Allergy to cephalosporins is common. Approximately 10% of patients who are allergic to penicillin will also be allergic to cephalosporins. Therefore, you should always inquire about all drug allergies when dispensing either one of these antibiotics.

Some suspension products, such as Omnicef, are high in sugar content, so patients with diabetes should be informed of this.

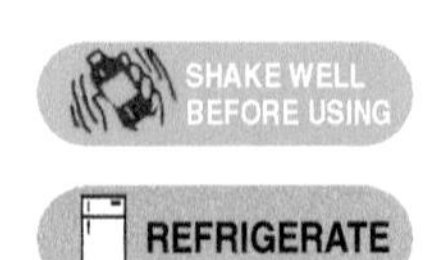

Most oral liquid dosage forms are suspensions and should be shaken well before every dose. Most of these suspensions must also be refrigerated. Suprax (cefixime) is one of the few that does not have to be refrigerated after reconstitution. When a suspension is prepared with water, it is good for only fourteen days from mixing. Any medication left over after treatment should be thrown away.

Some of the products in this class can be taken twice a day instead of three times a day. This feature is good for parents with children in daycare or school, where the ability to administer medications in the middle of the day can be problematic.

Carbapenems and Monobactams The two drug classes carbapenems and monobactams are grouped together here because they differ only slightly in their molecular structure from penicillins and cephalosporins. They kill bacteria by inhibiting the formation of the cell wall. **Monobactams** are used for gram-negative bacterial infections, and **carbapenems** are used for mixed infections that have both gram-positive and gram-negative bacteria. Both are used in special situations for serious nosocomial infections. Aztreonam is a monobactam, and carbapenems include ertapenem, imipenem, and meropenem. If you encounter these medications, please refer to other reputable resources for further details.

Vancomycin A single drug in a class by itself is **vancomycin (Vancocin)**. Its mechanism is not fully understood, but it probably works by inhibiting cell wall formation. Vancomycin has activity against gram-positive bacteria and is used primarily for MRSA infections. In fact, it is the drug of choice for this complicated infection. Unfortunately, some enterococci are resistant to vancomycin and are called **vancomycin-resistant *Enterococcus* (VRE)**.

Vancomycin is most frequently used in IV form because the oral form is poorly absorbed into the bloodstream. The oral dosage form is used, therefore, only for infections that are localized within the intestines. Doses range between 500 mg and 2 grams a day in divided doses.

Side Effects Vancomycin may commonly cause **nephrotoxicity** (kidney damage) and **ototoxicity** (hearing loss). With proper monitoring of blood levels and laboratory tests, these effects can be avoided or minimized. However, these side effects limit vancomycin use to difficult infections.

Cautions and Considerations Vancomycin must be administered slowly (usually over sixty minutes) to avoid an effect called **red man syndrome**. This syndrome involves hypotension, flushing, redness in the neck and face, and rash. Because the rate of infusion is particularly important for this medication, you should make sure that proper infusion rates are displayed prominently on the IV bag label.

Macrolides Another class of drugs, **macrolides**, works by blocking bacteria's ability to produce needed proteins for survival. At low doses, they are bacteriostatic, but at high doses can be bacteriocidal. Erythromycin is the most commonly used macrolide. Macrolides have a broad spectrum of activity in that they work against some gram-positive and gram-negative bacteria. Macrolides are used mainly for respiratory infections and pneumonia. They are also used with other drugs to treat *Helicobacter pylori*, the bacteria found in stomach ulcers. Azithromycin has an unusually short but convenient length of therapy (usually three to five days) as compared with other antibiotics (usually seven to fourteen days) (see Table 3.4 for more dosing information). Clindamycin is used for acne, female genital infections, intra-abdominal infections, and dental procedure prophylaxis. Sometimes antibiotics are taken prior to invasive dental work to prevent infection from introduction of bacteria into the bloodstream during the dental procedure.

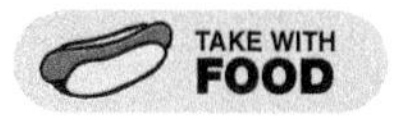

Side Effects Common side effects of macrolides include stomach upset, nausea, vomiting, heartburn, abdominal pain, and diarrhea. To reduce these effects, patients should take macrolides with food. If diarrhea or abdominal pain is severe, the patient should seek medical attention immediately because such pain could indicate a serious problem.

Liver toxicity has also occurred with the use of erythromycin. Patients with prior liver problems should not take this medication. If jaundice (yellowing of skin and eyes) occurs, medical attention should be sought immediately.

Cautions and Considerations Macrolides, especially erythromycin, have many drug interactions. Some of the effects caused by these interactions can be severe. You should heed any interaction warnings that appear in the computer system and alert the pharmacist.

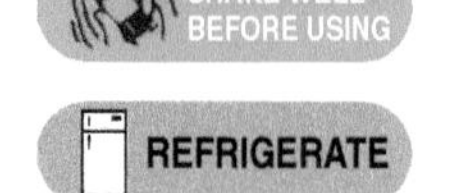

Oral suspension products should be shaken well before every dose. Most of these suspensions must also be refrigerated. Any of these suspensions prepared with water are good for only fourteen days from mixing. Any medication left over after treatment should be thrown away.

Table 3.4 Common Macrolides

Generic (Brand)	Dosage Form	Route of Administration	Common Dose
Azithromycin (Zithromax)	Tablet, oral suspension, injection	Oral, IV	PO: Pediatric: varies by age and weight of patient as well as type of infection Adult: 250–500 mg daily for 3–5 days IV: 500 mg daily for 2–10 days depending on type of infection
Clarithromycin (Biaxin)	Tablet, oral suspension	Oral	Pediatric: 15 mg/kg/day divided every 12 hours Adult: 250–500 mg every 12 hours
Clindamycin (Cleocin)	Tablet, oral solution, injection	Oral, IM, IV	PO: Pediatric: 8–20 mg/kg/day in 3–4 divided doses Adult: 150–300 mg every 6 hours IM/IV: 600–2,700 mg a day in divided doses
Erythromycin (EryC, Ery-Tab, EES, EryPed, Erythrocin, Pediazole)	Tablet, capsule, oral suspension, injection, solution, gel, ointment pledget	Oral, IM, IV, topical	Varies depending on age of patient and type of infection Usually given 3–4 times a day

Aminoglycosides A class of drugs called **aminoglycosides** kills bacteria by blocking their ability to make essential proteins for life. They are powerful bacteriocidal medications used for peritonitis, severe infection of the gums, and life-threatening infections such as sepsis. Aminoglycosides are often used in conjunction with other antibiotics (e.g., penicillins, cephalosporins, and vancomycin). Aminoglycosides work synergistically with these other drug classes. **Synergistic drug therapy** is when two or more drugs are used together because they employ different mechanisms of action (in this case, the inhibition of protein synthesis and cell wall lysis) that work better together than either drug works alone. The aminoglycosides gentamicin and tobramycin are used to treat eye infections in patients with immunodeficiency.

Many institutions have instituted pulse dosing, whereby aminoglycosides are given once a day instead of multiple times a day. Because the side effects of aminoglycosides can be serious, less exposure to the drug during the day seems to help reduce toxic effects. Special nomograms are used for dosing in these situations. Table 3.5 includes common aminoglycosides and their routes of administration.

Side Effects Common side effects of aminoglycosides include nephrotoxicity (kidney damage) and ototoxicity (tinnitus, hearing loss, and balance problems). With proper monitoring of blood levels and laboratory tests, these effects can be avoided or minimized. However, you can see why these drugs are saved for the most difficult of infections.

Cautions and Considerations Aminoglycosides have been known to cause neuromuscular blockade in some cases. If a patient complains of muscle weakness, difficulty breathing, numbness, tingling, twitching, or convulsions, the drug should be discontinued. Patients with muscular disorders, such as myasthenia gravis or Parkinson's disease, should not be given aminoglycosides. Caution must be used if aminoglycosides are given after surgery because they may interact with neuromuscular blockers, a class of drugs used in many surgical procedures.

Although aminoglycosides are often used in conjunction with other antibiotics such as cephalosporins or penicillins, they should not be mixed into the same IV bag. Ophthalmic preparations should be kept as sterile as possible. Do not touch the tip of the applicator to the eye or other surfaces.

Table 3.5 Common Aminoglycosides

Generic (Brand)	Dosage Form	Route of Administration
Amikacin (Amikin)	Injection	IM, IV
Gentamicin (Garamycin, Genoptic)	Injection, ophthalmic solution, ophthalmic ointment	IM, IV, ophthalmic
Tobramycin (TOBI, Tobrex)	Injection, solution for inhalation, ophthalmic solution, ophthalmic ointment	IM, IV, inhaled via nebulizer, ophthalmic

Tetracyclines

Another class of drugs for bacterial infections is **tetracyclines**, bacteriostatic drugs that inhibit protein synthesis within bacterial cells. Consequently, they require a functioning immune system to cure an infection.

Tetracycline itself is probably used most often for acne treatment. Tetracyclines as a class are also drugs of choice for Lyme disease and Rocky Mountain spotted fever. Doxycycline is used frequently for sexually transmitted diseases such as gonorrhea and chlamydia. Occasionally, they are used for RTIs and some abdominal infections. Table 3.6 contains dosage information for tetracyclines.

Side Effects Common side effects of tetracyclines include stomach upset, nausea, and vomiting. They can be taken with food (but not dairy products or antacids) to reduce

Table 3.6 Common Tetracyclines

Generic (Brand)	Dosage Form	Route of Administration	Common Dose
Doxycycline (Vibramycin, Doryx)	Tablet, capsule, oral suspension, syrup, injection	Oral, IV	100–200 mg twice a day
Minocycline (Minocin, Dynacin)	Tablet, capsule, oral suspension, injection	Oral, IV	100 mg every 12 hours
Tetracycline (Sumycin)	Capsule, oral suspension	Oral	250–500 mg 2–4 times a day

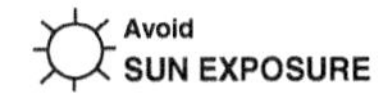

these effects. Tetracyclines also cause photosensitivity. Patients should be informed that their skin will burn faster when exposed to the sun and a rash may develop. Sunscreen and other protection should be worn when spending time outside.

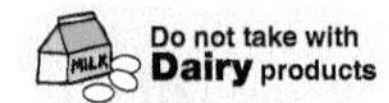

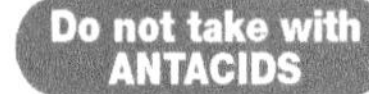

Cautions and Considerations Tetracyclines will bind with metals and ions, such as calcium, aluminum, and magnesium. When this occurs, they cannot be absorbed into the bloodstream. Therefore, you should apply warning labels to this effect and make sure the pharmacist counsels patients about avoiding food (cheese), drink (milk), and other products (antacids or laxatives) that contain these substances.

Tetracyclines accumulate in teeth and bones to cause discoloration. Consequently, children under eight years old and pregnant women cannot use tetracyclines because permanent teeth problems could occur.

Tetracycline breaks down over time to become toxic. Therefore, expired tetracycline should be discarded and never saved for future use. You should make sure expiration dates are accurate on all prescription vials containing tetracycline.

Fluoroquinolones The class of drugs known as **fluoroquinolones** (also called **quinolones**) kills bacteria by inhibiting the enzyme that helps DNA to coil. If DNA cannot coil, it is rendered useless, and the cell dies because it cannot function. Quinolones have strong activity against gram-negative bacteria. They tend to be used for bone and joint infections, eye infections, and serious RTIs and UTIs. Most of them work particularly well against difficult *Pseudomonas aeruginosa* infections. Quinolones also have a special use as treatment for anthrax, a potential bioterrorism agent.

Due to overprescribing, resistance to quinolones has developed. Therefore, their use is discouraged in ordinary and frequently seen infections. Quinolones should be saved for more serious and difficult gram-negative bacterial infections. Table 3.7 gives dosing information for common quinolones.

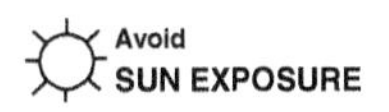

Side Effects Common side effects of quinolones include nausea, vomiting, dizziness, diarrhea, and an unpleasant taste. If the patient cannot tolerate these effects, different antibiotics will need to be chosen. Taking quinolones with food does not necessarily reduce these effects. These drugs also cause photosensitivity, so patients should wear sunscreen when outside. Less common but serious side effects include liver toxicity and alterations in glucose metabolism. Elongation of the QT interval on electrocardiogram reports has occurred with quinolone use. Consequently, these drugs may not be the best choice in patients with heart problems. Quinolones may also cause tendon ruptures, especially in younger patients.

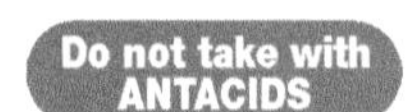

Cautions and Considerations Many drugs interact with quinolones, so technicians should heed interaction warnings that appear on the computer and alert the pharmacist. Quinolones should not be taken with antacids, dairy products, or calcium-fortified juices because their absorption will be reduced. You should be sure to affix appropriate auxiliary labels to the prescription vial when dispensing quinolones.

Table 3.7 Common Quinolones

Generic (Brand)	Dosage Form	Route of Administration	Common Dose
Ciprofloxacin (Cipro)	Tablet, oral suspension, injection	Oral, IV	PO: Pediatric: 6–20 mg/kg every 8–12 hours Adult: 250–750 mg every 12 hours IV: 200–400 mg every 12 hours
Gatifloxacin (Tequin, Zymar)	Ophthalmic solution	Ophthalmic	1–2 drops every 2 hours up to 8 times a day
Levofloxacin (Levaquin)	Tablet, oral solution, injection	Oral, IV	250–750 mg daily
Moxifloxacin (Avelox, Vigamox)	Tablet, injection	Oral, IV	400 mg daily

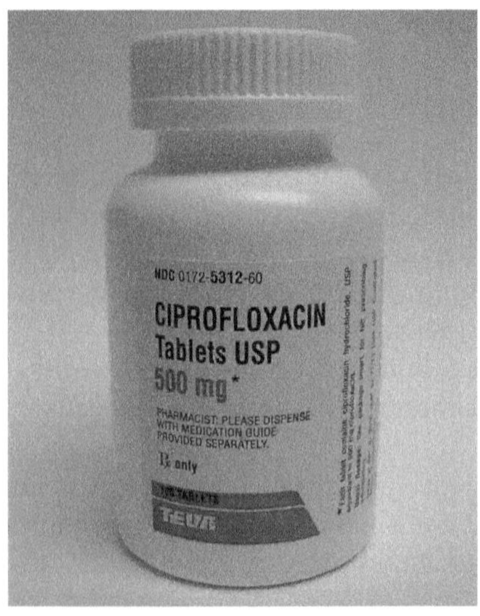

Stockpiles of Cipro (ciprofloxacin) have been accumulated in key locations around the country in anticipation of bioterrorist attacks. Pharmacies are sometimes asked to report their inventory of ciprofloxacin to assess readiness for homeland security.

Changes in mental function and convulsions have been reported with quinolones, especially ciprofloxacin. If a patient is exhibiting confusion, agitation, dizziness, hallucinations, insomnia, nightmares, or paranoia, stop the drug and seek medical attention immediately.

Sulfonamides and Nitrofurantoin Another common class of drugs is **sulfonamides**, or **sulfa drugs**, which are bacteriostatic and work by blocking bacteria from making folic acid, an essential substance for life. Although humans can absorb folic acid from food, bacteria cannot, and thus must make it. Sulfa drugs are used most often for UTIs. The most common sulfa drug is a combination containing trimethoprim. This combination is especially good for UTIs caused by *Escherichia coli*. Sulfa drugs are also used for community-acquired MRSA skin infections and as prophylaxis against *Pneumocystis carinii*, a common deadly lung infection in patients who have end-stage acquired immune deficiency syndrome (AIDS).

Like sulfa drugs, **nitrofurantoin** is used for UTIs. Its mechanism of action is not well understood, but it covers bacteria similar to those covered by sulfonamides. It works best if taken with food and plenty of fluids. Table 3.8 lists dosing information for common sulfonamides and nitrofurantoin.

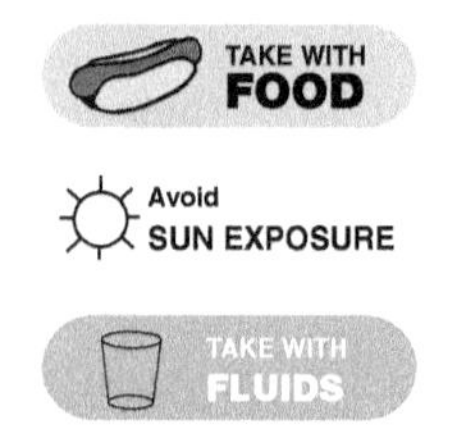

Side Effects Common side effects of sulfa drugs are nausea, vomiting, fever, and photosensitivity. Rarely, jaundice and Stevens-Johnson syndrome, a severe and possibly fatal skin rash condition, have occurred. Patients should know that if they have yellowing of their skin or eyes, or any kind of rash, they should stop taking the sulfa drug and notify their physician right away. Kidney damage has also occurred with sulfa drugs, so patients should be sure to drink six to eight glasses of water a day when taking these medications.

Common side effects of nitrofurantoin are nausea and vomiting. Taking it with food can help alleviate these effects.

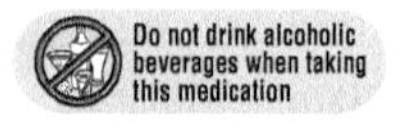

Cautions and Considerations Sulfa allergy is common, so you should always inquire about drug allergies when dispensing a sulfa drug. Sulfa drugs can possibly cause a disulfiram reaction if taken with alcohol. This reaction causes flushing, nausea, vomiting, and sweating. Therefore, patients should not drink any alcohol, including cough syrups and other OTC products containing alcohol, while taking and for a few days after taking a sulfa drug.

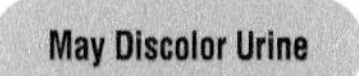

Nitrofurantoin turns urine brown, so be sure to use an appropriate warning label to alert patients to this harmless but sometimes alarming effect.

Table 3.8 Sulfonamides and Nitrofurantoin

Generic (Brand)	Dosage Form	Route of Administration	Common Dose
Nitrofurantoin (Macrobid, Macrodantin)	Capsule, suspension	Oral	Pediatric: 5–6 mg/kg a day in divided doses Adult: 5–100 mg 1–4 times a day
Trimethoprim/sulfamethoxazole (Bactrim, Cotrim, Septra)	Tablet, suspension, injection	Oral, IV	Varies depending on age and infection treated

Metronidazole The drug **metronidazole** is structured like an antifungal drug but works like an antibiotic. It also has activity on some protozoa. Common infections it is used for include *Giardia*, amebic dysentery, bacterial vaginosis, trichomoniasis, rosacea, and *H. pylori* ulcers. Metronidazole (Flagyl, MetroGel, or Vandazole) comes in tablet, lotion, cream, vaginal gel, and injectable dosage forms.

Side Effects The most common side effects of metronidazole are headache, anorexia, vomiting, diarrhea, and abdominal cramps. Taking it with food can help alleviate these effects.

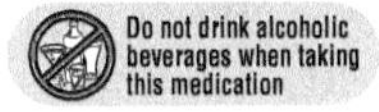

Cautions and Considerations One of the most important things to remember about metronidazole is that it interacts with alcohol to cause a severe reaction. Patients can become quite ill with nausea, vomiting, flushing, sweating, and headache if they ingest any alcohol while taking metronidazole and for three days after stopping it. Some cough medicines and other OTC products have alcohol in them. Patients should be warned not to use these products (in addition to alcoholic beverages) when taking metronidazole.

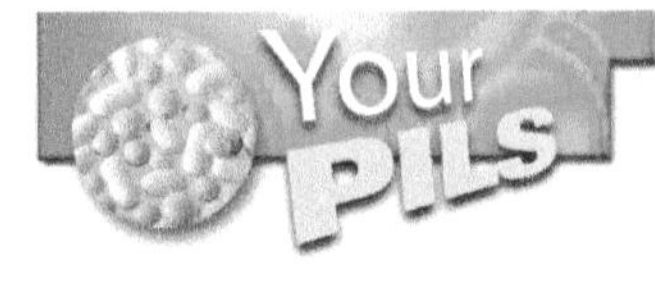

If you enjoy live-laboratory learning like Enactors do or practical application like Directors do, seek out someone who works with purchasing inventory in a retail and inpatient pharmacy. Which antibiotics do they dispense most often, and which ones cost them the most? Based on what you know about these drugs, postulate the types of infections these pharmacies are treating most often.

Viral Infections

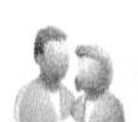

Professional Focus

Hepatitis B is a blood-borne pathogen passed by exposure to the body fluids of infected individuals. Accidental needle sticks when treating patients with hepatitis B are a common culprit. Therefore, most employers require patient care workers, including technicians, to get vaccinated against hepatitis B. The hep B vaccination series requires three shots spaced out over six months.

Viruses are not whole-cell organisms like bacteria. They are segments of nuclear material (DNA or RNA) surrounded by a capsule or protein coating. They attach to human cells and inject their nucleic material, which then alters that cell's function to instead begin replicating viruses. The cell's normal function is halted and it dies, releasing newly formed viruses that invade other cells. This process continues as the infection spreads.

Signs and symptoms of a viral infection depend on the type of cells destroyed by the virus. For example, a cold virus attacks cells in the respiratory mucosa, causing runny nose, sinus congestion, and coughing. The human immunodeficiency virus (HIV) attaches selectively to T cells, key components of the immune system. By infecting T lymphocytes, HIV promotes its own viability by destroying the very cells needed to detect and destroy it. When the disease progresses, patients are diagnosed with **acquired immunodeficiency syndrome (AIDS)**, a deadly disease that affects millions. In AIDS, even simple infections that normally would not cause any problems can become deadly.

Common viral infections include influenza and herpes, a family of viruses causing chicken pox (herpes varicella), shingles (herpes zoster), and sexually transmitted diseases (herpes simplex). Other viral infections include hepatitis (A, B, and C), measles, mumps, rubella, West Nile, rabies, respiratory syncytial virus (RSV), and rotavirus.

Drugs for Viral Infections

The number of **antiviral agents** is growing but does not rival the number of antibiotics available. Because viruses use a living cell to replicate, most drug therapy used to kill the virus also kills the cell. Antiviral drugs either prevent viruses from entering cells or alter their ability to replicate (see Figure 3.5). In most cases, it is preferable to prevent viral infections before they occur, using vaccines when possible.

For common viral infections such as influenza, cold sores, and shingles, drug therapy must be started as soon as the first symptoms begin. None of these agents eradicates the virus; they simply limit viral replication, which lessens the severity of symptoms and shortens the length of illness. Common side effects of antivirals include headache, malaise, fatigue, nausea, vomiting, diarrhea, cough, and rash. Usually, these effects are tolerable or indistinguishable from the viral infection being treated. Agents for influenza,

Figure 3.5

Mechanisms of Action for Antiviral Agents

Antiviral drugs either stop a virus from attaching to a cell, block its replication within the cell, or prevent its assembly into intact viruses for release.

Three methods to block viral infection or progression using medication:

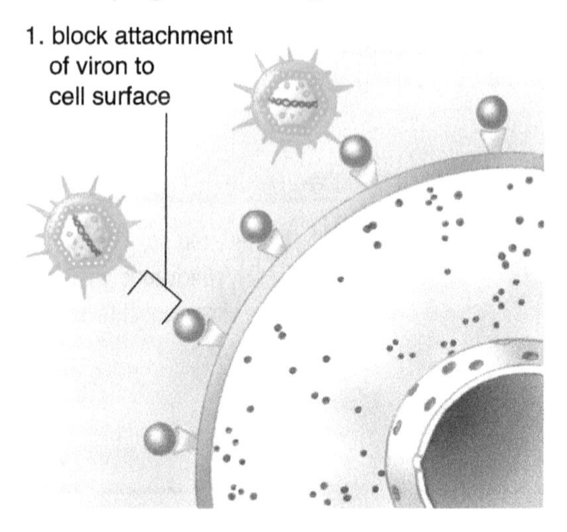

2. block viron replication and/or insertion into cell DNA (multiple methods, such as blocking enzymes that uncoil and splice DNA, are possible)

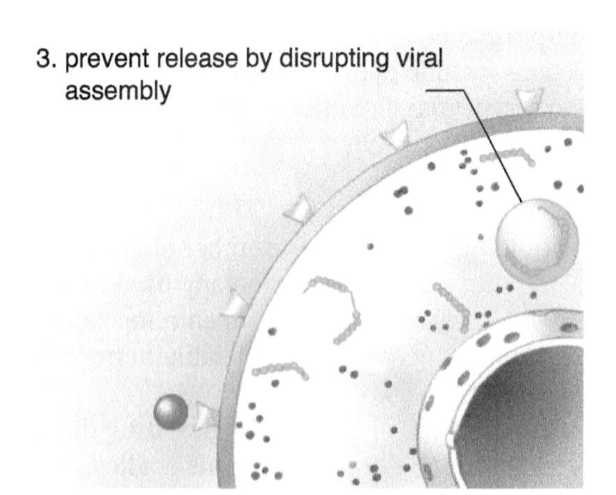

chickenpox, RSV, and shingles are taken only when symptoms indicate an infection has started and therapy is needed. Agents for hepatitis and genital herpes are taken on a chronic basis to suppress the virus and prevent or lessen outbreaks. Table 3.9 lists some common antivirals and their doses. Please refer to other resources for details on antiviral treatment specifically for hepatitis B.

Many antiviral agents are used to treat HIV and AIDS. HIV is a retrovirus that attaches to receptors on the surface of T cells and injects its contents. Once inside, an intracellular enzyme, reverse transcriptase, uses this material to make pro-DNA fragments. The pro-DNA fragments insert themselves into the host cell's DNA, which then alters the cell's function to produce parts of the HIV. Another enzyme, protease, then promotes assembly of the viral parts into intact HIVs, which are then released for further invasion.

The cadre of drugs used against HIV and AIDS saves lives but has numerous severe side effects and drug interactions, making them difficult medicines to take. These drugs can be combined into therapy, called a **"cocktail,"** to take advantage of the effects of synergistic drug therapy. By attacking the viral replication process in multiple stages, more viruses can be destroyed. Although these medications can reduce the number of viruses in the body to almost undetectable levels, patients must take the drugs throughout life to prevent progression of the illness and death and must strictly follow medication instructions to receive optimal effect.

Nucleoside and Nucleotide Reverse Transcriptase Inhibitors (NRTIs, NtRTIs) These HIV agents work by inhibiting reverse transcriptase, which forms pro-DNA molecules inside of T cells. Patients must pay attention to specific instructions about taking these drugs with or without food. Didanosine and zalcitabine must be taken on an empty stomach to work properly. Table 3.10 covers common dosing information for these drugs.

Take on an empty stomach

Side Effects Common side effects of these drugs are nausea and vomiting, which can be severe. Rarely, some of these agents can also cause lactic acidosis with liver enlargement, a life-threatening condition. These drugs can also cause pancreatitis, a painful inflammation of the pancreas, and peripheral neuropathy, a painful nerve condition in the legs and hands. Alcohol increases the incidence and severity of these toxicities. Avoiding alcohol is especially important when taking didanosine, emtricitabine, and abacavir.

Do not drink alcoholic beverages when taking this medication

Cautions and Considerations NRTIs and NtRTIs are metabolized in the liver, where many other drugs are also metabolized. Consequently, they can interact with other drugs. Didanosine cannot be taken with members

Table 3.9 **Antiviral Drugs for Common Infections**

Generic (Brand)	Dosage Form	Route of Administration	Indication and Common Dose
Acyclovir (Zovirax)	Tablet, capsule, oral suspension, ointment, IV	Oral, topical, IV	Herpes zoster (shingles) and chickenpox: 800 mg 5 times a day for 7–10 days Genital herpes (acute): 400 mg 5 times a day Genital herpes (chronic suppression): 400 mg twice a day for 1 year Chickenpox (pediatric): 20 mg/kg 4 times a day
Amantadine (Symmetrel)	Tablet, capsule, syrup	Oral	Influenza: 100–200 mg a day Influenza (pediatric): varies by age and weight of patient
Famciclovir (Famvir)	Tablet	Oral	Herpes zoster (shingles): 500 mg every 8 hours Genital herpes (acute): 1,000 mg twice a day for 1 day Genital herpes (chronic suppression): 250 mg twice a day for 1 year Herpes labialis (cold sores): 1,500 mg single dose
Oseltamivir (Tamiflu)	Capsule, oral suspension	Oral	Influenza (adult): 75 mg twice a day for 5 days Influenza (pediatric): varies by age and weight of patient
Ribavirin (Virazole, various)	Tablet, capsule, oral solution, inhalation	Oral, topical (inhaled)	RSV: 20 mg/mL inhaled for 12–18 hours a day
Rimantadine (Flumadine)	Tablet	Oral	Influenza (adult): 100 mg twice a day Influenza (pediatric): 5 mg/kg a day
Valacyclovir (Valtrex)	Tablet	Oral	Herpes zoster (shingles): 1 g 3 times a day for 7 days Genital herpes (acute): 1 g twice a day for 10 days Genital herpes (chronic suppression): 1 g a day Herpes labialis (cold sores): 2 g every 12 hours for 1 day
Zanamivir (Relenza)	Powder for inhalation	Topical (inhaled)	Influenza: 2 inhalations twice a day

Table 3.10 **Common NRTIs and NtRTIs**

Generic (Brand)	Dosage Form	Route of Administration	Common Dose
Abacavir/lamivudine (Epzicom)	Tablet	Oral	600 mg/300 mg a day
Abacavir/lamivudine/zidovudine (Trizivir)	Tablet		300 mg/150 mg/300 mg a day
Didanosine (Videx)	Tablet, capsule, powder for oral solution	Oral	125–200 mg twice a day or 250–400 mg once a day Oral solution: 167–250 mg twice a day
Emtricitabine (Emtriva)	Capsule, oral solution	Oral	200 mg a day Oral solution: 240 mg a day
Lamivudine (Epivir)	Tablet, oral solution	Oral	100 mg a day
Lamivudine/zidovudine (Combivir)	Tablet		150 mg/300 mg twice a day
Stavudine (Zerit)	Capsule, powder for oral solution	Oral	30–40 mg every 12 hours
Zalcitabine (Hivid)	Tablet	Oral	2.25 mg a day in divided doses
Zidovudine (Retrovir)	Tablet, capsule, oral solution, syrup, injection	Oral, IV	600 mg a day in divided doses IV: 1 mg a day/kg infused over 1 hour given 5–6 times a day

of its own class (zalcitabine and stavudine). You should heed any interaction warnings that appear on the computer and alert the pharmacist when filling prescriptions for these drugs.

Keep in AIRTIGHT Container

Zalcitabine must be stored in an airtight container or its potency will be affected.

Non-nucleoside Reverse Transcriptase Inhibitors (NNRTIs) These agents are used exclusively for HIV infection. NNRTIs inhibit reverse transcriptase, which forms pro-DNA molecules. Table 3.11 covers common doses of these drugs, as well as their side effects.

Table 3.11 Common NNRTIs

Generic (Brand)	Dosage Form	Common Dose	Side Effects
Delavirdine (Rescriptor)	Tablet	400 mg 3 times a day	Central obesity/weight gain, Stevens-Johnson syndrome
Efavirenz (Sustiva)	Tablet, capsule	600 mg a day	Dizziness, insomnia, drowsiness, abnormal dreams, hallucinations. CNS effects: depression, suicidal tendencies, paranoia, mania
Nevirapine (Viramune)	Tablet, oral suspension	200 mg 1–2 times a day	Liver problems, severe allergic reaction, Stevens-Johnson syndrome

Professional Focus

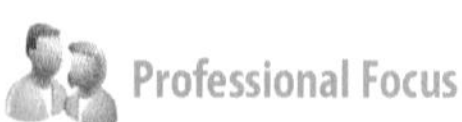

When needle sticks or exposure to body fluids of someone with HIV happens, prophylactic therapy can prevent infection if started within two hours of exposure. Healthcare workers, including pharmacy technicians, must report any such exposure immediately to their supervisors so that proper testing and preventive therapy can begin. If warranted, postexposure prophylaxis therapy will include a combination of agents for three to six months.

Cautions and Considerations Efavirenz cannot be taken with a high-fat meal, and delavirdine cannot be taken with antacids or it will not be absorbed properly.

Protease Inhibitors (PIs) Another class of drugs, **protease inhibitors**, works by blocking the enzyme that affects the assembly of proteins into working HIVs. In effect, the infection cycle is halted because nonfunctional and noninfectious viruses are produced. Table 3.12 covers common dosing.

Side Effects Many PIs can cause severe diarrhea, which usually decreases with use. Loperamide, an OTC diarrhea product, can be used to control diarrhea. Other side effects include headache, fatigue, dizziness, nausea, vomiting, bleeding problems, pancreatitis, depression, and Stevens-Johnson syndrome. Many patients also develop allergic reactions.

All of these agents cause fat redistribution, where fat and weight gain in the abdominal area is significant. In this process, normal fat and sugar metabolism is altered, causing many patients to get diabetes. Therefore, many patients with HIV and on these drugs will also have diabetes, for which other drugs are used (see Chapter 17).

Cautions and Considerations All of the PIs have numerous drug interactions, many of which are serious. One interaction involves antihistamines, a common OTC purchase. Pharmacy technicians should be mindful of this interaction, heed any additional drug interaction warnings that appear on the computer, and alert the pharmacist when filling prescriptions for these medications.

Most of these drugs cause liver and/or kidney problems. At times, these effects can be severe and life threatening. Patients with such conditions should work closely with their physicians when using these drugs.

Drink Plenty of
WATER
Do not take with grapefruit juice

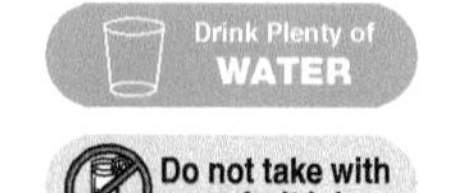

Patients taking indinavir should drink six to eight glasses of water a day to prevent kidney stones. This drug cannot be taken with food or grapefruit juice.

Some PIs should be taken with ritonavir to work properly. When dispensing one of these products, you should check to see that the patient is also receiving ritonavir.

Table 3.12 Common PIs

Generic (Brand)	Dosage Form	Common Dose
Atazanavir (Reyataz)	Capsule	400 mg twice a day with food
Darunavir (Prezista)	Tablet	600 mg twice a day with food (must be taken with ritonavir)
Fosamprenavir (Lexiva)	Tablet, oral suspension	700–1,400 mg twice a day (must be taken with ritonavir)
Indinavir (Crixivan)	Capsule	800 mg every 8 hours
Lopinavir/ritonavir (Kaletra)	Tablet, oral solution	400 mg/100 mg twice a day
Nelfinavir (Viracept)	Tablet, oral powder	1,250 mg 3 times a day with food
Ritonavir (Norvir)	Capsule, oral solution	600 mg twice a day
Saquinavir (Invirase, Fortovase)	Tablet, capsule	1,000 mg twice a day (must be taken with ritonavir)
Tipranavir (Aptivus)	Capsule	500 mg twice a day (must be given with ritonavir)

Miscellaneous New Therapies Currently, enfuvirtide (Fuzeon) is the only **fusion inhibitor** available. It works by blocking HIV from attaching to cellular membranes. Enfuvirtide can be quite costly and is usually used in advanced AIDS disease when other drugs have lost efficacy. It is given by subcutaneous injection and typically dosed at 90 mg twice a day. Side effects include diarrhea, nausea, fatigue, and injection site irritation.

Currently, maraviroc (Selzentry) is the only **chemokine coreceptor (CCR5) inhibitor** available. It works by blocking HIV from attaching to cellular membranes. It only works for certain strains of HIV, so special testing is performed to select appropriate patients for this therapy. It is given orally twice a day in combination with other antiviral agents. Side effects include abdominal pain, cough, dizziness, and fever. Severe allergic reactions and hepatotoxicity have also occurred.

Currently, raltegravir (Isentress) is the only **integrase inhibitor** available. It works by preventing HIV from inserting itself into the host DNA. It is given orally twice a day in combination with other antiviral agents. Side effects include headache, nausea, and fatigue.

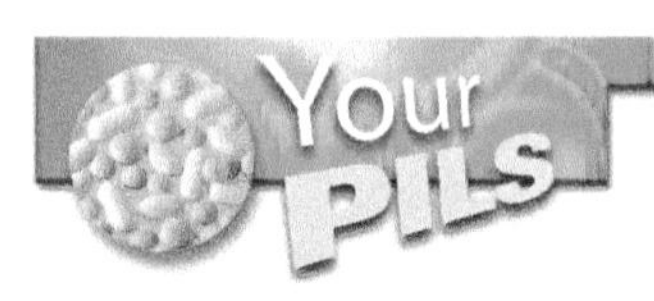

If you like to study on your own like Producers do, take time to do some research on the Internet for the newest combination antiviral products for HIV treatment. Because patients must take at least three agents to suppress the virus, several manufacturers have combined HIV drugs into combination products, making it easier for patients to adhere to their regimens. Make note of at least five of these products (brand name, generic name, and directions for use) and think about how they could improve a patient's ability to stick with therapy.

Fungal Infections

Fungi (or funguses) include **yeasts** and molds that are one-celled plant organisms. These organisms do not have chlorophyll, the substance that gives plants their green color. They do have a plant-like cell wall, the target for most antifungal medications. Usually, fungal infections are topical and mild in nature. **Dermatophytes**, fungi of the skin, cause some of the most frequent and ordinary infections, such as athlete's foot and ringworm. **Candidiasis** is another common fungus that causes vaginal yeast infections and oral thrush. However, when a fungus gains entry to the bloodstream or cannot be destroyed due to immunodeficiency, it can cause serious systemic infections. Table 3.13 lists common fungus organisms and related infections.

Drugs for Fungal Infections

Most antifungal drugs work on **ergosterol**, a substance in the cell wall of fungi. Without this molecule, the cell wall cannot form properly and the fungus cell dies. Many fungal infections and their treatments are topical in nature. Oral or IV drug therapy is needed

Table 3.13 Fungus Organisms and Common Infections

Organism	Associated Infection
Aspergillus spp.	Lung infection and other difficult-to-treat infections
Candida spp.	Oral or vaginal thrush (yeast infection), pneumonia, sepsis, meningitis
Cryptococcus	Meningitis and other difficult-to-treat infections
Histoplasma	Lung infection
Tinea spp.	Skin infections (athlete's foot and ringworm), toe-fingernail infections

for systemic fungal infections. However, most antifungal agents can be toxic to the liver when used systemically. **Pulse dosing**, in which the drug is given one week a month, is used to reduce the amount of time the drug comes in contact with the liver, which decreases the toxic effects. Laboratory tests are used periodically to check liver function in patients who take antifungal drugs systemically.

Amphotericin B is a drug that is particularly toxic to the liver and kidneys. Thus, its use is saved for the most serious and life-threatening fungal infections. This drug should be infused slowly or fever, chills, nausea, vomiting, and headache can occur. It should never be mixed or piggybacked with other drugs. It cannot be mixed using normal saline because precipitation will occur. It should be given through a central catheter IV line whenever possible to prevent local tissue inflammation. Amphotericin is also available in an IV **liposome** dosage form (see Figure 3.6), which surrounds the drug molecules with a fat/oil layer. This protective layer decreases the drug's ability to come into direct contact with body tissues and thus reduces its toxic effects. Table 3.14 lists common antifungal drugs and dosage information.

For TOPICAL use only
Keep away from HEAT or FLAME

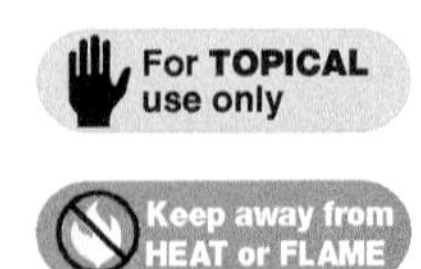

You should include an external use warning label on all topical antifungal prescriptions. Ciclopirox nail lacquer is flammable and should have an appropriate auxiliary warning label. Refer patients using a vaginal agent for the first time to the pharmacist for proper assessment and counseling.

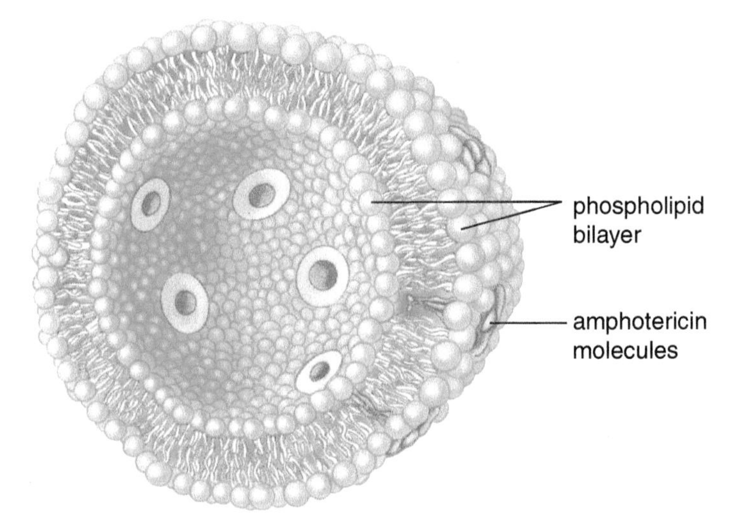

Figure 3.6
Liposome Dosage Form
Liposomal amphotericin comes as suspension or powder for injection, depending on the brand chosen. Be sure to remind patients to follow preparation instructions closely, for mistakes can be costly.

Table 3.14 Common Antifungal Drugs

Generic (Brand)	Dosage Form	Common Dose	Dispensing Status
Systemic Agents			
Amphotericin B	Powder for injection	Varies by patient and disease being treated	Rx
Caspofungin (Cancidas)	Powder for injection	70 mg as initial dose followed by 50 mg a day	Rx
Flucytosine (Ancobon)	Capsule	50–150 mg/kg/day in divided intervals every 6 hours	Rx
Itraconazole (Sporanox)	Capsule, oral solution	200–400 mg a day	Rx
Ketoconazole (Nizoral)	Tablet	200–400 mg a day	Rx
Liposomal amphotericin B (Abelcet, Amphotec, AmBisome)	Suspension and powder for injection	Varies by patient and disease being treated	Rx
Micafungin (Mycamine)	Powder for injection	Preventive therapy: 50 mg/day Active treatment: 150 mg/day	Rx
Voriconazole (Vfend)	Tablet, oral suspension, powder for injection	PO: 200 mg every 12 hours IV: 4–6 mg/kg every 12 hours	Rx

Table 3.14 Common Antifungal Drugs, *continued*

Generic (Brand)	Dosage Form	Common Dose	Dispensing Status
Skin/Nail Agents			
Butenafine (Lotrimin Ultra, Mentax)	Topical cream	Once a day for 2 weeks	OTC, Rx
Ciclopirox (Loprox, Penlac)	Cream, lotion, gel, shampoo, topical suspension, nail lacquer	Depends on dosage form and site of infection but can take up to 12 weeks for cure	Rx
Clotrimazole (Lotrimin AF, Desenex)	Cream, lotion, topical solution	Twice a day for 2–4 weeks	OTC
Clotrimazole/betamethasone (Lotrisone)	Cream, lotion, ointment	Twice a day for 4 weeks	Rx
Griseofulvin (Fulvicin, Gris-PEG)	Tablet, capsule	Varies depending on age and weight of patient (4 weeks for athlete's foot, 4–6 months for nail infections)	Rx
Ketoconazole (Nizoral)	Cream, foam, gel, shampoo	200–400 mg a day for 2–4 weeks	Rx
Miconazole (Micatin, Neosporin AF, Lotrimin AF)	Topical cream, powder, ointment, spray, solution, gel	Twice a day for 2 weeks	OTC
Nystatin (Mycostatin)	Cream, ointment, powder	Twice a day until lesions heal	Rx
Terbinafine (Lamisil AT)	Cream, gel, spray	Once a day for 1–2 weeks	OTC
Vaginal Agents			
Butoconazole (Mycelex-3)	Vaginal cream	Once a day for 1–3 days	Rx, OTC
Clotrimazole (Gyne-Lotrimin)	Vaginal suppository and cream	100 mg a day for 7 days 200 mg a day for 3 days	OTC
Fluconazole (Diflucan)	Oral tablet, oral suspension, IV	PO: 150 mg in 1 dose IV: varies depending on infection being treated	Rx
Miconazole (Monistat)	Vaginal cream	1,200 mg at bedtime for 1 day 200 mg a day for 3 days 100 mg a day for 7 days	OTC
Tioconazole (Monistat-1)	Vaginal ointment	1 applicator at bedtime for 1 day	OTC
Oral Thrush Agents			
Clotrimazole (Mycelex)	Lozenge	Dissolve in mouth 5 times a day	Rx
Nystatin (Mycostatin)	Tablet, oral suspension, lozenge, powder	500,000–1 million units 3 times a day 1–2 lozenges 5 times a day	Rx
Posaconazole (Noxafil)	Oral suspension	100–400 mg twice a day	Rx

Parasitic and Protozoan Infections

Parasites are organisms that live off of a host. Most parasites do not kill their host, but they can create great discomfort and severe symptoms. Some examples of parasites include pinworms, hookworms, roundworms, and tapeworms. **Protozoa** are single-celled parasites that cause infection, usually through the oral–fecal route. These parasites are passed along when hands, food, or water are contaminated with feces from an infected human or animal. *Giardia*, an intestinal infection caused by protozoa in humans and dogs, can be carried in bird droppings, deposited in water or on vegetation, and cause diarrhea when ingested. In tropical areas where mosquitoes thrive, the sporozoan infection malaria affects millions of people. Table 3.15 covers common parasitic and protozoan infections.

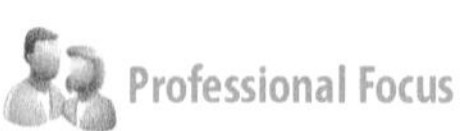

Professional Focus

Some pharmacies offer travel clinics for patients going to countries where specialized immunization or preventive medication is needed. Personnel working in travel clinics must become familiar with such vaccines and drugs. Although people living in the United States are not routinely vaccinated against hepatitis A and yellow fever, these vaccines are needed for travel to an area where these infections are more common. Technicians in such pharmacies will handle these vaccines and dispense malaria prevention medications.

Table 3.15 Common Parasitic and Protozoan Organisms and Infections

Parasite or Protozoa	Associated Infection
Giardia lamblia	Intestinal infection
Plasmodium vivax	Malaria
Toxoplasma gondii	Toxoplasmosis
Pneumocystis carinii (PCP) or *P. jiroveci*	Lung infection
Trichomonas vaginalis	Vaginal infection

Drugs for Parasitic and Protozoan Infections

Most of the drugs used for parasitic and protozoan infections have already been covered in this chapter. For example, metronidazole is used for several common intestinal infections caused by protozoa such as *Giardia*. Malaria, however, is treated using several other drugs. Therapy often combines two or three drugs, including quinine, chloroquine, primaquine, doxycycline, tetracycline, clindamycin, atovaquone, proguanil, and mefloquine. Because malaria is not a common disease in the United States, pharmacy technicians do not dispense many of these prescriptions. Such prescriptions will be filled only when a patient is traveling to or from a country where malaria is common. For these reasons, greater detail on these agents is not provided in this text.

Herbal and Alternative Therapies

Echinacea is an herb some patients use for the common cold, RTIs, and even vaginal yeast infections. It has been found to reduce the severity and length of symptoms. Echinacea does not cure infections, but it may be used to augment drug therapy. Echinacea increases phagocytosis, the process by which immune system cells "eat up" foreign cells such as bacteria. It also enhances lymphocyte activity. A variety of products contain echinacea and have varying dosages. A standard dose has not been established. However, for echinacea to be effective, patients must use it multiple times a day and start it at the very first signs of infection. Dosing is heaviest during the first five days of infection but continues for up to ten days.

Zinc is a cofactor in many biological processes in the body, including protein synthesis. It also boosts immune function. Like echinacea, zinc can be used for infections including the common cold, flu, and RTIs. Patients take it orally, by pill or lozenge. Doses vary but range from 24 mg to 200 mg multiple times a day. Zinc should not be taken with coffee because coffee reduces its absorption by up to 50%. Zinc also interacts with several other prescription medications, so patients should check with their pharmacists and healthcare providers about taking zinc along with other medications.

Vitamin C is ascorbic acid, a substance that boosts the immune system and has antioxidant effects. It can be taken in high doses but can cause diarrhea, stomach upset, and kidney stones. Vitamin C is best taken during cold and flu season, when the likelihood of encountering infection is greatest. Doses for fighting infection are in the range of 1–3 g a day. For details on vitamin C and other vitamins, see Chapter 16.

Many sham herbal products and remedies are promoted and sold to patients with HIV and AIDS. These products do not cure this disease, but patients with this terminal illness often look for "miracle cures." Encourage patients to talk with their pharmacists and healthcare providers about herbal products they want to take.

Chapter Summary

Infections are caused by pathogenic organisms or normal floras that go out of control. Organisms that cause disease are bacteria, viruses, fungi, and protozoa. Most infections can be treated with medication. Unfortunately, some pathogens have developed resistance to the drugs typically used. When this happens, more expensive therapies must be tried, and in some cases we do not have effective drug therapy.

Common classes of antibiotics used for bacterial infections are penicillins, cephalosporins, vancomycin, aminoglycosides, tetracyclines, sulfonamides, and metronidazole. These agents are chosen based on the type, site, and severity of infection. Viral diseases such as influenza and herpes are treated with antiviral agents. These drugs do not eradicate the infection but can lessen the symptoms and length of sickness. Several antiviral drugs, including NRTIs, NNRTIs, and PIs, are available for HIV and AIDS. These drugs are usually taken in combinations of two or three and can be difficult to take due to side effects and toxicities. Antifungal drugs are used for simple fungal infections, such as athlete's foot, as well as for life-threatening systemic infections.

These drugs come in a wide variety of dosage forms. Pharmacy technicians dispense drugs for various infections on a daily basis, no matter the setting in which they work. Becoming familiar with this large set of medications can be challenging but is valuable because you will see them every day in practice.

Chapter Review

For the following sets of exercises, write the exercise heading, exercise numbers, and your answers on a separate sheet of paper. Your instructor may direct you to turn in the sheet of paper or discuss your answers as a class.

REVIEW THE BASICS

Choose a, b, c, or d as the correct answer to each multiple-choice question.

1. Which of the following involves a body-wide immune response that attacks cells that have already been infected with viruses?
   a. cellular immunity
   b. humoral immunity
   c. innate immunity
   d. all of the above

2. Which of the following cells directly produces antibodies for fighting infection?
   a. mast cells
   b. neutrophils
   c. T cells
   d. B cells

3. Many healthcare employers (including pharmacies) require employees to get vaccinated against hepatitis B. What type of pathogenic organism causes this infection?
   a. bacteria
   b. virus
   c. fungus
   d. protozoa

4. *Staphylococcus aureus* (a common skin bacteria) is shaped most like which of the following?
   a. chains of rod-shaped cells
   b. grape-like clusters of spherical cells
   c. flat cells
   d. spiral-shaped cells

5. Which of the following drugs is a patient most likely to be allergic to if he or she is also allergic to penicillin?
   a. cephalosporins
   b. macrolides
   c. sulfonamides
   d. tetracyclines

6. Which of the following drugs is used most frequently for MRSA infections?
   a. ceftriaxone
   b. levofloxacin
   c. metronidazole
   d. vancomycin

7. Which drug is used most commonly with the sulfonamide antibiotic, sulfamethoxazole, for urinary tract infections (UTIs)?
   a. tioconazole
   b. trimethoprim
   c. ticarcillin
   d. tetracycline

8. Which of the following cannot be used by pregnant women and by children under eight years old, due to tooth discoloration problems?
   a. cephalexin
   b. levofloxacin
   c. metronidazole
   d. tetracycline

9. Which of the following is most likely to be used to treat herpes zoster (shingles)?
   a. indinavir
   b. acyclovir
   c. amantadine
   d. zidovudine

10. Which of the following is a PI agent used for HIV and can cause fat redistribution and diabetes?
    a. acyclovir
    b. atazanavir
    c. efavirenz
    d. lamivudine

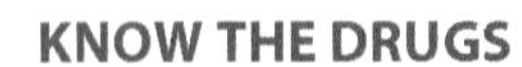

KNOW THE DRUGS

Match each brand name drug with its corresponding generic name and most common use. Your answers should follow this example format: Generic Name: 1. a; 2. b; 3. c; etc. Most Common Use: 1. g; 2. h; 3. i; etc.

Brand Name	Generic Name	Most Common Use
1. Epivir	a. azithromycin	g. bacterial infection
2. Crixivan	b. clotrimazole	h. viral infection
3. Lotrimin AF	c. lamivudine	i. fungal infection
4. Zithromax	d. indinavir	
5. Suprax	e. cefixime	
6. Biaxin	f. clarithromycin	

PUT IT TOGETHER

For each item, write down either a short answer or a single term to complete the sentence.

1. Name three antimicrobial drugs to which you should attach a warning label about avoiding drinking alcohol.
2. Name the generic and brand names of a drug in each of the four generations of cephalosporins.
3. Prescriptions for ______________ should have a warning label on the vial to alert patients against drinking milk or taking antacids at the same time.
4. A prescription for ______________ should have a warning label to caution patients that it may turn their urine brown.
5. How soon after the onset of symptoms should an antiviral drug be taken to decrease the symptoms and severity of an influenza infection?
6. ______________ is an antibiotic and ______________ is an antifungal that are given primarily by IV infusion.

THINK IT THROUGH

Read and think through each numbered scenario carefully and then write several sentences in reply to the question(s) presented. Question 4 requires you to do some Internet research before completing your answer(s).

1. Explain how each of the following situations can contribute to antibiotic resistance in bacteria.
   a. Overuse of antibiotics (prescribing them when not needed)
   b. Inappropriate duration of treatment with antibiotics (not taking until gone)
2. You take a call from the floor nurse complaining that you must have sent up the wrong drug or mixed something incorrectly. She explains she just started an IV drip fifteen minutes ago for her patient, based on an order from the physician for vancomycin. She states the patient has a red rash on the neck and his blood pressure is dropping. She asks whether this could be an allergic reaction. What might be happening and what should you do?
3. A patient comes to the pharmacy to pick up a prescription for metronidazole for a vaginal infection. Along with her prescription, she is purchasing Tylenol Sinus and Nyquil for the cold symptoms she has also been experiencing. What should you notice and what should you do?

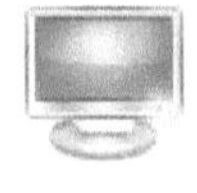

4. **On the Internet**, find the Web site for Centers for Disease Control and Prevention (CDC), and once there, look up information on HIV and AIDS in the United States. In particular, review the fact sheets on HIV and AIDS. Describe the trends seen in HIV and AIDS diagnosis and treatment. Find a classmate or health professional to discuss your take on these trends. How are advances in antiviral drug therapy changing the course of HIV disease and the health of people living with it in our country?

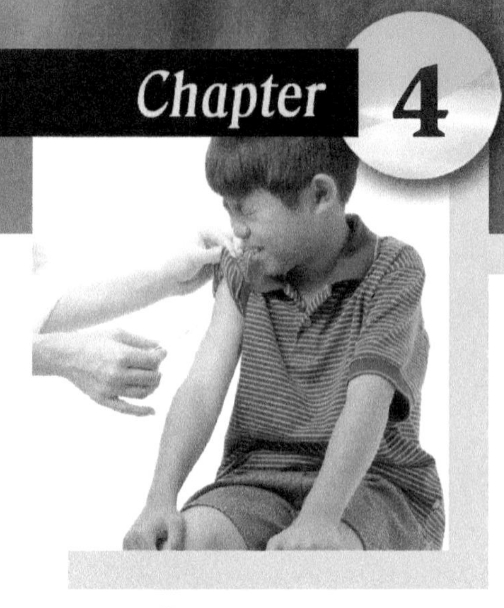

Chapter 4 Immunologic Drugs and Vaccines

LEARNING OBJECTIVES

- Explain the basic physiology of acquired immunity and immunization.
- Explain the therapeutic effects of vaccines and immunologic medications commonly used to prevent and treat diseases of the immune system.
- Describe the adverse effects of vaccines and immunologic medications commonly used to prevent and treat diseases of the immune system.
- Identify the brand and generic names of vaccines and immunologic medications commonly used to prevent and treat diseases of the immune system.
- State the common doses, dosage forms, and routes of administration for vaccines and immunologic medications used to prevent and treat diseases affecting the immune system.

Interactive self-quizzes, games, audio files, and glossaries help you to learn drug names and facts.

While Chapter 3 covered the conventional treatment of infectious diseases, this chapter delves into drug therapies that prevent infection and provide immunosuppression. As mentioned in Chapter 3, viral infections are difficult to treat once they have already occurred. Antiviral drugs have their limitations, so preventive strategies are preferred whenever possible. Vaccines are given to prevent diseases that have high rates of mortality or result in significant illness. Immunization is a way to boost the immune system in advance of exposure to a disease that has great impact on public health and productivity. Recently, pharmacy participation in immunization efforts has evolved significantly. Pharmacists now give millions of immunizations, mostly in the form of flu shots, in community pharmacies around the country. Your role as a pharmacy technician is expanding in operating immunization clinics because technicians are often called on to organize and manage them.

The body's immune system is also supplemented by medications to fight diseases such as multiple sclerosis, hepatitis, and cancer. These immunologic agents are costly and not often seen in traditional practice settings. But they are an important lifeline to patients with these debilitating diagnoses. These agents require special handling, so you should appreciate their unique requirements. In the field of organ transplantation, the immune system can become the body's own enemy and attack a transplanted organ because it sees the tissue as foreign. Immunosuppressants are used to prevent organ rejection. As organ transplantation becomes more common, pharmacy technicians should be aware of these agents and their implications for the healthcare of patients they serve.

Physiology of Acquired Immunity

The immune response is a complex system that protects and fights against infectious disease. In **acquired immunity**, pathogens are carried to the lymph nodes where lymphocytes detect and destroy them. As shown in Figure 4.1, **helper T cells** detect specific antigens (molecules on foreign pathogens) and stimulate killer T cells and B cells to become active. **Killer T cells** start killing any cells of the body infected with the foreign antigens. Interestingly, killer T cells can also help rid the body of cancerous cells in a similar manner. In organ transplantation, this part of the body's immune system must be suppressed to keep it from attacking new tissue.

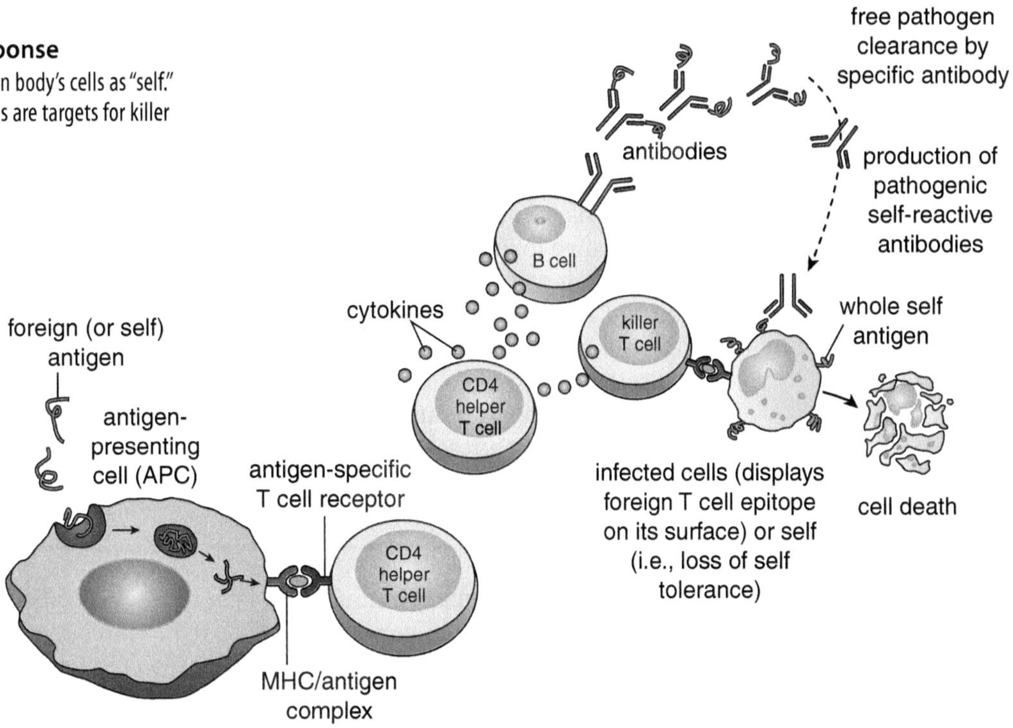

Figure 4.1
Acquired Immune Response
Lymphocytes recognize their own body's cells as "self." Cells infected with a foreign virus are targets for killer T cells.

B cells begin to produce antibodies, which are also called **immunoglobulins (Ig)**. Immunoglobulins have a variety of jobs that affect the immune system (see Table 4.1). They fight infection by binding viruses and prevent them from infecting healthy cells. Sometimes, the immune system can malfunction and begin producing antibodies against normal, healthy cells (see Figure 4.1). **Autoimmune disorders** are defined by such activity and include systemic lupus erythematosus (SLE), myasthenia gravis, rheumatoid arthritis, and **multiple sclerosis (MS)**. Each disorder affects specific tissues, depending on the type of antibodies produced and the cells they attack. Type 1 diabetes is caused by an autoimmune process that destroys the beta cells that produce insulin in the pancreas. MS is covered here because its only treatment involves immunologic therapy. Other autoimmune disorders, such as rheumatoid arthritis (Chapter 6) and myasthenia gravis (Chapter 10), are covered elsewhere.

The immune system also mediates **allergic reactions**, which are cases of **hypersensitivity**. Hypersensitivity is categorized into four types. **Type I hypersensitivity** reactions

Table 4.1 Immunoglobulins (Ig)

Type	Function
IgA	Most prominent in mucous membranes of digestive system and respiratory tract, tears, sweat, and saliva. Defends these surfaces against exposure to external pathogens. Found in breast milk and passes immunity to child when breast-feeding.
IgD	Found in plasma and on surface of lymphocytes. Function not fully understood. May be involved in B cell maturation.
IgG	Most common antibody in blood. Passes from mother to fetus through placenta, giving baby passive immunity. Small amounts produced after first exposure to a pathogen, large amounts produced on subsequent exposures.
IgE	Found in basophils and mast cells. Responsible for mounting allergic response and fighting parasites.
IgM	First antibody to be produced after exposure to a pathogen. Responsible for natural defense against bacteria. Activates complement system. Found on surface of red blood cells and responsible for A, B, and O blood typing.

are anaphylactic reactions that can be life threatening. **Anaphylaxis** is a process mediated by antibodies, basophils, and mast cells and causes swelling of the airways, blood vessel dilation, and shock, if not treated quickly. Some drugs can cause anaphylaxis. **Type II hypersensitivity** reactions stimulate the complement system, another component of the immune system. Antibodies attach to foreign cells and attract complement molecules, which in effect poke holes in these cells and kill them. This kind of reaction occurs when blood of the wrong type is given to a patient. **Type III hypersensitivity** reactions involve toxins and antibodies. Normally, this process occurs in the spleen but if severe enough can cause inflammation of blood vessels. A **Type IV hypersensitivity** reaction is the immune response mediated by killer T cells. Type IV reactions are called delayed responses, because they take 12–72 hours to occur. A tuberculin skin test for tuberculosis is an example of a Type IV reaction. When drugs cause this type of allergy, patients will have hives or an itchy rash. This hypersensitivity is not harmful if the drug is stopped but can progress to anaphylaxis if the drug continues to be given.

Immunization

Immunization uses acquired immunity to fight against specific diseases. **Natural immunization** occurs when your body is exposed to foreign antigens in normal daily life and produces antibodies against them. When you next encounter that disease, the body quickly builds a defense and protects you from getting sick again. **Artificial immunization** occurs when an antigen is intentionally introduced to the body via vaccination. It builds a defense in advance of disease exposure.

Artificial immunity can be accomplished through active or passive means. **Active immunity** exposes the body to an antigen or part of an antigen, which then uses the body's natural immune response to make antibodies. Vaccinations use active immunity to prevent disease by introducing the body to killed, weakened, or partial antigens. Some vaccines (called live attenuated vaccines) use live but weakened pathogens to produce an immune response. **Passive immunity** occurs when antibodies themselves are introduced into the bloodstream. This occurs either naturally (such as from mother to fetus during pregnancy) or artificially (through injecting immunoglobulin agents).

Although people could wait for natural immunization to fight disease, many lives would be lost in the process. **Vaccination** reduces and prevents life-threatening diseases such as polio when used widely. For example, vaccination practices have effectively eliminated smallpox worldwide. Vaccination also reduces many other diseases that cause great sickness and disability, especially among children. For instance, the impacts of measles, polio, and influenza have all been reduced with vaccination practices.

Several vaccines require multiple doses to produce an adequate immune response and confer full immunity to a disease. The **Centers for Disease Control and Prevention (CDC)** publishes a **schedule for childhood and adult vaccines** (see Figure 4.2). Certain immunizations are recommended for children, whereas others are more appropriate for adults. In most cases, specific vaccines are required for children to enter public school. When the dosage is complete, most childhood vaccinations afford lifetime immunity. Others, for example the tetanus vaccine, must be readministered periodically as booster shots to continue immunity protection.

Healthcare professionals, including pharmacy technicians, should be informed of immunization schedules and be certain they are personally up to date. Working in the field of healthcare without being properly vaccinated increases risk of exposure to diseases and promotes disease transmission. Certain vaccines are recommended for those who work in healthcare. These immunizations include hepatitis B and an annual influenza shot. Those workers with high risk of exposure to active tuberculosis may consider the BCG vaccine as well. Many employers require technicians to get these vaccinations and keep all others current as part of employment.

Figure 4.2

CDC Immunization Schedule for Adults

From this schedule, you can see that adults aged 50 and older should get an annual flu shot, and adults aged 60 and older should get the zoster vaccine. The current immunization schedules for children aged 0–6 years, 7–18 years, and adults with special medication indications can be found on the CDC Web site.

<table>
<tr><th>Vaccine ▼ Age Group ▶</th><th>19–26 years</th><th>27–49 years</th><th>50–59 years</th><th>60–64 years</th><th>≥ 65 years</th></tr>
<tr><td>Tetanus, diphtheria, pertussis (Td/Tdap)</td><td colspan="4">Substitute 1-time dose of Tdap for Td booster; then boost with Td every 10 years</td><td>Td booster every 10 years</td></tr>
<tr><td>Human papillomavirus (HPV)</td><td>3 doses</td><td></td><td></td><td></td><td></td></tr>
<tr><td>Varicella</td><td colspan="5">2 doses</td></tr>
<tr><td>Zoster</td><td></td><td></td><td></td><td colspan="2">1 dose</td></tr>
<tr><td>Measles, mumps, rubella (MMR)</td><td colspan="2">1 or 2 doses</td><td colspan="3">1 dose</td></tr>
<tr><td>Influenza</td><td colspan="2"></td><td colspan="3">1 dose annually</td></tr>
<tr><td>Pneumococcal (polysaccharide)</td><td colspan="4">1 or 2 doses</td><td>1 dose</td></tr>
<tr><td>Hepatitis A</td><td colspan="5">2 doses</td></tr>
<tr><td>Hepatitis B</td><td colspan="5">3 doses</td></tr>
<tr><td>Meningococcal</td><td colspan="5">1 or more doses</td></tr>
</table>

For all persons in this category who meet the age requirements and who lack evidence of immunity (e.g., lack documentation of vaccination or have no evidence of prior infection)

Recommended if some other risk factor is present (e.g., on the basis of medical, occupational, lifestyle, or other indications)

No recommendation

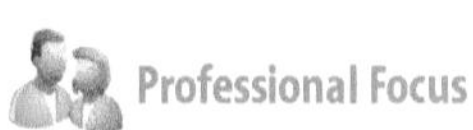
Professional Focus

Although pharmacy technicians do not administer vaccinations, they order the inventory, oversee storage and quality control, and obtain consent and medical histories directly from patients for immunization clinics in pharmacies. As part of your storage and quality control duties, you may be asked to chart the daily refrigerator temperature where vaccines are stored.

Common Vaccines

Many **vaccines** are administered in the physician's office or inpatient settings where you as a technician may not encounter them. But greater numbers of vaccines are administered in pharmacies every day. Some pharmacies do not administer childhood vaccinations but commonly give flu shots, travel vaccines, and immunizations for pneumonia and shingles to adults. Many patients now get their annual **flu shot** at their local pharmacy.

Many pharmacies operate travel **immunization clinics** where they provide immunizations and advice about what vaccines are appropriate for various areas of the world. Examples of travel vaccines include those for hepatitis and cholera. These diseases are not common enough to warrant mass vaccination in the United States but are found in other areas of the world. **Travel vaccines** must be given well in advance of travel to allow the immune system enough time to mount the appropriate response and confer full immunity. Time to level of immunity differs between vaccines. Many immunizations should be given two or more weeks prior to travel. Helping patients prepare for travel in this way is a valuable resource that community pharmacies can provide.

Vaccines are fragile proteins that usually must be given by injection. Only a few are available in other dosage forms (see Table 4.2). Therefore, healthcare workers must be trained and certified to give injections before they may administer vaccines. Pharmacists in most states can obtain this training and certification, but technicians cannot. Technicians, however, are involved in ordering, storing, and preparing vaccines for injection.

Side Effects Common side effects of vaccines include fever, headache, stomach upset, local injection site irritation, mild rash, and irritability. These symptoms are related to

Table 4.2 Vaccines Commonly Handled by Pharmacy Technicians

Generic (Brand)	Route of Administration	Storage	Use
BCG	Injection	Refrigerate Protect from light	Recommended for patients at high risk of exposure to tuberculosis Recommended for healthcare workers in high-risk settings only
Diphtheria, tetanus, and pertussis (various combinations available)	Injection	Refrigerate (do not freeze)	Diphtheria, tetanus, and/or pertussis (whooping cough) in children or adults
Haemophilus influenza B or HIB (HibTITER, ActHIB, PedvaxHIB)	Injection	Refrigerate (do not freeze)	*Haemophilus influenza* type B in children
Hepatitis A or HAV (Havrix, Vaqta)	Injection	Refrigerate (do not freeze)	Recommended for patients at high risk of exposure to hepatitis A
Hepatitis B or Hep B (Recombivax HB, Engerix-B)	Injection	Refrigerate (do not freeze)	Hepatitis B in children Recommended in adults at high risk of exposure to hepatitis B Recommended for healthcare workers
Human papilloma virus or HPV (Gardasil)	Injection	Refrigerate (do not freeze) Protect from light	Recommended for girls/boys and women/men 9–26 years old to prevent cervical cancer in females and genital warts due to HPV
HIB + Hep B (Comvax)	Injection	Refrigerate (do not freeze)	*Haemophilus influenza* and hepatitis B in children
Influenza (Afluria, Fluarix, FluLaval, Fluvirin, Fluzone)	Injection	Refrigerate (do not freeze) Protect from light	Influenza in children and adults Recommended for healthcare workers
Influenza (FluMist)	Intranasal	Refrigerate (do not freeze)	Influenza in patients 2–50 years old Recommended for healthcare workers
Japanese encephalitis (JE-VAX)	Injection	Refrigerate (do not freeze)	Recommended for patients at high risk of exposure to Japanese encephalitis
Measles, mumps, rubella (M-M-R II)	Injection	Room temperature during shipping Refrigerate during storage in pharmacy Protect from light	Measles, mumps, and rubella in adults and children
Meningococcal (Menomune, Menactra)	Injection	Refrigerate (do not freeze)	Recommended for patients at high risk of exposure to *Neisseria meningitidis*
Pneumococcal, conjugate (Prevnar)	Injection	Refrigerate (do not freeze)	Pneumonia and otitis media (ear infections) in children
Pneumococcal, polyvalent (Pneumovax)	Injection	Refrigerate	Pneumonia in patients < 2 years old or > 50 years old
Polio, inactivated or IPV (IPOL)	Injection	Refrigerate (do not freeze)	Poliovirus in children
Rotavirus (Rotarix, RotaTeq)	Oral	Refrigerate (do not freeze) Protect from light	Rotavirus in infants and children
Typhoid (Vivotif Berna, Typhim Vi)	Oral, injection	PO: refrigerate or freeze Injection: refrigerate (do not freeze)	PO: *Salmonella typhi* in adults and children Injection: recommended for patients at high risk of exposure to typhoid fever
Varicella (Varivax)	Injection	Frozen (refrigerated for 72 hours only)	Chickenpox in children
Yellow fever (YF-Fax)	Injection	Frozen during shipping Refrigerate (do not freeze) during storage in pharmacy	Recommended for patients at high risk of exposure to yellow fever
Zoster (Zostavax)	Injection	Room temperature or refrigerate	Herpes zoster (shingles) in patients > 60 years old

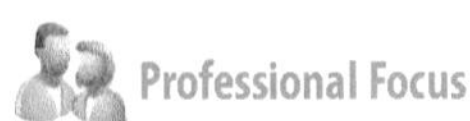

Professional Focus

You must wait one month between the first and second hepatitis B vaccine injections and six months between the second and third injections to allow the body to build an appropriate immune response. People sometimes do not realize how long it will take to finish this series of shots before they are fully immune.

the humoral, or systemic, immune response (see Chapter 3), which makes a person feel generally tired and achy. It can feel like the onset of the flu, which is why many patients claim that the influenza shot itself gave them the flu. This is not true, and such symptoms can also occur after injection of other vaccines. All guidelines state specifically that taking acetaminophen for twenty-four to forty-eight hours after immunization usually alleviates these symptoms. If patients are already sick or feeling poorly, it is usually recommended that they wait to receive a vaccine so as not to exacerbate their symptoms. Receiving the vaccine is not necessarily harmful, but waiting avoids additional undesired effects.

Some media reports have perpetuated a fear that immunization increases the risk of developing autism. This idea stems from limited studies done years ago that suggested a possible link between autism and the preservatives contained in some vaccines. Although subsequent studies have not proven this connection, vaccine makers have eliminated use of these preservatives. Some parents continue to be concerned about exposing their children to a potential cause of harm.

Cautions and Considerations Like any drug therapy, immunization is not without risk. Patients must receive written information about risks before getting a vaccination. A **vaccine information sheet (VIS)** is available from the CDC for all vaccines on the market. You can find a copy of these sheets on the CDC Web site. Patients must sign a consent form stating that they are making an informed decision to receive vaccination and verifying they have received a VIS for the appropriate vaccine. Obtaining these signatures and maintaining this paperwork are usually the responsibilities of pharmacy technicians. These responsibilities should not be taken lightly, because the patient consent form is required by law.

The influenza vaccine is grown in chicken eggs, so patients who are allergic to eggs cannot receive this injection. Asking all patients whether they are allergic to eggs is an essential step in processing patients before they receive a vaccine. Those giving immunizations must be trained in administering cardiopulmonary resuscitation (CPR) and other necessary treatments in case an anaphylactic reaction occurs.

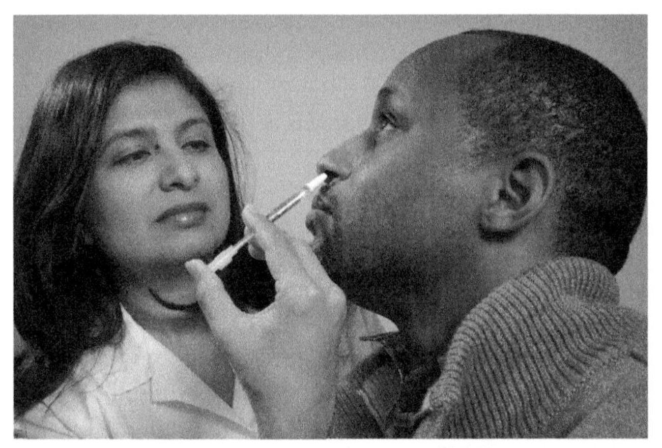

FluMist is a nasal spray option for those who want to get the influenza (flu) vaccine without a shot. This dosage form is only for patients two to fifty years old and contains **live attenuated virus**, rather than **deactivated virus**. Using FluMist instead of the flu shot has extra precautions and limitations, of which patients must be aware.

Each vaccine offered at a pharmacy may have its own unique requirements for storage and preparation. Most require storage in either the refrigerator or freezer. The temperature range appropriate for storing vaccines is tight and strict. The recommended temperature range can differ from vaccine to vaccine, too. Most vaccine products cannot be used if frozen. If allowed to warm to room temperature, most must be used right away (not refrigerated again). In most cases, daily temperature measurement of refrigerators and freezers is required to ensure that vaccines stored there are kept appropriately and do not spoil. Vaccines that come as powder for injection usually must be used within minutes to hours after reconstitution. Advance mixing and preparation of multiple doses is not recommended. Technicians responsible for maintaining stock must be familiar with the specific storage and preparation instructions associated with each vaccine.

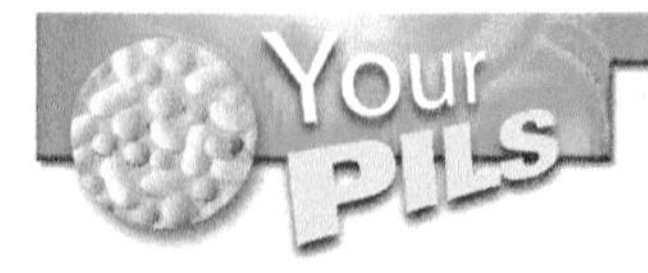

If you like working independently like Producers do, make a list of the vaccines that must be refrigerated and put it in your home refrigerator along with a thermometer. Each day, pick a disease for which you would need a vaccine and look in the refrigerator to locate the appropriate brand name on your list. As you look inside to locate the appropriate drug name, check the refrigerator temperature and chart it on a piece of paper. Continuing this activity for a couple of weeks at home not only mimics your duties as a technician but also helps you associate the disease, brand name, refrigeration requirements, and particular storage temperature for the vaccines in the pharmacy.

Interferon Therapy

Interferons are used for a variety of conditions affecting the immune system, including MS and hepatitis. They work in different ways for these various conditions, so they are described separately in relation to the condition they treat. Interferon therapy is quite costly (thousands of dollars a year) and usually dispensed only in specialty pharmacies.

Interferons are easily degradable protein products, so special storage procedures must be followed. Additionally, these agents should be stored in the refrigerator. However, the patient should wait until the product reaches room temperature before injecting it. The product can be slowly rolled between the palms to increase the temperature before use. Refer patients to the pharmacist if self-injection training is necessary. You should also make sure patients know how to dispose of needles properly. Specific laws and procedures for needle disposal vary from state to state.

Multiple Sclerosis (MS)

MS is an autoimmune disorder in which antibodies destroy the myelin sheath surrounding many nerve cells. Damaged myelin tissue forms scars (sclerosis) that interfere with coordinated signal conduction along these nerves. Symptoms usually start with numbness in the limbs. Eventually, tissue destruction leads to loss of nerve axons and white matter in the brain. Severe symptoms range from vision loss to paralysis. Disease progression and symptoms are variable among individual patients and can be difficult to predict. Of the four main types of MS, relapsing-remitting MS is the most frequently diagnosed. In relapsing-remitting MS, severe symptoms flare up, followed by periods of remission. Secondary progressive MS usually happens after relapsing-remitting MS and for this type of MS, remissions disappear and symptoms steadily worsen.

Drugs for MS Interferons are used to prevent progression and relapse of MS so as to postpone disability and preserve cognitive function. Currently, they are the only treatment option for patients with this condition, and they do not work for everyone. Although they do not cure the disorder, interferons can help preserve a patient's level of function and delay progression to full disability. Because these agents are injectable and very costly, they are usually carried only in specialty pharmacies. If you work in such a pharmacy, you should know that any patients taking immunologic suppressive therapies such as interferons should not get the flu shot. These patients will be unable to mount an appropriate immune response to the vaccine.

Hepatitis

Hepatitis literally means inflammation of the liver. It can be caused by viral disease, alcohol use, medications, poisons, or autoimmune diseases. The three types of viral hepatitis include hepatitis A, B, and C. Each of these viruses exhibits different symptoms and disease patterns, and they all infect liver cells exclusively.

Hepatitis A is transmitted through ingestion of contaminated food or liquids. It is a short-term, acute infection that does not become a chronic disease. Once the immune system develops antibodies, symptoms resolve and the patient is resistant for life. Although rare in the United States, hepatitis A is common in less developed countries. Therefore, the hepatitis A vaccine is recommended as a preventive measure prior to travel to these areas.

Hepatitis B is transmitted via sexual activity; use of contaminated needles, or receipt of blood products infected with hepatitis B; or from mother to infant. Hepatitis B begins as an acute infection that either mimics flu-like symptoms or is asymptomatic. In some patients, it leads to a chronic infection of the liver. The longer a person has the disease, the greater the chance it will convert to a chronic infection and cause permanent liver damage. Infants who are infected at birth have the highest likelihood of getting a chronic form of the disease. Chronic infection can lead to complications such as cirrhosis, liver cancer, and liver failure.

Hepatitis C is primarily spread by blood-to-blood contact. Although transmission through sexual intercourse is possible, it is much less common than is true for hepatitis B. In the United States, high-risk populations include injection drug users, the homeless, and prison inmates. Hepatitis C is known for its very high rate of mutation. This means that the immune system has a tough time destroying the virus, and nearly all patients who contract the disease develop a chronic infection. As is true with hepatitis B, a chronic infection can lead to cancer, cirrhosis, or liver failure.

Drugs for Hepatitis Because hepatitis A does not cause chronic disease, treatment is limited to supportive care, allowing the immune system to clear the infection on its own. Vaccines are available for both hepatitis A and B, but they are not effective if a person already has the disease. Hepatitis B is more common than hepatitis A in the United States, and routine vaccination of children and healthcare workers is now recommended. The hepatitis B vaccine is a three-injection series. Hepatitis B and C can lead to chronic infection and can be treated by using interferon therapy. Interferons work by boosting the patient's immune system, allowing it to fight and suppress the infection.

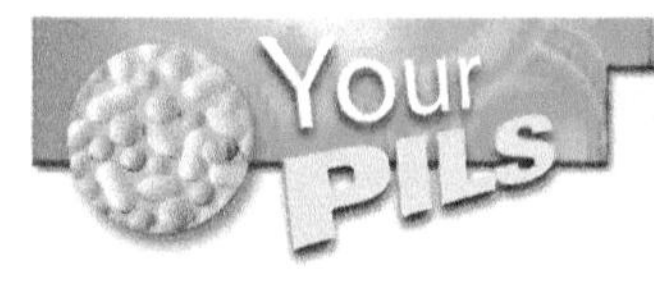

No matter what learning style(s) you prefer, you can learn from applying vaccination concepts to your own life. Look up your own vaccination records and determine your immunization status for hepatitis A and B. Depending on your age, you may have been vaccinated against them as a child as is recommended currently. Did you get all three doses of the hepatitis B series? Did you get boosters of the hepatitis A vaccine? This practical application exercise is useful for remembering vaccinations and completes a task that is necessary for anyone hoping to be employed in healthcare.

Immunosuppression

When someone receives an **organ transplant**, T cells detect and attack the foreign tissue, and B cells make antibodies against it. Unless **immunosuppression** is begun, the body will reject an implanted organ in this way. Prior to transplant surgery, tissue typing is performed to find a good match for organ donation, which helps reduce the chance of **organ rejection** but never completely eliminates this risk. If nothing is done to prevent this natural immune response to foreign tissue, the new organ will be destroyed. In addition, T cells remaining in the transplanted organ can mount an attack against the recipient's body after transplant, a reaction called **graft versus host disease**.

Immunosuppressants

Medications that suppress immune system activity are used to prevent organ rejection after someone has received a transplant. Although some agents mentioned here are used short term, **immunosuppressant** therapy of some kind must be taken for life after receiving a transplant to prevent rejection of the new organ.

Immunosuppressants are also used to suppress autoimmune disorders such as rheumatoid arthritis or SLE. A few are used for psoriasis, an autoimmune disorder that is not well understood but that causes dry skin patches, pain, and itching. Immunosuppressants work by inhibiting T cell and B cell activity. See Table 4.3 for common immunosuppressants and their dosing information.

Side Effects Common side effects of immunosuppressants include sore throat, cough, dizziness, nausea, muscle aches, fever, chills, itching, and headache. Most of the time, these effects are mild to moderate. Taking acetaminophen can alleviate some of these effects if they are bothersome.

Rare but serious effects include changes in heart rhythm or blood pressure, chest pain, unusual bleeding, bruising, anemia, and hyperlipidemia. Therefore, patients taking these agents need close monitoring for cardiac function and periodic blood tests. Some evidence in studies also shows that long-term immunosuppressant use may increase cancer risk.

Muromonab can cause severe pulmonary edema (fluid accumulation in the lungs) on the first dose. Patients must be given corticosteroids before taking this agent to prevent this potentially severe effect from occurring. The intensity of this effect diminishes with each dose.

Cautions and Considerations Because these agents suppress the immune system, patients taking them are at increased risk of infection. Patients are often instructed to take special precautions to minimize exposure to infection. They may be directed to wear face masks and stay out of crowded public areas. Of course, frequent hand washing to prevent disease is recommended.

Keep in refrigerator
but DO NOT FREEZE
Protect medication
from exposure
to light

DO NOT
SHAKE

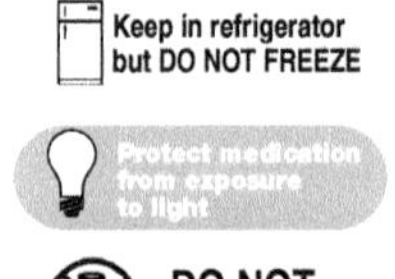

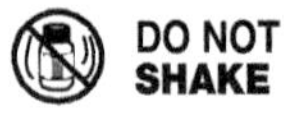

The IV dosage forms of these agents have special handling and mixing instructions. Some agents must be refrigerated, and others should be protected from light. They cannot be shaken and must be used within a limited time from mixing. Cyclosporine must be prepared in glass containers.

Table 4.3 Commonly Used Immunosuppressants

Generic (Brand)	Dosage Form	Route of Administration	Common Use	Common Dose
Alefacept (Amevive)	Injection	IM	Psoriasis	15 mg once a week
Azathioprine (Imuran)	Tablet, injection	Oral, IV	Organ transplant Rheumatoid arthritis	1–3 mg/kg a day
Cyclosporine (Neoral, Sandimmune, Gengraf)	Capsule, oral solution, injection	Oral, IV	Organ transplant Rheumatoid arthritis	Depends on product and use
Efalizumab (Raptiva)	Injection	Subcutaneous injection	Psoriasis	0.7 mg/kg followed by 1 mg/kg a week
Muromonab (Orthoclone)	Injection	IV	Organ transplant	5 mg a day
Mycophenolate (CellCept, Myfortic)	Tablet, capsule, IV	Oral, IV	Organ transplant SLE	Depends on product, route of administration, and type of organ transplant
Sirolimus (Rapamune)	Tablet, oral solution	Oral	Organ transplant Psoriasis	2–5 mg a day
Tacrolimus (Prograf)	Capsule, injection	Oral, IV	Organ transplant Rheumatoid arthritis	Depends on type of organ transplant

Special administration instructions apply to each of these agents. For instance, oral tacrolimus cannot be taken with antacids. Sirolimus can be taken with or without food, but once one method is chosen, the patient should stick with it. Read labels carefully because some agents must be given as an IV infusion, whereas others must be given as an IV bolus injection. They usually cannot be given both ways.

A few of these agents have serious drug interactions. You must heed computer alerts and notify the pharmacist when interactions are detected. Alerts should not be taken lightly.

Oral Corticosteroids

Systemic (oral) corticosteroids are used for their anti-inflammatory and immunosuppressant properties. Oral corticosteroids are glucocorticoids that have potent anti-inflammatory effects. They work by modifying the immune response. They slow leukocyte function and decrease fever, redness, and swelling. They are frequent choices for treating hypersensitivity and allergic reactions. They also help reduce inflammation and improve breathing during asthma exacerbations. When used for allergic reactions or asthma, they are used short term in high doses. Oral corticosteroids can be used over long periods of time to protect against organ transplant rejection. They are even used in rheumatic and some autoimmune disorders because they slow immune system activity. Topical and inhaled corticosteroids are covered in Chapters 5 and 14, respectively. Table 4.4 includes commonly used oral corticosteroids.

Side Effects Common side effects of corticosteroids include headache, dizziness, insomnia, and hunger. Taking oral corticosteroids first thing in the morning will mimic the typical daily cycle of cortisol in the bloodstream, which may lessen these effects, especially insomnia. Long-term therapy can affect normal metabolism in the body, involving facial swelling ("moon face"), significant weight gain, fluid retention, and fat redistribution to the back and shoulders ("buffalo hump"). For these reasons, these agents are taken on a short-term basis whenever possible. Severe effects include high blood pressure, loss of bone mass (osteoporosis), electrolyte imbalance, cataracts or glaucoma, and insulin resistance (diabetes). In some cases, long-term use of high-dose corticosteroids may cause steroid-induced psychosis. Patients taking corticosteroids long term will need special monitoring and treatment for these effects.

Table 4.4 Commonly Used Oral Corticosteroids

Generic (Brand)	Dosage Form	Route of Administration	Common Dose
Betamethasone (Celestone)	Oral solution, injection	Oral	Varies depending on preparation and indication
Budesonide (Entocort EC)	Capsule	Oral	9 mg a day
Cortisone	Tablet	Oral	25–300 mg a day
Dexamethasone (Decadron)	Tablet, elixir, oral solution	Oral	0.75–9 mg a day
Hydrocortisone (Cortef, Solu-Cortef, A-Hydrocort)	Tablet, injection	Oral, IM, IV	PO: 20–240 mg a day IV/IM: 100–500 mg
Methylprednisolone (Medrol, Depo-Medrol, Solu-Medrol, A-Methapred)	Tablet, injection	Oral, IM, IV	Varies depending on preparation and indication
Prednisolone (Prelone, Flo-Pred, Orapred, Pediapred)	Tablet, suspension, solution, syrup	Oral	Varies depending on preparation and indication
Prednisone (Sterapred)	Tablet, oral solution	Oral	5–60 mg a day

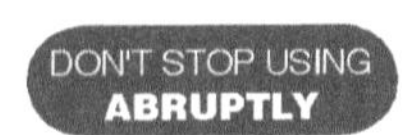

Cautions and Considerations Patients taking corticosteroids longer than a couple of weeks should slowly decrease the dose over time when stopping therapy. Abruptly changing corticosteroid levels can cause untoward and even life-threatening effects. Technicians dispensing these medications should use an auxiliary warning label informing patients not to stop taking the medication abruptly and to talk with their prescribers before stopping.

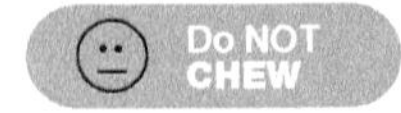

Because corticosteroids suppress the immune system, patients taking them are at increased risk of infection. Patients may have to follow similar precautions as for other immunosuppressants.

Budesonide should be swallowed whole, not crushed or chewed.

With prolonged use, corticosteroids have been found to stunt growth in children. Again, therapy should be as brief as possible but is often necessary to properly treat conditions such as asthma.

Immunoglobulins, Antitoxins, and Antivenoms

Immunoglobulins are administered when rapid immunity is needed for a specific disease for a defined period of time. For instance, a patient recently exposed to a disease for which immunity status is uncertain may be given an immunoglobulin product. Immunoglobulin therapies provide artificial passive immunity through injected exogenous antibodies. The onset of immunity is quick and does not require repeated boosters because the body does not need to produce its own antibodies. The length of immunity, however, is short and usually lasts only a few months. Immunoglobulin products are available for rabies, tetanus, chickenpox, shingles, and respiratory syncytial virus (RSV). Immunoglobulin therapies are specialized and usually administered in inpatient and physician clinic settings, so they are not covered here.

Antitoxins and **antivenoms** use injected antibodies to reduce effects from toxins and venoms in the bloodstream. The antibodies in these agents combine with the toxin or venom and neutralize it. For instance, Rh factor immune globulin is used to bind up antigens in the bloodstream of a negative-blood-type pregnant woman carrying a child with a positive blood type. This immunoglobulin inactivates the antibodies the mother makes to the foreign antigens from the positive-blood-type baby. Otherwise, these antibodies would build up and harm the developing fetus. Rh factor antitoxin is administered in physicians' offices.

Antivenoms (also called **antivenins**) are used for spider bites and snakebites. If you work in the inpatient setting, you may encounter antivenins for black widow spiders and snakes, including rattlesnakes, copperheads, and North American coral snakes. Most antivenins must be administered intravenously within four hours of the bite to be effective. Therefore, these antivenins are kept for use in the emergency room (ER). Orders for these products must be prepared immediately and rushed to the ER for administration. Preparation can be difficult because most products are stored cold in the refrigerator but must warm to room temperature before administration, a difficult process to do quickly without harming the fragile proteins in the product. Gently roll the vial between the palms of your hands to warm the reconstituted product.

Herbal and Alternative Therapies

Limited herbal and alternative therapies are available for autoimmune disorders, hepatitis, or immunosuppression. Along with other benefits on heart function and bone health, vitamin D supplementation may help decrease the risk of MS in women, according to some reports. However, no particular dose has been determined.

Chapter Summary

The acquired immune response is specific to exposure to certain diseases and mediated by T cells and B cells. T cells detect specific foreign antigens and trigger B cells to produce antibodies against them. Immunization uses acquired immunity to protect against disease. Vaccinations trigger a specific, cell-mediated immune response to produce antibodies that will protect a patient when encountering that specific disease. Immunization is increasingly taking place in pharmacies, and technicians are called on to assist. Pharmacy technicians are frequently in charge of ordering, storing, and preparing vaccines and managing patient intake for immunization clinics. Familiarity with the vaccines is imperative.

Interferon therapy is used to treat autoimmune disorders such as MS and viral infections such as hepatitis. MS is an autoimmune disease in which the myelin sheath around nerves becomes damaged, causing numbness, paralysis, and vision loss. No cure exists for this debilitating condition. Special storage and patient education must be provided for these products. Multiple types of hepatitis (A, B, and C) exist, and drug treatment varies for each. Vaccines are available to prevent hepatitis A and B. Interferon therapy is used to treat hepatitis B and C once they occur.

Immunosuppression inhibits the immune system from attacking transplanted tissue after organ transplant. Specialized immunosuppressant medications and oral corticosteroids are used for this purpose. These therapies are riddled with side effects and increase the risk of infection, so risks versus benefits must be weighed. Other immunologic therapies that affect the immune system include immunoglobulins, antivenins, and antitoxins.

✔ Chapter Review

For the following sets of exercises, write the exercise heading, exercise numbers, and your answers on a separate sheet of paper. Your instructor may direct you to turn in the sheet of paper or discuss your answers as a class.

REVIEW THE BASICS

Choose a, b, c, or d as the correct answer to each multiple-choice question.

1. Which of the following cells of the immune system produce immunoglobulins?
   a. B cells
   b. killer T cells
   c. helper T cells
   d. all of the above
2. Which of the following antibodies are found in mucous membranes and pass from mother to baby during breast-feeding?
   a. IgA
   b. IgE
   c. IgG
   d. IgM
3. Which of the following is the brand name of an injectable vaccine for influenza?
   a. Pneumovax
   b. FluMist
   c. Fluzone
   d. Varivax
4. Where should most vaccines be stored in the pharmacy?
   a. on the shelf
   b. in the refrigerator
   c. in the freezer
   d. in a cabinet, protected from light
5. Which of the following is true of MS?
   a. Patients taking drug therapy for MS should be sure to get an annual flu shot.
   b. MS is an autoimmune disorder that affects the myelin sheath on nerve tissue.
   c. Immunosuppressants are the cornerstone of treatment for MS.
   d. all of the above
6. Which side effects are common after receiving a vaccine or other immunologic therapy and can be relieved by taking acetaminophen?
   a. abdominal pain and diarrhea
   b. fever and headache
   c. gas and bloating
   d. dizziness and drowsiness
7. Which of the following viral diseases can be prevented with a vaccine?
   a. hepatitis A
   b. hepatitis B
   c. hepatitis C
   d. a and b
8. For which of the following is cyclosporine used?
   a. immunization against shingles
   b. treating MS
   c. preventing organ rejection after transplant
   d. immunization against hepatitis
9. Interferons are available in which of the following dosage forms?
   a. capsule
   b. tablet
   c. injection
   d. a and b
10. Which of the following immunologic therapies are given in advance to protect against infection?
    a. antivenins
    b. immunoglobulins
    c. interferons
    d. vaccines

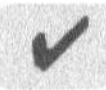

KNOW THE DRUGS

Match each brand name drug with its corresponding generic name and most common use. Your answers should follow this example format: Generic Name: 1. a; 2. b; 3. c; etc. Most Common Use: 1. f; 2. g; 3. h; etc.

Brand Name	Generic Name	Most Common Use
1. Varivax	a. Varicella vaccine	f. Immunization for shingles
2. Zostavax	b. Tacrolimus	g. Immunization for influenza
3. Afluria	c. Human papilloma virus vaccine	h. Immunosuppressant
4. Gardasil	d. Zoster vaccine	i. Immunization for HPV
5. Prograf	e. Influenza vaccine	j. Immunization for chickenpox

PUT IT TOGETHER

For each item, write down true or false, a short answer, or a single term to complete the sentence.

1. True or False: All vaccines are given by injection.
2. Which vaccine is indicated for patients under two and over fifty years old?
3. Name three drugs that are used for allergic reactions and as immunosuppressant therapy.
4. Over what age is the shingles vaccine usually given?
5. Cyclosporine and tacrolimus are given by ____________ and ____________.

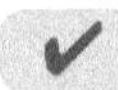

THINK IT THROUGH

Read and think through each numbered scenario carefully and then write several sentences in reply to the question(s) presented. Question 4 requires you to do some Internet research before completing your answer(s).

1. A frequent customer, Mrs. Patterson, tells you that she does not want to get the flu shot. She heard from some friends that they got the flu right after getting the vaccine. Even though she is a certified nursing assistant who works in a long-term care facility and also has diabetes, she refuses to get the flu shot this year. What should you tell her?
2. Most vaccines and immunologic products are fragile proteins that must be kept in the refrigerator, but then injected at room temperature. Explain how you should warm the product to room temperature to mix, prepare, and inject these drug products.
3. A client purchasing some Tylenol confides in you that she is feeling awful, with a fever, chills, and headache. She is worried that she is coming down with the flu because she just started on immunosuppressant therapy. She knows that this drug therapy inhibits her immune system's ability to fight off infection. What should you tell her?

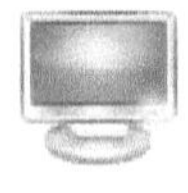

4. **On the Internet,** look up some reports on the alleged association between vaccines and autism. See whether you can find reports from both sides of this controversy. Research shows that vaccines do not cause autism, but some outspoken parents continue to believe that they do. Explain the rationale and reasons behind some parents' reluctance to allow their children to get vaccinations. Can you discern the differences between hype and fact, and between truth and fear?

unit 3

Drugs for the Integumentary and Skeletal Systems

Chapter 5 The Skin and Dermatologic Drug Therapy

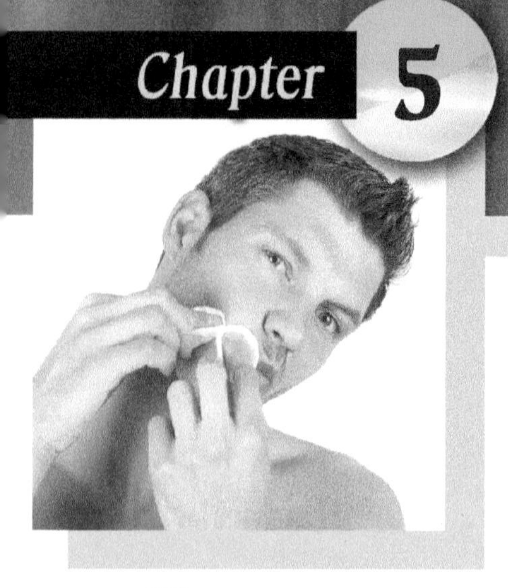

LEARNING OBJECTIVES

- Describe the basic anatomy and physiology of the dermatologic system.
- Explain the therapeutic effects of prescription medications, nonprescription medications, and alternative therapies commonly used to treat diseases of the dermatologic system.
- Describe the adverse effects of prescription medications, nonprescription medications, and alternative therapies commonly used to treat diseases of the dermatologic system.
- Identify the brand and generic names of prescription and nonprescription medications commonly used to treat diseases of the dermatologic system.
- State the common dosage forms and routes of administration of prescription and nonprescription medications commonly used to treat diseases of the dermatologic system.

Interactive self-quizzes, games, audio files, and glossaries help you to learn drug names and facts.

Most medications for skin conditions are applied topically and are available over the counter. Thus, pharmacists consult frequently with patients in need of treatment for skin problems. Acne, sunburn, and skin rashes, for example, are common issues seen by pharmacy professionals. Self-treatment is the norm for most minor skin conditions, but a few of them can potentially be dangerous if not recognized and referred to a healthcare provider for proper diagnosis. In some cases, prescription drugs are needed. Pharmacy technicians can serve as a liaison between patients, pharmacists, and other healthcare providers to improve patient care.

After describing the normal structure and function of the dermatologic system, this chapter discusses the most common pathologic conditions for which drug therapy is needed. Such conditions include skin damage due to sun exposure; acne; burns, wounds, and ulcers; hair loss; and dermatitis. Skin infections caused by bacteria, fungi, viruses, and even insects are covered. This chapter discusses topical anti-infectives and anti-inflammatory agents as well as specialized products for damaged and inflamed skin tissue. Some adverse and allergic reactions to drug therapy manifest as skin problems. These reactions can include Stevens-Johnson syndrome, drug allergy rash, heparin-induced thrombocytopenia (HIT), and photosensitivity. Topical antihistamines or corticosteroids may be used to treat these problems, but often more involved medical treatment is needed. Signs and symptoms of these problems must be recognized early so that patients can seek proper medical care. You can help identify when these problems arise and alert the pharmacist.

Anatomy and Physiology of the Skin

The **integumentary system** refers to the dermatologic tissue that covers the body and includes skin, nails, and hair. This system protects the body from exposure to harmful pathogens and harsh substances as well as helping to regulate body temperature. The **skin** is the largest body organ, accounting for 10% of body weight. The skin has three layers: the epidermis, dermis, and subcutaneous tissue (see Figure 5.1). The **epidermis**, the outermost layer, is made up of dead and dried cells generated from the next layer down, the dermis. The **dermis** comprises the living, functioning layer of skin where **hair follicles** and **nail beds** form, arteries and veins circulate blood, and nerves provide sensation. **Melanocytes** provide skin pigmentation. The dermis also contains sweat, sebaceous, and ceruminous glands. **Sweat glands** are found all over the body and produce watery secretions, including pheromones and other odorous material.

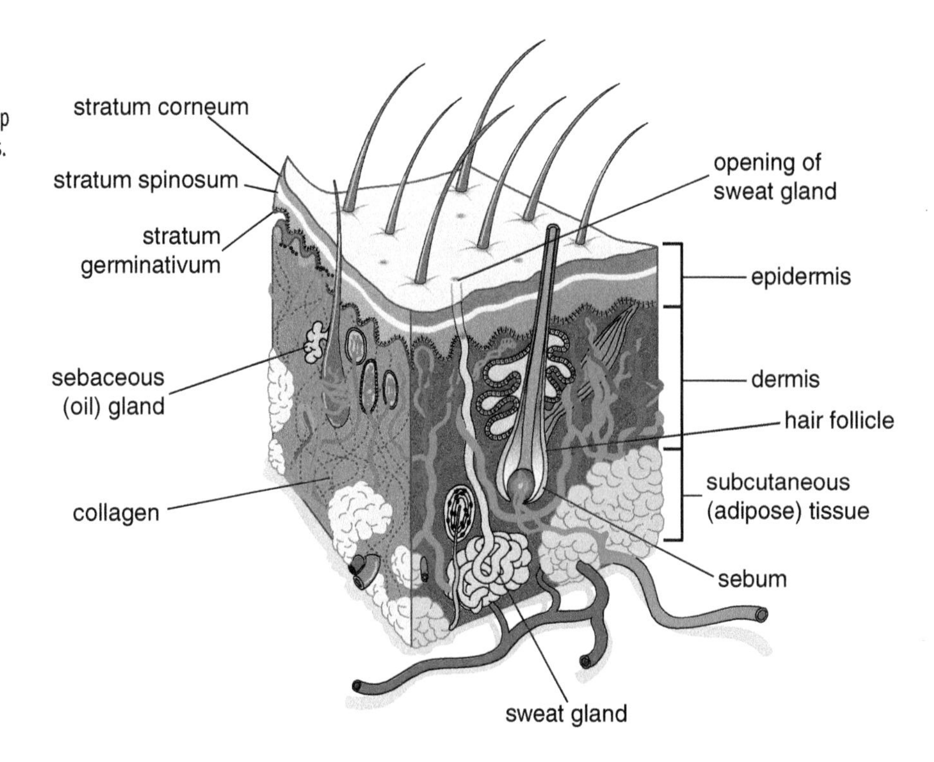

Figure 5.1
Normal Skin Structure
Collagen, a material used cosmetically to plump up lips and facial features, is part of the dermis.

Sebaceous glands secrete oil for hair and skin lubrication. **Ceruminous glands** in the ear canal release waxy material.

The **subcutaneous tissue** is the innermost layer and connects the dermis to underlying organs and tissues. This layer is composed of elastic fibers, also called fascia, and adipose tissue (fat cells). The thickness of this layer varies, depending on the region of the body. Female breast tissue arises from the subcutaneous layer.

Unlike most body organs, which are internal, the skin is external and easy to examine in the pharmacy setting. A pharmacist can inspect the area of skin that a patient is concerned about to determine whether self-treatment will suffice or the patient should be referred to a primary care provider or dermatologist. Pharmacy technicians can help identify patients with likely problems but should get the pharmacist involved in physically assessing a particular skin problem.

Sun Exposure, Aging, and Skin Cancer

Natural skin aging involves loss of **collagen** and **elastin** in the dermis. Without these fibrous structures, fine lines and wrinkles form. Over time, glands produce less oil, leading to dryness. Subcutaneous tissue shrinks, skin thins, and sagging occurs as gravity pulls on dermal tissue, which is less elastic and pliable. This **intrinsic aging** process cannot be stopped, but good skin care can slow it.

Extrinsic aging is caused by external factors such as sun exposure (which accelerates the loss of collagen and elastin), air pollutants, smoking, and skin irritation. **Lesions**, or injuries to the skin, are caused by external factors, genetic predisposition, or a combination of the two. Skin is constantly exposed to sunlight and the oxidizing chemicals that cause DNA mutation. DNA damage not only results in benign tumors, such as moles and skin tags, but can also cause precancerous conditions such as **actinic keratosis** and skin cancer including **squamous cell carcinoma**, **basal cell carcinoma**, and **melanoma**. Squamous and basal cell carcinomas grow slowly. Melanoma, however, is fast-growing and should be diagnosed and treated early to prevent it from spreading quickly and becoming life-threatening.

One thing that pharmacists and technicians can help patients understand is how to identify signs of dangerous skin lesions. Signs of skin cancer are categorized into the

"**ABCDs**." When patches of skin, for example moles, appear to have any of the following characteristics, a patient should be evaluated medically:

- **A**symmetry (one half unlike the other half)
- **B**order irregularity (edges are jagged, not smooth in shape)
- **C**olor variation (patches of tan, brown, black, red, and/or white)
- **D**iameter (larger than 6 mm or the top of a pencil eraser)

Drugs for Sun Exposure

Drug therapy can be used to limit **sun exposure** and prevent damage from **ultraviolet radiation.** It can also be used to treat damage once it has occurred. Because ultraviolet radiation has been strongly linked to skin cancer, treating damage once it has occurred is not as effective as limiting sun exposure in the first place. In a pharmacy, sunscreen and sun block products are encountered often. Products for skin damage such as actinic keratosis, or for skin cancer itself, are usually applied in a physician's office by trained personnel.

Sunscreens and Sun Blocks These products work by either limiting ultraviolet radiation in the case of **sunscreens** or completely occluding ultraviolet light from reaching the dermis with **sun blocks**. Ultraviolet radiation is divided into two types: A, which produces tanning (but can burn with prolonged exposure), and B, which leads to burning. Most sunscreen products are aimed at reducing type B ultraviolet rays while allowing type A rays to continue tanning the skin. A variety of active ingredients can be found in these OTC lotions, creams, sprays, and gels. For practical purposes, they are not all listed here. An example is para-aminobenzoic acid (PABA). Some patients are allergic to PABA. Zinc oxide is a sun block that completely occludes any radiation from reaching the skin.

Pharmacy technicians can help patients understand how the rating system for sunscreens and sun blocks works. The **Sun Protection Factor (SPF)** estimates the amount of resistance to burning that a product provides. In effect, the SPF number estimates how much longer a person can be in the sun and receive the same amount of radiation effects. For instance, an SPF of 8 generally means a patient can spend eight times longer in the sun than the normal time it would take to burn. Table 5.1 shows which factor is recommended for someone with each type of skin and burning tendency. Patient skin type is based on exposure to unprotected sun for forty-five to sixty minutes. Products with a rating of 50 or higher can be considered sun blocks, which occlude ultraviolet radiation completely and do not allow tanning to occur.

Table 5.1 Recommended Sunscreen Product Guide

Patient Skin Type	Minimum Suggested SPF Product
Always burns, rarely tans	20–30
Burns easily, tans minimally	12–20
Burns moderately, tans gradually	8–12
Burns minimally, tans well	4–8
Rarely burns, tans profusely	2–4
Never burns, deeply pigmented	None needed

Acne and Dandruff

Acne is probably the most common skin condition for which treatment, either OTC or prescription, is sought. Acne is initiated by the overproduction of **sebum**, which is produced from glands around hair follicles. Such overproduction is most often stimulated by the hormonal changes encountered during puberty. **Pimples**, **blackheads**, and

whiteheads appear as pores and follicles clog with oily material, dead skin cells, and dirt from the skin's surface. Mild forms of acne can be treated with OTC products. However, acne in its most severe forms such as **nodular acne** or **acne vulgaris** can cause deep cysts that permanently damage the dermis layer. Visible scars and pockmarks can form. Prescription drug therapy is needed for moderate to severe acne.

Rosacea is categorized as acne (and is also called adult acne) but arises from a different physiologic process entirely. Rosacea is a chronic inflammatory disorder seen in adults and characterized by redness, visible surface blood vessels, and raised bumps or pustules on the face and cheeks. Exposure to sunlight or extreme temperatures can worsen this condition.

Dandruff is a malfunction of the oil-producing glands around hair follicles on the scalp. Cell proliferation in the scalp is also accelerated. Overproduction of sebum and cells results in layers of epidermis sticking together and flaking off as they dry. Specks of skin become visible in the hair and on the scalp. Although unsightly, dandruff is not harmful.

Drugs for Acne

First-line treatment for mild to moderate acne is to cleanse the affected area daily. Although daily cleansing will not eliminate acne, it can help prevent new blackheads and pimples from forming. Mild soap or cleanser is used twice a day to remove excess oil, dirt, and dead skin cells that build up and clog pores.

Treating repeated acne lesions starts with OTC products, such as benzoyl peroxide. Moderate to severe acne conditions require prescription products, starting with topical agents then progressing to oral agents when needed. Oral agents include oral contraceptives in some females (see Chapter 18) and antibiotics such as erythromycin, tetracycline, doxycycline, minocycline, and clindamycin (see Chapter 3). Metronidazole and azelaic acid are also used for rosacea. Because oral agents have more side effects, they are saved for patients who do not gain adequate control with topical treatments.

Topical Acne Agents These acne agents are used alone for mild acne and may be used in combination with oral agents for moderate to severe acne. **Benzoyl peroxide** and **salicylic acid** are the mainstays of treatment for mild acne. If they do not work, prescription topical agents will be used.

Benzoyl peroxide is a bleaching agent that promotes cell turnover in follicles. It produces oxygen, which is toxic to the bacteria that cause pimples. Benzoyl peroxide is available in both OTC and prescription strengths. Salicylic acid is a **keratolytic** agent that breaks down and peels off dead skin cells, preventing them from clogging pores. Both of these active ingredients can be found in numerous facial cleansers, washes, and masks in a variety of strengths (see Table 5.2).

Table 5.2 Common Acne Products

Generic (Brand)	Dosage Form	Route of Administration
OTC Products		
Benzoyl peroxide (Benzac, Brevoxyl, Clearasil, Desquam, NeoBenz, Neutrogena, Oxy, PanOxyl, Triaz, ZoDerm)	Liquid, bar, cleanser, cream, gel	Topical
Salicylic acid (Clearasil, Sal-Clens, Stridex, Fostex, PROPA pH, Oxy, others)	Cream, lotion, cleanser, pads, stick	Topical
Prescription Products		
Azelaic acid (Azelex, Finacea)	Cream, gel	Topical
Benzoyl peroxide (Benzac, Triaz, Brevoxyl, ZoDerm, PanOxyl, NeoBenz)	Liquid, bar, cleanser, lotion, cream, gel	Topical
Clindamycin (Cleocin T, Clindagel, ClindaMax, Clindets, Evoclin)	Gel, lotion, topical solution, foam	Topical
Erythromycin (Eryderm, Emgel, Akne-Mycin, Ery Pads)	Solution, gel, ointment, pads	Topical
Metronidazole (MetroLotion, MetroCream, MetroGel)	Lotion, cream, gel	Topical

Side Effects Common side effects of topical acne products include dryness, redness, burning, and flaking or peeling skin. Moisturizers can be applied to control these side effects. In general, less frequent use of these products is recommended if side effects are bothersome.

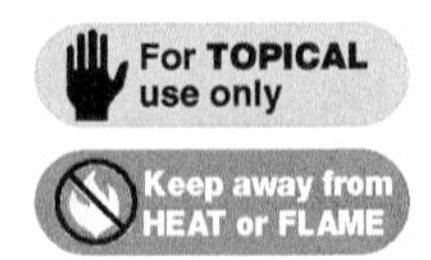

For TOPICAL use only
Keep away from HEAT or FLAME

Cautions and Considerations All of these products are for external use only. An auxiliary warning label should be applied when dispensing these products.

Some of the topical antibiotic products are flammable. Patients should keep them away from intense heat. You should apply an auxiliary warning label to this effect.

Retinoids Vitamin A derivatives including **retinoids** (see Table 5.3) work by increasing cell turnover in follicles, which pushes clogged material out of the pores. In acne vulgaris, retinoids alter cell development and inflammatory processes to reduce swelling and redness.

Retinoids are used for moderate to severe acne as well as to reduce the appearance of fine lines and wrinkles from aging. Acitretin is used exclusively for psoriasis. Because of severe side effects and toxicities, oral retinoid agents are saved for use in the most severe forms of acne or psoriasis.

Table 5.3 Retinoid Agents

Generic (Brand)	Dosage Form	Route of Administration
Acitretin (Soriatane)	Capsule	Oral
Adapalene (Differin)	Cream, gel	Topical
Isotretinoin (Accutane, Amnesteem, Claravis, Sotret)	Capsule	Oral
Tazarotene (Avage, Tazorac)	Cream, gel	Topical
Tretinoin (Altinac, Avita, Renova, Retin-A, Atralin)	Cream, gel	Topical

Professional Focus

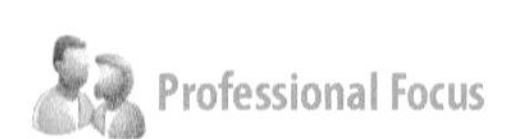

Many insurance companies consider retinoid use for reducing fine lines and wrinkles caused by aging a cosmetic indication and do not cover its cost. You may have to enter specific information into the profile for patients using retinoids for acne for the claim to process smoothly and without rejection.

Side Effects Common side effects of topical retinoid agents include burning, peeling, dry skin, redness, and itching. These effects are quite common. Care should be taken not to apply topical retinoid products close to the eyes or around the mouth. Sensitive skin may be especially prone to these effects. If severe or bothersome, the patient should stop using the product. Retinoids also should not be used along with topical antibiotics such as tetracycline because the antibiotics can increase these side effects.

Oral agents, such as isotretinoin, have systemic side effects that can include depression, psychosis, pancreatitis, high triglycerides, and hepatotoxicity. Patients who already have these conditions should not take isotretinoin. Patients must be monitored closely for mental status changes, and regular laboratory tests must be drawn to watch for pancreas or liver problems.

Cautions and Considerations Isotretinoin cannot be used by women who are or might become pregnant. Severe birth defects are highly likely if a woman becomes pregnant while taking isotretinoin. For this reason, isotretinoin is prescribed and dispensed through a special distribution program approved by the U.S. FDA. This program, **iPLEDGE**, requires pharmacies, wholesalers, and patients to be registered. Women must agree to use effective contraception and submit to regular pregnancy tests as part of the program. Anyone taking isotretinoin should not donate blood for up to one month after taking it so that possible recipients are not exposed. More information about this program is available by finding the iPLEDGE program Web site or tollfree phone number.

Dandruff Products The active ingredients used most in dandruff products are **selenium sulfide** and **pyrithione zinc**. Both are available over the counter in shampoo, such as head & shoulders® and Selsun Blue®. They are used daily or on a regular basis to control dandruff. **Coal tar** shampoos including Neutrogena® T/Gel® are also available over the counter but tend to be used in severe cases. Coal tar is safe but messy and odorous to use, and most patients find long-term use unpleasant. Nizoral® shampoo is available in OTC and prescription strengths. It contains ketoconazole, which is typically considered an antifungal agent. All of these active ingredients work by slowing cell and oil production, resulting in reduced skin flaking. They also have antipruritic properties that reduce the itching associated with dry, flaking skin. Side effects of dandruff products are rare and mild in nature. However, possible effects include contact dermatitis, photosensitivity, and aggravation of prior skin conditions such as acne or psoriasis. If such effects occur, the patient should stop using the product and these effects will subside.

Skin Infections

Fungal infections of the skin are commonly caused by **dermatophytes** and *Candida albicans,* a yeast. They infect skin, nail beds, and even mucous membranes such as those inside the mouth. **Tinea** is a dermatophyte that causes **ringworm**, **athlete's foot**, and **jock itch**. Agents that treat fungal infections in skin and nails are covered (along with other antifungal agents) in Chapter 3.

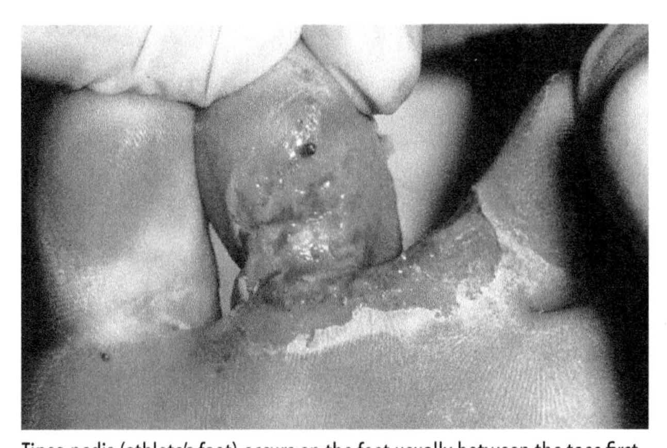

Tinea pedis (athlete's foot) occurs on the feet usually between the toes first.

Few viruses affect the skin, but the herpes virus family causes many skin problems. **Herpes simplex virus, type 1** causes cold sores, and **herpes zoster** causes shingles (see Chapter 3). **Shingles** is an inflammation and reemergence of a systemic viral infection, but it affects nerve pathways near the skin and manifests as painful skin lesions. **Genital herpes** is a sexually transmitted disease that manifests in chancre sores on the skin (see Chapter 18). Many different viruses cause warts on the skin. Most are harmless, but **human papillomavirus (HPV)** is particularly problematic. HPV causes genital warts and has been linked to cervical cancer in women (see Chapter 18).

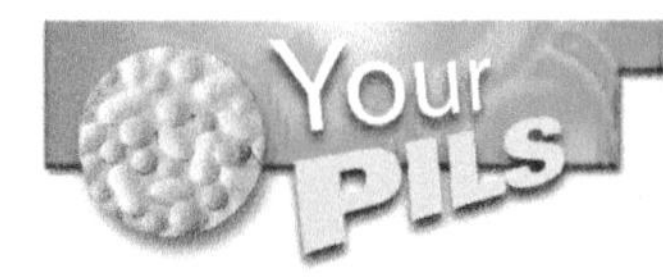

If you like to reflect on learning like Creators do, go back to Chapter 3 and review the lengths of treatment for topical antifungal agents. Recall how often and long they must be applied for athlete's foot versus ringworm. Take another look at the oral agents. How long will a patient have to use them to cure a dermatophyte infection under the nails versus on the feet?

Bacterial Skin Infections

Bacterial skin infections most frequently involve *Staphylococcus aureus*. *S. aureus* is considered normal flora and is not generally harmful unless overgrowth occurs or it is introduced internally through a cut or sore. For that reason, systemic antibiotics are given prior to surgery to prevent infection from incision through the skin. **Impetigo** is an example of a skin infection caused by *S. aureus*. Impetigo typically occurs in children and is characterized by pus-filled blisters that break to form a yellow crust. When infection is

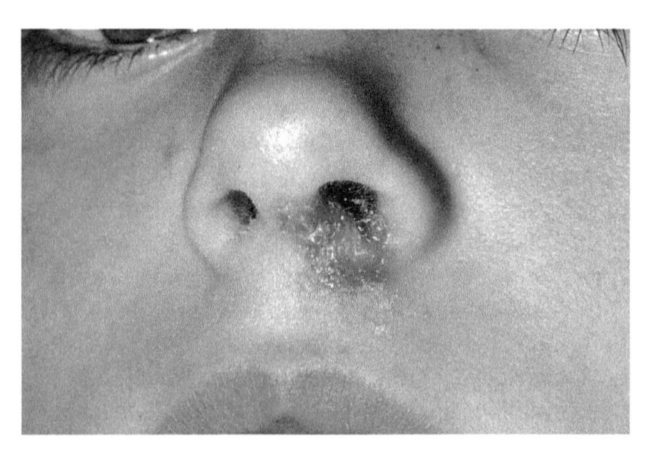

Impetigo frequently occurs on the face, particularly around the nose and mouth in children.

localized to the superficial layers of the skin, topical agents are appropriate. When skin infections become severe and spread to other soft tissues, systemic agents are needed (see Chapter 3).

Topical Antibiotics Most antibiotic medications are covered in Chapter 3, along with other anti-infective agents. However, mention of **topical antibiotic** drugs is warranted here. Generic names are different for topical agents, so familiarity with oral antibiotics does not confer knowledge of these products. Topical antibiotics are used for local skin infections such as cuts or scrapes, impetigo, and diaper rash. Mupirocin is used most often for impetigo and rosacea. These agents work by a variety of mechanisms, depending on their drug class (see Table 5.4).

Table 5.4 Common Topical Antibiotics

Generic (Brand)	Dosage Form	Dispensing Status
Bacitracin	Ointment	OTC
Bacitracin+neomycin+polymyxin B (triple antibiotic ointment)	Ointment	OTC
Clindamycin (Cleocin T, ClindaMax)	Gel, lotion, solution, foam	Rx
Erythromycin (Eryderm, Erygel, Ery Pads)	Solution, gel, ointment, pledgets	Rx
Mupirocin (Bactroban)	Ointment, cream	Rx
Neomycin, polymyxin B (Neosporin)	Ointment, irrigation	OTC
Retapamulin (Altabax)	Ointment	Rx

Side Effects Side effects of topical antibiotic products include burning, stinging, pain, rash, dry skin, swelling, and redness. If used near the nose, headache, runny nose, respiratory congestion, and sore throat can occur. Keep these products away from the eyes and other mucous membranes.

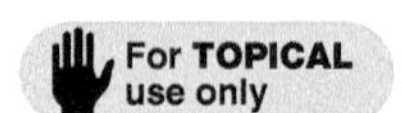

Cautions and Considerations These products are for external use only. Appropriate auxiliary warning labels should be used when dispensing. They should not be applied over large areas of skin because systemic absorption can occur.

Lice and Scabies Infestation

Two types of parasitic insects, lice and scabies, use the human body as a host. **Lice** feed on human blood, which causes intense itching. The normal life cycle for lice is forty to forty-five days. They lay eggs (nits) on hair follicles next to the skin, which hatch in about eight days. Three different species of lice affect humans: head lice, body lice, and pubic lice. Table 5.5 shows common products to treat lice and scabies.

Table 5.5 Common Lice and Scabies Products

Generic (Brand)	Dosage Form	Route of Administration
Lindane	Lotion, shampoo	Topical
Permethrin (Nix, Elimite, Acticin)	Cream, lotion	Topical
Pyrethrin (Tisit, Rid, Pronto)	Lotion, gel, shampoo, mousse	Topical

Head lice are passed from person to person through direct contact or by sharing hats, hairbrushes/combs, clothing, or sometimes bedding. Children tend to get head lice most often because they play in close contact with each other and share personal items frequently. **Pubic lice** ("crabs") are very small and passed only through sexual contact. Symptoms include intense itching that may resemble dermatitis.

Scabies are insects that burrow into the epidermal layer of the skin and feed on cellular material there. Scabies are very small and difficult to see, but the burrows they make into the skin are visible as grayish-white wavy lines that are slightly raised. As they burrow, they secrete substances that disintegrate skin cells. The intense itching the host experiences is most likely from the fecal pellets the scabies leave behind. Scabies are spread through skin-to-skin contact or by sharing a bed (even without sexual contact). They are more common in urban, crowded areas where hygiene is not ideal.

Treatment for lice and scabies is primarily over the counter, so pharmacists and technicians are involved on a regular basis in helping patients select and use self-treatment products. Many patients are embarrassed about these infections because they carry a stigma. Pharmacy personnel need to be sensitive to these concerns but forthright with accurate information so that patients can use these products with success.

In addition to treating lice and scabies with drugs, patients should wash all clothing, underwear, pajamas, pillows, towels, and bed linens in hot water. Hair should be combed with a fine-toothed comb to remove dead lice and nits. Stuffed animal toys may be washed or enclosed in airtight bags or containers for four weeks. Rooms should be thoroughly vacuumed. Hairbrushes, combs, and other personal items that could contain insects should be washed in hot water or treated with a pediculicide, discussed below.

Pediculicides and Scabicides In conjunction with the washing regimen described above, treating lice and scabies involves applying a drug that kills insects. **Pediculicides** kill lice, and **scabicides** are used against scabies. They have similar activity to insecticides such as DDT. They impair the central nervous system of insects, causing seizure and death. These agents are used to treat infestations but should not be used to prevent them.

These products are spread on the hair or body, left on for a specified amount of time, and then washed off. For body lice, the patient must first bathe from the neck down, and then the product is applied and allowed to remain on the skin overnight. Treatment is repeated, if needed, in one week. For head lice, the product is applied to the hair and scalp, allowed to remain for ten minutes, and then rinsed off. Repeat treatment is recommended in one week to kill newly hatched lice. For pubic lice, the product is applied from the thighs to the trunk of the body and allowed to remain on the skin overnight. Treatment is repeated, if needed, in one week. For scabies, the product is applied to the skin from the neck down and allowed to remain on the skin overnight, and then washed off. Repeat treatment is rarely needed.

Pyrethrin and **permethrin** are considered first-line therapies because they are available over the counter. Pyrethrin is used, however, only for head lice. Permethrin, depending on the formulation, can be used for either lice or scabies and has residual activity for up to fourteen days. Thus, repeat application may not be needed with this product.

Lindane lotion is used for scabies, and the shampoo is used for lice. It has significant central nervous system toxicities and can cause seizures, so it is limited to prescription use only. It should not be used on children or infants. Patients must follow instructions closely and avoid getting it in the eyes or on mucous membranes. Lindane should be washed off in eight to twelve hours. Repeat applications can cause dermatitis, so reapplication is not recommended. Patients or caregivers applying lindane should wear gloves or wash their hands thoroughly after application.

Side Effects Side effects of pyrethrin and permethrin include mild itching, burning, tingling, numbness, and rash in the area of application. They can also cause headache, dizziness, diarrhea, nausea, and vomiting. These effects can be avoided or lessened by using only the recommended amount for only the time period indicated on the package.

Side effects of lindane are significant and possibly life-threatening, so patients must follow application instructions carefully. Seizures and even death have occurred from lindane use, usually when used incorrectly. Patients should not use more than two ounces, as prescribed, and should wash the product off in eight to twelve hours to reduce systemic absorption. Other side effects include dermatitis, itching, headache, pain, and hair loss. Other OTC products should be tried first, if at all possible, to avoid these potential toxic effects.

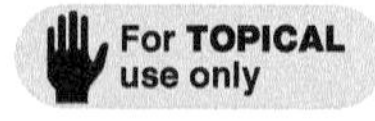

Cautions and Considerations All pediculicide products are for external use only. Ingestion is very dangerous, especially for lindane. Ingestion is considered a poisoning situation. If it is swallowed, patients should call a poison center. In case of contact with the eyes, flush well with water immediately.

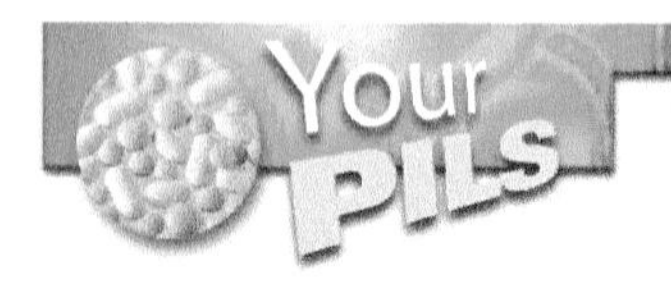

If you like active experimentation like Enactors do, try this homework. Look up the Web sites for Nix and Rid lice treatments. Investigate the information provided, watch the demonstration videos, and then find a classmate with whom to discuss your findings. What are the advantages and disadvantages of these products? What other nondrug therapy measures are necessary to eliminate head lice?

Hair Loss

Two major types of **hair loss** include androgenic alopecia and alopecia areata. **Androgenic alopecia** is more common, affecting both men and women, even though it is often referred to as male-pattern baldness. It is genetically related and hormonally mediated. Hair follicles shrink in size and produce finer hair. **Alopecia areata** is a chronic inflammatory disorder affecting hair follicles and may cause areas of complete hair loss. It can affect nail beds as well.

Drugs for Hair Loss

Used for androgenic alopecia in both men and women, **minoxidil** (Rogaine) works for hair loss by improving blood flow to the scalp and stimulating resting hair follicles. It is available over the counter, so pharmacy personnel are involved in advising patients about its use. Applied to the scalp twice a day, minoxidil is available as a 2% or 5% strength solution or foam. Although men can use either strength, the 2% strength is recommended for women. Hair regrowth, should it occur, takes four months or longer to become noticeable. You should inform patients that the amount applied is small (only 1–2 mL) and using more does not improve results. Patients should be sure to wash their hands after application.

In addition to minoxidil, treatment for hair loss may include finasteride, a 5-alpha reductase inhibitor also used for prostate enlargement (see Chapter 19). Finasteride is contraindicated in women because it affects testosterone production and may affect a developing fetus if the patient is pregnant. Treatment for alopecia areata includes potent topical corticosteroids.

Side Effects Side effects of minoxidil are rare but can include dermatitis, redness, itching, skin flaking, and possibly worsening of hair loss. If any of these effects occur, the patient should stop using the treatment and seek medical care if such effects are severe.

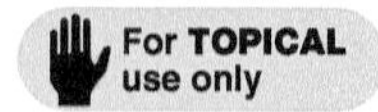

Cautions and Considerations Patients should be aware that minoxidil does not work for everyone. If no hair regrowth is seen after four to six months, patients should talk with their healthcare providers about alternative treatments. Also, once treatment is stopped, hair regrowth will stop and newly grown hair will be shed within a few months.

Dermatitis, Eczema, and Psoriasis

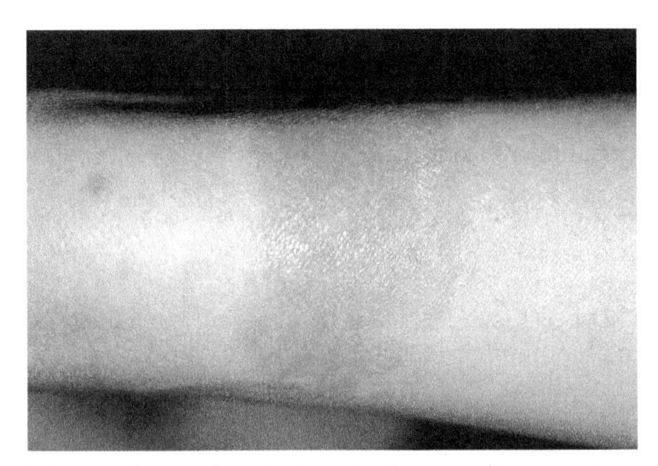

This contact dermatitis is an allergic reaction that occurred in response to the leather of a wristwatch band.

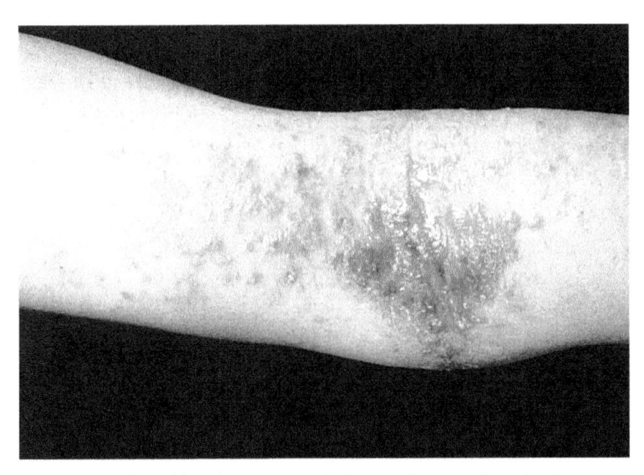

Areas most affected by atopic dermatitis (eczema) are eyelids, cheeks, ears, trunk, naval, and the crooks of the elbows (as in this photo) and knees.

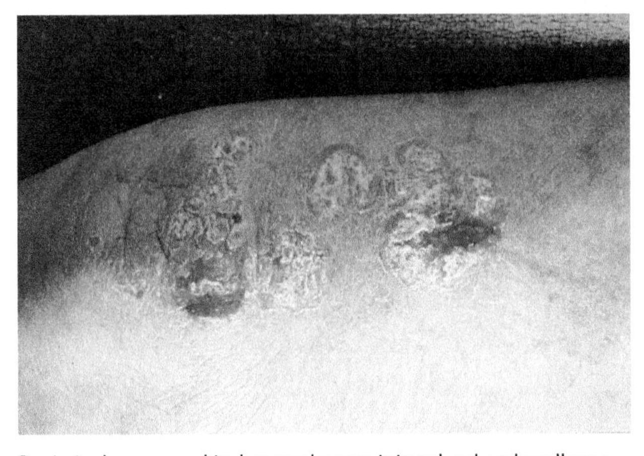

Psoriasis plaques are white but may become irritated, red, and swollen as are those shown in this photo.

Dermatitis is **pruritic** (itchy), inflamed skin that can be caused by a variety of factors. The most severe cases can result in blisters and oozing erosions on the skin, but typical symptoms include areas of redness, dry flaky skin, raised or bumpy skin, and pruritus. **Contact dermatitis** occurs in response to exposure to irritants or allergenic substances. Rash appears wherever skin has come into contact with the offending substance, such as soaps, detergents, or poison ivy. Poison ivy, poison oak, and other plants can cause redness, itching, rash, and blisters when their oils come in contact with the skin.

Seborrheic dermatitis, also called **cradle cap**, is a greasy, scaly area on the skin and is sometimes colored red, brown, or yellow. It usually first shows up in infants and occurs in areas where sebaceous follicles are concentrated, such as the scalp, ears, upper trunk, eyebrows, and around the nose. In adult men, it can occur in the beard area on the face. This type of dermatitis can be treated with attention to good hygiene and topical antihistamines, anti-inflammatory agents, and moisturizing creams.

Atopic dermatitis, also called **eczema,** is a chronic condition that usually first occurs in childhood and can continue into adulthood. Atopic dermatitis is not well understood but has an immunologic component in that patients tend to have elevated levels of IgE in their blood. Patients with atopic dermatitis have a greater tendency to develop asthma or hay fever sometime in life. Eczema appears as dry, flaky, red skin that is very itchy. Patients sometimes scratch enough to cause secondary skin infections. Unlike other types of dermatitis that are usually curable, atopic dermatitis is a chronic condition. Periods of severe symptoms (exacerbation) can cycle with periods of remission. Common triggers for exacerbations include stress, exposure to skin irritants, and food allergies. Treatment involves constant maintenance of skin condition with moisturizers to prevent exacerbations, along with topical corticosteroids for flare-ups.

Psoriasis is an immunologic condition affecting T cell activity in the skin. It manifests on the skin as well-defined plaques (patches) that are raised, silvery or white, flaky, and pruritic. The plaques can appear anywhere on the body and may be very small or quite large and painful. Like eczema, psoriasis is characterized by periods of exacerbation that cycle with times of remission. Stress and exposure to environmental factors that dry out skin can trigger exacerbation. Psoriasis can be difficult to treat and does not always respond well to drug therapy.

Diaper rash occurs most frequently in children who are not yet toilet trained, but it can also occur in incontinent adults who must wear absorbent undergarments. When skin remains wet for long periods of time, tissue breakdown allows bacteria on the surface to gain entry to deeper tissues. Diaper rash products are used for irritation and redness when skin comes in frequent contact with urine and/or feces. They contain a variety of ingredients that combine to promote healing, protect skin from further insult, and prevent infection. Individual ingredients include the following:

- eucalyptol (eucalyptus oil) for antimicrobial activity
- zinc oxide, a drying agent
- camphor or menthol to provide local anesthetic action to relieve pain and itching
- balsam of Peru for wound healing and tissue repair
- talc or kaolin for moisture absorption

These agents should be used as soon as redness appears in order to protect the skin from further damage and prevent infection from bacteria or fungus.

Drugs for Dermatitis, Eczema, and Psoriasis

Corticosteroids are usually the first choice for therapy for dermatitis, eczema, and psoriasis. Therapy starts with topical medications but may include oral corticosteroids (see Chapter 4) if severe. When adequate treatment cannot be achieved with corticosteroids, immunosuppressants and immunomodulators are used. Immunosuppressants include azathioprine, cyclosporine, and methotrexate. Immunomodulators include biological therapies such as adalimumab (Humira) and etanercept (Enbrel) (see Chapter 4). Biological agents (also called TNF-alpha inhibitors) are a costly but effective treatment for severe psoriasis.

Calamine Mild itching from insect bites, rashes, hives, poison ivy or oak, and other allergic reactions can be relieved with **calamine**. It can be used frequently without many side effects or limitations. If itching and rash are not relieved within a few days, patients should see their healthcare providers. Stronger prescription products may be needed, or there may be a problem that needs medical treatment.

Topical Corticosteroids Anti-inflammatory agents that work by inhibiting redness, swelling, itching, and pain in the dermal layer of the skin, **topical corticosteroids** are used for contact dermatitis, eczema, psoriasis, and allergic reactions. A thin layer of medication is applied to affected skin for a limited amount of time.

Because corticosteroids can penetrate the skin and be absorbed systemically, they should be used sparingly. Systemic absorption can cause **hypothalamus-pituitary axis (HPA) suppression**, which is associated with appetite changes, weight gain, fat redistribution, fluid retention, and insomnia. Treatment with topical corticosteroids starts with OTC-strength products, such as 0.5% or 1% hydrocortisone. Both strengths are usually effective for poison ivy and diaper rash (the lower strength should be used for infants and children). Combination products that contain an antifungal along with a corticosteroid can be useful for severe diaper rash.

Corticosteroid products vary in potency, depending on the formulation (see Tables 5.6 and 5.7). Ointments are typically more potent than creams. Ointments are best for dry, scaly lesions, whereas creams are most effective for moist or oozing lesions. When using gels, patients should follow package and prescription instructions. Creams, gels, and ointments are not interchangeable and should not be substituted for each other.

Side Effects Common side effects of topical corticosteroids include burning, itching, dryness, hair growth, dermatitis, acne, hypopigmentation, and skin thinning. Using the least amount over the smallest area for the shortest length of time possible is recommended to minimize these effects.

Table 5.6 Common Topical Corticosteroids

Generic (Brand)	Dosage Form	Dispensing Status	Strength
Alclometasone (Aclovate)	Ointment, cream	Rx	0.05%
Hydrocortisone (Cortizone 10, Dermolate, HydroSKIN, Cortaid, Scalpicin, Procort)	Stick, spray, gel, liquid, lotion, cream, ointment	OTC	0.5%, 1%
Hydrocortisone (Hycort, Hytone, Ala-Cort, Cort-Dome, Hi-cor, Synacort, Eldecort, Hydrocort, Cetacort, Acticort, LactiCare, Penecort, Texacort)	Cream, ointment, lotion, liquid, solution	Rx	1%, 2.5%
Hydrocortisone acetate (Lanacort, Corticaine, Cortaid, Cortef, Tucks, Gynecort)	Ointment, cream	OTC, Rx	0.5%, 1%
Hydrocortisone butyrate (Locoid)	Ointment, cream, lotion, solution	Rx	0.1%
Hydrocortisone probutate (Pandel)	Cream	Rx	0.1%
High Potency			
Betamethasone dipropionate (Diprosone, Maxivate)	Ointment, cream, lotion, aerosol	Rx	0.05%, 0.1%
Betamethasone valerate (Psorion, Beta-Val, Luxiq)	Ointment, cream, lotion, foam	Rx	0.05%, 0.1%
Clocortolone (Cloderm)	Cream	Rx	0.1%
Desoximetasone (Topicort)	Ointment, cream, gel	Rx	0.05%, 0.25%
Fluocinolone acetonide (Synalar, Capex, Derma-Smoothe)	Ointment, cream, solution, shampoo, oil	Rx	0.01%, 0.025%
Fluocinonide (Lidex, Vanos)	Cream, ointment, solution, gel	Rx	0.05%, 0.1%
Fluticasone (Cutivate)	Cream, ointment, lotion	Rx	0.05%
Halcinonide (Halog)	Ointment, cream, solution	Rx	0.1%
Hydrocortisone valerate (Westcort)	Ointment, cream	Rx	0.2%
Mometasone (Elocon)	Ointment, cream, lotion, solution	Rx	0.1%
Triamcinolone (Kenalog, Flutex, Kenonel)	Ointment, cream, lotion, aerosol	Rx	0.025%, 0.1%, 0.5%
Very High or Super Potency			
Betamethasone dipropionate, augmented (Diprolene)	Ointment, cream, gel, lotion	Rx	0.05%
Clobetasol propionate (Temovate, Cormax, Olux, Clobex)	Ointment, cream, lotion, gel, foam, shampoo, spray, solution	Rx	0.05%
Desonide (DesOwen, LoKara, Verdeso)	Ointment, cream, lotion, gel, foam	Rx	0.05%
Halobetasol propionate (Ultravate)	Ointment, cream	Rx	0.05%

Table 5.7 Combination Antifungal and Corticosteroid Products

Generic (Brand)	Dosage Form	Dispensing Status	Strength
Clotrimazole and betamethasone (Lotrisone)	Cream, lotion	Rx	0.05%, 1%
Triamcinolone and nystatin (Nystatin, Mycogen, Myconel, Tri-Statin, Mycolog, Myco-Triacet)	Cream, ointment	Rx	0.1%, 100,000 units/g

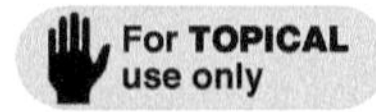

Cautions and Considerations Super-potent corticosteroid products are restricted in the length of treatment or total amount used, in order to reduce the potential for systemic absorption and HPA suppression. They should not be used for longer than two consecutive weeks. The total amount used in one week should not exceed 45–50 g. They should not be applied close to eyes or mucous membranes.

Occlusive wound dressings should not be applied over topical corticosteroid products, especially the more potent ones.

Calcineurin Inhibitors These medications are immunomodulators that work by inhibiting T cell activation, which prevents release of chemical mediators that promote inflammation. **Calcineurin inhibitors**, such as pimecrolimus (Elidel) and tacrolimus (Prograf, Protopic), are used for severe eczema, especially when topical corticosteroids have not worked. They are available as cream, ointment, solution, and capsules.

Side Effects Common side effects of calcineurin inhibitors include burning, itching, tingling, acne, and redness at the site of application. Other effects can include headache, muscle aches and pains, sinusitis, and flu-like symptoms. Therefore, these agents should be used sparingly for a short treatment period to reduce these effects.

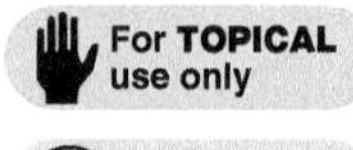

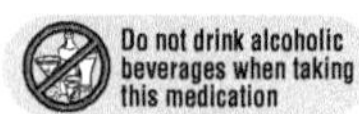

Cautions and Considerations Calcineurin inhibitors have been associated with increased occurrence of cancer (skin cancer and lymphoma). Topical application is less likely to cause malignancy, but patients must be informed of this risk. Pharmacists need to provide adequate counseling for patients using these agents.

Use of calcineurin inhibitors, even topical application, can cause alcohol intolerance. Facial flushing can occur when drinking alcohol and using calcineurin inhibitors. Appropriate auxiliary warning labels for avoiding alcohol use should be included.

Vitamin D Analogs A synthetic form of vitamin D, **calcipotriene** (Dovonex, Taclonex) regulates cell growth and development of skin cells. In psoriasis, skin cells reproduce abnormally and rapidly to form plaques. Vitamin D naturally regulates this cell process. Calcipotriene is a **vitamin D analog** used for psoriasis. Some dosage forms can be used on the scalp, which is useful for psoriatic lesions in the hair when other creams and ointments are too greasy and thick. Vitamin D analogs come as ointment, cream, solution, and suspension.

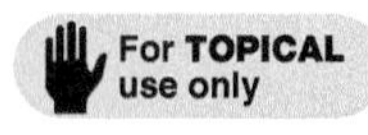

Side Effects Common side effects of calcipotriene include burning, itching, and redness at the site of application. Less common effects include inflamed hair follicles (folliculitis), skin irritation, change in skin color at site of application, and skin thinning. Patients who experience these problems should stop using calcipotriene and contact their healthcare providers.

Cautions and Considerations Vitamin D analogs can cause alterations in calcium metabolism, so patients who have had problems with too much calcium in the blood (such as kidney stones) should not use them. Periodic blood tests may be performed to monitor calcium levels.

Wounds and Burns

Decubitus ulcers, also called **pressure sores**, are severe **wounds** that involve tissue damage through the epidermis and dermis layers. Decubitus ulcers are caused by constant pressure applied to an area of skin, usually from lying down in one position for a long time. Such ulcers are referred to as **bedsores** because they are prominent in patients who are bedridden. They tend to appear in areas where skin covers bony protrusions that receive constant pressure when lying or sitting down or from frequent friction and rubbing on sheets, casts, or braces. This pressure and friction cut off blood flow to dermal layers, allowing necrosis (decay) to begin. Areas most affected are the coccyx (tailbone), heels, hips, spine, and elbows. Patients who have mobility problems, such as those confined to a bed or wheelchair, are most at risk. Decubitus ulcers are categorized into stages, depending on the depth of tissue damage. Wounds that are not cared for will progress in severity.

Decubitus ulcers can be prevented through aggressive nursing care involving turning and repositioning immobile patients every two hours and applying skin protection to high-risk areas. Two hours is the maximum amount of time tissue can withstand constant pressure before breakdown and damage occur. Special air beds that minimize pressure points can be used for patients at high risk. Maintaining good hydration and nutrition also helps. Once an ulcer has developed, treatment involves wound cleaning and removal of necrotic (dead) tissue (called **debridement**) while the wound heals on its own. These wounds, especially deep ones, can take significant time to heal. Some drugs promote **regranulation**, which is the process of building new skin layers over a wound area.

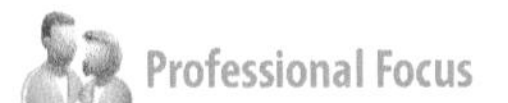

Technicians who work in pharmacies that supply long-term care facilities will handle wound products most often, because many patients in skilled nursing care settings are bedridden.

Burn wounds are caused by heat and thermal injury or by electrical and chemical sources. When burns are extensive, treatment and prognosis depend on the severity and amount of body surface area affected. Surface area affected is estimated by dividing the body into major sections, each representing approximately 9% of total surface area (see Figure 5.2). Severity of burns is categorized by how deeply the tissue damage penetrates skin layers (see Table 5.8). Treatment at a burn center is needed for third-degree burns over a significant portion of the body. Prognosis for survival gets worse as a greater percentage of body surface area is affected. Patients with burns over 80% or more of their bodies are not likely to survive long term.

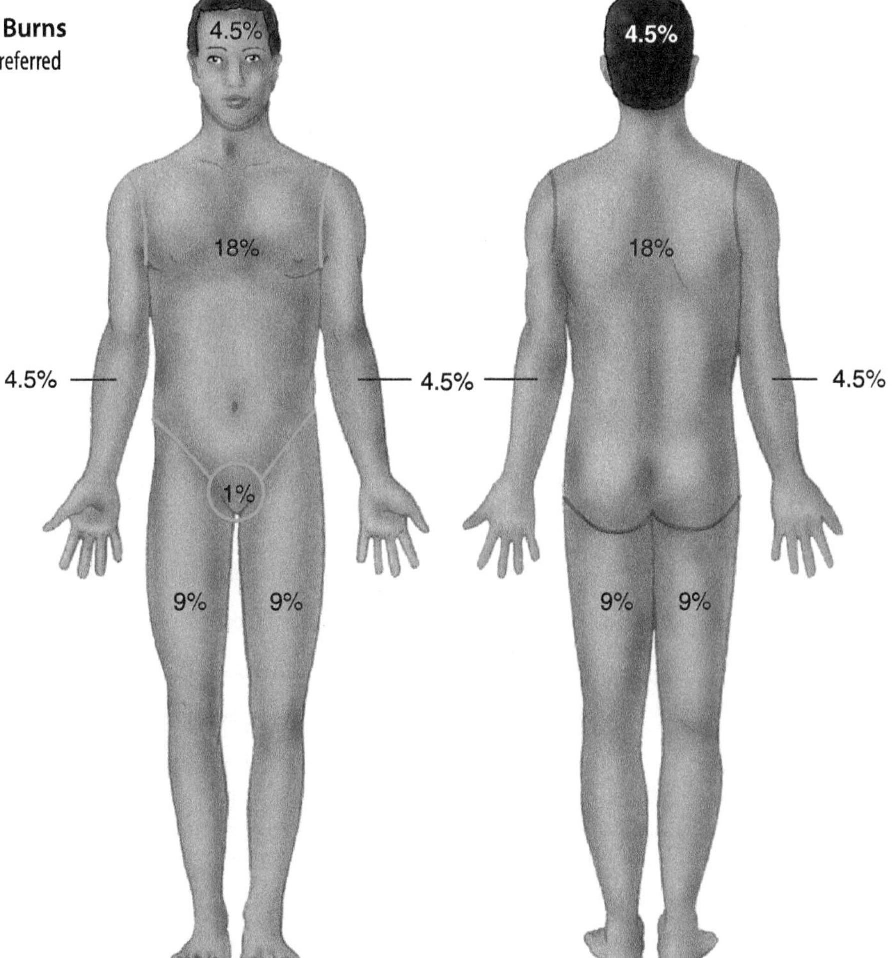

Figure 5.2
Estimating Body Surface Area for Burns
Estimating body surface area in this manner is referred to as the "rule of 9s."

Table 5.8 Burn Wound Staging

Degree	Damage
First-degree burn	Surface epidermal layers damaged, causing redness and possibly peeling, but no blisters.
Second-degree burn	Epidermis and dermis skin layers damaged, causing redness, blisters, swelling, and pain. Scarring is possible.
Third-degree burn	Destruction of epidermis and dermis layers, with possible damage to tissue underneath. Permanent scarring is problematic. Pain may not be present immediately because sensory nerve endings are typically damaged or destroyed. Management requires medical treatment.

Adverse Drug Reactions on the Skin

A couple of the most common reactions to medication manifest on the skin, so it is useful to be familiar with drug-induced skin problems. Pharmacists counsel patients on these potential side effects frequently. You should take special care to ask each patient about drug allergies because skin rash is the most prominent sign of allergy. Just because a patient has received prescriptions in the past with no allergies documented does not mean that she or he has not developed a new allergy since that time. Technicians must diligently ask about and document any drug allergies (and the nature of the symptoms) so that patient safety is maintained.

Photosensitivity

Avoid
SUN EXPOSURE

A frequent side effect of many drug therapies is photosensitivity. **Photosensitivity** is an excessive response to solar exposure, wherein skin easily burns after a short time in the sun. Patients taking drugs with this side effect may find they get sunburned more quickly or more severely than usual. Education should be provided and precautions taken to avoid severe sunburns. Sun block and clothing should be used to protect skin from sun exposure when taking such drug therapies. Drugs that are most associated with this reaction are shown in Table 5.9. During the dispensing process, auxiliary warning labels should be affixed to medications with this potential. Applying warning labels is often a responsibility of pharmacy technicians.

Table 5.9 Drugs Most Associated with Photosensitivity

Drug Class	Drug Example
ACE inhibitors	all agents
antibiotics	griseofulvin, quinolones, sulfas, tetracyclines
antidepressants	clomipramine, maprotiline, sertraline, tricyclic antidepressants (TCAs)
antihistamines	cyproheptadine, diphenhydramine
antipsychotics	haloperidol, phenothiazines
cardiovascular drugs	amiodarone, diltiazem, quinidine, simvastatin, sotalol
chemotherapeutic agents	dacarbazine, fluorouracil, 5-FU, methotrexate, procarbazine, vinblastine
diuretics	acetazolamide, furosemide, metolazone, thiazides
hypoglycemics	sulfonylureas
NSAIDs	all agents

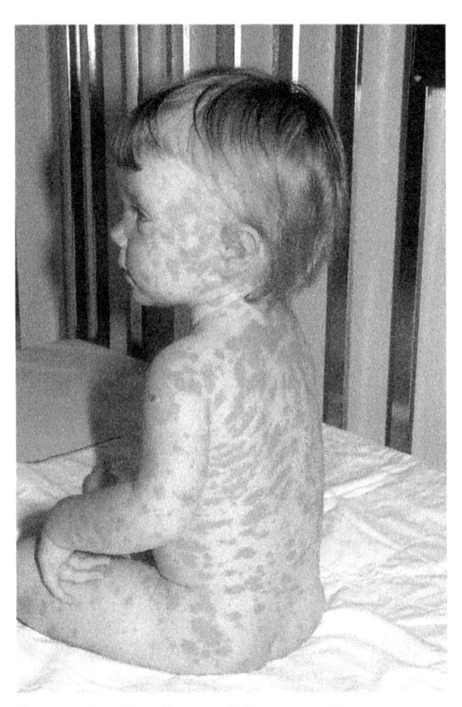

The reaction from Stevens-Johnson syndrome starts as a diffuse red rash that, if left untreated, spreads deeper, causing the dermis to slough off.

Drug Allergy Rashes

Rashes from **drug allergies** appear as **urticaria** (**hives**) and pruritus, or as a diffuse redness on the trunk of the body that may not be pruritic at all. The reaction typically shows up soon after starting to take a new medication, but occasionally it can occur after taking a drug for a while. Patients should inform their prescribers and pharmacists if they get either of these types of rash while taking any drug therapy. Allergic reactions can progress in severity and become life threatening if the patient continues to take the drug. **Anaphylaxis** is a severe and potentially fatal reaction to drug therapy, causing airway swelling and affecting one's ability to breathe (see Chapter 4). Therefore, the offending drug should be stopped immediately and proper documentation of the allergy made in the patient's medical record. Antihistamines, corticosteroids, and even epinephrine are used to treat allergic reactions to drugs.

One rare but potentially life-threatening skin reaction is **Stevens-Johnson syndrome**. This drug reaction begins as a localized rash but, if not treated, can progress to a generalized condition in which layers of skin slough off, exposing vulnerable tissues beneath. If skin integrity is lost over a large enough area of the body, severe infection and temperature regulation problems can ensue. Although this reaction is rare, it tends to occur with specific drug therapies such as antiepileptic agents, penicillin, and some antibiotics including sulfonamides and tetracyclines. If caught early and the offending drug stopped, this syndrome can be treated without life-threatening consequences.

Heparin-induced thrombocytopenia (HIT) is an allergic reaction to the anticoagulant heparin. It can be life threatening as well. This reaction involves a severe and dangerous drop in platelet count in the blood, which can put a patient at risk for bleeding. The reaction first appears as a diffuse red, pruritic rash on the trunk and/or upper legs after a patient receives the anticoagulant drug heparin. Heparin should be stopped immediately and alternative anticoagulation started. Heparin is used frequently in hospitals to keep IV lines open and for various clotting disorders encountered in the inpatient setting. Therefore, pharmacy technicians in hospitals will be involved in dispensing heparin to many patients. Special attention should be given to recognizing and documenting HIT reactions.

Herbal and Alternative Therapies

Numerous herbal and natural substances are added to topical skin care products and cosmetics. Many natural substances, such as **lanolin**, **cocoa butter**, and **vegetable** or **seed oils**, are added as moisturizers to creams and lotions. They work in conjunction with the base vehicle to promote moisture in the epidermis. They supply added oils and cover the skin, preventing moisture evaporation from within. Together, these actions keep skin hydrated and soft. **Vitamins E, A, and D** are emollients added to moisturizers to promote skin health and healing.

Aloe vera is another frequent ingredient in skin care products. It contains a variety of active compounds that have several proven healing and anti-inflammatory properties. When used in concentrated form on a regular basis, aloe vera has been effective for mild psoriasis and burn wound healing. To have significant effects, it needs to be applied three times a day for up to four weeks. Concentrations of aloe vera in many lotions and oils may not be high enough to produce measurable effects beyond moisturizing properties.

Chapter Summary

The skin, the largest body organ, is made up of three layers: epidermis, dermis, and subcutaneous tissue. The dermis comprises the living layer where most glands, hair follicles, blood vessels, and nerves are located. Skin damage can arise from sun exposure, natural aging, wounds, burns, and infections. Damage from wounds and burns is staged, based on the layer of skin affected. Sunscreens and sun blocks are worn to reduce the risk of sunburn. Acne is probably the most common skin condition for which drug therapy is sought. Acne is the overproduction of sebum produced from glands around hair follicles, which clogs pores and forms blackheads, pimples, and even cysts. In addition to daily cleansing, OTC topical agents and retinoids are used to promote clearing and reduce bacterial buildup in pores. Topical antibiotics are used for acne as well as for skin infections such as impetigo. Fungal infections on the skin include athlete's foot and ringworm. Pediculicides are used for head, body, and pubic lice. Another indication for topical drug therapy is dermatitis. Contact dermatitis occurs when skin comes in contact with an allergen or irritant. Atopic dermatitis is eczema, an inflammatory condition that causes dry skin, scaling, and itching. Psoriasis is an immunologic condition that causes scaly patches on the skin that are pruritic and painful. Topical corticosteroids and calcineurin inhibitors are used for dermatitis and eczema, and vitamin D analogs are used for psoriasis. Some drug reactions, for example drug allergies, photosensitivity, and Stevens-Johnson syndrome, manifest on the skin. Technicians play a key role in interviewing patients about drug allergies, so you are the first line of defense for patient safety. Because the skin is so visible, the pharmacy is a place where skin-related inquiries from patients are encountered regularly. Technicians can help identify when patients are having noticeable skin problems and prompt the pharmacist to get involved.

Chapter Review

For the following sets of exercises, write the exercise heading, exercise numbers, and your answers on a separate sheet of paper. Your instructor may direct you to turn in the sheet of paper or discuss your answers as a class.

REVIEW THE BASICS

Choose a, b, c, or d as the correct answer to each multiple-choice question.

1. Which of the following is a characteristic of the dermis?
   a. dead or dying cells and contains skin pigment (melanin)
   b. living tissue and contains blood vessels (supply)
   c. layer made up of mostly fatty adipose tissue
   d. all of the above
2. A burn involving the dermis and including blisters and possible scarring is what type of burn?
   a. first degree
   b. second degree
   c. third degree
   d. fourth degree
3. Which of the following is an infection of the skin and caused by bacteria?
   a. warts
   b. impetigo
   c. scabies
   d. tinea
4. Which of the following is a severe dry skin condition that often appears in the crooks of the elbows and knees?
   a. epidermis
   b. eczema
   c. psoriasis
   d. urticaria
5. Which of the following is caused by pressure (such as the pressure caused by lying in bed in one position too long)?
   a. pruritus
   b. urticaria
   c. decubitus ulcer
   d. squamous cell carcinoma
6. Which of the following is true about topical antibiotics?
   a. Triple antibiotic ointment contains clindamycin, erythromycin, and metronidazole and is available over the counter.
   b. Tetracycline topical is available only by prescription.
   c. Neosporin ointment contains neomycin and polymyxin B and is available only by prescription.
   d. Clotrimazole cream is available only by prescription.
7. What is the most common drug in OTC acne products?
   a. pyrethrin
   b. benzoyl peroxide
   c. erythromycin
   d. minoxidil
8. Which of the following topical corticosteroids is available without a prescription?
   a. betamethasone
   b. fluocinonide
   c. halog
   d. hydrocortisone
9. For which of the following would you most likely use aloe vera?
   a. impetigo
   b. shingles
   c. sunburn
   d. psoriasis
10. Which of the following is a super-potent topical corticosteroid?
    a. Diprolene
    b. hydrocortisone
    c. Topicort
    d. triamcinolone

KNOW THE DRUGS

Match each brand name drug with its corresponding generic name and most common use. Your answers should follow this example format: Generic Name: 1. a; 2. b; 3. c; etc. Most Common Use: 1. h; 2. i; 3. j; etc.

Brand Name	Generic Name	Most Common Use
1. Prograf	a. minoxidil	h. acne
2. Bactroban	b. triamcinolone	i. bacterial skin infection
3. Elocon	c. tacrolimus	j. hair loss
4. Retin A	d. mupirocin	k. dermatitis
5. Cleocin T	e. clindamycin	
6. Rogaine	f. mometasone	
7. Kenalog	g. tretinoin	

PUT IT TOGETHER

For each item, write down either a short answer or a single term to complete the sentence.

1. How long does it take before changes in hair growth will be noticeable with minoxidil?
2. _______________ is a prescription medication used for both lice and scabies, but it is contraindicated in _____________________.
3. Name an oral agent used for severe acne that can only be obtained via the iPLEDGE program, under which dispensing is limited and patients must agree to regular pregnancy tests.
4. What burn wound stage is reached when epidermis and dermis layers are destroyed, exposing tissue underneath?
5. Name two drug classes and generic names for the drugs that cause photosensitivity.

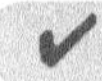

THINK IT THROUGH

Read and think through each numbered scenario carefully and then write several sentences in reply to the question(s) presented. Question 4 requires you to do some Internet research before completing your answer(s).

1. A young woman approaches you at the counter to ask about treating diaper rash. She shows you a tube of Diprolene. She says that she uses it for her eczema flare-ups and it works great. She wants to use this for her six-month-old, who has had diarrhea and now has a bad diaper rash. The child is screaming next to you. What should you do? Why?

2. While you are stocking the OTC aisle, a man with a bottle of Rogaine approaches you to ask your take on its effectiveness. He wants to know how well it works and how soon it will take to grow hair. What should you do?

3. You are on the medicine floor, stocking the electronic drug cabinet with unit dose medication, and a nurse stops you. She asks you how to enter an order for some hydrocortisone cream for a patient who has developed a rash. You just finished stocking this patient's drawer with heparin. What should you do?

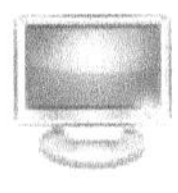

4. **On the Internet,** look up use of biological agents such as adalimumab (Humira), etanercept (Enbrel), infliximab (Remicade), and golimumab (Simponi) for psoriasis. Even though these injectable agents are covered later in Chapter 6, they bear mention here because they are used for both rheumatoid arthritis and psoriasis. What are the costs associated with these agents? Check Web sites for on-line drug stores to locate price information. What are the beneficial effects and side effects patients can expect from them? What can you conclude about how health insurance plans are debating their cost-effectiveness?

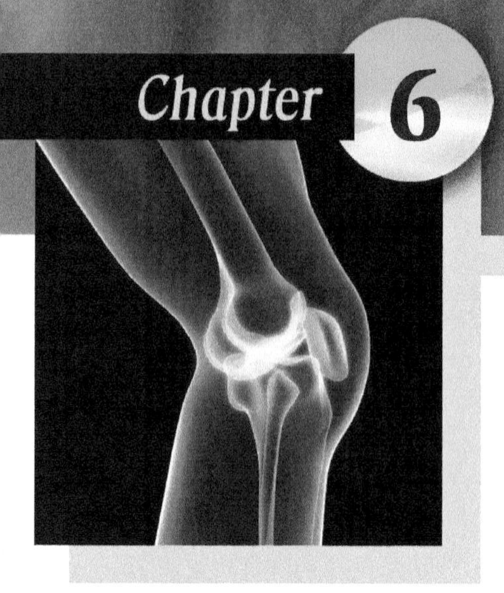

Chapter 6 The Skeletal System and Drug Therapy

LEARNING OBJECTIVES

- Describe the basic anatomy and physiology of the skeletal system (bones and joints).
- Explain the therapeutic effects of prescription medications, nonprescription medications, and alternative therapies commonly used to treat diseases of the skeletal system.
- Describe the adverse effects of prescription medications, nonprescription medications, and alternative therapies commonly used to treat diseases of the skeletal system.
- Identify the brand and generic names of prescription and nonprescription medications commonly used to treat diseases of the skeletal system.
- State the doses, dosage forms, and routes of administration of prescription and nonprescription medications commonly used to treat diseases of the skeletal system.

Interactive self-quizzes, games, audio files, and glossaries help you to learn drug names and facts.

Conditions of the **skeletal system**, such as arthritis and osteoporosis, are quite common. As the population's average age increases, the number of patients with these conditions is growing. In fact, drugs for arthritis are among the top fifty drugs dispensed in pharmacies. Osteoporosis treatment and prevention are frequently advertised and promoted throughout the healthcare arena, especially to those who serve women, the population most affected by this condition.

This chapter discusses the normal and abnormal physiology of the skeletal system (bones and joints). Bone homeostasis and joint function are the most important concepts to learn. Risk factors for osteoporosis and strategies for prevention and treatment of it are covered first. Next, the difference between osteoarthritis and rheumatoid arthritis is explained. The treatment approach differs for these distinct physiologic processes. Acute and chronic drug treatments for gout are also discussed. Last, common dietary supplement products such as glucosamine and chondroitin are covered.

Anatomy and Physiology of Bones and Joints

Bones serve multiple functions beyond the most obvious, which is providing structure and support for the body (see Figure 6.1). Without bones to attach to and pull on, muscles would have a difficult time moving parts of the body effectively. Some bones, including the ribs and pelvis, do not produce movement but serve as protection for delicate organs. Long bones, such as the femur, contain marrow, the birthplace for blood cells. Consequently, bones are important for the normal functioning of multiple body systems.

All bones store calcium and maintain its balance in the body, a constant process of buildup and breakdown called **bone remodeling**. **Osteoclasts** break down bone tissue and release calcium into the bloodstream, whereas **osteoblasts** take calcium from the blood to build bone tissue (see Figure 6.2). Bones grow and increase in density at the greatest rate during childhood and continue to build into the thirties. After that time, a gradual decrease in **bone density** occurs, with the greatest decline later in life, especially for women after menopause. Estrogen is a strong supporter of osteoblast activity and promotes bone density maintenance. After menopause, a woman's estrogen level decreases dramatically, which leads to a natural decline in bone density.

Articulations, the **joints** between bones, are necessary for fluid and efficient movement. As shown in Figure 6.3, the ends of bones are coated with **cartilage** and cushioned from friction by the **synovial membrane** and **synovial fluid**.

Figure 6.1

Anatomy of the Skeletal System

Bones are grouped into two categories: appendicular, which are found in the extremities, and axial, which includes the skull, spine, and thorax (ribs).

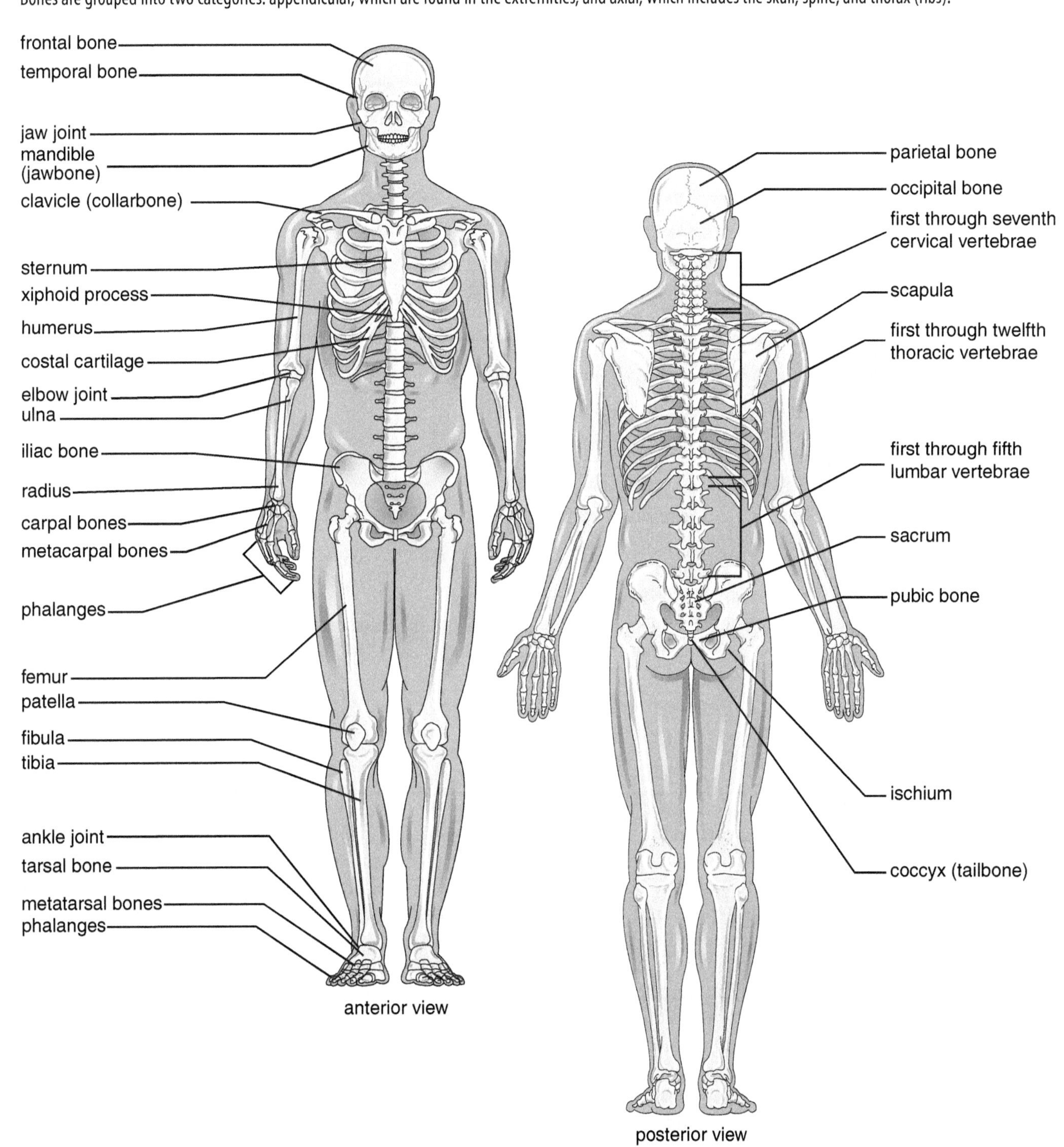

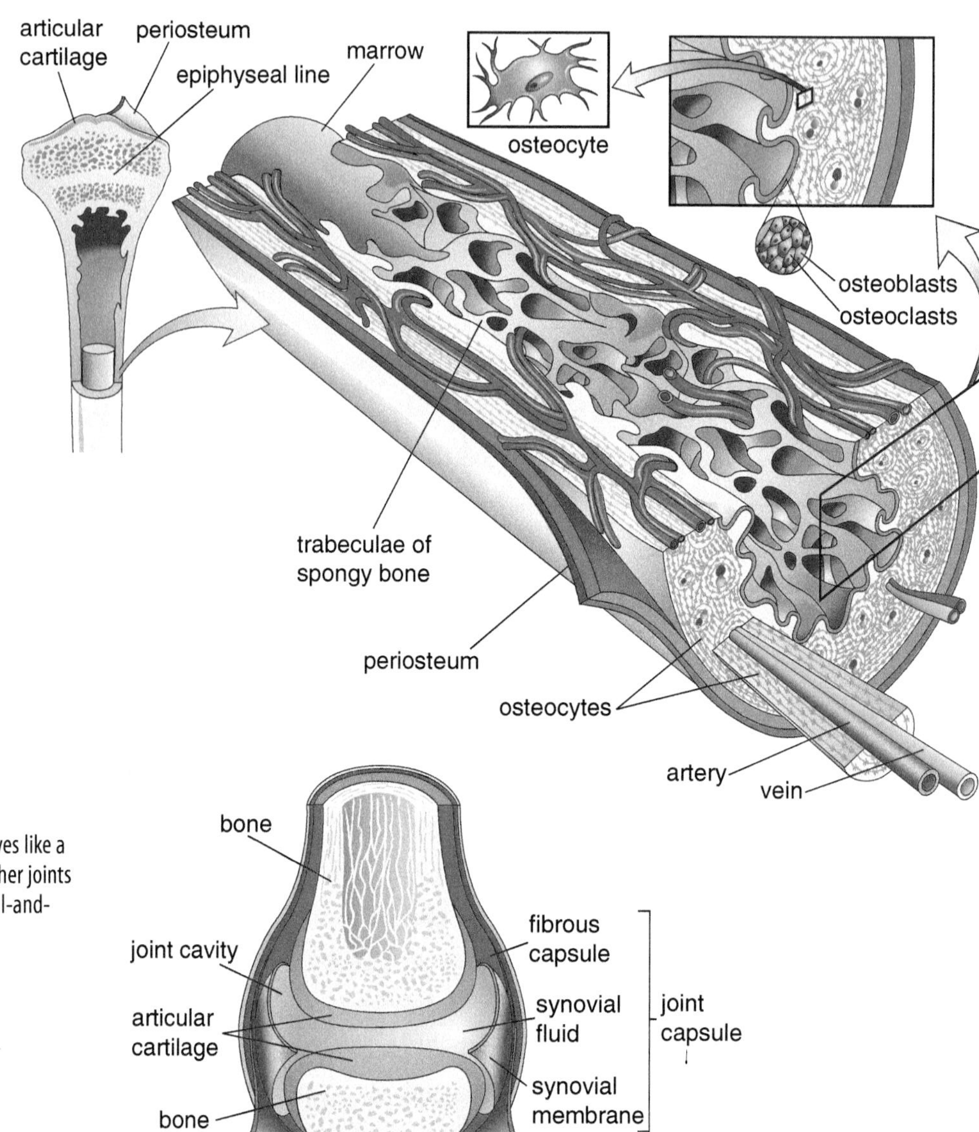

Figure 6.2
Microscopic View of Bone
Osteoclasts and osteoblasts provide bone homeostasis, a continual process that grows and repairs bone.

Figure 6.3
Anatomy of a Joint
Although the joint shown here moves like a hinge (as do knees and elbows), other joints have different functions such as ball-and-socket and pivot movements.

Osteoporosis

Osteoporosis is a reduction in bone density that results in weakened bones and fractures. Although a decline in bone density is expected later in life, osteoporosis occurs when this decline accelerates beyond the normal rate. This condition causes fractures in the hips, spine, and wrists, which cause pain and debilitation. **Hip fractures** can even be life threatening, because the subsequent hip replacement surgery, recovery, and any complications are often dramatic. Older patients may never return to normal function after a hip fracture. Ninety percent of patients with osteoporosis are women. Risk factors for this condition are:

- being female
- being Caucasian
- family history of osteoporosis
- small body frame
- smoking
- heavy caffeine intake
- poor nutrition (i.e., low calcium intake)

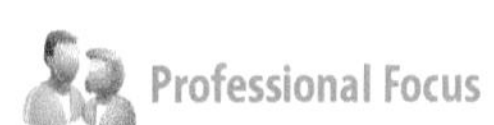

Professional Focus

If you are asked to help with an osteoporosis screening in your pharmacy, check what type of technology the BMD machine employs. Some states require special certifications and registrations for machines using x-ray radiation (labeled DEXA and SXA). Ultrasound machines do not require such measures.

Many pharmacies provide screening tests for osteoporosis. **Bone mineral density (BMD)** machines use x-ray and ultrasound technology. Usually the heel bone is measured because it is a good estimate of hip and spine bone density. Pharmacists and technicians can be trained to perform this test. The result of a BMD screening yields a **T-score**, which is an estimate of risk, not a diagnosis. Armed with such information, patients can make changes in their lives, such as adding weight-bearing exercise, eating foods high in calcium, quitting smoking, and decreasing caffeine intake, which are all ways to increase bone density. If diagnosis of osteoporosis is made by a healthcare provider, drug therapy may be prescribed.

Drugs for Osteoporosis

It would seem to make sense that supplementing estrogen in women whose levels are declining would stave off drastic drops in bone mineral density. However, increases in heart disease, cancer, and stroke associated with estrogen replacement have been found to outweigh this benefit. Consequently, **hormone replacement therapy (HRT)** with estrogen has fallen out of favor as treatment for osteoporosis. However, HRT continues to be used for perimenopausal symptoms such as hot flashes but is taken at the lowest dose for the shortest time possible to alleviate menopausal symptoms only.

Calcium and Vitamin D Normal, healthy adults should get around 1,000 mg of calcium a day to maintain bone strength. Patients with osteoporosis, individuals over age sixty-five, and women after menopause should get 1,500 mg of calcium a day. This daily total can be obtained from diet and dietary supplement products. When diet alone does not provide enough calcium, a variety of calcium-containing products is available in several dosage forms. Only 500–600 mg of calcium is absorbed at a time, so the total daily requirement must be given in divided doses.

When patients take prescription drugs for osteoporosis, they should also take **calcium** and **vitamin D**. Without calcium, osteoblasts cannot build more bone. Vitamin D improves calcium absorption from the gastrointestinal (GI) tract. Therefore, calcium and vitamin D supplementation help other osteoporosis agents work more effectively. Supplementation of these substances is also useful for patients with **osteopenia** (bone weakening), who are at high risk for developing osteoporosis.

The exact amount of calcium absorbed varies among calcium salts (see Table 6.1). Only **elemental calcium** (dissociated calcium ions) gets absorbed with the help of vitamin D into the bloodstream. You can help patients choose appropriate products to deliver a dose of elemental calcium to meet their needs.

Often, vitamin D comes as a combination product with calcium. Vitamin D can be found in fish and is added to milk and breakfast cereals. Exposure to sunlight activates vitamin D in the skin to a form that can be used by the body. Published recommended daily requirements for vitamin D are 400 international units (IU) a day, but many clinicians prescribe up to 1,100 IU a day to replenish and maintain vitamin D stores. One microgram (mcg) of vitamin D equals 1 IU.

Table 6.1 Calcium Salts and Elemental Absorption

Salt	Brand Name	Typical Dose	Elemental Calcium Absorbed
Calcium acetate	Calphron, Eliphos, PhosLo	667 mg	167 mg (~25% of dose)
Calcium carbonate	Caltrate, Os Cal, Tums	500 mg	200 mg (~40% of dose)
Calcium citrate	Citracal, Cal-Citrate, Cal-Cee	Varies	180–250 mg (~20% of dose)
Calcium gluconate	Cal-G	500–1,000 mg	50–100 mg (~10% of dose)
Calcium lactate	Cal-Lac	500–650 mg	100 mg (~10% of dose)

Side Effects Common side effects of calcium supplements are nausea, vomiting, and constipation. Taking calcium with food or a meal helps alleviate these problems. The citrate form of calcium can often be easier on the stomach, but it does not offer as much elemental calcium as do other salts.

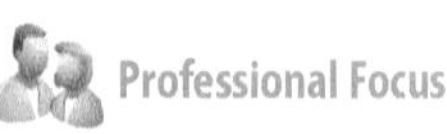

Calcium and vitamin D are dietary supplements ordered regularly as cornerstones in osteoporosis treatment. You should be prepared to answer patient questions about these OTC items, especially about differences among calcium salts and proper dosing for vitamin D.

Common side effects of vitamin D supplements are nausea, vomiting, and edema (swelling). These effects are usually mild. Occasionally, fever/chills, flulike symptoms, lightheadedness, and pneumonia can occur. If patients experience any of these effects, they should stop taking vitamin D and talk with their healthcare providers. Since vitamin D is a fat-soluble vitamin, excessive amounts can accumulate and lead to a condition called hypervitaminosis D.

Cautions and Considerations Taking too much calcium can lead to kidney stones, which are usually caused by crystallization of excess calcium in the urine. Patients with a history of kidney stones should not take calcium supplements.

Calcium supplements should not be taken at the same time as quinolone antibiotics, tetracyclines, or iron supplements. Calcium binds to these other drugs and keeps them from being absorbed. Patients should avoid taking these drugs within two hours of taking a calcium supplement. Calcium has also been found to decrease the effects of verapamil, a medication used to treat hypertension and angina. Patients should speak with their prescribers if they would like to take a calcium supplement while taking verapamil.

Taking too much vitamin D can lead to hypercalcemia and kidney problems. Patients should follow labeling closely to avoid taking more than recommended. Patients with prior kidney problems should talk with their doctors before taking vitamin D.

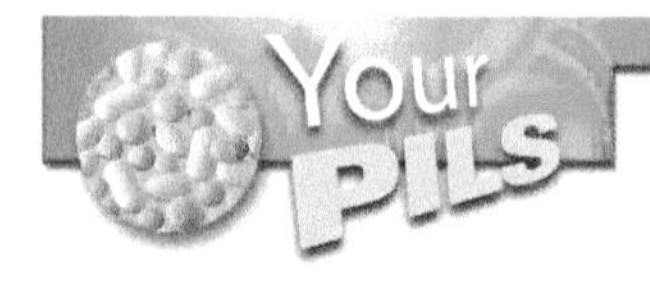

Directors and Enactors who prefer hands-on, real-life learning may find this exercise useful. Pretend you have osteoporosis and go to a pharmacy to shop for calcium supplements. Calculate how much elemental calcium you would absorb from the recommended dose for each product you find. How many tablets would you need to take of each a day to absorb a total of 1,500 mg of calcium?

Bisphosphonates This class of drugs inhibits osteoclasts from removing calcium from bone tissue. **Bisphosphonates** prevent bone breakdown so that stronger bones are maintained. Over time, bone density can be maintained and, hopefully, fractures can be prevented. Bisphosphonates are used primarily for osteoporosis but can treat Paget's disease (another bone-remodeling disorder). Sometimes bisphosphonates are used in bone and spinal injury cases to promote bone regrowth and strengthening. Depending on the product chosen, bisphosphonates can be taken orally once a day, once a week, or once a month. They can even be infused intravenously every month, three months, or annually. This variety of choices creates a great opportunity to individualize treatment for every patient's needs.

Side Effects Common side effects of bisphosphonates include headache, nausea, vomiting, diarrhea, constipation, abdominal pain, and indigestion. Taking oral dosage forms with a full glass of water and remaining upright afterward can decrease some of these effects. Other side effects include insomnia and anemia, for which patients must seek medical advice to manage. A less common yet severe side effect is osteonecrosis (bone tissue death) of the jaw. The IV dosage forms can cause fever, so acetaminophen is given.

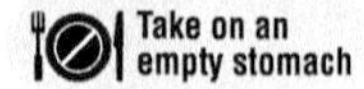

Cautions and Considerations Oral bisphosphonates are poorly absorbed from the GI tract and are adversely affected by food. Therefore, they must be taken on an empty stomach (preferably first thing in the morning) with water. After taking a bisphosphonate,

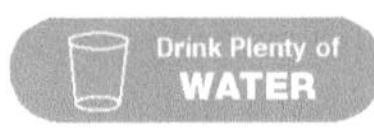

patients should wait at least thirty minutes before eating. Bisphosphonates are highly irritating to the GI tract, so they must be taken with a full glass of water to ensure they are not caught in the esophagus. Patients must remain upright for at least thirty minutes to prevent reflux.

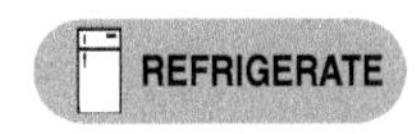

In most cases, bisphosphonate infusions are administered in a physician's office or clinic, so preparation often occurs outside of the pharmacy. If prepared in the pharmacy for later use, infusions should be refrigerated and then used within twenty-four hours. Table 6.2 lists agents for treating osteoporosis and dosing information.

Table 6.2 Osteoporosis Agents

Generic (Brand)	Dosage Form	Route of Administration	Common Dose
Alendronate (Fosamax)	Tablet, oral solution	Oral	5–10 mg a day 70 mg once a week
Calcitonin (Miacalcin)	Nasal spray	Nasal	1 spray per day, alternate nostrils
Etidronate (Didronel)	Tablet	Oral	800 mg a day for 2 weeks in a 15-week cycle
Ibandronate (Boniva)	Tablet, injection	Oral, IV	PO: 2.5 mg a day or 150 mg once a month IV: 3 mg infused every 3 months
Pamidronate (Aredia)	Injection	IV	30 mg infused every 4 weeks
Risedronate (Actonel)	Tablet	Oral	5 mg a day 35 mg once a week 75 mg on 2 consecutive days once a month
Tiludronate (Skelid)	Tablet	Oral	400 mg a day
Zoledronic acid (Reclast)	Injection	IV	5 mg infusion once a year
Selective Estrogen Receptor Modulator (SERM)			
Raloxifene (Evista)	Tablet	Oral	60 mg a day
Tamoxifen (Nolvadex)	Tablet, solution	Oral	10–40 mg a day
Toremifene (Fareston)	Tablet	Oral	60 mg a day

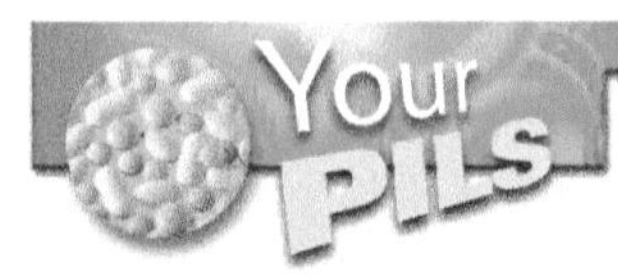

If you are detail-oriented like Producers are, or learn to apply new knowledge from completing homework exercises like Enactors do, make a list of the osteoporosis agents, ranked from longest to shortest dosing interval. Be sure to include both brand and generic names. Although infusions are more invasive, the dosing interval for them is the longest. Think about which patients would benefit from the longer versus the shorter dosing intervals and who would prefer an oral over an injectable route.

Selective Estrogen Receptor Modulator (SERM) Raloxifene (Evista), tamoxifen (Nolvadex), and toremifene (Fareston) are all **SERMs** currently available. SERMs work as estrogen receptors by mimicking the beneficial effects of estrogen on bone mineral density. However, they do not increase the risk of breast or uterine cancer the way regular estrogen can. In fact, they can improve cholesterol, although they are not used for hyperlipidemia.

Common side effects of raloxifene are hot flashes, headache, diarrhea, joint pain, leg cramps, and flulike symptoms. The most serious side effect is deep vein thrombosis or blood clots. Raloxifene should not be taken if prolonged immobility is anticipated. If patients experience pain, swelling, or bruising in one leg or difficulty breathing, they should seek medical care immediately.

Human Parathyroid Hormone Teriparatide (Forteo) supplements the body's production of **parathyroid hormone**, which regulates the calcium–phosphate balance and stimulates new bone growth. It is used in patients with especially severe osteoporosis as a short-term therapy. It has been associated with osteosarcoma, so patients with Paget's disease or others with increased risk for bone cancer should not use teriparatide. Patients must be taught how to use the injector device, and the drug must be kept in the refrigerator.

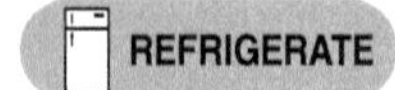

Arthritis

Arthritis is the most common joint disorder, and it affects millions. Drug therapy is used for three main types of arthritis: osteoarthritis, rheumatoid arthritis, and gouty arthritis. **Osteoarthritis (OA)** occurs more frequently than the other types and is caused by the wear and tear on joints that comes with age. In fact, its onset is usually after age forty or fifty. The cartilage that normally coats the ends of bones inside joints erodes, resulting in painful rubbing. The large joints (e.g., the knees, shoulders, and hips) are affected first because the majority of body weight and force is placed on these joints. Fingers and hands can also be affected because they get daily stress throughout life. Symmetry (same joint affected on both sides of the body) is often not present, at least not in the beginning stages of OA. Although morning stiffness is prominent, it fades within an hour and is relieved by activity.

Rheumatoid arthritis (RA) is an entirely different disease from OA. RA involves an abnormal process in which the immune system destroys the synovial membrane and produces inflammation within the joint itself. Small joints, such as those in the fingers, wrists, and elbows, are affected first. Usually symmetry is present. Signs of RA are morning pain and stiffness that last longer than an hour and are not relieved by activity. The resulting deformation of the joints can be disabling. Erythrocyte sedimentation rate (ESR) and rheumatoid factor (RF) are two laboratory tests used to help diagnose RA. This disease is not curable but can be slowed with drug therapy.

Finally, **gouty arthritis** is a condition in which excessive uric acid accumulates in the blood. Next, urate crystals form in the synovial fluid and irritate joints. Usually, joint pain and swelling first occur in the big toe. Other joints may also be affected, especially in the elbows and heels. If the condition is allowed to continue, urate crystals can eventually cause kidney damage. Drugs that predispose someone to gout include diuretics, salicylates, nicotinic acid (niacin), ethanol, and cytotoxic agents such as those used for cancer treatment. Certain foods rich in the amino acid purine, such as red meat, are also implicated in gout. Acute gout attack is treated with drug therapy. Chronic preventive therapy is warranted if a patient has a particularly severe acute attack or more than two to three attacks in one year.

Drugs for OA

Drug therapy for OA reduces pain and inflammation but does not remove the underlying causes. If OA is severe enough, surgery and joint replacement are performed. Nonpharmacologic therapy for arthritis includes physical therapy techniques, such as cold/hot packs and massage. Rest to the affected joint(s) is usually helpful, but prolonged immobility is not recommended because it will worsen arthritis symptoms.

Acetaminophen The drug of choice for OA is **acetaminophen** because it treats pain but does not have as many side effects as do other agents. OA is not an inflammatory condition; instead, it is a structural problem that creates pain and discomfort. Although anti-inflammatory drugs are frequently used for arthritis, they are not necessary. Many patients do not take acetaminophen for arthritis, even though it is considered the drug of choice, because it must be taken multiple times a day to maintain pain control. Arthritis pain can become bad enough that acetaminophen no longer controls it. Acetaminophen is covered in greater detail in Chapter 9.

Nonsteroidal Anti-inflammatory Drugs (NSAIDs) The class of drugs known as **NSAIDs** blocks pain by inhibiting **cyclooxygenase I (COX-1)** and **II (COX-2)**. Cyclooxygenase is an enzyme that converts arachidonic acid to prostaglandins (see Figure 6.4). **Prostaglandins** are produced in response to various stimuli. They promote inflammation and connect to pain receptors to trigger the pain response. NSAIDs are good analgesics when inflammation is the primary cause of pain or acetaminophen no longer works.

In the stomach and intestines, prostaglandins protect against erosion from gastric acid. This beneficial effect is eliminated when NSAIDs block prostaglandin production. Therefore, NSAIDs have a deleterious effect on the GI lining when taken in high doses or over a long time. NSAIDs are used for mild to moderate pain, including arthritis. They also reduce inflammation associated with injury. Some are used to treat dysmenorrhea (painful menstrual cycle) and fever as well. NSAID therapy is kept as short as possible to address immediate needs. In arthritis, however, long-term therapy is needed to control chronic pain. Table 6.3 lists commonly used NSAIDs and dosing information.

Side Effects Common side effects of NSAIDs are headache, diarrhea, nausea, constipation, and occasionally dizziness and drowsiness. These effects are dose-dependent and usually mild. Because NSAIDs block prostaglandins, they are associated with GI side effects, such as indigestion, heartburn, abdominal pain, bleeding, and even ulcer. Taking NSAIDs with food is recommended to avoid this GI irritation. Patients should alert their prescribers and pharmacists to any abdominal pain, heartburn, blood in the stool, or black and tarry stools because these are signs of GI bleeding. If someone taking NSAIDs is losing blood in the GI tract, they can become mildly anemic. Therefore, patients taking NSAIDs on a long-term basis, such as for arthritis, should be monitored by their healthcare providers.

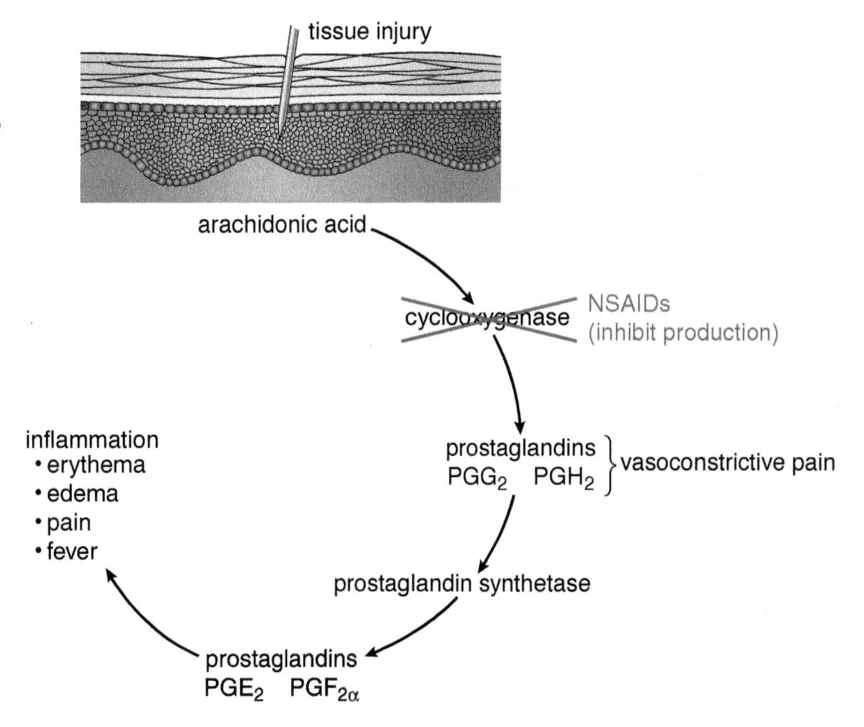

Figure 6.4
Pain Pathway
Prostaglandins also stimulate fever in the central nervous system, so some NSAIDs such as ibuprofen are used as antipyretics or agents that treat fever.

Table 6.3 Commonly Used NSAIDs

Generic (Brand)	Dosage Form	Dispensing Status	Route of Administration	Common Dose
Diclofenac (Voltaren)	Tablet	Rx	Oral	100–200 mg a day
Etodolac (Lodine)	Tablet, capsule	Rx	Oral	600–1,000 mg a day
Ibuprofen (Motrin, Advil)	Tablet, chewable tablet, capsule, oral suspension, oral drops	Rx, OTC	Oral	OTC: 200 mg taken 3 or 4 times a day Rx: 400–800 mg taken 3 or 4 times a day
Indomethacin (Indocin)	Capsule, oral suspension, suppository	Rx	Oral, rectal	150–200 mg a day
Ketoprofen (Orudis)	Capsule	Rx	Oral	200–300 mg a day
Ketorolac (Toradol)	Tablet, injection	Rx	Oral, IM, IV	PO: 10–20 mg every 4–6 hours but not to exceed 40 mg in 24 hours* IM/IV: 30–60 mg every 4–6 hours*
Meloxicam (Mobic)	Tablet, oral suspension	Rx	Oral	7.5–15 mg a day
Nabumetone (Relafen)	Tablet	Rx	Oral	1,000–2,000 mg a day
Naproxen (Aleve, Naprosyn)	Tablet, oral suspension	Rx, OTC	Oral	250–550 mg twice a day
Oxaprozin (Daypro)	Tablet, capsule	Rx	Oral	600–1,200 mg a day
Piroxicam (Feldene)	Capsule	Rx	Oral	20 mg a day
Sulindac (Clinoril)	Tablet	Rx	Oral	150–200 mg a day

*Ketorolac is meant for short-term use only (5 days maximum).

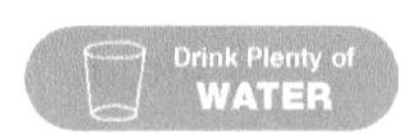

Cautions and Considerations NSAIDs can cause renal (kidney) problems and fluid accumulation, especially if the patient becomes dehydrated. Patients should drink plenty of water and immediately report any edema/swelling or difficulty urinating.

NSAIDs interact with a few other drugs, some of which can add to potential kidney problems. Taking NSAIDs with diuretics or methotrexate can increase the risk of kidney damage. Warfarin (Coumadin) and cyclosporine can interact with NSAIDs as well. The pharmacist can help determine whether a patient should continue taking these drugs with NSAIDs or whether a referral to a healthcare provider is in order.

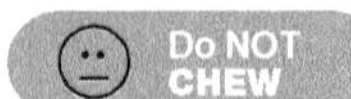

Some tablets such as etodolac are enteric coated or extended-release forms and should not be crushed or chewed. Appropriate warning labels should be used.

Pharmacy technicians should assist patients to avoid duplication of therapy with OTC products such as Advil. Patients should not take aspirin with other NSAIDs because it will decrease their effectiveness by competing for similar sites of action. If an OTC analgesic or antipyretic is needed, patients should use acetaminophen with a prescription NSAID, instead of using aspirin. Document all known, regular OTC drug use in the patient profile to prevent such interactions.

Cyclooxygenase-II (COX-2) Inhibitors Celecoxib (Celebrex) is the only **COX-2 inhibitor** currently available on the market. It works by selectively inhibiting **cyclooxygenase-II (COX-2)**, an enzyme that promotes production of the prostaglandins that cause pain and inflammation but not those that protect the GI lining. NSAIDs and aspirin block both COX-1 and COX-2, which cuts off prostaglandins in the GI lining. Celecoxib is taken for arthritis pain and other pain in patients with a history of ulcers or GI bleeding. It can be taken on a short- or long-term basis.

Side Effects Common side effects of celecoxib are headache, abdominal pain, heartburn, and nausea. Taking it with food can reduce these effects. Occasionally, upper respiratory tract infections can occur. Although COX-2 inhibitors do not ordinarily cause as much GI irritation and bleeding as do NSAIDs or aspirin, they occasionally produce such effects. Patients should report blood in the stool, black tarry stools, and abdominal pain to their healthcare providers because these are signs of GI bleeding and irritation.

Cautions and Considerations Other COX-2 inhibitor agents were removed from the market due to adverse effects involving heart problems and death from cardiac complications. Some patients recall the news coverage of this event and are hesitant to take a COX-2 inhibitor. Celecoxib has not been associated with such effects, but patients should work with their prescribers to monitor heart function.

Drugs for RA

The goal of drug therapy in RA is to maintain mobility and delay disability for as long as possible. Medication cannot cure RA, but it can improve pain symptoms and slow the disease progression that eventually erodes and distorts joints. Some of the drugs used for RA, such as NSAIDs, are used to treat symptoms, whereas other drugs actually modify the course and progression of the disease.

Disease-Modifying Antirheumatic Drugs (DMARDs) In treating RA, **DMARDs** are used to improve functional status by slowing the disease progression. They do this through a variety of mechanisms, depending on the agent chosen. Many work by inhibiting the immune system to slow down the destruction of joint tissue. DMARDs are taken on a chronic basis to maintain disease and symptom control. If one agent does not generate a response, others are tried or combinations of multiple DMARDs are used. They work best when started within the first three months from diagnosis. Disease remission can sometimes be achieved. At a minimum, early therapy slows the joint destruction that creates disability. Azathioprine (Imuran) and cyclosporine (Neoral, Sandimmune) have dual indications—as immunosuppressants after transplant and DMARDs for RA (see Chapter 4). The injectable biological response modifiers, including etanercept, infliximab, adalimumab, and anakinra, are made through recombinant DNA technology and work by inhibiting either interleukin-1 (IL-1) or tumor necrosis factor (TNF), two substances that cause inflammation and joint damage. See Table 6.4 for commonly used DMARDs.

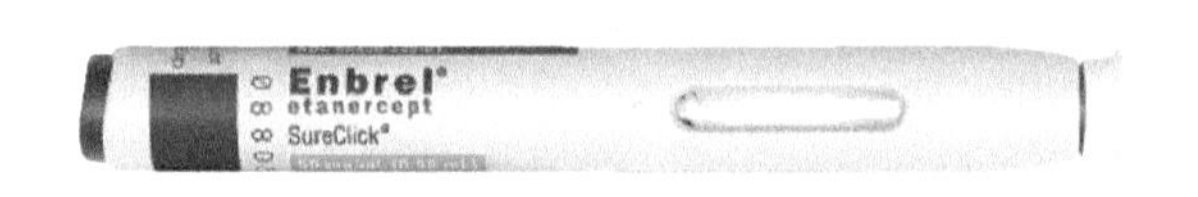

Subcutaneous (SC) injectable DMARDs are more convenient than IM or IV dosage forms, but patients must be trained on how to self-administer them.

Side Effects Side effects for DMARDs vary among agents (see Table 6.4). In many cases, these effects mimic those of chemotherapy and are unpleasant. Quite a few of these effects can have severe consequences and become barriers to treatment. Patients must work closely with their pharmacists and healthcare providers to manage such effects. At times, patients will have to stop one drug and try another simply due to the side effects.

Sometimes these agents (especially auranofin) can cause severe diarrhea, which is treated with antidiarrheal agents. Patients should be instructed to purchase an OTC antidiarrheal product when getting a new prescription for auranofin, so that they are prepared if diarrhea occurs.

Cautions and Considerations Liver, kidney, and blood problems caused by many of the DMARDs can be serious. Laboratory tests should be conducted periodically to gauge these effects.

Because many DMARDs are immunosuppressants, they can increase a patient's risk of getting infections. In fact, increased incidence of infection is common with the biological response modifiers. Patients may be instructed to avoid people who are ill

Table 6.4 Commonly Used DMARDs

Generic (Brand)	Dosage Form	Route of Administration	Usual Dose	Side Effects
Auranofin (Ridaura)	Capsule	Oral	3 mg 1–2 times a day	Diarrhea, nausea, vomiting, abdominal pain, anorexia, indigestion, gas, constipation, itching, rash, hair loss, photosensitivity, blood disorders, kidney and liver damage, lung problems (serious but rare)
Cyclophosphamide (Cytoxan)	Tablet, injection	Oral	1–2 mg/kg a day	Anorexia, nausea, vomiting, hair loss, blood disorders, kidney damage, infertility, fluid imbalance, secondary malignancy (cancer), heart problems, lung problems (serious but rare)
Hydroxychloroquine (Plaquenil)	Tablet	Oral	200–300 mg a day	Nausea, vomiting, abdominal pain, diarrhea, anorexia, headache, dizziness, confusion, seizures, blurred vision or vision changes, allergy, skin rash, muscle weakness/pain, anemia, blood disorders, hearing loss, heart problems
Leflunomide (Arava)	Tablet	Oral	100 mg a day for 3 days, then 10–20 mg a day	Headache, dizziness, diarrhea, abdominal pain, indigestion, weight loss, liver problems, peripheral neuropathy (nerve pain), hair loss, high blood pressure, anemia, blood disorders, lung disease
Methotrexate (Rheumatrex)	Tablet, injection	Oral, IM, IV, SC	7.5–15 mg a week	Mouth sores, nausea, vomiting, abdominal distress, anemia and blood disorders, liver and kidney damage, Stevens-Johnson syndrome, eye irritation, heart problems
Sulfasalazine (Azulfidine)	Tablet	Oral	500 mg twice a day, then increase to 1 g twice a day	Anorexia, diarrhea, abdominal pain, indigestion, headache, nausea/vomiting, colitis, blood disorders, rash, Stevens-Johnson syndrome, liver and kidney problems, hair loss, male infertility
Biological Agents				
Adalimumab (Humira)	Injection	SC	40 mg every 2 weeks	Headache, nausea, vomiting, flulike symptoms, rash, itching, heart problems, anemia and blood disorders, secondary malignancy, nephrotic syndrome, confusion, tremor, reactivation of hepatitis B
Anakinra (Kineret)	Injection	SC	100 mg a day	Headache, nausea, vomiting, diarrhea, redness and pain at injection site, flulike symptoms, blood disorders
Certolizumab (Cimzia)	Injection	SC	400 mg every 2-4 weeks	Headache, runny nose, upper respiratory tract and urinary tract infections, rash, heart failure, high blood pressure, back pain
Etanercept (Enbrel)	Injection	SC	25 mg twice a week or 50 mg every 7 days	Pain, itching, and swelling at injection site; headache; nausea; vomiting; hair loss; cough; dizziness; abdominal pain; rash; indigestion; swelling; mouth sores; blood disorders; secondary lymphoma; Stevens-Johnson syndrome; seizures; heart problems; pancreatitis; difficulty breathing
Infliximab (Remicade)	Injection	IV	3 mg/kg at 0, 2, and 6 weeks, then every 8 weeks	Nausea, vomiting, headache, diarrhea, abdominal pain, cough, indigestion, fatigue, back pain, fever/chills, chest pain, flushing, dizziness, heart failure, nerve problems, seizures, Stevens-Johnson syndrome
Golimumab (Simponi)	Injection	SC	50 mg once a month	Upper respiratory tract infections, runny nose, fever/chills, dizziness, redness at injection site

and follow special precautions to prevent infection. An individual's tuberculosis status should be ascertained prior to the use of immunosuppressant therapy. When infection and illness occur, patients on these drugs should seek medical attention.

Some of the DMARDs, such as sulfasalazine, are enteric coated and should not be crushed or chewed. An appropriate auxiliary warning label should be applied.

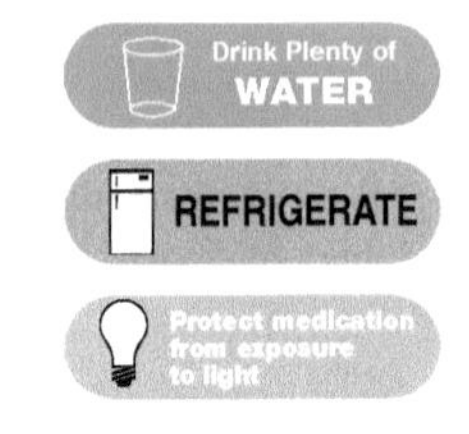

Many of the DMARDs can cause kidney damage. Patients are instructed to drink plenty of water to counteract this effect. An auxiliary label about drinking fluids is suggested for those agents that have side effects related to kidney problems or damage.

Some DMARDs have special instructions for mixing and storage. For example, leflunomide tablets must be protected from light to preserve their potency. The injectable forms of DMARDs must be refrigerated.

Drugs for Gouty Arthritis

Treatment during an **acute gout attack** differs from **chronic gout prophylaxis** (see Table 6.5). If a patient has a particularly severe attack or repeated gout exacerbations within a year, chronic low-dose therapy will be used to prevent future attacks. Medications for gout work by lowering uric acid levels in the bloodstream and reducing inflammation within the joints, which is caused by urate crystal formation.

Colchicine is the drug of choice used to lower uric acid levels in both acute and chronic attacks, and it is also used in preventive therapy at a lower dose. Triamcinolone injection is a corticosteroid administered directly into the joint to relieve pain and swelling. Treatment for acute attacks typically lasts for a few days to a week or two. Indomethacin, an NSAID mentioned previously in this chapter, and prednisone (see Chapter 4) are used frequently in combination with these agents to reduce the pain and inflammation of a gout attack. **Allopurinol** is the most frequently prescribed drug for gout prophylaxis and is usually one of the top 200 drugs dispensed in pharmacies.

Side Effects Common side effects for gout drugs are listed in Table 6.5. If a patient experiences diarrhea when taking colchicine, he or she should stop taking it and contact a doctor about alternative therapy. For an acute attack, colchicine may be given until the patient has diarrhea, and then stopped.

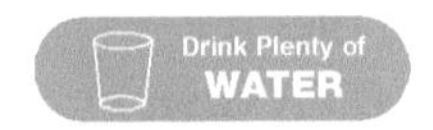

Cautions and Considerations When taking probenecid, patients should take care to drink plenty of water because this drug can be harmful to the kidneys. An appropriate auxiliary warning label should be used. Patients should also avoid taking aspirin with this agent because aspirin can decrease probenecid's effectiveness.

Table 6.5 Gout Agents

Generic (Brand)	Dosage Form	Route of Administration	Usual Dose	Side Effects
Acute Treatment				
Colchicine	Tablet	Oral	0.6–1.2 mg initially then 0.6 mg every hour or 1.2 mg every 2 hours (8 mg max)	Diarrhea, nausea, vomiting
Triamcinolone (Aristospan)	Injection	Intra-articular	20–40 mg injected into joint	Rash, fluid retention, allergic reaction, pain, redness, swelling in joint where injected
Preventive (Prophylactic) Treatment				
Allopurinol	Tablet	Oral	200–600 mg a day	Skin rash, nausea, diarrhea
Colchicine	Tablet	Oral	0.6 mg twice a day	Diarrhea, nausea, vomiting, blood disorders
Febuxostat (Uloric)	Tablet	Oral	80–120 mg a day	Diarrhea, headache, angioedema
Probenecid	Tablet	Oral	250 mg BID for 1 week, then 600 mg BID for 2 weeks, increase 500 mg/day every other week until 3,000 mg/day	Nausea, vomiting, anorexia

Herbal and Alternative Therapies

Glucosamine is used by some to improve pain and stiffness from OA. However, studies do not necessarily support the effectiveness of glucosamine for OA. It is derived from the exoskeleton of shellfish and is thought to slow joint degeneration. If patients want to take glucosamine, typical dosing is 1,500 mg a day, in divided doses. Side effects are usually mild and include nausea, heartburn, diarrhea, and constipation. Taking glucosamine with food can decrease these effects. Although glucosamine has not proven to be harmful in studies, it is recommended that patients with shellfish allergies avoid taking it.

Chondroitin is taken by some in combination with glucosamine for hip and knee OA. However, studies do not clearly show that chondroitin taken with glucosamine is effective for OA. Chondroitin is derived from shark cartilage and bovine (cow) sources and is thought to work by inhibiting an enzyme that promotes inflammation. If patients want to take chondroitin, typical dosing is 200–400 mg twice or three times a day. Common side effects tend to be mild and include nausea, heartburn, diarrhea, and constipation. Rare side effects include eyelid swelling, lower limb swelling, hair loss, and allergic reaction. If patients experience any of these effects, they should stop taking chondroitin.

Chapter Summary

Bones support the body frame and maintain calcium balance. Bone density builds early in life but drops off with increasing age. Osteoporosis occurs when bone density drops lower than the average level. Several drugs are now available to treat and prevent osteoporosis and the bone fractures it causes. The most frequently used medications for osteoporosis are bisphosphonates and selective estrogen receptor modulators (SERMs). A variety of dosage forms is available, from monthly oral therapy to annual infusions. Consequently, patients have many choices. Patients with osteoporosis should also take calcium and vitamin D to promote bone strength.

Osteoarthritis (OA) is common and is caused by age and joint stress over time. Although acetaminophen is considered the first-line choice of therapy for OA, many patients progress to needing nonsteroidal anti-inflammatory drugs (NSAIDs) on a long-term basis to control pain symptoms. Glucosamine and chondroitin are two natural products also used for OA.

Rheumatoid arthritis is an abnormal immune process in which joint tissue is inflamed and damaged. The pain and resulting joint deformation can be disabling to patients. Disease-modifying antirheumatic drugs (DMARDs), in addition to NSAIDs for analgesia, are used to halt the destructive immune process and improve function. These drugs have many side effects and are difficult for patients to take but can keep patients from becoming disabled.

Gout is a joint disorder resembling arthritis, in which uric acid accumulates in the bloodstream, causing urate crystals to form in joint spaces. Drugs such as colchicine and allopurinol are used to treat this condition.

Chapter Review

For the following sets of exercises, write the exercise heading, exercise numbers, and your answers on a separate sheet of paper. Your instructor may direct you to turn in the sheet of paper or discuss your answers as a class.

REVIEW THE BASICS

Choose a, b, c, or d as the correct answer to each multiple-choice question.

1. Which of the following is responsible for the formation/building of new bone?
   a. cartilage
   b. osteoblasts
   c. osteoclasts
   d. marrow
2. Which of the following is a risk factor for developing osteoporosis?
   a. female gender
   b. small frame
   c. smoking
   d. all of the above
3. Some pharmacies screen for osteoporosis with a bone mineral density test on what part of the body?
   a. elbow
   b. heel
   c. hip
   d. spine
4. Which of the following drugs is used for osteoporosis?
   a. etanercept
   b. indomethacin
   c. meloxicam
   d. risedronate
5. Which of the following drugs is a selective estrogen receptor modulator?
   a. Fosamax
   b. Evista
   c. Forteo
   d. Relafen
6. Which of the following is an abnormal immune process that breaks down joint tissue and results in joint deformation?
   a. osteoporosis
   b. osteoarthritis
   c. rheumatoid arthritis
   d. gout
7. NSAIDs block which of the following substances in the pain pathway in order to reduce pain and inflammation?
   a. arachidonic acid
   b. cyclooxygenase
   c. prostaglandins
   d. rheumatoid factor
8. Which of the following drugs is used to slow disease progression in rheumatoid arthritis?
   a. diclofenac
   b. colchicine
   c. methotrexate
   d. all of the above
9. What is the most frequently used drug for chronic prevention of gout?
   a. colchicine
   b. probenecid
   c. indomethacin
   d. allopurinol
10. Which of the following is derived from shark cartilage and is used for osteoarthritis?
    a. glucosamine
    b. colchicine
    c. chondroitin
    d. calcium

KNOW THE DRUGS

Match each brand name drug with its corresponding generic name and most common use. Your answers should follow this example format: Generic Name: 1. a; 2. b; 3. c; etc. Most Common Use: 1. h; 2. i; 3. j; etc.

Brand Name	Generic Name	Most Common Use
1. Voltaren	a. infliximab	h. osteoporosis
2. Boniva	b. ketoprofen	i. osteoarthritis
3. Remicade	c. sulindac	j. rheumatoid arthritis
4. Arava	d. ibandronate	k. gout
5. Orudis	e. leflunomide	
6. Clinoril	f. raloxifene	
7. Evista	g. diclofenac	

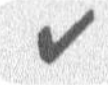

PUT IT TOGETHER

For each item, write down either a short answer or a single term to complete the sentence.

1. List an important auxiliary warning label you should put on a prescription for Voltaren.
2. Which of the following drugs or drug classes interacts with NSAIDs?

diuretics	tiludronate
etidronate	chondroitin
methotrexate	warfarin
naproxen	cyclosporine

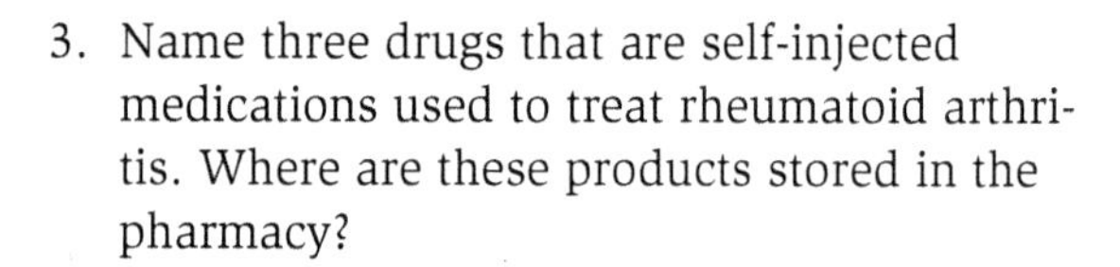

3. Name three drugs that are self-injected medications used to treat rheumatoid arthritis. Where are these products stored in the pharmacy?
4. ________________ is the drug of choice for acute gout attack, and ________________ is the drug of choice for chronic gout prevention.
5. ________________ is an NSAID that should be used for a maximum of five days only.

THINK IT THROUGH

Read and think through each numbered scenario carefully and then write several sentences in reply to the question(s) presented. Question 4 requires you to do some Internet research before completing your answer(s).

1. If a patient did not have insurance to cover a prescription for 400 mg Motrin, what could be done to save the patient some money and still allow him or her to get this medication? How should this situation be handled with the patient?
2. An eighty-year-old woman comes to the pharmacy to pick up a new prescription for Nexium (a drug used to reduce gastric acid production in treating and preventing ulcers) and asks to refill her Relafen while she is here. When you look up the refill in her computer profile, you notice she also takes Fosamax. She is discouraged because now her doctor thinks she is developing an ulcer, and she states she just got over the pain of a vertebral fracture in her back. What could be going on here? What might you alert the pharmacist to when filling this prescription?
3. A woman finds you in the OTC aisle and tells you that her nurse practitioner told her to take a calcium supplement. She asks you which one she should get to obtain the total daily dose of 1,000 mg. What will you recommend?

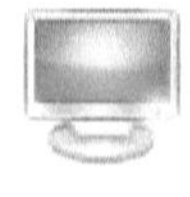

4. **On the Internet,** go to the ".org" Web site for the Arthritis Foundation and review the patient and healthcare provider information on managing arthritis. Note the different types of arthritis covered and the information about self-management tools and techniques. Think about how this organization and its site could be a resource to which your pharmacy can refer patients. What information presented here would you find most useful as a patient yourself?

unit 4

Drugs for the Nervous, Muscular, and Sensory Systems

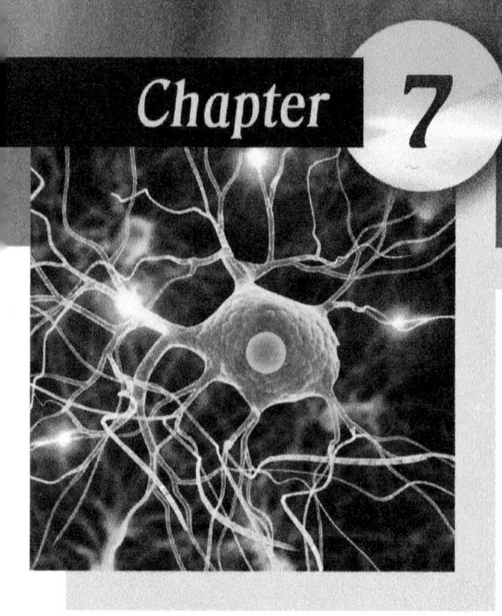

Chapter 7 The Nervous System and Drug Therapy

LEARNING OBJECTIVES

- Describe the basic anatomy and physiology of the nervous system.
- Explain the therapeutic effects of prescription medications, nonprescription medications, and alternative therapies commonly used to treat diseases of the nervous system.
- Describe the adverse effects of prescription medications, nonprescription medications, and alternative therapies used to treat diseases of the nervous system.
- Identify the brand and generic names of prescription and nonprescription medications commonly used to treat diseases of the nervous system.
- State the doses, dosage forms, and routes of administration for prescription and nonprescription medications commonly used to treat diseases of the nervous system.

Interactive self-quizzes, games, audio files, and glossaries help you to learn drug names and facts.

After an overview of the anatomy and physiology of the nervous system, common conditions affecting the central and autonomic nervous systems are discussed. Nervous system conditions such as Parkinson's disease, Alzheimer's disease, and attention-deficit hyperactivity disorder (ADHD) are well known and dramatically portrayed in the media. Parkinson's disease is not curable, but various choices for drug therapy can mean the difference between being active and being bedridden. Alzheimer's disease is increasingly encountered as the U.S. population ages. Unfortunately, few drugs effectively treat it. ADHD, on the other hand, has several drug treatments. Pharmacists and technicians work daily with the stimulants used to treat ADHD. You have a unique role in assisting parents of children with ADHD in understanding these medications. Be aware that most of these agents are controlled substances and require special handling and procedures.

Few disorders of the autonomic nervous system exist, but drug therapy is frequently used to affect this system, which controls heart rate, blood pressure, breathing, pupil dilation, and digestion. These agents are important to know because they are used to treat common conditions such as high blood pressure and glaucoma and because many of them cause anticholinergic side effects. Therefore, you should understand drug activity on the autonomic nervous system because you will encounter such medications regularly.

Anatomy and Physiology of the Nervous System

The **nervous system** senses and interprets our surroundings and controls vital bodily functions (see Figure 7.1). The nervous system is divided into the central and peripheral systems and the somatic and autonomic systems. The **central nervous system (CNS)**, including the brain and spinal cord, is responsible for processing information received from the body. The **peripheral nervous system**, made up of all nerves outside the brain and spinal cord, is responsible for bringing signals to the CNS for interpretation. Signals from the brain are then conducted back through the peripheral system to direct movement and other responses. The **somatic nervous system** controls intentional, voluntary movement. The **autonomic nervous system** controls involuntary and automatic body functions, such as heart rate, respiration, and digestion. The autonomic system is further divided into the **sympathetic nervous system** (which uses adrenergic receptors and some cholinergic receptors) and the **parasympathetic nervous system** (which uses cholinergic receptors only).

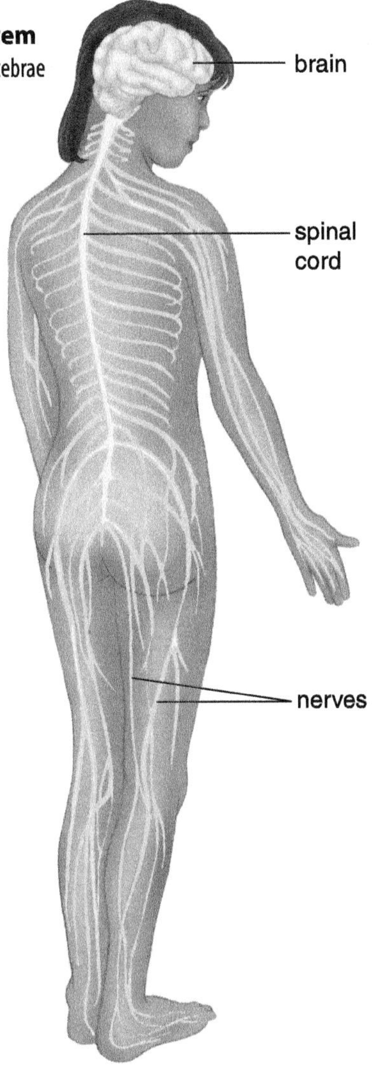

Figure 7.1
Anatomy of the Nervous System
Pinched nerves from dislocated spinal vertebrae and the disks between them can cause significant pain.

The brain is divided into sections, and each section is responsible for different functions. The **cerebrum**, including the **cerebral cortex**, performs higher cognitive functions, such as thinking and memory (see Figure 7.2). The **cerebellum** coordinates movement and balance. The **pons** and **medulla** in the **brain stem** regulate automatic and reflex functions of the body. In the middle of the brain are the **thalamus** and **hypothalamus**, which control various functions, including hormone regulation and body temperature. The neighboring **pituitary gland** also helps regulate hormones and controls the growth cycle throughout life (see Chapter 18).

The cell structure along the border of the CNS is different from elsewhere in the body. Oxygen, carbon dioxide, small molecules (e.g., glucose), and small lipid-soluble drugs pass easily from the blood to CNS tissue, but larger water-soluble molecules, including drugs and most pathogens, do not easily enter the brain or spinal cord. The **blood-brain barrier (BBB)** protects this delicate tissue from potentially harmful chemicals. It must be overcome, however, when drug therapy should enter the CNS to exert its action.

Neurotransmitters are chemicals that carry signals from one nerve cell to the next (see Table 7.1). These chemicals are released from the end of one nerve, cross the **synaptic space** between nerve cells, and connect to receptors on the adjoining cell so that the signal is passed (see Figure 7.3).

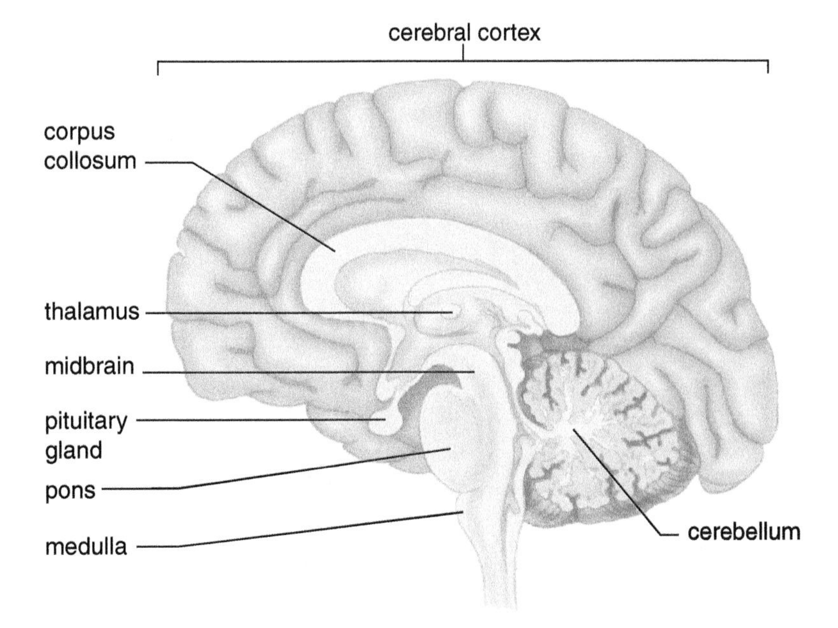

Figure 7.2
Anatomy of the Brain
The cerebrum and cerebral cortex contain tissue called white and gray matter.

Table 7.1 Neurotransmitters and Their Actions

Neurotransmitter	Action
Acetylcholine (ACh)	Used in the parasympathetic nervous system. Acts on receptors in smooth muscle to control blood pressure and digestion, in cardiac muscle to control heart rate, and in exocrine glands.
Dopamine (DA)	Used primarily in the CNS to control mood and coordinated movement.
Epinephrine	Used in the sympathetic nervous system. Acts on receptors to regulate cardiac function and bronchodilation. Also called adrenaline.
GABA (gamma-aminobutyric acid)	Used in the brain to regulate signal delivery.
Norepinephrine	Used in the CNS and the sympathetic nervous system. In the brain, involved in mood and emotions. In the periphery, acts on receptors to control blood pressure, cardiac function, and digestion.
Serotonin (5-HT)	Used in the peripheral nervous system and the CNS. In the periphery, acts on receptors in smooth muscle (blood vessels and the lining of the gastrointestinal tract). In the brain, involved in mood and emotions.

Altered production, release, or metabolic breakdown of neurotransmitters appears to be at the core of many nervous system conditions. Deficiencies in certain neurotransmitters are assumed to underlie mood disorders (e.g., depression) or psychiatric problems (e.g., schizophrenia or bipolar disorder) (see Chapter 8). In fact, most drugs for these conditions supplement, mimic, or block the actions of specific neurotransmitters.

Individual nerve cells consist of a cell body, where the nucleus resides, and other cell parts. **Dendrites** bring signals into the cell body. **Axons** carry signals away from the nucleus to neighboring cells. **Schwann cells** in the peripheral nervous system and oligodendrocytes in the CNS form a **myelin sheath** that surrounds and protects axons. Without this sheath, signal conduction from cell to cell is not well coordinated and becomes sporadic. Sporadic nerve conduction makes coordinated muscle movement, including walking and talking, difficult. Destruction of this myelin sheath occurs in diseases such as multiple sclerosis.

Figure 7.3
Neurotransmission
Nerve signals are carried from cell to cell by neurotransmitters.

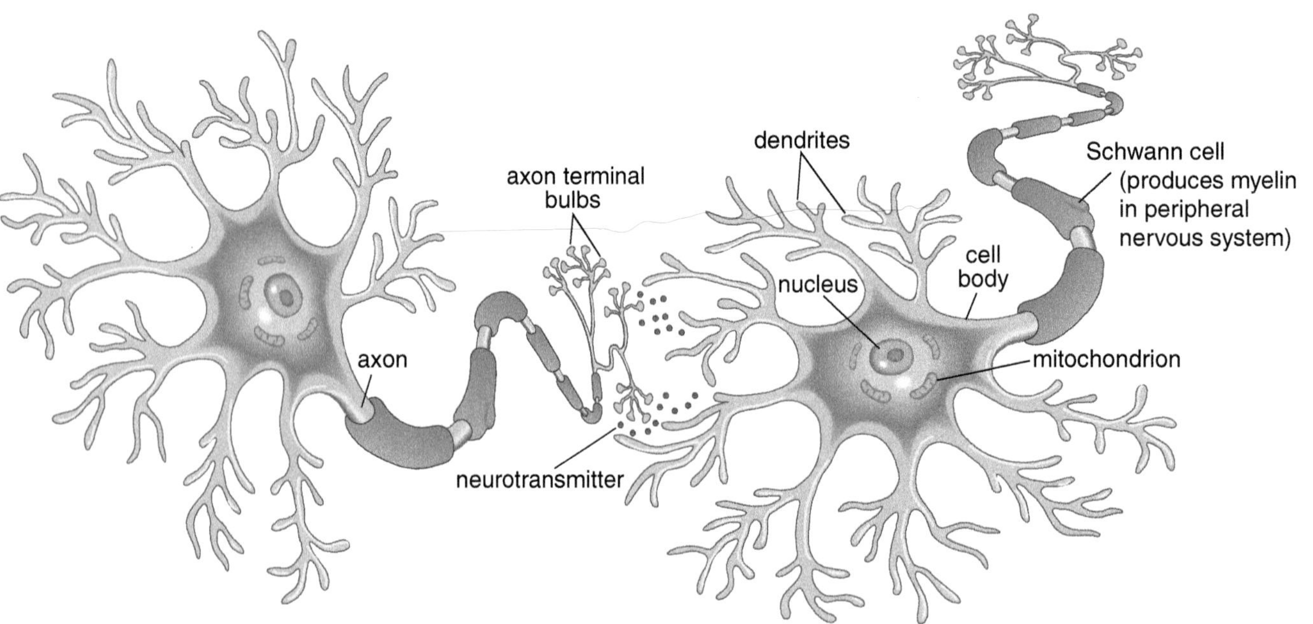

Autonomic Nervous System

Autonomic nerves (located close to the spinal column) regulate functions of the body that we do not consciously control. This system is responsible for a set of responses to stressful stimuli, which are collectively called the **"fight or flight" response** (see Figure 7.4). **Sympathetic nerves** regulate this response. For example, when confronted with a scary or surprising situation, the body's response is to increase the heart and respiration rates, and dilate the pupils in anticipation of the need to physically fight or flee immediately. Blood pressure also rises to increase circulation for a burst of physical activity. We do not think about or choose these reactions; they simply happen automatically. Sympathetic nerves release **norepinephrine** as part of the "fight or flight" response. (The one exception occurs at the sweat glands, where acetylcholine is the neurotransmitter). The adrenal medulla, another element in the autonomic nervous system, releases epinephrine into the circulation. Epinephrine is often referred to as adrenaline, and hence the term **adrenergic**.

The **parasympathetic nerves** regulate restful body functions. When you are relaxed or resting, your heart rate and breathing slow, digestion occurs, and the bladder and rectum are able to relax and release their contents. These functions are not desired during a frightening situation. Parasympathetic nerves are called **cholinergic** because of their type of receptor, and their primary neurotransmitter is **acetylcholine (ACh).** In a general sense, sympathetic and parasympathetic stimulation have opposite effects on body functions (see Figure 7.4).

Two subsets of adrenergic receptors include alpha receptors and beta receptors. Both are activated by norepinephrine and epinephrine in the sympathetic part of the autonomic

Figure 7.4
Autonomic Nervous System Anatomy and Effects
The autonomic nervous system regulates sweating (among other responses), which is decreased with parasympathetic activity and increased with sympathetic activity.

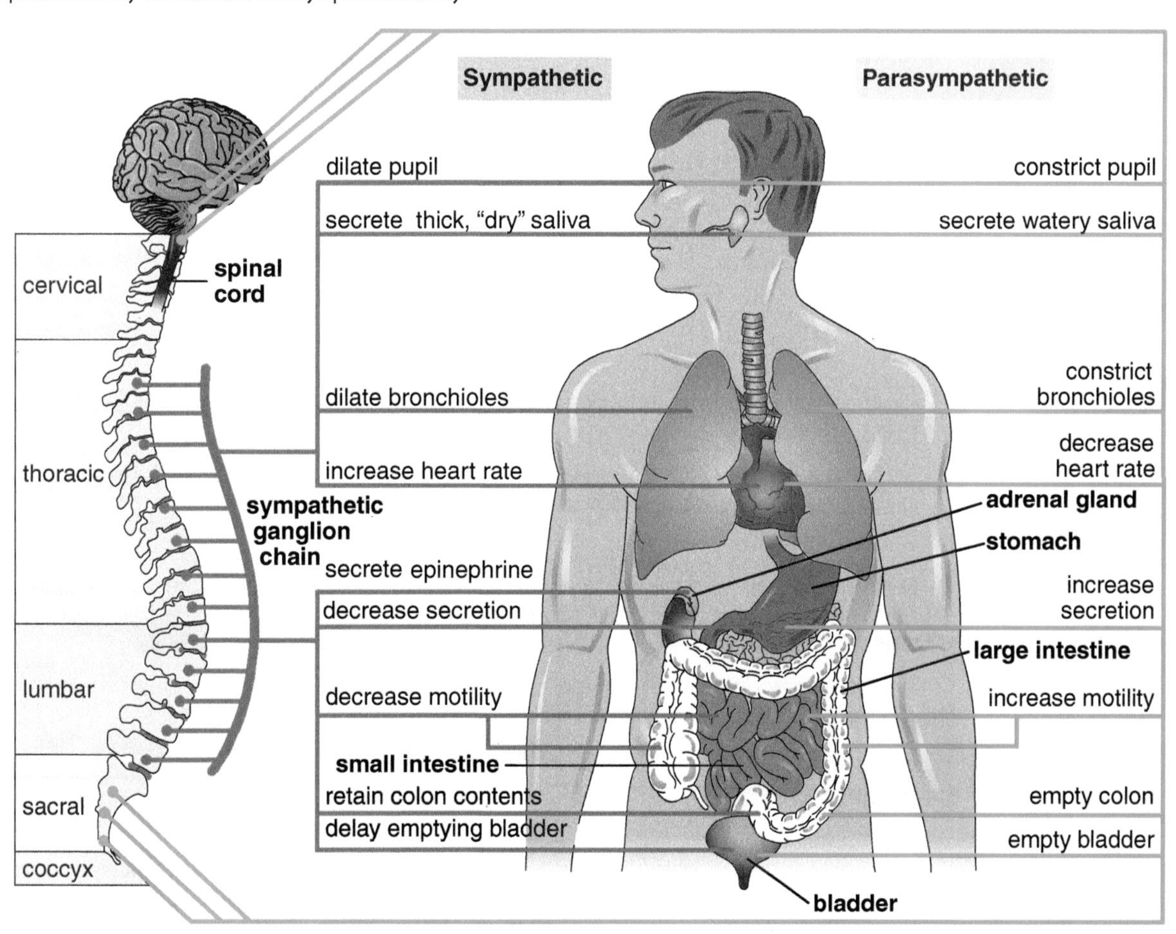

nervous system. **Alpha receptors** are found in the blood vessels. When stimulated, they constrict blood vessels, raising blood pressure. When they are blocked by drugs, blood pressure lowers. Consequently, alpha receptor blockers are used to treat hypertension.

Beta receptors are divided into two types: beta-one receptors and beta-two receptors. **Beta-one receptors** are found mostly within the heart. When stimulated, they increase heart rate and contraction force. **Beta-two receptors** are found in the smooth muscle of arteries and bronchioles in the lungs and also in other tissues. When stimulated, these receptors cause blood vessels and bronchioles to dilate. When beta receptors are blocked with drug therapy, heart rate slows and the demand for oxygen within the heart decreases. Beta-blocking medications decrease contractility in the heart, thus lowering blood pressure.

Sometimes, the goal of drug therapy is to stimulate both alpha and beta receptors. During cardiac arrest, severe shock, or anaphylactic reactions, it is necessary to increase heart rate, raise blood pressure, or dilate airways. Adrenergic agonist agents are used to exert these effects in urgent situations.

Seizure Disorders

Seizures (convulsions) are uncoordinated bursts of neuronal activity that result in brain dysfunction. Depending on the extent of the seizure and the area of the brain affected, symptoms can be as mild as staring or twitching to as severe as a total loss of consciousness and whole-body convulsions. **Epilepsy** is a chronic seizure disorder that causes a variety of different types of seizures (see Table 7.2). All patients with epilepsy have seizures, but not all patients with seizures have epilepsy. Although only 1 to 2% of U.S. residents have epilepsy, almost one in ten individuals will have a single unprovoked seizure within his or her lifetime. Common causes for seizure include:

- alcohol or drug withdrawal
- high fever
- stroke
- electric shock
- hypoglycemia or hyperglycemia (low or high blood sugar)
- hyponatremia (low sodium in the blood)
- hypocalcemia (low calcium in the blood)
- infection (meningitis)
- brain tumors or scar tissue
- head injury or trauma

Table 7.2 Types of Seizures

Partial	
Simple	Localized area of the body is affected in movement. May result in twitching, tightness, or contortion of specific body parts. No loss of consciousness.
Complex	Localized area of the body is affected in movement. May result in twitching, tightness, or contortion of specific body parts. Impaired consciousness may occur, but not complete loss.
Generalized	
Absence (petit mal)	Begins with interruption of normal activity, such as blank stare, rolling or blinking eyes, uncontrolled facial movements, or arm/leg jerking. No whole-body convulsions occur. Attacks are short (≈30 seconds) but occur frequently, usually multiple times a day. Common in children with epilepsy and can progress to tonic-clonic seizures later in life.
Tonic-clonic (grand mal)	Tonic phase happens first: the body goes rigid, and the patient usually falls down. Clonic phase happens next: whole body convulsions occur and may be accompanied by altered breathing rhythm, loss of bladder control, and excessive salivation.
Atonic	Sudden loss of muscle tone and consciousness. Appears as if the patient has fainted.
Myoclonic	Sudden massive muscle jerks, which may throw the patient down or wake him or her from sleeping. Consciousness is often not lost.
Status epilepticus	Continuous tonic-clonic convulsions with or without loss of consciousness for at least 30 minutes. Usually characterized by high fever and a lack of oxygen severe enough to cause brain damage or death. This type of seizure is a medical emergency because 10% of patients die regardless of treatment.

Sometimes, drug therapy can reduce the seizure threshold in the brain. If drug therapy is combined with one of the other causes listed above, a seizure can more easily occur.

The most common type of seizure is a **partial seizure,** in which a localized area of the brain is affected. The patient usually does not lose consciousness. Instead, a defined area of the body is affected. A partial seizure may manifest as twitching or muscle tightness in a specific area of the body; some patients may, at the same time, experience visual disturbances or hallucinations. Even so, a patient can usually communicate during a partial seizure. **Generalized seizures** do not occur as often but tend to be the type of seizure that is dramatized in movies and other media. During a generalized seizure, loss of consciousness usually occurs. Afterward, the patient experiences a period of memory loss, confusion, and tiredness that may last for a few minutes or up to a few hours.

Antiepileptic Drugs (AEDs)

Drugs used to treat seizure disorders are called **anticonvulsants**. They vary in their mechanisms of action and can work via multiple mechanisms at once. Therefore, they can be difficult to categorize into specific classes and are covered together as one group in this chapter. Collectively, **AEDs** affect the influx of sodium, calcium, or chloride ions across the nerve cell membrane in some way. This effect slows the transmission of erratic nerve impulses because membranes are less excitable. **Glutamate** is an excitatory neurotransmitter that affects sodium and calcium influx; **GABA** is an inhibitory neurotransmitter that affects chloride influx. Some anticonvulsants work directly on ion channels, whereas others inhibit glutamate or enhance GABA. Some AEDs work in multiple ways. For instance, topiramate blocks sodium channels, inhibits glutamate, and enhances GABA, all at the same time.

Drug therapy regimens for seizures must be individualized for each patient. Monotherapy with one drug is tried first, and other agents may be added to control seizure activity. It can take up to a month of treatment to see the full benefit from these drugs.

Treatment for **status epilepticus**, an emergency situation, includes one of two benzodiazepines (diazepam or lorazepam, see Chapter 8) plus phenytoin or fosphenytoin. Phenobarbital may also be used. This drug combination may be stored in crash cart kits, which pharmacy technicians often maintain.

Several AEDs have other uses (see Table 7.3). Gabapentin is frequently used to treat nerve pain related to diabetic neuropathy, nerve injury (such as back and spinal cord injuries), and shingles. The dosing range varies widely for these various conditions and must be individualized for each patient.

Side Effects Many side effects of AEDs (as listed in Table 7.3) are dose-dependent, so blood levels are monitored for highest (peak) and lowest (trough) concentrations. Dosing AEDs is highly individualized. Phenytoin, valproate, and carbamazepine undergo what is called zero-order pharmacokinetics: a patient's metabolism becomes saturated with the drug to a point after which even slight dose increases result in dramatic increases in blood concentrations. Severe toxicity and side effects necessitate close monitoring of drug concentrations with blood tests.

May Cause DROWSINESS
Use Caution while Driving

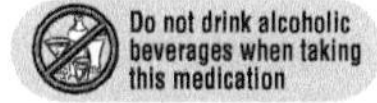

Many AEDs cause drowsiness, dizziness, and mental confusion to varying extents. These effects improve with time, but when patients first start taking one of these medications, they should be careful when driving or making important decisions. An auxiliary label warning of sedation should be used on most of the AEDs. Patients should also avoid drinking alcohol when taking these drugs, because alcohol creates additive effects when mixed with AEDs.

Many patients are concerned about the dulling effect these medications can have on their ability to think. This effect is a common reason for discontinuing treatment with an AED. This issue is especially sensitive for children in school trying to learn and keep up with classmates.

Several AEDs can cause rare but serious side effects such as Stevens-Johnson syndrome (a severe and sometimes fatal rash) and blood abnormalities. Patients should

Table 7.3 Commonly Used AEDs

Generic (Brand)	Dosage Form	Route of Administration	Common Dose	Side Effects
Sodium Channel Blockers				
Carbamazepine (Tegretol)	Tablet, capsule, suspension	Oral	Tonic-clonic, partial seizure (No effect on absence)	Dizziness, drowsiness, nausea, unsteadiness, vomiting, abnormal vision, hyponatremia, hepatotoxicity, arrhythmias, increased suicide risk
Fosphenytoin (Cerebyx)	Injection	IM, IV	Status epilepticus (Short-term use until phenytoin can be given)	Dizziness, itching, numbness, headache, tiredness, decreased movement, hypotension, cardiovascular collapse (rare but serious)
Oxcarbazepine (Trileptal)	Tablet, suspension	Oral	Partial seizure (Alternative uses: bipolar disorder, diabetic neuropathy, neuralgia)	Abdominal pain, headache, trouble walking, abnormal or double vision, difficulty moving, dizziness, fatigue, nausea, tremors, vomiting, hyponatremia
Phenytoin (Dilantin)	Tablet, capsule, suspension, injection	Oral, IV	Tonic-clonic, partial seizure, status epilepticus	Decreased coordination/movement, mental confusion, slurred speech, dizziness, headache, insomnia, twitches, nervousness, hepatotoxicity, gingival hyperplasia, hair growth
Calcium Channel Blockers				
Ethosuximide (Zarontin)	Capsule, syrup	Oral	Absence seizure	Drowsiness, headache, dizziness, hiccups, aggression, fatigue, difficulty moving, loss of appetite, stomach upset, diarrhea, nightmares
Valproate (Depakote)	Tablet, capsule, syrup, injection	Oral, IV	Partial and absence seizure, tonic-clonic (Alternative use: bipolar disorder)	Dizziness, headache, nausea, vomiting, tremor, diarrhea, tiredness, weight gain, hair loss, hepatotoxicity
Valproic acid (Depakene)	Tablet, capsule, syrup, injection	Oral, IV	Partial and absence seizure	Dizziness, headache, nausea, vomiting, tremor, diarrhea, tiredness, hair loss, hepatotoxicity
Zonisamide (Zonegran)	Capsule	Oral	Partial seizure (Alternative uses: binge eating disorder, obesity)	Tiredness, dizziness, loss of appetite, headache, nausea, irritability, difficulty thinking, sulfa allergy, kidney stones
GABA Enhancers				
Gabapentin (Neurontin)	Tablet, capsule, oral solution	Oral	Partial seizure (Alternative uses: diabetic neuropathy, neuralgia, shingles, fibromyalgia, hot flashes, hiccups, restless legs syndrome, others)	Dizziness, drowsiness, tiredness, nausea, vomiting, diarrhea, dry mouth, swelling in legs/arms, abnormal thinking, difficulty moving, weight gain
Mephobarbital (Mebaral)	Tablet	Oral	Tonic-clonic, absence seizure	Tiredness, drowsiness, hepatotoxicity, aggression or mood changes, hypotension
Phenobarbital (Barbital)	Tablet, capsule, elixir, injection	Oral, IV	Tonic-clonic, status epilepticus (Alternative uses: sedative for anxiety and insomnia)	Tiredness, drowsiness, hepatotoxicity, aggression or mood changes, hypotension
Primidone (Mysoline)	Tablet	Oral	Tonic-clonic seizure (Alternative use: tremor)	Difficulty moving, dizziness, nausea, loss of appetite, vomiting, fatigue, mood changes, impotence, double vision
Glutamate Inhibitors				
Felbamate (Felbatol)	Tablet, suspension	Oral	Tonic-clonic, partial seizure	Insomnia, loss of appetite, weight loss, nausea, vomiting, headache, dizziness, tiredness, acne, rash, constipation, diarrhea
Lamotrigine (Lamictal)	Tablet	Oral	Tonic-clonic, partial seizure (Alternative use: bipolar disorder)	Rash, decreased coordination/movement, dizziness, headache, insomnia, tiredness, rash, nausea, vomiting, blurred or double vision
Tiagabine (Gabitril)	Tablet	Oral	Partial seizure (Alternative use: bipolar disorder)	Dizziness, tiredness, nausea, nervousness, tremor, abdominal pain, abnormal thinking, depression
Topiramate (Topamax)	Tablet, capsule	Oral	Tonic-clonic, partial seizure (Alternative use: migraine)	Dizziness, numbness, memory problems, depression, kidney stones, insomnia, nausea, tiredness, appetite loss, weight loss
Unknown Mechanism				
Levetiracetam (Keppra)	Tablet, oral solution, injection	Oral, IV	Partial seizure	Dizziness, tiredness, lack of energy, depression, behavior changes and/or psychosis

be advised to alert their prescribers if any type of rash appears. Blood tests are taken periodically to check for abnormalities in blood cells.

Phenytoin can cause gingival hyperplasia, which is overgrowth of gum tissue in the mouth. Patients should maintain good oral hygiene when using this drug.

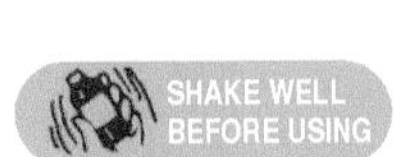

Cautions and Considerations Abrupt withdrawal of AEDs should always be avoided, because sudden discontinuation may trigger seizures. The dose should be slowly decreased over time if a patient needs to stop taking an anticonvulsant.

Several anticonvulsants are classified in pregnancy category D, meaning they are harmful to a developing fetus if taken while the patient is pregnant. However, seizures can also pose life-threatening effects for the mother and baby. Anticonvulsants are carefully selected for pregnant women.

Zonisamide is similar to sulfa drugs. Therefore, patients who are allergic to sulfa antibiotics should not take this medication.

Phenytoin is highly bound to protein in the bloodstream, and it interacts with many other medications that are also bound to protein. All alerts for drug interactions should be taken seriously, and the pharmacist must evaluate each one carefully. Phenytoin can adhere to nasogastric tubing. If it is given through a tube into the stomach, it must be mixed well with normal saline and separated by two hours from feedings given through the same tube. Intravenous (IV) phenytoin should be mixed or prepared using only normal saline. Suspensions of phenytoin must be shaken well—as should any medication in suspension form.

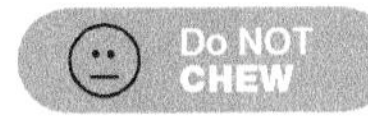

Valproate and valproic acid tablets should be swallowed whole, not crushed or chewed. They should not be taken with aspirin or carbonated beverages. Aspirin competes with valproic acid for protein-binding sites, and carbonated beverages can break it down before absorption can occur.

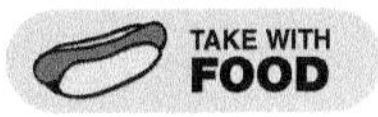

The extended-release form of carbamazepine works as an osmotic pump and leaves an empty pill casing in the stool. Patients should not be alarmed by the appearance of this "ghost tablet" in their stool. The drug is released while going through the digestive system. This product works best when taken along with a fatty meal.

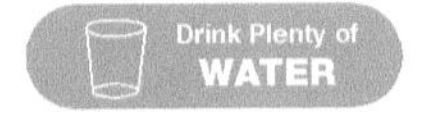

Ethosuximide works best when taken with food. An auxiliary label informing the patient to take this medication with food is recommended.

Barbiturates (phenobarbital, amobarbital, and mephobarbital) and primidone are controlled substances, thus special storage and handling are needed. Some pharmacies require double and triple counting of controlled substances. Refills are limited on controlled substances. Patients can develop tolerance and dependence, and they need more of the drug to get the same effects.

Drink Plenty of WATER

Topiramate and zonisamide can cause kidney stones, so patients should drink plenty of fluids to avoid this effect. An auxiliary warning label informing patients to take with fluids is often used on these medications.

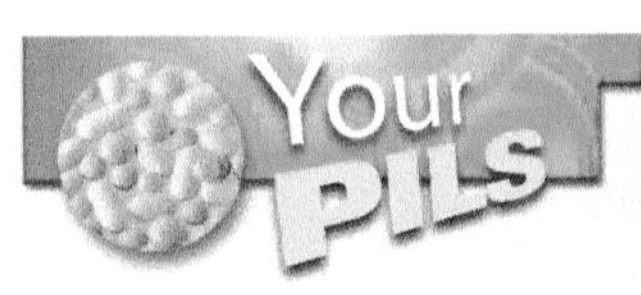

To become familiar with the many side effects of AEDs, make a list of the effects from Table 7.3 that would pose a personal barrier for you. Which effects would you consider intolerable or would affect your ability to remain adherent to therapy? If you enjoy details and working alone as Producers do, make a list of the AEDs associated with each side effect you find particularly difficult. If you enjoy reflection as Creators do, think about which AEDs are associated with these particularly difficult side effects and discuss your thoughts with a classmate.

Parkinson's Disease

Parkinson's disease (PD) was first described by James Parkinson in 1817. The condition is characterized by tremors, muscle rigidity, difficulty moving, and balance problems. It can be quite debilitating and is most common among elderly patients. In fact, 1% of people in the United States over the age of sixty have PD. However, PD can develop in middle age. For instance, Michael J. Fox, a popular actor and activist, announced he had PD in his forties.

PD is a CNS disorder of the central nervous system in which cells are lost in the **substantia nigra**, a region in the midbrain. These cells produce dopamine, a neurotransmitter used in initiating and coordinating muscle movement. Most patients with PD walk with a shuffling gait, lean forward, and are somewhat off-balance. Tremors and inability to move make activities of daily life difficult. The disease is progressive and has no cure. Drug therapy can relieve symptoms, allowing patients freedom to move instead of being wheelchair-bound.

Other symptoms associated with PD include anxiety, depression, fatigue, slow thinking, dementia, fragmented sleep, and hallucinations. Abnormalities of the autonomic nervous system can cause night sweating, orthostatic hypotension (low blood pressure on standing), sexual dysfunction, and constipation. Some patients also experience tingling sensations, lack of energy, loss of sense of smell, and diffuse pain. PD is a major reason for nursing home admissions.

Pharmacists and technicians should be aware that some drugs cause PD-type symptoms. Usually, these effects are reversible on discontinuation of the medications. Occasionally, these effects are permanent. Drugs that can cause PD-type symptoms include:

- antipsychotic agents
- metoclopramide
- phenothiazine antiemetics
- pimozide
- amoxapine
- lithium
- serotonin reuptake inhibitors (antidepressants)

Patients with movement problems should have their drug regimens evaluated. If a drug can be eliminated, PD-type symptoms may also disappear.

Drugs for Parkinson's Disease

As PD progresses from early symptoms to advanced disease, the approach to drug therapy changes. Initial therapy starts with one drug, such as an anticholinergic agent or a dopaminergic agent such as levodopa. Eventually, adjunct therapy is added to improve symptom control. Adjunctive treatments include COMT inhibitors, selegiline, apomorphine, and amantadine. Surgical options are available, but the risks of brain surgery limit its use to the most severely affected patients.

Dopamine Agents The mainstay of treatment for PD are **dopaminergic agents**. **Levodopa** is widely recognized as the most effective treatment for PD because it significantly improves movement and significantly restores normal function. Unfortunately, the effects of this drug (that is, its ability to provide movement control, or "on" time to patients) wear off over time. Dopamine agonists offer another alternative without some of the movement effects that levodopa causes, but they are not always as effective as levodopa. The average amount of time for which a dopaminergic drug will work without significant side effects is about five years.

This group of drugs either replaces dopamine or mimics its action in the brain. In effect, these agents either give the brain more dopamine or provide a drug that has the same action. Dopamine itself cannot cross the BBB, so its prodrug, levodopa, is given. Once levodopa enters the brain, it is broken down into dopamine. Carbidopa is usually given in combination with levodopa (see Table 7.4) because it slows the breakdown of levodopa before it reaches the CNS, allowing more of it to enter.

Apomorphine is a self-injected agent used for acute treatment of intermittent "off" time or inability to move. Despite its name, apomorphine is not an opioid drug. It should not be used regularly; instead, it is saved for when levodopa wears off more quickly than anticipated. It boosts the effects of levodopa until the next dose can be taken. If repeated doses of apomorphine are needed, adjustments in other therapies should be made to avoid frequent "off" times.

Side Effects Common side effects of levodopa/carbidopa include nausea and **dyskinesias**, which are abnormal, involuntary writhing movements of the arms, legs, neck, and mouth. Dyskinesias are associated with peak concentrations of levodopa in the bloodstream. They tend to occur sixty to ninety minutes after taking a dose. Taking levodopa with food can help with nausea; the only way to alleviate movement symptoms is to lower the dose or add adjunct drug therapy.

Common side effects of dopamine agonists include dizziness, constipation, nausea, insomnia, daytime sleepiness, "sleep attacks," yawning, hallucinations, and mood elevations that increase risk-taking behavior, such as gambling. Taking these medications with food can alleviate stomach upset, but other side effects are difficult to treat.

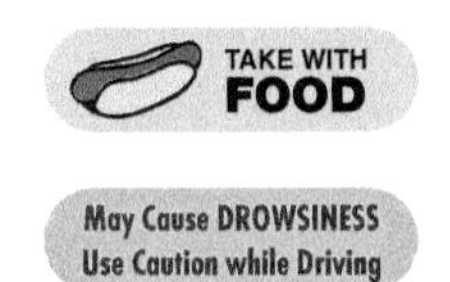

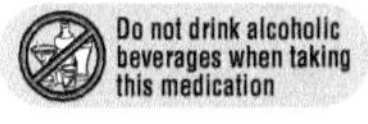

Daytime sleepiness and sleep attacks may impair a patient's ability to drive or participate in daily activities. An auxiliary warning label about drowsiness and driving or operating machinery should be affixed to the prescription vial. Patients should also avoid drinking alcohol because it will intensify this effect. Dopamine agonists should be used with caution in patients with preexisting sleep disorders.

Bromocriptine is associated with soft tissue fibrosis, which can affect the heart valves and lung function. Thus, it is not used much. Apomorphine can cause significant drops in blood pressure. Patients with orthostatic hypotension should not use this agent. A test dose may be given in a physician's office to see how the drug will affect a patient's blood pressure before self-injection at home.

Cautions and Considerations Apomorphine should not be taken along with antiemetic agents such as ondansetron, granisetron, or alosetron. If a patient complains of nausea and drug treatment is needed, other antiemetic medications should be used.

Apomorphine comes in a self-injector pen. The pharmacist needs to teach the patient how to use the pen if she or he has not been instructed already. Ampules and cartridges for the injector can be stored at room temperature. If syringes are prefilled with apomorphine, they can be stored in the refrigerator for one day.

Table 7.4 Dopaminergic Drugs

Generic (Brand)	Dosage Form	Route of Administration	Common Dose
Apomorphine (Apokyn)	Injection	SC injection	2–6 mg
Bromocriptine (Parlodel)	Tablet, capsule	Oral	2.5–100 mg a day
Levodopa/carbidopa (Sinemet)	Tablet	Oral	Levodopa: 400–1,600 mg a day Carbidopa: 70–100 mg a day
Pramipexole (Mirapex)	Tablet	Oral	0.375–4.5 mg a day
Ropinirole (Requip)	Tablet	Oral	0.75–3 mg a day

Anticholinergics and Amantadine These agents are used early in PD for mild symptoms (primarily tremors). They are used later in the disease progression as adjunct therapy for the movement side effects caused by levodopa. **Anticholinergics** work by blocking muscarinic receptors in the brain, which helps balance cholinergic activity and reduces tremors. **Amantadine**, an antiviral drug used for influenza, inhibits the reuptake of dopamine into presynaptic nerve endings. This inhibition allows reduced dopamine to accumulate in the synaptic cleft and stimulate more dopamine receptors. (See Table 7.5 for information on these drugs.)

Table 7.5 Anticholinergics and Amantadine

Generic (Brand)	Dosage Form	Route of Administration	Common Dose
Amantadine (Symmetrel)	Tablet, capsule, syrup	Oral	200–400 mg a day
Anticholinergics			
Benztropine (Cogentin)	Tablet, injection	Oral, IV, IM	1–2 mg a day
Trihexyphenidyl (Trihexy)	Tablet, elixir	Oral	6–15 mg a day

Side Effects Common side effects of anticholinergics are anxiety, confusion/memory impairment, drowsiness, dry nose and mouth, blurred vision, constipation, fast heartbeat, and difficulty urinating. These drugs also decrease sweating, making body heat regulation a potential problem. Heatstroke can occur easily.

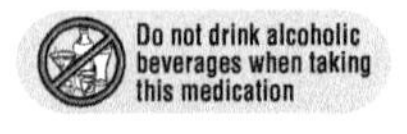

May Cause DROWSINESS
Use Caution while Driving

Cautions and Considerations Because these agents can cause drowsiness and confusion, patients should avoid alcohol because these effects will intensify. An auxiliary warning label about drowsiness and driving may also be used to emphasize that patients should be cautious and monitor how these drugs affect them. Patients may also be advised to drink plenty of fluids and eat foods high in fiber to counteract the constipation these agents can cause.

COMT Inhibitors An adjunct therapy (not monotherapy), **catechol-o-methyltransferase (COMT) inhibitors** help when levodopa starts to wear off at the end of each dosing interval. Typically, one of these agents (see Table 7.6) is given with each dose of levodopa to increase the amount of "on" time by 1 to 2 hours each day. Usually, the levodopa dose is decreased by approximately 100 mg a day when one of these drugs is added. This class of drug works by blocking an enzyme that metabolizes dopamine. COMT inhibitors boost the effects of levodopa and dopamine by allowing dopamine to remain present longer.

Table 7.6 COMT Inhibitor

Generic (Brand)	Dosage Form	Route of Administration	Common Dose
Entacapone (Comtan)	Tablet	Oral	200–1,600 mg a day
Tolcapone (Tasmar)	Tablet	Oral	100–200 mg a day

Side Effects Common side effects of entacapone include worsening of dyskinesia, nausea, diarrhea, and abdominal pain. Postural hypotension (a drop in blood pressure on sitting or standing up) can also occur. Patients should rise slowly from a sitting position. They should take care in driving until they know how this drug will affect them. These effects may decrease over time.

May Discolor Urine

Cautions and Considerations Entacapone can cause urine discoloration. Technicians should use an auxiliary label warning patients of this effect when dispensing this medication.

MAOIs Mild dopamine-boosting drugs that are used early on in disease progression or as adjunct therapy in advanced PD are **monoamine oxidase inhibitors (MAOIs)**. Rasagiline is often used for mild PD symptoms. Selegiline is usually used as adjunct therapy when levodopa begins wearing off (see Table 7.7 for information on these drugs). These agents block MAO, an enzyme that breaks down dopamine in neurons.

Table 7.7 MAOIs

Generic (Brand)	Dosage Form	Route of Administration	Common Dose
Rasagiline (Azilect)	Tablet	Oral	0.5–1 mg a day
Selegiline (Eldepryl, Zelapar)	Tablet, capsule	Oral	2.5–5 mg twice a day

Side Effects Common side effects of MAOIs include insomnia, confusion, hallucinations, euphoria, dizziness, and postural hypotension. If a second dose is prescribed, patients should take it early in the afternoon to avoid insomnia. Rasagiline does not produce as much insomnia, so it is a good alternative to selegiline.

Cautions and Considerations MAOIs block the metabolism of **tyramine,** a substance in many aged and pickled foods. If tyramine concentrations rise high enough in the blood, they can raise the blood pressure to dangerous levels. Therefore, patients should be instructed to limit their intake of tyramine-rich foods, including:

- aged cheese
- red wine
- beef
- peppers
- sausage
- sauerkraut
- tap beer

Pharmacy technicians who work in the food store setting should be mindful of the food in patients' shopping carts and remind them that these foods should be eaten in moderation when taking an MAOI.

Dementia and Alzheimer's Disease

Alzheimer's disease is a form of **dementia** that affects many in the United States. Up to 250,000 people are diagnosed each year. No clear cause of Alzheimer's disease has been identified, so it is diagnosed by ruling out all other causes of dementia. Alzheimer's disease is a degenerative brain disorder leading to loss of memory, intellect, judgment, orientation, and speech. Losing these higher brain functions causes patients with this disease to wander, become irritable or hostile, and experience changes in personality. Depression and anxiety are common in patients with Alzheimer's disease. Eventually, patients reach a "failure to thrive" level that causes death. This disease has no cure and poses difficult challenges to family members as they care for their loved ones.

Drugs for Alzheimer's Disease

Drug therapy for Alzheimer's disease does not alter the disease's progression. The goal of drug therapy is to maintain cognitive function and alertness for as long as possible. Several drugs are used for this disease (see Table 7.8). These drugs are used for mild symptoms early in disease progression but will not work once severe memory and functional loss has occurred. These agents work by inhibiting enzymes that break down acetylcholine, a neurotransmitter thought to be deficient in early Alzheimer's disease. Later in the disease, antidepressants can be used for depression, and benzodiazepines can be used for anxiety and sleep problems. Hallucinations may be treated with antipsychotic medications such as haloperidol.

Side Effects Common side effects of cholinesterase inhibitors include nausea, vomiting, agitation, rash, loss of appetite, weight loss, and confusion. These effects can be significant, so doses must be started low and increased slowly. If these effects do not ease with time or are particularly bothersome, the drug should be discontinued.

Table 7.8 Alzheimer's Disease Drugs

Generic (Brand)	Dosage Form	Route of Administration	Common Dose
Memantine (Namenda)	Tablet, oral solution	Oral	5–20 mg a day
Cholinesterase Inhibitors			
Donepezil (Aricept)	Tablet, oral solution	Oral	5–10 mg once a day
Galantamine (Razadyne)	Tablet, capsule, oral solution	Oral	8–24 mg a day
Rivastigmine (Exelon)	Capsule, oral solution, transdermal patch	Oral, transdermal	3–12 mg a day
Tacrine (Cognex)	Capsule	Oral	10–40 mg taken four times a day

Cautions and Considerations Tacrine is broken down in the liver by the cytochrome P450 system, an enzyme system that works to eliminate many drugs. Therefore, tacrine interferes with many other drugs. Drug interaction warnings on the computer should be heeded and properly evaluated by the pharmacist. Tacrine can also affect results of liver function tests.

Donepezil can interact with nonsteroidal anti-inflammatory drugs, theophylline, and nicotine (through smoking). These substances should be avoided while taking donepezil. Patients with cardiac disease, liver problems, or Parkinson's disease should not take donepezil.

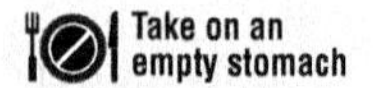

Tacrine should be taken on an empty stomach. You should be aware, however, that tacrine is taken four times a day—a difficult regimen to adhere to while also ensuring that all doses are on an empty stomach.

Attention-Deficit Hyperactivity Disorder (ADHD)

Attention-deficit hyperactivity disorder (ADHD) has received a lot of media attention and carries many misconceptions about diagnosis and treatment. The condition is characterized by inattention, impulsivity, and hyperactivity. To be diagnosed with ADHD, an individual must exhibit six or more symptoms of inattention and six or more hyperactivity/impulsivity symptoms that impair daily life in at least two settings for at least six months. Although many think environment and stressors cause someone to have ADHD, research has shown that they merely exacerbate the condition rather than cause it.

Some estimate that 3 to 10% of school-aged children have some aspect of the disorder, whereas 5% of adults have ADHD. Onset occurs by age three and is more prevalent in boys. Although hyperactivity symptoms decline with age, the inattention and impulsivity can persist into adulthood for half of those who have this condition. Several other disorders often coexist with ADHD. These include bipolar disorder, learning disabilities, depression, anxiety, and substance abuse. Therefore, ADHD and its coexisting conditions can be a difficult mix to treat effectively.

Drugs for ADHD

Controversy around the use and misuse of drugs to treat ADHD has been a public argument. Some believe that ADHD is overdiagnosed and overmedicated. However, studies have shown drug therapy to be effective, if approached appropriately. The best results occur when drugs are used in conjunction with counseling or behavioral therapy. A dual approach also helps identify and treat coexisting conditions. Drug therapy for ADHD has its risks and should never be entered into lightly.

Central Nervous System (CNS) Stimulants The first-line drug therapy for children and adults with ADHD is the use of **CNS stimulants**. These agents work best when used in conjunction with behavioral therapy. Dosing starts low and is increased until optimal improvement in symptoms is seen without side effects. Immediate-release products are usually tried first. The first dose is given before school (for children); if a second dose is needed, it will be given after school (see Table 7.9 for more specific dosing information). If longer effects are needed, extended-release products are used. Transdermal patches are applied in the morning, worn for nine hours, and then removed.

CNS stimulants work by enhancing the release and blocking the reuptake of dopamine and norepinephrine in presynaptic nerve cells. Increasing levels of these neurotransmitters enhances executive functions, increases inhibition, improves attention, and allows for better focus. In effect, boosting these neurotransmitters dampens the "noise" patients with ADHD experience with thought and allows them to focus and concentrate. Stimulants can also help with self-control, aggression, and productivity. However, these agents may not help with reading skills, social skills, or academic achievement.

Table 7.9 Drugs for ADHD

Generic (Brand)	Dosage Form	Route of Administration	Maximum Dose
Stimulants			
Amphetamine salts (Adderall, Adderall XR, Microtel)	Tablet, capsule	Oral	40 mg a day
Dexmethylphenidate (Focalin, Focalin XR)	Tablet, capsule	Oral	20 mg a day
Dextroamphetamine (Dexedrine, DextroStat)	Tablet, capsule	Oral	40 mg a day
Methylphenidate immediate-release (Ritalin)	Tablet	Oral	2 mg/kg/day or 60 mg
Methylphenidate extended-release (Concerta, Ritalin LA, Metadate, Methylin, Daytrana)	Tablet, capsule, transdermal patch	Oral, transdermal	72 mg a day
Nonstimulants			
Atomoxetine (Strattera)	Capsule	Oral	40–100 mg a day

Side Effects Common side effects of CNS stimulants include headache, stomachache, loss of appetite, weight loss, insomnia, and irritability. Growth suppression in children has also been found to occur, so it is recommended that the prescriber monitor patient height and weight every three to six months. To minimize these effects, children are given a therapeutic holiday, where the drug is stopped when school is not in session. Although rare, liver dysfunction can occur with these agents. The drug should be stopped immediately if a patient develops jaundice or yellowing of the eyes and skin.

Cautions and Considerations Rare but serious (even fatal) cardiac abnormalities have occurred with use of CNS stimulants. Adderall XR should not be used in patients with cardiac abnormalities.

All CNS stimulants are controlled substances (Schedule II) and have addiction and abuse potential. Therefore, no refills are allowed, and limited supplies can be given at a time. Because these medications will be taken long term, patients and their parents must be informed that a new written prescription is needed each time they need a refill. A plan between the prescriber, patient, and pharmacy should be established to address this issue. Pharmacy technicians can help by reminding patients or caregivers about this refill requirement when dispensing the first prescription. Taking a proactive attitude toward this limitation can alleviate problems later.

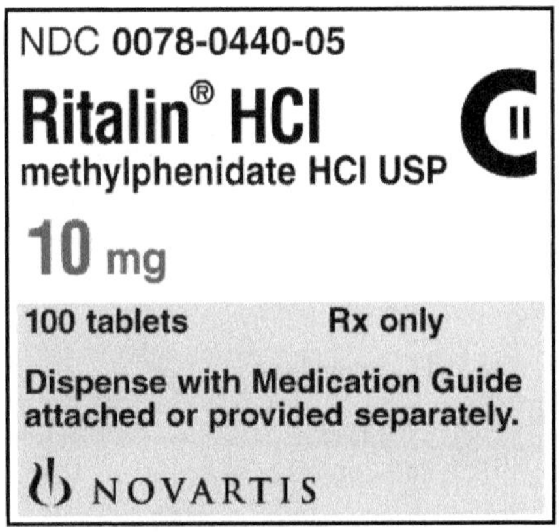

NDC 0078-0440-05
Ritalin® HCl
CII
methylphenidate HCl USP
10 mg
100 tablets Rx only
Dispense with Medication Guide attached or provided separately.
NOVARTIS

The CII mark on the label indicates the medication is a controlled substance that must be stored separate from other inventory and locked.

Nonstimulant Drugs for ADHD An alternative to CNS stimulants is atomoxetine, which is not a controlled substance and can help with behavioral management. It is a good choice for addressing ADHD in a patient who has substance abuse problems. Atomoxetine (Strattera) works by potentiating norepinephrine and/or dopamine in the brain, which, alone or in combination with CNS stimulants, helps increase focus and curb impulsivity. Typical dose is 100 mg a day. Patients should be aware that it can take up to two to four weeks to see the full effect. Other nonstimulant agents, including antidepressants such as bupropion, desipramine, nortriptyline, and venlafaxine, may also be used (see Chapter 8). Clonidine and guanfacine are used when a patient has tics or insomnia as part of ADHD.

Common side effects with atomoxetine are nausea, heartburn, fatigue, and decreased appetite. Atomoxetine can cause severe liver injury; therefore, lab tests will be conducted and results monitored. Patients with preexisting liver problems cannot use atomoxetine.

Drugs that Affect the Autonomic Nervous System

Most drugs that affect the autonomic nervous system are used to control blood pressure and heart rate. **Adrenergic inhibitors** block alpha and beta receptors; **adrenergic agonists** stimulate these receptors. Sometimes these medications and their indications can be confusing to understand. Once you know what happens when alpha and beta receptors are stimulated, you can reason what happens when they are blocked and predict why specific agents are chosen. In many ways, blocking sympathetic action appears to cause parasympathetic effects.

Adrenergic Inhibitors

Because alpha and beta receptors are found in the heart and blood vessels, stimulating those causes increased heart rate, vasoconstriction, and elevated blood pressure. Activating alpha receptors also delays bladder emptying. Blocking these receptors with drugs causes the opposite (i.e., slowed heart rate and lowered blood pressure) to occur.

Alpha Blockers The class of drugs known as **alpha blockers** is used primarily to treat hypertension (HTN). They are especially useful in men who also have benign prostatic hyperplasia (BPH), a condition in which the prostate enlarges with age. Because alpha blockers delay bladder emptying, they are used to relieve urinary urgency and frequency associated with BPH (see Table 7.10).

Side Effects Common side effects seen with alpha blockers include headache, dizziness, nausea, and fatigue/tiredness. Patients should avoid driving until they know how tired these medications can make them. Luckily, these effects usually improve over time, as a patient gets used to the medication.

May Cause DROWSINESS
Use Caution while Driving

Although rare, male patients have also experienced priapism (erection lasting longer than four hours). If this occurs, the patient should seek medical help right away because this can cause permanent impotence if left untreated.

Cautions and Considerations Patients should be warned of significant hypotension and heart palpitations that can happen with the first few doses of these agents. Symptoms of this effect are dizziness, lightheadedness, and fainting. Patients should work with family members or others who can monitor them as they begin taking one of these medications. They should not drive or undertake hazardous tasks for twelve to

Table 7.10 Alpha Receptor Blockers

Generic (Brand)	Dosage Form	Route of Administration	Use and Common Dose
Doxazosin (Cardura)	Tablet	Oral	BPH: 1–2 mg a day HTN: 1–16 mg a day
Prazosin (Minipress)	Capsule	Oral	HTN: 2–20 mg a day taken in divided doses
Terazosin (Hytrin)	Tablet, capsule	Oral	BPH: 1–10 mg once a day HTN: 1–5 mg a day

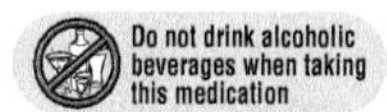

twenty-four hours after taking their first dose. Drinking alcohol or taking verapamil can intensify the hypotensive effects and should be avoided when possible. If these symptoms occur, the patient should lie down until they pass and notify a physician. Doses can be adjusted slowly to minimize or avoid this effect.

Beta Blockers The **beta blockers** class of drugs (see Table 7.11) is used for hypertension, **angina**, and arrhythmias. In fact, beta blockers make up the entire **Class II of antiarrhythmic agents** (see Chapter 12). The volume of published research that supports their use and their low cost makes them an attractive and frequent choice for treating high blood pressure. Beta blockers are also recommended for heart attack patients because these agents reduce oxygen demands and stress on the heart. This benefit has been found to help prevent subsequent heart attacks. **Cardioselective beta blockers** (e.g., atenolol, esmolol, bisoprolol, betaxolol, and metoprolol) inhibit only beta-one receptors in the heart. They are useful in treating angina and certain arrhythmias without causing bronchoconstriction. Another, less common use for beta blockers is as prophylaxis against migraine headache and mild anxiety. Ophthalmic formulation beta blockers are used to treat glaucoma (see Chapter 11).

Side Effects Common side effects for beta blockers include headache, dizziness, lightheadedness, nausea, and fatigue/weakness. Patients should avoid driving until they know how these medications affect them. Luckily, these effects generally improve over time as a patient gets used to the medication. This class of drugs has been associated with an increased incidence of depression. Patients who complain of depression symptoms should be referred to their physicians for appropriate evaluation.

Beta blockers can sometimes slow the heart rate too much and exacerbate cardiac conditions such as angina, arrhythmia, and heart failure. Patients who experience difficulty breathing (especially with physical activity or when lying down), night coughing, or swelling of the extremities should seek medical attention right away.

Table 7.11 Beta Blockers

Generic (Brand)	Dosage Form	Route of Administration	Common Dose
Acebutolol (Sectral)	Capsule	Oral	400–800 mg a day
Atenolol (Tenormin)	Tablet	Oral	50–100 mg a day
Betaxolol (Kerlone)	Tablet	Oral	10–20 mg a day
Bisoprolol (Zebeta)	Tablet	Oral	5–20 mg a day
Carteolol (Cartrol)	Tablet	Oral	2.5–5 mg a day
Carvedilol (Coreg)	Tablet, capsule	Oral	Tablet: 6.25–25 mg twice a day Capsule: 10–80 mg once a day
Esmolol (Brevibloc)	Injection	IV	Varies depending on patient weight Infused over 1–4 minutes
Metoprolol (Lopressor, Toprol)	Tablet, injection	Oral, IV	Tartrate oral: 100–450 mg a day Succinate oral: 50–100 mg a day
Nadolol (Corgard)	Tablet	Oral	40–320 mg a day
Nebivolol (Bystolic)	Tablet	Oral	5–40 mg a day
Penbutolol (Levatol)	Tablet	Oral	20–80 mg a day
Pindolol (Visken)	Tablet	Oral	10–60 mg a day in divided doses
Propranolol (Inderal)	Tablet, capsule, oral solution, injection	Oral, IV	Dose and frequency vary depending on indication/use
Sotalol (Betapace)	Tablet	Oral	80–160 mg twice a day
Timolol (Blocadren)	Tablet	Oral	10–40 mg twice a day

Cautions and Considerations Blocking beta-two receptors constricts airways in the lungs in addition to lowering blood pressure. This effect can be harmful to patients with impaired respiratory function, for example, those with asthma or chronic obstructive pulmonary disease (COPD). For these people, care must be taken to choose drugs that selectively block beta-one receptors only. Beta blockers that can be used by patients with asthma or COPD include metoprolol, acebutolol, betaxolol, bisoprolol, and atenolol.

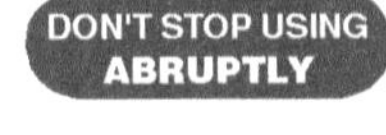

Abrupt withdrawal from a beta blocker can cause severe cardiac problems, such as heart attack, angina, or arrhythmia. Thus, patients should not stop taking a beta blocker suddenly. If a change in medication is made, the dose will be decreased slowly until it is discontinued.

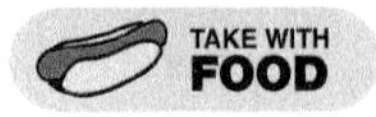

Patients with diabetes should use beta blockers with caution. These drugs can inhibit the usual signs and symptoms of a reaction to low blood sugar. The only symptom of low blood sugar that a patient taking a beta blocker may have is sweating. The pharmacist should counsel patients with diabetes who are taking beta blockers.

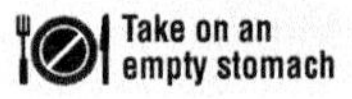

Propranolol and metoprolol work best when taken with food, whereas sotalol is best on an empty stomach. Corresponding auxiliary warning labels should be used.

Over-the-counter decongestants are vasoconstrictors that can raise blood pressure. Patients taking beta blockers for high blood pressure should avoid taking oral decongestants. Technicians can help identify these situations and provide information or have the pharmacist counsel the patients at the checkout counter.

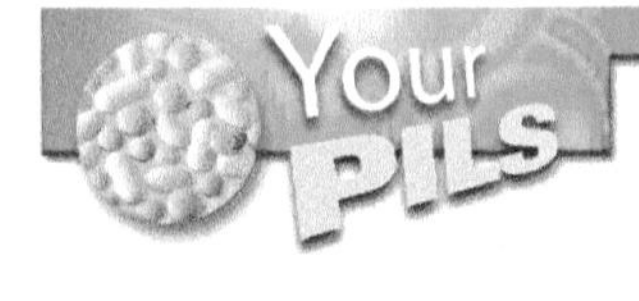

If you are a visual learner or enjoy learning in a group atmosphere, you might find creating a graphical diagram of the adrenergic drugs with classmates and then quizzing each other a good way to learn these drugs. Draw three circles: one for alpha receptors, one for beta-one receptors, and one for beta-two receptors. On scrap paper, write down and then cut out all brand and generic drug names for alpha blockers, beta blockers, and adrenergic agonists. Work with a classmate to put each drug name into the circle it is associated with and explain your reasoning out loud. Does a drug go in the beta-two receptor circle because it stimulates or blocks their activity? Which drugs could be put into multiple circles? Explain why.

Adrenergic Agonists

Adrenergic agonists stimulate the autonomic nervous system to produce sympathetic activity, such as increased heart rate, bronchodilation, and elevated blood pressure. Depending on how they are used, these drugs can stimulate the heart to start beating again, open airways that are constricted, raise blood pressure when large amounts of blood have been lost, and constrict blood vessels to treat the swelling that occurs during sinus infections and severe allergic reactions.

Vasopressors and Sympathomimetics Adrenergic agonists are sympathomimetics in that they mimic the effect of stimulating the sympathetic nervous system. Therefore, they are used in respiratory distress, allergic reactions, and sinus congestion. Ophthalmic versions of these agents are used to treat glaucoma. Many adrenergic agonists also have vasopressor action, which increases the heart rate and blood pressure. They are used for cardiac arrest and shock situations. Dosing ranges vary, depending on how and why they are used (see Table 7.12).

Epinephrine is used as a sympathomimetic agent in severe allergic reactions. It opens airways to assist in breathing and constricts blood vessels to treat swelling during anaphylactic reactions. Patients with life-threatening allergies (such as to peanuts or bee stings) can keep a prefilled autoinjector with this medication on hand for when they are exposed and begin to have allergy symptoms. Epinephrine is used for anaphylactic reactions, during which swelling and closure of airways is possible, but not for simple rash, hives, or itching allergies.

Table 7.12 Adrenergic Agonists

Generic (Brand)	Dosage Form	Route of Administration	Use
Dobutamine	Injection	IV	Cardiac stimulation during cardiac arrest, shock, or surgery
Dopamine	Injection	IV	Cardiac stimulation during cardiac arrest or shock
Ephedrine	Capsule, injection	Oral, IV	Bronchodilation for asthma
Epinephrine (Adrenaline, EpiPen, Nephron, Primatene)	Solution for injection, inhalation, or nasal aerosol	SC injection, IV, inhalation, nasal	Bronchodilation for asthma Cardiac stimulation during cardiac arrest Anaphylactic reactions Nasal decongestant
Isoproterenol (Isuprel)	Injection	IV	Cardiac stimulation during cardiac arrest or shock Bronchospasm during anesthesia
Metaraminol (Aramine)	Injection	IM, IV	Hypotension due to hemorrhage or spinal anesthesia
Midodrine (ProAmatine)	Tablet	Oral	Orthostatic hypotension
Norepinephrine (Levophed)	Injection	IV	Restoration of blood pressure during cardiac arrest or shock

Ephedrine and phenylephrine are used topically in the nose as decongestants to reduce sinus swelling during respiratory infections (see Chapter 11). Ephedrine is also used intravenously during surgery to support blood pressure and respiration.

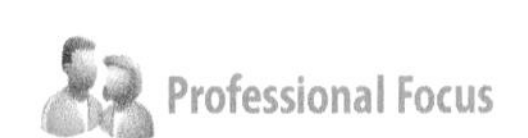

Professional Focus

Dopamine and dobutamine have sound-alike, look-alike names. Be sure to select the correct drug when preparing and dispensing these products. Double-check expiration dates, too. You don't want to find out in an emergency situation that your available drug stock is no longer effective.

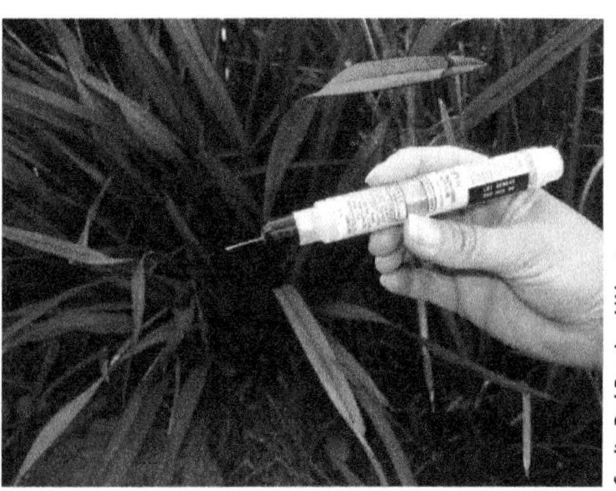

The EpiPen autoinjector can be used through clothing.

Credit: Rod Brouhard/About.com

Side Effects Common side effects of adrenergic agonists include headache, excitability, fast heart rate, restlessness, and insomnia. Rarely, they can cause arrhythmia. Due to these side effects, these medications are used only when needed.

Cautions and Considerations Pharmacy technicians may handle IV forms of these agents only if they supply the emergency room or critical care unit. These agents are often mixed as needed in the unit for cardiac code situations. If you work with these agents, be aware that they are mixed in dextrose solution, not normal saline. Some may be stocked in the emergency drug kits that technicians maintain.

Epinephrine in the autoinjector form is increasingly prescribed and dispensed in an outpatient setting. The pharmacist will need to counsel patients or their caregivers on how to inject this medication in times of severe allergic reaction. It should be injected into the thigh, not the buttocks. The autoinjector contains only one dose, so a refill will be needed once it is used. When dispensing, alert patients or caregivers to the expiration date. If they do not use it by the expiration date, they should return for a refill so they always have one on hand for urgent situations.

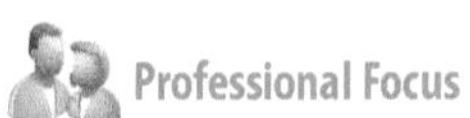

Professional Focus

When stocking the shelf with EpiPen autoinjectors, check the expiration date. If the date is upcoming, return it to the wholesaler. You do not want to be left with an expired drug before you have a chance to dispense it or sell one that expires soon after the patient gets it. An expiration date at least six months away is a good rule to follow.

Anticholinergic Drug Effects

When a drug blocks cholinergic activity in the parasympathetic system, dry mouth, dry eyes, constipation, and urinary retention may occur. Blood pressure also rises. Surprisingly, many drugs exert these **anticholinergic side effects**. Depending on a patient's medical condition, these effects could be problematic. For instance, patients with urinary difficulty (e.g., prostatic hyperplasia) or bowel problems (e.g., irritable bowel syndrome or constipation) should not use drugs with anticholinergic side effects.

Opioid pain medications (see Chapter 9) and bladder spasticity agents (see Chapter 19) are drugs that cause significant anticholinergic side effects—constipation and dry mouth, respectively. These side effects are the basis for many drug–disease interactions. You should heed such interaction warnings when prompted by the computer and alert the pharmacist.

Herbal and Alternative Therapies

Ginkgo biloba may have a modest benefit for patients with early Alzheimers disease, but serious side effects (e.g., bleeding, seizures, and coma) have occurred with it. Results in studies are controversial and do not necessarily show dramatic improvement in memory or thinking. It is questionable whether taking ginkgo biloba actually prevents Alzheimers disease, although many patients take it for this purpose. If patients choose to take it, they should clearly realize the risks and benefits. Typical doses are 120–720 mg ginkgo extract, and commercially available products vary in their content. Ginkgo biloba has antiplatelet effects that affect bleeding. Patients taking warfarin or aspirin for coagulation effects should not use ginkgo biloba without medical supervision. It also interacts with several other prescription medications, particularly anticonvulsants. Therefore, patients who take other prescription medications should discuss taking ginkgo biloba with their prescriber and pharmacist before doing so.

Dietary supplements that contain **ephedra**, also called ***ma huang***, were banned from sale in the United States in April 2004. This plant contains ephedra alkaloids (like ephedrine), which boost physical activity, suppress appetite, and promote weight loss. Ephedra can also cause heart palpitations, tremors, and insomnia. Deaths from cardiac arrest have occurred as a result of using this dietary supplement.

Chapter Summary

The nervous system is categorized into the CNS and the peripheral system as well as the somatic and autonomic systems. Seizure disorders are conditions of the CNS in which signals in the brain become sporadic. Seizures vary in their presentation, and a variety of antiepileptic drug therapies is used to control them. Side effect profiles are significant for antiepileptic drugs. Parkinson's disease (PD) is a deficiency in dopamine in the brain and usually occurs with increasing age. Drugs for PD include dopamine agonists, anticholinergics, and COMT inhibitors. Alzheimer's disease is a type of dementia. Cholinesterase inhibitors and memantine are drugs that can be used to enhance cognitive function early in the disease, but their effects are usually short-lived. Attention-deficit hyperactivity disorder is usually diagnosed during childhood and involves symptoms of inattention, impulsivity, and hyperactivity. CNS stimulants are used to control brain activity and allow patients to focus and learn. These agents are controlled substances and require special handling.

The autonomic nervous system controls functions of the body normally considered to be reflexive or automatic. This system is broken into sympathetic and parasympathetic actions. Sympathetic actions are associated with increased heart rate, bronchodilation, elevated blood pressure, and pupil dilation. Parasympathetic actions include digestion, urination, and relaxation. The drugs used on this system, alpha and beta blockers, are usually used to control blood pressure, heart rate, and airway openness. Adrenergic agonists (such as dobutamine and isoproterenol) stimulate sympathetic action and are used to stimulate the heart in cardiac arrest or shock situations. Epinephrine is used in anaphylactic reactions to open airways and treat severe swelling. When parasympathetic activity is inhibited, anticholinergic effects including constipation and dry mouth can occur. Many drugs have these side effects.

Ginkgo biloba is used for memory loss and may be helpful in Alzheimer's disease. Ephedra (*ma huang*) is an herbal product that has sympathomimetic activity and was banned from sale in the United States. It was used for weight loss, but it caused severe cardiac problems and even death in some patients.

Chapter Review

For the following sets of exercises, write the exercise heading, exercise numbers, and your answers on a separate sheet of paper. Your instructor may direct you to turn in the sheet of paper or discuss your answers as a class.

REVIEW THE BASICS

Choose a, b, c, or d as the correct answer to each multiple-choice question.

1. Which of the following is responsible for cognitive thinking and memory?
   a. thalamus
   b. cerebral cortex
   c. cerebellum
   d. pituitary gland
2. Which of the following neurotransmitters is found primarily in the CNS and controls mood and coordinated movement?
   a. acetylcholine
   b. dopamine
   c. epinephrine
   d. GABA
3. Which of the following seizure types is characterized by muscle rigidity and jerks, loss of bladder control, and typically, loss of consciousness?
   a. grand mal
   b. petit mal
   c. partial
   d. myoclonic
4. Which of the following is used as a first-line treatment for ADHD?
   a. methylphenidate
   b. amantadine
   c. donepezil
   d. metoprolol
5. Which of the following drugs can cause "sleep attacks," for which an auxiliary warning label about drowsiness should be used?
   a. lamotrigine
   b. levodopa/carbidopa
   c. atomoxetine
   d. benztropine
6. Which of the following medications is available in a transdermal patch?
   a. amantadine
   b. apomorphine
   c. fosphenytoin
   d. methylphenidate
7. Which of the following drugs can cause gingival hyperplasia, requiring attention to good oral hygiene?
   a. Dilantin
   b. Trileptal
   c. Adderall
   d. all of the above
8. Which of the following would happen if beta-one receptors are blocked with drug therapy?
   a. vasoconstriction
   b. decreased heart rate
   c. bronchodilation
   d. all of the above
9. Which of the following drugs is used for BPH as well as for HTN?
   a. Hytrin
   b. Levophed
   c. Inderal
   d. Ephedra
10. Which of the following drugs would be used for preventing a second heart attack for a patient who has already had one?
    a. atenolol
    b. terazosin
    c. dobutamine
    d. ephedrine

KNOW THE DRUGS

Match each brand name drug with its corresponding generic name and most common use. Your answers should follow this example format: Generic Name: 1. a; 2. b; 3. c; etc. Most Common Use: 1. h; 2. i; 3. j; etc.

Brand Name	Generic Name	Most Common Use
1. Sinemet	a. propranolol	h. seizure disorder
2. EpiPen	b. topiramate	i. Parkinson's disease
3. Topamax	c. methylphenidate	j. ADHD
4. Ritalin	d. levodopa/carbidopa	k. hypertension
5. Zarontin	e. ethosuximide	l. anaphylaxis
6. Inderal	f. epinephrine	
7. Cardura	g. doxazosin	

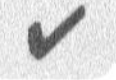

PUT IT TOGETHER

For each item, write down either a single term to complete the sentence or a short answer.

1. ________ is an herbal supplement used to combat memory loss and early stages of Alzheimer's disease.
2. PD develops from a deficiency in the neurotransmitter ______________.
3. List the drugs that are used for status epilepticus. Explain why they may be stocked in a crash cart or emergency drug kit.
4. Children often have difficulty swallowing pills. Epilepsy and ADHD are both conditions for which drug therapy is frequently needed in the pediatric setting. List the AEDs and ADHD drugs that should not be chewed or crushed.
5. Name the four primary anticholinergic side effects that many drugs cause.
6. What auxiliary warning label(s) should be affixed to a prescription for Toprol?

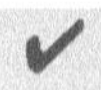

THINK IT THROUGH

Read and think through each numbered scenario carefully and then write several sentences in reply to the question(s) presented. Question 4 requires you to do some Internet research before completing your answer(s).

1. Mrs. Taylor drops off a new prescription for Tenormin. You notice on her profile that she also takes glyburide and metformin. As you fill the prescription, the computer displays a drug interaction warning. Why? What should you do, and what concern should you bring up to the pharmacist for counseling?
2. All but one of the CNS stimulants used to treat ADHD are controlled substances. In what control schedule are these medications categorized? What limitations does this put on storage and security of these products within the pharmacy? What limitations does this put on patients for getting such prescriptions filled? Brainstorm ways you could address these potential barriers to care.
3. A new patient in your pharmacy drops off a prescription for Toprol 50 mg QD #30 and requests a box of pseudoephedrine for his sinus headaches. What should you notice about this situation, and what should you do?
4. 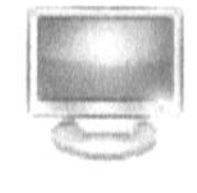

   On the Internet, look up news reports and other information about why the Food and Drug Administration (FDA) withdrew ephedra from the market. What was it used for, and what were the circumstances that prompted this FDA action? What other names might ephedra be found under? Are these products legal to sell in the United States?

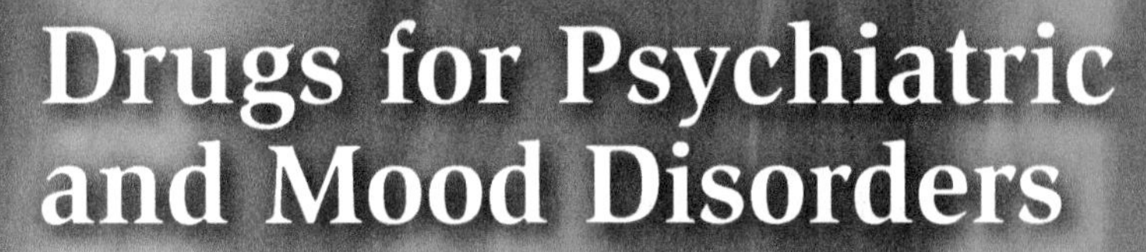

Chapter 8 Drugs for Psychiatric and Mood Disorders

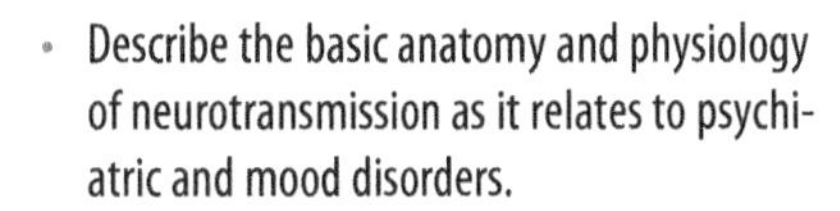

LEARNING OBJECTIVES

- Describe the basic anatomy and physiology of neurotransmission as it relates to psychiatric and mood disorders.
- Explain the therapeutic effects of prescription medications, nonprescription medications, and alternative therapies commonly used to treat psychiatric and mood disorders.
- Describe the adverse effects of prescription medications, nonprescription medications, and alternative therapies commonly used to treat psychiatric and mood disorders.
- Identify the brand and generic names of prescription and nonprescription medications commonly used to treat psychiatric and mood disorders.
- State the doses, dosage forms, and routes of administration for prescription and nonprescription medications commonly used to treat psychiatric and mood disorders.

Interactive self-quizzes, games, audio files, and glossaries help you to learn drug names and facts.

Psychiatrists, counselors, and therapists are not the only healthcare professionals who see and treat patients with mental illness. Pharmacists and pharmacy technicians in all settings dispense medications for psychiatric and mood disorders on a regular basis. Dealing with these patients can sometimes require special care and sensitivity. The chapter begins with a description of how neurotransmitters work and the abnormalities that result in mental illness. Next, specific disorders, including depression, anxiety, bipolar disorder, and schizophrenia, are described. Drug therapies used in the treatment of these various conditions include selective serotonin reuptake inhibitors, sedatives, and atypical antipsychotic agents. Even though it is not considered a mental illness, insomnia is often a sign of depression and anxiety. Therefore, similar drug classes are used to treat both insomnia and anxiety, and the drugs used for both of these conditions are covered in this chapter.

Anatomy and Physiology of Neurotransmission

Neurotransmitters are chemicals that are responsible for transmitting signals from nerve cell to nerve cell within the brain. Neurotransmitters such as **serotonin**, **norepinephrine**, and **dopamine** are released from one cell, cross the **synaptic cleft** between cells, and connect with receptors on the membranes of adjacent cells to create **signal conduction** (see Figure 8.1). Neurotransmitters are then either taken back up into the presynaptic nerve cell (a process called **reuptake**) or broken down by metabolic enzymes while in the cleft. **Monoamine oxidase** is one enzyme that breaks down neurotransmitters in neurons.

We know that disorders affecting mood and mental function are related to deficiency or dysfunction of neurotransmitters, although research is ongoing to elucidate brain pathophysiology. For instance, depression is related to a deficiency or dysfunction of neurotransmitters such as serotonin and norepinephrine. We know that dopamine is a neurotransmitter involved in psychoses, including schizophrenia. Drug therapy is used to manipulate levels of neurotransmitters by either mimicking their actions or altering the processes that eliminate them from the synaptic cleft.

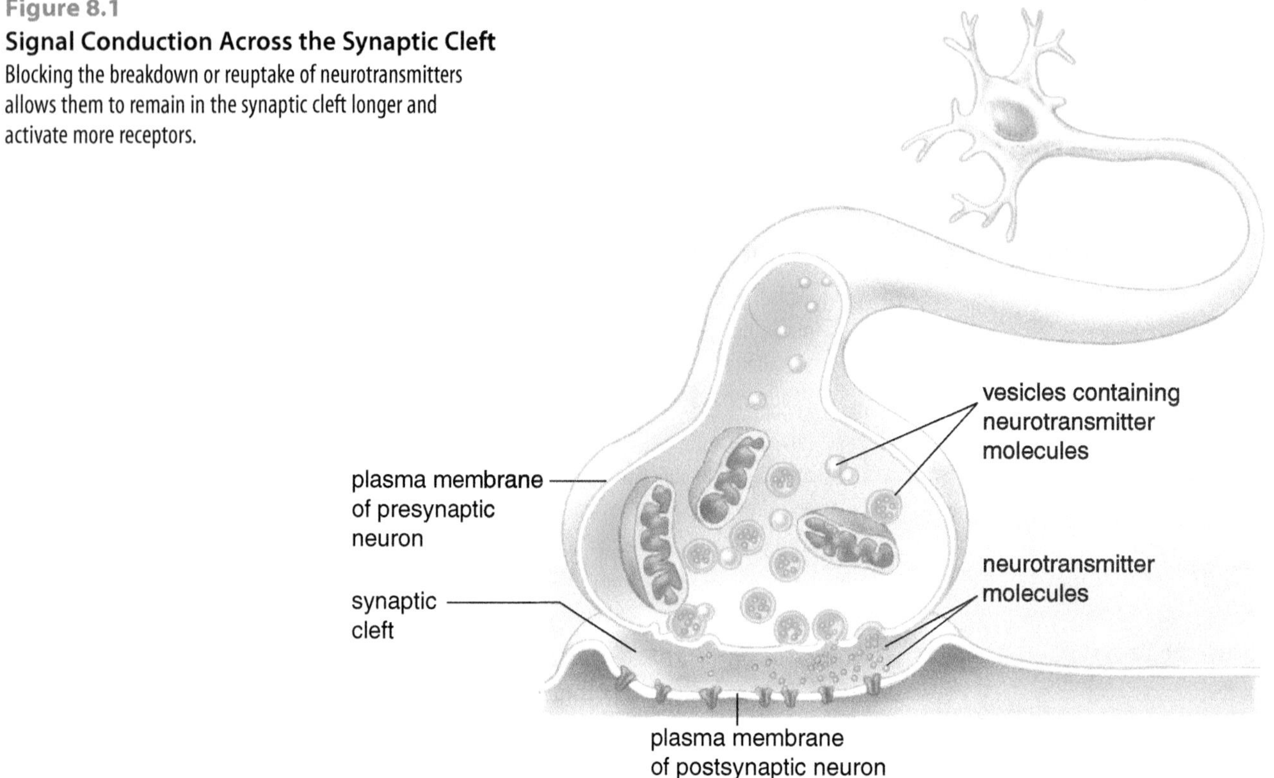

Figure 8.1
Signal Conduction Across the Synaptic Cleft
Blocking the breakdown or reuptake of neurotransmitters allows them to remain in the synaptic cleft longer and activate more receptors.

Depression

Depression is a leading health concern; treatment for this condition accounts for several of the top fifty prescription medications in the United States. Depression can be caused by external (exogenous) sources, such as a response to the death of a loved one, or by internal (endogenous) causes that lack logical, observable reasons for happening. In both cases, counseling can be helpful and necessary. **Endogenous depression** is more likely to require drug therapy to control. Neurotransmitters involved in mood include norepinephrine, serotonin, and probably dopamine. Signs of depression include crying (often without obvious cause), loss of interest in life or social activities, increased focus on death, and significant weight loss or gain. Symptoms patients express are low self-esteem, pessimism, sleep disturbances (insomnia or hypersomnia), loss of energy and ability to think, feelings of worthlessness and guilt, confusion, poor memory, and thoughts of **suicide**.

Antidepressants

Drug therapy for depression includes **selective serotonin reuptake inhibitors (SSRIs)**, **serotonin-norepinephrine reuptake inhibitors (SNRIs)**, **tricyclic antidepressants (TCAs)**, **monoamine oxidase inhibitors (MAOIs)**, **bupropion**, and **trazodone**. It takes three to six weeks for a patient to feel the effects of one of these antidepressants because it takes time for the number of receptors for neurotransmitters to increase and cells to adapt. Therefore, a genuine drug therapy trial should last at least three to four weeks, and doses should be changed only once a month under guidance by the prescriber. Patients should understand that mood does not change and symptoms do not subside immediately.

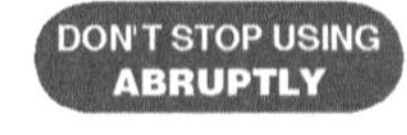

Antidepressants should not be stopped abruptly. Patients may experience worsened depression symptoms if they stop taking an antidepressant without gradually decreasing the dose. Some agents are associated with acute withdrawal symptoms when stopped abruptly. If patients want to stop therapy, they should talk with their prescribers to determine an appropriate plan.

SSRIs and SNRIs First-line therapy for depression includes SSRIs and SNRIs (see Table 8.1). SSRIs block serotonin reuptake into the presynaptic neuron, and SNRIs block reuptake of both serotonin and norepinephrine. SSRIs are also used for **obsessive-compulsive disorder (OCD)** and **premenstrual dysphoric disorder (PMDD)**. OCD is a form of anxiety wherein obsessive thoughts intrude daily consciousness and impair function. Patients engage in repetitive behaviors, such as hand washing and counting, in an attempt to relieve fears and anxiety. PMDD is marked by emotional and behavioral changes in the second half of a woman's menstrual cycle. Although some symptoms are similar to premenstrual syndrome (PMS), PMDD is more severe and life altering. SSRIs may also be used for anxiety and panic disorder. Duloxetine is used primarily for the nerve pain that accompanies depression.

Side Effects Common side effects of SSRIs include nausea, vomiting, dry mouth, drowsiness, insomnia, headache, and diarrhea. These effects can subside over time, but if bothersome, a different agent may be prescribed. Most of these agents can also cause sexual dysfunction, including decreased libido, inability to achieve orgasm, or impaired ejaculation. These effects are a frequent reason that patients stop therapy. Fluoxetine can also cause weight loss and is sometimes used for eating disorders, including bulimia. Patients should not use this agent simply to lose weight.

Cautions and Considerations SSRIs have been associated with an increased risk of suicide in the first few weeks of therapy, especially in pediatric and adolescent patients. Patients should be monitored closely, particularly until the drug's full effects are felt. Patients should be offered counseling and psychotherapy in addition to medication.

Because SSRIs increase serotonin levels, they increase the risk for **serotonin syndrome**, a potentially fatal medical condition. This syndrome occurs when too much serotonin is present, causing changes in cardiovascular function and even heart attack, in severe cases. The risk for serotonin syndrome is particularly high for patients taking more than one antidepressant or taking **St. John's wort**, an herbal product sold for depression. If patients experience the combination of racing heart rate, fever, high blood pressure, and headache, which may be signs of serotonin syndrome, they should seek immediate medical attention.

Table 8.1 Common SSRIs and SNRIs

Generic (Brand)	Dosage Form	Route of Administration	Common Dose
SSRIs			
Citalopram (Celexa)	Tablet, capsule, oral solution	Oral	20–40 mg a day
Escitalopram (Lexapro)	Tablet, oral solution	Oral	10–20 mg a day
Fluoxetine (Prozac, Sarafem)	Tablet, capsule, oral solution	Oral	20–80 mg a day
Fluvoxamine (Luvox)	Tablet	Oral	50–300 mg a day
Paroxetine (Paxil)	Tablet, suspension	Oral	10–60 mg a day
Sertraline (Zoloft)	Tablet	Oral	50–200 mg a day
SNRIs			
Desvenlafaxine (Pristiq)	Tablet	Oral	50 mg a day
Duloxetine (Cymbalta)	Capsule	Oral	40–60 mg a day
Venlafaxine (Effexor)	Tablet, capsule	Oral	75–375 mg a day

Tricyclic Antidepressants (TCAs) These antidepressants get their name from their chemical structure, which contains three rings. TCAs block reuptake of norepinephrine and/or serotonin. TCAs are sometimes prescribed for insomnia because their primary side effect is drowsiness. Consequently, they can be an effective choice for therapy when a patient's depression symptoms include insomnia. TCAs also have effects on neuropathic pain and are used to treat selected nerve conditions. A tetracyclic agent is also included in this class. As the name indicates, there is in fact a fourth ring in the chemical structure. Drug activity and properties, however, are similar (see Table 8.2 for dosing information on tricyclic and tetracyclic agents). Prior to the availability of SSRIs, TCAs were the most widely prescribed class of antidepressants.

Table 8.2 Common TCAs

Generic (Brand)	Dosage Form	Route of Administration	Common Dose
Amitriptyline (Elavil)	Tablet, injection	Oral, IM	30–300 mg a day
Desipramine (Norpramin)	Tablet, capsule	Oral	75–200 mg a day
Doxepin (Adapin)	Capsule	Oral	25–150 mg a day
Imipramine (Tofranil)	Tablet, capsule	Oral	100–300 mg a day
Nortriptyline (Aventyl, Pamelor)	Tablet, oral solution	Oral	25–100 mg a day
Tetracyclic Agent			
Mirtazapine (Remeron)	Tablet, orally disintegrating tablet	Oral	15–45 mg a day

May Cause DROWSINESS
Use Caution while Driving

Side Effects The most common side effect of TCAs is drowsiness, so patients should take these drugs at bedtime. Other common side effects include anticholinergic effects (e.g., dry mouth, blurred vision, constipation, and urinary retention). Some of these agents can cause **priapism**, an erection lasting longer than four hours. If this occurs, the patient should seek medical attention immediately.

Cautions and Considerations TCAs can cause cardiotoxicity and heart arrhythmias. Patients with preexisting heart conditions or who have recently had a heart attack should not take TCAs. They can also cause postural hypotension (a drop in blood pressure on sitting or standing up). Patients should take care to sit and stand up slowly.

TCAs can lower seizure threshold, so most patients with seizure disorders should not take these drugs. They can also cause liver toxicity, so those with liver problems should not take TCAs. Periodic blood tests will be taken to monitor liver function.

TCAs should not be taken with MAOIs because serotonin syndrome could develop. If a TCA is not working and an MAOI must be tried, the two therapies must be completely separated by two weeks. This time in between therapies is called **washout**. An overdose of TCAs can be fatal, so many pharmacists are uncomfortable dispensing a large supply to a patient for fear of suicidal behavior. Pharmacists may also be resistant to warning patients that an overdose could be lethal, because that message could suggest a pathway to suicide.

Monoamine Oxidase Inhibitors (MAOIs) These agents are not used as often as they used to be. Other drug therapies with fewer side effects and drug interactions are available, so these agents are saved as a last resort for intractable depression symptoms. MAOIs work by inhibiting one of the primary enzymes that metabolizes neurotransmitters. In effect, neurotransmitter levels rise in the synaptic cleft (see Table 8.3 for common dosing information).

Table 8.3 Common MAOIs

Generic (Brand)	Dosage Form	Route of Administration	Common Dose
Isocarboxazid (Marplan)	Tablet	Oral	10–60 mg a day
Phenelzine (Nardil)	Tablet	Oral	45–90 mg a day
Tranylcypromine (Parnate)	Tablet	Oral	30–60 mg a day

Side Effects MAOIs can cause heart palpitations and postural hypotension. Patients should sit and stand up slowly. Other side effects include dizziness, headache, tremors, insomnia, anxiety, restlessness, agitation, and anticholinergic effects (i.e., dry mouth, blurred vision, constipation, and urinary retention). These side effects frequently cause patients to stop therapy.

Cautions and Considerations These agents interact with numerous other drugs. Whenever patients are taking an MAOI, they should work closely with their physicians and pharmacists to manage any additional prescription or over-the-counter (OTC) medications they want to take.

MAOIs interact with **tyramine**, a substance found in aged and pickled foods. This interaction causes serotonin syndrome, a life-threatening condition involving a rapid heart rate, high blood pressure, headache, and fever. Patients who take MAOIs should avoid eating foods such as aged cheeses, beer, wine, sauerkraut, and pickled foods.

Bupropion This antidepressant blocks the reuptake of dopamine, primarily, but it also weakly blocks the reuptake of serotonin and norepinephrine. In addition to treating depression, it is used as adjunct therapy for **smoking cessation** and anxiety. The extended-release tablets should not be chewed or crushed. Bupropion can cause headache, agitation, weight gain, and insomnia. Taking doses early in the day can help with insomnia. Patients with seizure disorders should not take bupropion. It also should not be taken with alcohol or other drugs that cause central nervous system (CNS) depression (such as opiate pain medicines). The bupropion generic product and the brand-name versions Wellbutrin and Zyban are all produced as tablets for oral administration, with common dosage at 300 mg a day.

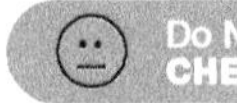

Trazodone This antidepressant is widely used, but its mechanism of action is not fully understood. It may affect serotonin reuptake. It is used for depression with insomnia because its predominant side effect is drowsiness. Trazodone is often used for neuralgic pain and sometimes anxiety that affects sleep. Doses typically range between 50 mg and 150 mg a day.

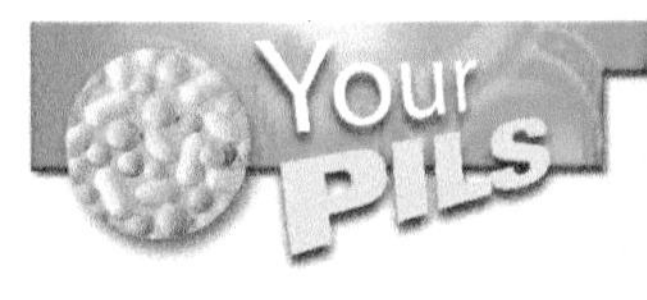

Learners who prefer to work with concrete information and details, like Producers and Directors, may find creating a table of antidepressants useful. Make one column for each major drug class of antidepressants. Include a row for the mechanism of action and list the neurotransmitter(s) on which each class works. List all generic and brand drug names under each class; then use this table as a reference for studying and memorizing.

Anxiety

Anxiety is associated with the abnormal function of the neurotransmitters that regulate brain activity, mood, and the fear response. The brain has natural benzodiazepine receptors that help regulate neurotransmitters. Serotonin and norepinephrine are also involved.

Anxiety is a constellation of symptoms categorized into two main types: **panic disorder** and **generalized anxiety disorder**. Other types, including phobic disorders and OCD, are treated with similar drugs. Panic disorder is characterized by symptoms such as chest pain, difficulty breathing, palpitations, dizziness, sweating, a choking sensation, trembling, and unrealistic feelings of doom. These feelings and symptoms occur in the absence of typical stimuli such as physical activity, life-threatening situations, or fearful events. The onset of these symptoms is sudden and quick, often described as an "attack." A formal diagnosis of panic disorder is made when a patient experiences at least three panic attacks in three weeks.

Generalized anxiety disorder is defined as excessive worry that causes significant distress or disturbance to work or social functioning and that continues for at least six months. Symptoms of worry include restlessness, irritability, difficulty concentrating, muscle tension, sleep disturbances, and fatigue. Unlike panic disorder, these symptoms are constant and do not subside. They can become debilitating and interfere with a patient's normal life activities.

Post-traumatic stress disorder (PTSD) is a variation of anxiety. It is prevalent with military personnel returning from combat zones. PTSD occurs in response to a traumatic event after which a reexperiencing syndrome continues for at least a month. Reexperiencing symptoms include avoidance behavior in which the patient avoids thoughts, conversations, activities, people, or places they would normally enjoy. This behavior has a numbing effect, allowing the patient to remain unemotional (flattened affect). Avoidance behavior is coupled with hyperarousal symptoms including sleep disturbances, an exaggerated startle reflex, irritability, outbursts, and difficulty concentrating. Treatment for PTSD is similar to therapy for other anxiety disorders in that both counseling and drug therapy are used to maintain control and normal function.

Sedatives and Hypnotics

Anxiety often requires drug therapy, but counseling is useful to address contributing factors. **Hypnotic** is a term for medication that causes sedation and relaxation. **Sedatives**, another word for hypnotics, are used to induce sleep. For panic disorder, agents with sedatives or hypnotices such as benzodiazepines may be useful for short-term treatment. For generalized anxiety disorder, benzodiazepines typically are necessary. SSRIs are also used for PTSD and anxiety.

Benzodiazepines The drugs of choice for generalized anxiety disorder are **benzodiazepines**. They are also used for panic disorder and PTSD. They are regularly used as preanesthetic medications to calm patients prior to procedures such as colonoscopy or surgery (see Chapter 9). Benzodiazepines are also part of the standard treatment for alcohol withdrawal symptoms and status epilepticus (see Chapter 7).

Benzodiazepines work by stimulating omega receptors in the CNS, causing drowsiness and relaxation. When used to treat anxiety, they have a calming and sometimes euphoric effect. When used for sleep, they reduce the time it takes to fall asleep, decrease early morning wakening, and generally improve sleep quality (see Table 8.4 for dosing information).

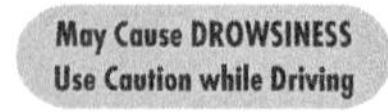

Side Effects Common side effects of benzodiazepines include constipation, muscle weakness, and impaired reflexes. Patients may also experience difficulty waking up in

Table 8.4 Common Benzodiazepines

Generic (Brand)	Dosage Form	Route of Administration	Common Dose
Alprazolam (Xanax)	Tablet	Oral	1–6 mg a day
Chlordiazepoxide (Librium)	Capsule, injection	Oral, IM, IV	24–300 mg a day in divided doses
Clonazepam (Klonopin)	Tablet, orally disintegrating tablet	Oral	1.5–20 mg a day
Clorazepate (Tranxene)	Tablet	Oral	15–60 mg a day
Diazepam (Valium)	Tablet, oral solution, rectal gel, injection	Oral, rectal, IM, IV	5–40 mg a day
Lorazepam (Ativan)	Tablet, oral solution, injection	Oral, IM, IV	1–10 mg a day
Quazepam (Doral)	Tablet	Oral	7.5–15 mg a day
Temazepam (Restoril)	Capsule	Oral	7.5–30 mg a day
Triazolam (Halcion)	Tablet	Oral	0.25–0.5 mg a day

the morning and leftover drowsiness the following day. A warning label about drowsiness should be used when dispensing a benzodiazepine.

Other concerning effects include oversedation and respiratory depression (slowed breathing). Patients should be informed of these effects and notify their physicians if they occur. In settings where the patient can be observed, such as inpatient or long-term care, caregivers should monitor for slowed breathing and excessive sleepiness. Patients should not drink alcohol or take other medications that cause sedation (e.g., opiate pain medications) because excessive sedation and drastically slowed breathing can occur. Breathing can slow to the point of causing death.

Cautions and Considerations All benzodiazepines have dependence and abuse potential. Consequently, they are scheduled as controlled substances Schedule IV. Patients can become both physically and emotionally dependent on benzodiazepines, making it difficult to stop therapy. Patients should be aware of this potential and should understand that benzodiazepines should be used only for a short time. If used for longer than a couple of weeks, doses must be slowly tapered to avoid withdrawal symptoms. As controlled substances, benzodiazepines are limited in refills and may have storage limitations. You should be familiar with regulations and follow policies and procedures for dispensing benzodiazepines at your practice site.

These drugs can increase heart rate. Patients with heart conditions may not be able to take benzodiazepines and should be monitored closely.

Buspirone A preferred antianxiety medication, **buspirone** works by blocking serotonin receptors in the brain. It is preferred because it is not a controlled substance and does not cause euphoria as do benzodiazepines. Buspirone (BuSpar) is available as tablets for oral administration and is commonly dosed at 15–60 mg a day. Unlike benzodiazepines, which can be taken episodically, buspirone must be taken on a regular basis to be effective.

Professional Focus

Patients who consistently request refills of benzodiazepines a few days early could be exhibiting physical or psychological dependence. Point out these patients to the pharmacist so they can be evaluated. Some patients may need help to stop taking these drugs and may benefit from intervention.

Side Effects Common side effects of buspirone include drowsiness, dizziness, headache, and nausea, all of which may decrease over time. More serious effects include hostility, depression, serotonin syndrome, and extrapyramidal symptoms (see the section on antipsychotics later in this chapter). Patients who experience these effects should see their healthcare providers right away.

Cautions and Considerations Buspirone has been associated with depression and increased suicidal tendencies. Patients should be monitored closely. Counseling should accompany buspirone therapy when warranted. Buspirone interacts with MAOIs and should not be taken with them.

Insomnia

Insomnia is the inability to fall asleep (sleep latency) or stay asleep (sleep maintenance). It often is a symptom of depression, anxiety, and other mental disorders. Sometimes other medical conditions, such as gastric reflux disease, have an impact on the ability to sleep. Other disorders that affect sleep include obstructive sleep apnea, restless legs syndrome, and narcolepsy. However, insomnia is usually a reaction to a stressful situation and simply a disruption in the normal sleep cycle.

Drugs for Insomnia

Treatment for insomnia begins with identifying and eliminating external or medical causes, followed by implementing good **sleep hygiene** (bedtime habits that promote quality sleep). Drug therapy is a last resort, and even then medications should be used short term. The intention is for patients not to use medications on a regular basis.

Drug therapy options begin with OTC antihistamines. Diphenhydramine and hydroxyzine (see Chapter 11) cause drowsiness as a side effect. They may be useful for someone who needs short-term assistance to feel drowsy and fall asleep. However, these agents are not necessarily effective long-term treatment choices for insomnia. TCAs also cause drowsiness and are sometimes used for insomnia, especially if it accompanies depression.

Nonpharmacologic therapy for insomnia includes setting a consistent time for going to bed and waking; using the bedroom only for sleeping; increasing physical activity during the day but not close to bedtime; reducing alcohol, cigarette, and caffeine consumption; eliminating naps; and stopping medications that can affect sleep. If sleep problems continue for longer than two weeks, the patient should see a healthcare provider.

Sleep Aids Ramelteon, a sleep aid, is a selective melatonin agonist that works by mimicking melatonin, one of the body's natural sleep/wake cycle hormones. Eszopiclone, zaleplon, and zolpidem are all sleep aids that are used exclusively for insomnia. They are shorter acting than are benzodiazepines and do not cause as much leftover drowsiness the next day. In some cases, they can be taken in the middle of the night when frequent awakening is a problem (see Table 8.5 for dosing information).

Table 8.5 Common Prescription Sleep Aids

Generic (Brand)	Dosage Form	Route of Administration	Common Dose	Controlled Substance Class
Eszopiclone (Lunesta)	Tablet	Oral	2–3 mg a day	CIV
Ramelteon (Rozerem)	Tablet	Oral	8 mg 30 min prior to bed	Rx
Zaleplon (Sonata)	Capsule	Oral	5–20 mg a day	CIV
Zolpidem (Ambien)	Tablet	Oral	5–12.5 mg	CIV

Side Effects Common side effects of eszopiclone, zaleplon, and zolpidem include headache, drowsiness, dry mouth, dizziness, nausea, hallucination, and memory loss. These agents should be used only short term so that such effects do not pose a problem for long. Some can cause swelling of the face and tongue and difficulty breathing. If patients experience swelling, they should seek medical attention right away. A warning label about drowsiness and caution when driving should be used when dispensing these sleep aids. Although rare, sedatives can cause sleepwalking, and talking and eating while sleepwalking.

May Cause DROWSINESS
Use Caution while Driving

Cautions and Considerations Like the benzodiazepines, eszopiclone, zaleplon, and zolpidem are controlled substances. They should be prescribed for two weeks or less. Ramelteon is not a controlled substance, but it should not be taken with or immediately following a high-fat meal. It interacts with many other prescription drugs that are metabolized through the liver. Pharmacy technicians should take care to get a thorough medication history for all patients taking ramelteon. Patients with liver problems should discuss use of ramelteon with their healthcare providers before taking it.

Bipolar Disorder

Bipolar disorder is related to the dysfunction of neurotransmitters such as GABA, serotonin, and norepinephrine. It is characterized by periods of depression with times of **mania**, during which the patient exhibits irritability, elevated mood, excessive involvement in work or other activities, grandiose ideas, racing thoughts, and a decreased need for sleep. Patients vary in how much they experience mania versus depression. Frequently, other psychoses coexist with bipolar disorder.

Drugs for Bipolar Disorder

Lithium is the primary drug therapy used for bipolar disorder. Some anticonvulsants, such as carbamazepine, lamotrigine, and valproic acid, are used for treating bipolar disorder, but lithium is the drug of choice and is usually prescribed first. Lithium is available in tablet, capsule, and syrup forms for oral administration and commonly dosed at 900–2,400 mg a day. Several atypical antipsychotic agents may be used instead of lithium for bipolar disorder. Lithium is an important mood stabilizer. In patients with bipolar disorder, mood stabilizer therapy must accompany antidepressants during depressive episodes.

Side Effects Common side effects of lithium include nausea, vomiting, dizziness, tremors, fatigue, muscle weakness, a dazed sensation, and increased thirst and urination due to sodium retention. Significant weight gain is also a concern. Serious effects include hypothyroidism, heart arrhythmias, and leukocytosis (an increase in white blood cells). Therefore, patients taking lithium must get regular lab tests to monitor these conditions.

Schizophrenia and Psychosis

The pathophysiology of **schizophrenia** is not fully understood. Although it is related to an imbalance of various neurotransmitters, the processes associated with dopamine and serotonin have been studied the most. In general, schizophrenia is comprised of **positive symptoms** (including hallucinations and delusions) and **negative symptoms** (including withdrawal, ambivalence, behavior changes, memory loss, and confusion). Negative symptoms are associated with thought disorders in which the patient displays language and communication that is illogical, contradictory, irregular, distracting, and tangential. Onset of symptoms usually occurs in the teenage or early adult years. Most often, drug therapy is necessary for patients to maintain normal thought and function. Drugs are usually successful at treating positive symptoms but may not always completely eliminate negative symptoms.

Schizophrenia is one of a variety of psychotic disorders. A few of these related conditions include (1) **reactive psychosis,** which occurs briefly, lasting from only a few hours to just under a month, and then subsides; (2) **delusional disorder,** which is characterized by delusional (but not necessarily illogical) thoughts that last longer than a month but do not impair normal function; and (3) **schizophreniform disorder,** which involves symptoms that are similar to those of schizophrenia but occur for less than six months. When symptoms continue for more than six months and are not the result of illicit or prescription drug use, a formal diagnosis of schizophrenia is made.

Patients with bipolar disorder can struggle with thought disorders, hallucinations, or delusions. For example, half of patients with bipolar disorder will have at least one psychotic symptom at least once in their lifetime. Patients with dementia can also display psychotic symptoms. Psychosis can also be caused by drugs.

Drugs for Schizophrenia and Psychosis

Drug therapy for schizophrenia is highly individualized and often requires changing therapies over time. Doses are slowly increased over weeks to months and then adjusted to achieve a balance between the control of symptoms and minimal side effects. Typical antipsychotics are discussed first in the following section, because they have been available longer than have atypical agents. However, their side effect profiles are problematic and often dose-limiting. Usually, patients are given atypical agents first.

Typical Antipsychotics The mechanisms of action of **typical antipsychotic agents** vary and are not fully elucidated. However, many drugs in this category are phenothiazines or thioxanthenes, which block dopamine receptors that control emotion and thought. Blocking dopamine activity reduces abnormal thoughts and hallucinations but does not always affect other behavior characteristics of schizophrenia, such as withdrawal and ambivalence. Haloperidol is also used for Tourette's syndrome. Prochlorperazine is also used in low doses for nausea and vomiting (see Table 8.6 for more information).

Many of these medications are used for agitation and delirium in patients who do not have schizophrenia. In these cases, lower doses are prescribed to minimize side effects. However, prescribers must be careful about giving these agents to elderly patients in long-term care. This population commonly deals with dementia and its related effects, such as irritability, confusion, and delirium. Antipsychotics can cause excessive dizziness, drops in blood pressure, and falling down. Reduced kidney and liver functions in elderly patients also slow the elimination of the drug. Thus, smaller doses are necessary, and patients must be monitored closely for falls. Laws and regulations govern the use of antipsychotic agents in long-term care settings and limit giving them to patients who are simply wandering, calling out, or agitated. A true medical need, such as behavior that is harmful to the patient or to others, should be present for these agents to be used appropriately in this population.

May Cause DROWSINESS
Use Caution while Driving

Side Effects Common side effects of typical antipsychotics include sedation, dizziness, constipation, dry mouth, blurred vision, weight gain, photosensitivity, and changes in sexual desire or function. Taking these medications at bedtime can help with drowsiness, an effect that gets better with time. Decreases in blood pressure, especially on standing or sitting up, can occur. Patients should rise slowly after sitting or lying down. Older patients should be especially careful until they know how these medications will affect them. When dispensing antipsychotics, an auxiliary label should be used to warn patients about drowsiness.

Typical antipsychotics can cause **extrapyramidal symptoms (EPS) or EPS side effects**. Such effects include tremors, muscular rigidity, and difficulty initiating movement (akinesia). Women tend to have motor restlessness and constant movement of the limbs. These odd movements can make normal activities difficult and embarrassing. Because EPS side effects occur mostly at higher doses, dose amounts are slowly increased. The intention is to gain relief of schizophrenia symptoms without occurrence of significant EPS effects. If necessary, anticholinergic drugs such as dimenhydrinate (Dramamine), diphenhydramine (Benadryl), or benzodiazepines are given to reduce EPS effects.

Another concerning side effect is **tardive dyskinesia**. This late-onset effect causes uncontrollable tongue thrusting and lip smacking. This effect is not always dose-dependent and can even show up months after stopping therapy with a typical antipsychotic. It is sometimes permanent, so typical antipsychotic agents are saved as second-line therapy for schizophrenia.

Table 8.6 Typical Antipsychotics

Generic (Brand)	Dosage Form	Route of Administration	Common Dose
Chlorpromazine (Thorazine)	Tablet, oral solution, syrup, injection	Oral, IM, IV	100–800 mg a day
Haloperidol (Haldol)	Tablet, oral solution, injection	Oral, IM	2–20 mg a day
Mesoridazine (Serentil)	Tablet, oral solution, injection	Oral, IV	50–400 mg a day
Molindone (Moban)	Tablet	Oral	50–225 mg a day
Perphenazine (Trilafon)	Tablet, oral solution, injection	Oral, IM, IV	10–64 mg a day
Prochlorperazine (Compazine)	Tablet, capsule, syrup, injection	Oral, IM	12.5–200 mg a day
Thioridazine (Mellaril)	Tablet, oral solution	Oral	100–800 mg a day
Trifluoperazine (Stelazine)	Tablet, oral solution, injection	Oral, IM	5–40 mg a day

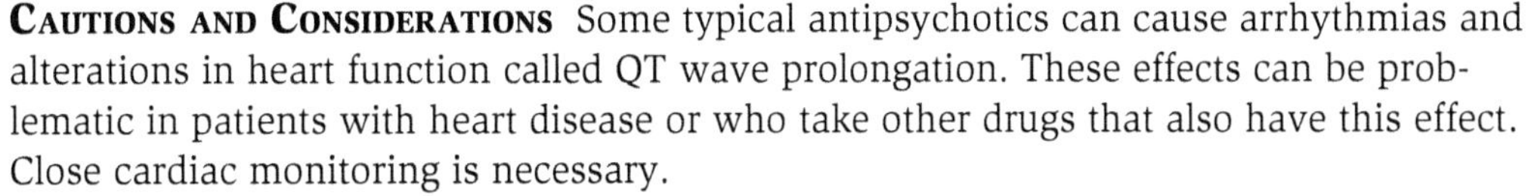

Cautions and Considerations Some typical antipsychotics can cause arrhythmias and alterations in heart function called QT wave prolongation. These effects can be problematic in patients with heart disease or who take other drugs that also have this effect. Close cardiac monitoring is necessary.

Do not drink alcoholic beverages when taking this medication

Patients with liver or kidney problems should not take typical antipsychotics if possible. Typical antipsychotics may also cause bone marrow suppression, a rare but serious effect that may result in underproduction of blood cells. Regular laboratory tests are necessary to monitor for this effect.

Patients should not drink alcohol while taking antipsychotic medications because excessive sedation and hallucinations can occur. An auxiliary warning label to this effect should be used when dispensing these medications.

Atypical Antipsychotics The mechanisms of action for **atypical antipsychotics** are not fully elucidated and vary among agents. Some block dopamine and others enhance it. Atypical antipsychotics are first-line therapy for schizophrenia and other psychoses. Each agent has a variable effectiveness for individual patients. If one agent does not work, others are tried until a medication and dose is found to provide symptom control (see Table 8.7). Side effects are similar to those of typical antipsychotics, but their incidence is lower. They may be effective for the negative symptoms of schizophrenia.

Table 8.7 Atypical Antipsychotics

Generic (Brand)	Dosage Form	Route of Administration	Common Dose
Aripiprazole (Abilify)	Tablet, oral disintegrating tablet, oral solution, injection	Oral, IM	15–30 mg a day
Clozapine (Clozaril)	Tablet, oral disintegrating tablet	Oral	50–500 mg a day
Olanzapine (Zyprexa, Zydis)	Tablet, oral disintegrating tablet, injection	Oral, IM	5–20 mg a day
Paliperidone (Invega)	Tablet	Oral	6–12 mg a day
Quetiapine (Seroquel, Seroquel XR)	Tablet	Oral	150–800 mg a day
Risperidone (Risperdal)	Tablet, oral solution, injection	Oral, IM	1–12 mg a day IM: 25–50 mg every 1–2 weeks
Ziprasidone (Geodon)	Capsule, oral suspension, injection	Oral, IM	40–160 mg a day

May Cause DROWSINESS
Use Caution while Driving

Side Effects Common side effects of atypical antipsychotics include drowsiness, headache, constipation, dry mouth, urinary incontinence or retention, rash, excitation, and occasionally hiccups. Taking these medications at bedtime can help with drowsiness, an effect that gets better with time. Atypical antipsychotic agents can cause EPS side effects, but to a much lesser extent than do typical antipsychotic agents. Quetiapine can increase a patient's risk for cataracts, so regular eye exams are necessary.

Decreases in blood pressure, especially when standing or sitting up, can also occur. Patients should rise slowly after sitting or lying down. Older patients should be especially careful until they know how these medications will affect them.

Significant weight gain occurs for many patients on these medications. This weight gain is often associated with high cholesterol levels and new-onset diabetes. Many patients on atypical antipsychotic agents will need medication for type 2 diabetes.

Some atypical antipsychotics can cause arrhythmias and QT wave prolongation. These effects can be problematic in patients with heart disease. Close cardiac monitoring is necessary.

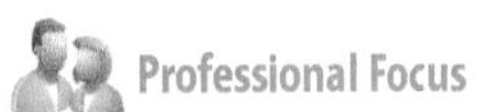

Professional Focus

Zyprexa (an atypical anti-psychotic agent) and Celexa (an SSRI antidepressant) have sound-alike drug names. Be sure you select the correct product when dispensing. A mix-up with these drugs could pose undesirable consequences for the patient.

Cautions and Considerations Atypical antipsychotics can lower seizure threshold, so patients with seizure disorders must be monitored closely when taking these medications. Patients with liver or kidney problems should not take atypical antipsychotics if possible. Some atypical antipsychotics can cause bone marrow suppression, a rare but serious effect. Regular laboratory tests are necessary to check for this condition.

Atypical antipsychotics should be used with caution in elderly patients because excessive dizziness, drops in blood pressure, and sedation can cause falls. Due to reduced kidney and liver functions, elderly patients cannot eliminate these medications well. Smaller doses are necessary, and patients must be monitored closely for falls.

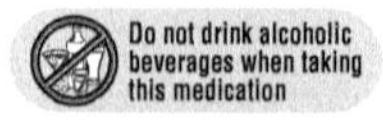

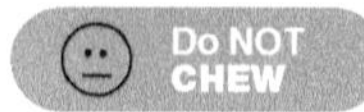

Because patients with schizophrenia or psychosis, at any age, can have thought disorders, it is important for patients to be monitored closely and offered counseling or psychotherapy in addition to drug treatment.

Patients should not drink alcohol while taking atypical antipsychotic medications because excessive sedation and hallucinations can occur. An auxiliary warning label to this effect should be used when dispensing these medications.

Paliperidone comes in extended-release formulations only, so it should not be chewed or crushed.

Clozapine is associated with severe blood disorders affecting blood cell growth and development, so its distribution is limited, and laboratory monitoring of blood work is mandatory. Only certain pharmacies and distributors are allowed to dispense clozapine.

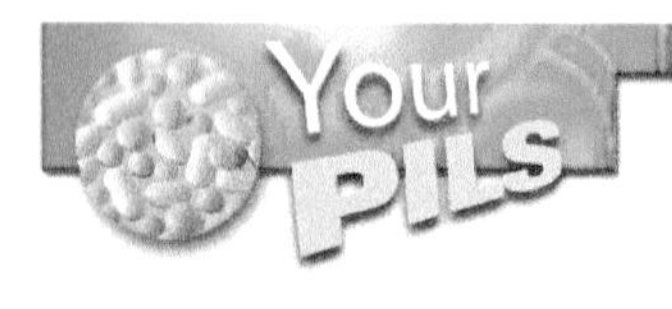

For learners who enjoy group discussion and problem solving, as do Creators and Enactors, find a few classmates and name all side effects for typical and atypical antipsychotic agents. Have you ever witnessed these effects? Share which ones would be most concerning if you had to take one of these drugs yourself.

Herbal and Alternative Therapies

Melatonin is used for a variety of sleep and insomnia disorders as well as for benzodiazepine and nicotine withdrawal. It is used occasionally for a variety of other disorders including headache. Melatonin is a naturally produced hormone that helps regulate circadian rhythms (the sleep–wake cycle). People generally take 0.3–5 mg prior to bedtime to induce sleep. Common side effects include drowsiness, headache, and dizziness. It can also cause mild tremor, anxiety, abdominal cramps, irritability, confusion, nausea, and low blood pressure. Melatonin has interactions with other medications. It should never be taken with CNS depressants or excessive sedation could occur.

Kava is used for anxiety and insomnia. It has been found to be effective but dangerous. Kava can induce hepatotoxicity and liver failure, so patient self-treatment is not recommended. Kava lactone is the active ingredient and is thought to work by affecting GABA and dopamine in the brain. Other side effects include stomach upset, headache, dizziness, drowsiness, dry mouth, and EPS. Patients should also realize that herbal and dietary supplements are not subject to standardization among manufacturers as are prescription and OTC drugs.

St. John's wort is taken orally for mild depression with some success. It has also been used to relieve the psychological symptoms of menopause when used with black cohosh (Remifemin). The active ingredient in St. John's wort is hypericin, which has similar activity to SSRIs. Common doses are 250 mg twice a day or 300 mg three times a day. Side effects include insomnia, vivid dreams, restlessness, anxiety, irritability, stomach upset, diarrhea, fatigue, dry mouth, dizziness, and headache. Usually these effects are mild. St. John's wort can cause photosensitivity, so proper skin protection should be used. St. John's wort should not be taken with other antidepressants because serotonin syndrome could develop. It also should not be taken with CNS depressants, digoxin, phenytoin, or phenobarbital. St. John's wort can alter the effectiveness of these and other drugs, including warfarin and some HIV/AIDS drugs. Patients should discuss St. John's wort with their healthcare providers before taking it.

SAMe is used for mild depression and osteoarthritis. It may also be effective for fibromyalgia. SAMe is produced naturally in the body and supports neurotransmitter formation. It also has anti-inflammatory effects. For depression, dosing is 400–1,600 mg a day. For osteoarthritis, the dose is 200 mg three times a day. Common side effects include gas, nausea, vomiting, diarrhea, constipation, dry mouth, headache, mild insomnia, anorexia, sweating, dizziness, and nervousness. However, this product is usually well tolerated. It should never be taken with other antidepressants.

Patients taking natural products for mood disorders or insomnia should work with their healthcare providers. Symptoms of mental illness should be evaluated by a physician—they should not be self-treated. Herbal and dietary supplements may not adequately treat symptoms of depression or insomnia. Encourage patients to communicate with their healthcare providers.

Chapter Summary

Mental illness is pervasive throughout healthcare, and medications used for these conditions are frequently handled in pharmacy practice. Depression is so common that drugs to treat it are among the top fifty most commonly dispensed drugs in the United States. Medications used for depression primarily include SSRIs, TCAs, and MAOIs. Anxiety is categorized into panic disorder and generalized anxiety disorder. Benzodiazepines, controlled substances with addiction and abuse potential, are used most often for anxiety. They can also be used for insomnia, but normally nonpharmacologic and OTC remedies are tried first. Ramelteon is a new prescription agent for insomnia and enhances melatonin. Other prescription sleep aids include eszopiclone, zaleplon, and zolpidem. Lithium is the drug of choice for bipolar disorder. Drugs for schizophrenia and psychosis are categorized as typical and atypical antipsychotics. These agents have significant side effects, such as those of EPS and tardive dyskinesia. Side effects must be managed in patients who need these valuable drugs for normal life function. Herbal products used for anxiety and insomnia include melatonin and kava. St. John's wort and SAMe are used for mild depression.

✔ Chapter Review

For the following sets of exercises, write the exercise heading, exercise numbers, and your answers on a separate sheet of paper. Your instructor may direct you to turn in the sheet of paper or discuss your answers as a class.

REVIEW THE BASICS

Choose a, b, c, or d as the correct answer to each multiple-choice question.

1. Which of the following responses lists a neurotransmitter and an enzyme that breaks down neurotransmitters in the brain?
   a. norepinephrine, serotonin
   b. dopamine, GABA
   c. norepinephrine, monoamine oxidase
   d. all of the above
2. Someone who has hallucinations, delusions, ambivalence, and withdrawal from reality would most likely have which of the following?
   a. anxiety
   b. mania
   c. bipolar disorder
   d. schizophrenia
3. Paroxetine works by which of the following mechanisms of action?
   a. inhibiting serotonin reuptake
   b. inhibiting reuptake of norepinephrine and serotonin
   c. inhibiting monoamine oxidase from breaking down norepinephrine and serotonin
   d. inhibiting dopamine reuptake
4. Amitriptyline is used for which of the following conditions?
   a. depression
   b. insomnia
   c. bipolar disorder
   d. a and b
5. Which of the following side effects apply to TCAs?
   a. anticholinergic effects
   b. arrhythmias
   c. priapism
   d. all of the above
6. Which of the following antidepressants is also used for smoking cessation?
   a. selegiline
   b. trazodone
   c. bupropion
   d. Celexa
7. Which of the following is the drug of choice for bipolar disorder?
   a. venlafaxine (Effexor)
   b. lithium
   c. valproic acid (Depakote)
   d. phenelzine (Nardil)
8. Which of the following is an atypical anti-psychotic agent?
   a. Ativan
   b. fluoxetine
   c. Haldol
   d. olanzapine
9. Which of the following medications is most likely to cause EPS side effects?
   a. Mellaril
   b. Sonata
   c. trazodone
   d. venlafaxine
10. Which of the following is recommended for mild, short-term insomnia before prescription sedatives are given?
    a. Stelazine
    b. temazepam
    c. diphenhydramine
    d. lithium

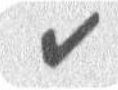

KNOW THE DRUGS

Match each brand name drug with its corresponding generic name and most common use. Your answers should follow this example format: Generic Name: 1. a; 2. b; 3. c; etc. Most Common Use: 1. h; 2. i; 3. j; etc.

Brand Name	Generic Name	Most Common Use
1. Seroquel	a. amitriptyline	h. depression
2. Zoloft	b. diazepam	i. anxiety
3. Elavil	c. quetiapine	j. schizophrenia
4. Celexa	d. olanzapine	k. bipolar disorder
5. Zyprexa	e. citalopram	
6. Ativan	f. lorazepam	
7. Valium	g. sertraline	

PUT IT TOGETHER

For each question, write down either a short answer or a single term to complete the sentence.

1. Which atypical antipsychotic agent is distributed only through select pharmacies and requires strict adherence to laboratory testing to check for blood cell problems? List the drug class and brand/generic names of the other drugs in it.
2. List the brand name and dosage forms in which diazepam is available. What are all of the uses for benzodiazepines?
3. Special laws and regulations limit the use of ____________ for elderly patients in the long-term care setting who exhibit the dementia symptoms of wandering and calling out.
4. Most antidepressant medications take ____________ for the full effect to be felt.
5. List five drugs from this chapter that are controlled substances under Schedule IV.
6. In order to prevent serotonin syndrome, someone taking __________ should not take other antidepressants at the same time or eat foods containing tyramine.

THINK IT THROUGH

Read and think through each numbered scenario carefully and then write several sentences in reply to the question(s) presented. Question 4 requires you to do some Internet research before completing your answer(s).

1. Mrs. Corey comes to the counter to pick up a new prescription for Zoloft 50 mg a day. She started taking Zoloft two weeks ago when her doctor gave her some samples. She also has a bottle of Aleve and St. John's wort in her basket. She says that her new antidepressant is not working that well, and she heard St. John's wort is good for mood. She wants to see whether it will help. What should you do?

2. You call Mr. Johnson to the counter for his new prescription for amitriptyline. When verifying the prescription is for him, you mention the drug name. As you go get the pharmacist for counseling, Mr. Johnson stops you, alarmed at what the prescription is for. He states, "I am getting a prescription for my back pain, not a tranquilizer like amitriptyline. I've heard of that one before. You better clean up your mistake, because that prescription can't be for me." How should you handle this situation?

3. Prochlorperazine is dispensed frequently in low doses in the inpatient setting. If you work in that setting, you will probably handle it often. To what do you contribute the high use of this drug in the hospital setting? What is it being used for, and when should you become concerned about potential overuse?

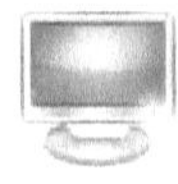

4. **On the Internet**, look up two important organizations that advocate for and work with mental illness. The first is the National Alliance on Mental Illness (NAMI), a grassroots organization for patients and people affected by mental illness. The second is the American Psychiatric Association (APA), where the *Diagnostic and Statistical Manual of Mental Disorders* is published. This reference is the authority in healthcare for diagnosing mental illness.

   Find out how the drugs covered in this chapter are used for other mental illnesses besides those discussed here. As you look through the information provided by these groups, think about their different perspectives (patients versus clinicians). What is mental illness, and what does it mean to patients suffering from it and their healthcare providers treating it? Consider also what some different cultures and religions think about mental illness. As a pharmacy technician dispensing medications for mental illness, you should be aware of the confluence of beliefs and treatments for mental illness. You must be aware of your own stereotypes and preconceptions as you become sensitive to other perspectives.

Chapter 9 Drugs for Pain, Headache, and Anesthesia

LEARNING OBJECTIVES

- Describe the basic anatomy and physiology of the nervous system as it relates to pain, headache, and sensation.
- Explain the therapeutic effects of prescription medications, nonprescription medications, and alternative therapies commonly used for pain, headache, and anesthesia.
- Describe the adverse effects of prescription medications, nonprescription medications, and alternative therapies commonly used for pain, headache, and anesthesia.
- Identify the brand and generic names of prescription and nonprescription medications commonly used for pain, headache, and anesthesia.
- State the doses, dosage forms, and routes of administration of prescription and nonprescription medications commonly used for pain, headache, and anesthesia.

Interactive self-quizzes, games, audio files, and glossaries help you to learn drug names and facts.

Pain is a physiological process regulated by the nervous system. Peripheral nerves sense painful stimuli, and the central nervous system (CNS) perceives and responds to it. Pain is so pervasive in healthcare that it is considered the "fifth vital sign," something that should be assessed in all patients. Whereas acute pain is often the reason patients seek care, chronic pain usually coexists with other conditions. Treating pain is challenging because it is subjective in nature and sometimes involves drug therapy that can promote dependence and addiction. The goal is to gain adequate pain relief without undue misuse, abuse, and addiction.

This chapter explains the physiological process of pain perception, including migraine headache. It also discusses analgesic options for drug therapy, including narcotic medications. Pharmacy technicians should be aware of the desired and undesired effects of pain medications in order to assist patients, pharmacists, and prescribers in achieving overall pain relief. Because many pain drugs are controlled substances, you must be familiar with the legal and ethical ramifications of dispensing them.

Last, this chapter covers anesthesia. Anesthetic drugs work on the sensory nervous system, but they do more than treat pain. Local anesthetic drugs temporarily block or reduce pain, and general anesthetics produce a loss of the conscious sensation of pain. Anesthetic agents produce a total lack of sensation so that procedures including surgery can be performed without discomfort. Pharmacy technicians working in inpatient settings and surgical satellites prepare anesthetic agents on a daily basis.

Anatomy and Physiology of Pain and Sensation

Pain is an unpleasant sensation and an emotional response with an important biological function. It is a normal physiological response to stimuli and usually associated with tissue damage of some kind. The **peripheral nervous system** is responsible for detecting temperature and touch as well as pain. **Sensation** starts with heat, cold, pressure, or chemical stimulus to sensory receptors and nerve endings in the peripheral nervous system. These signals travel up the spinal cord to the cerebral cortex, where sensation is perceived (see Figure 9.1). The peripheral nervous system is also responsible for the five senses (sight, smell, hearing, taste, and touch). Pain alerts the body to harmful injury or inflammation.

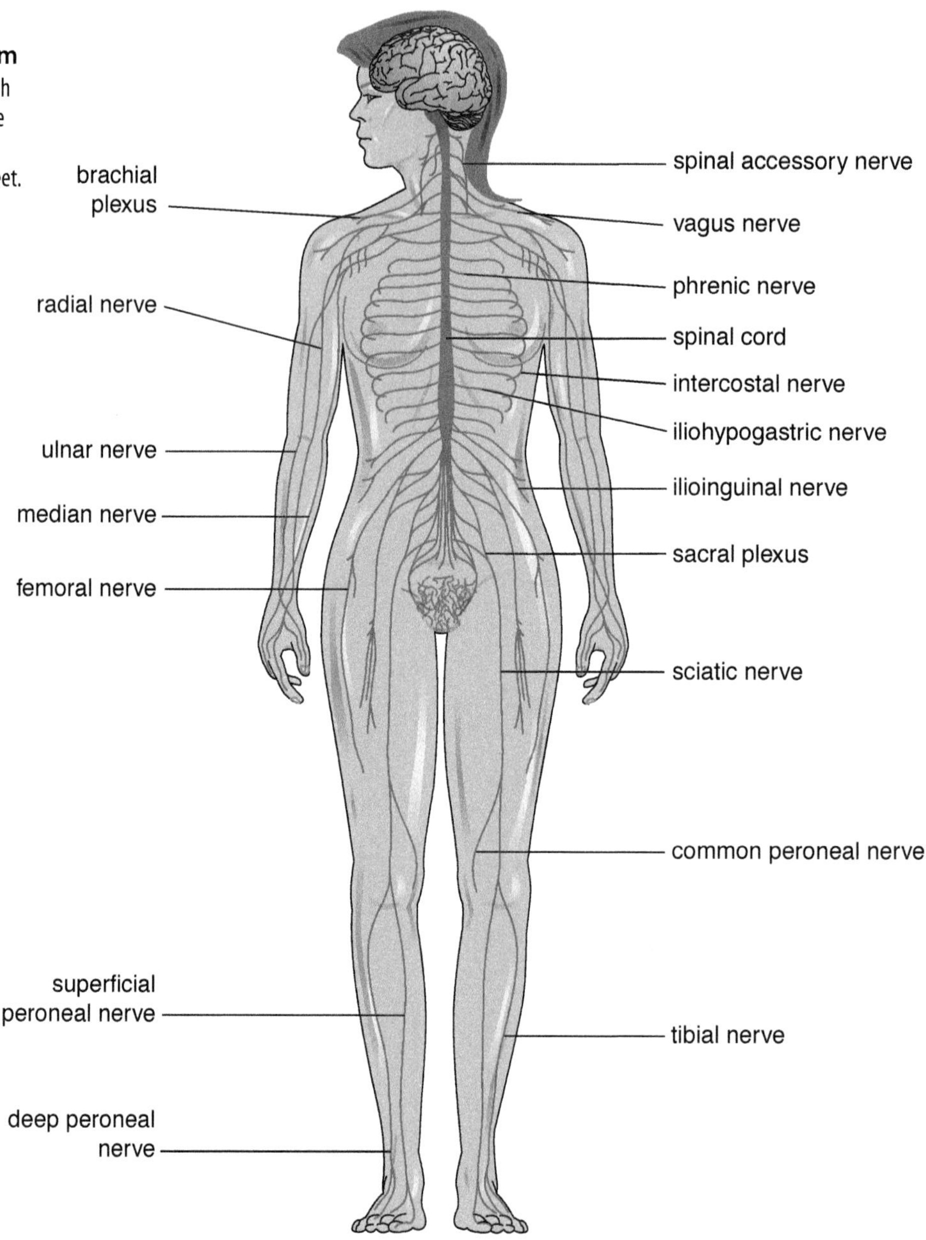

Figure 9.1

Anatomy of the Nervous System

Peripheral nerves commonly associated with neuropathic pain are the sciatic nerve in the legs, the trigeminal nerve in the face (not pictured), and the peroneal nerves in the feet.

Inflammation causes a cascade of events starting with the release of **arachidonic acid**, which is acted upon by the enzyme **cyclooxygenase** to form **prostaglandins** (refer to Figures 3.1 and 6.4). Prostaglandins are chemical triggers for pain and cause local redness and swelling. They are also **pyrogens** (substances that produce fever). Some pain medications, including aspirin and nonsteroidal anti-inflammatory drugs (NSAIDs), treat pain and fever by inhibiting prostaglandin production.

When **pain receptors** are stimulated, and the signal is strong enough to surpass the threshold, the sensation is perceived as pain. Response to **acute pain** involves the sympathetic nervous system: pulse increases, blood pressure rises, breathing speeds up, muscles tense, and pupils dilate (see Chapter 7). Other **physiological responses** include altered stomach and bowel functions, impaired immune response, and even water retention.

Chronic pain lasts longer than three months and may not be associated with sympathetic manifestations such as acute pain. Instead, chronic pain produces a **compensatory response** that involves depression and behavioral adaptation over time. When someone first experiences acute pain, they focus on it, talk about it, cry, moan, rub the painful area, and grimace. Someone with chronic pain may suffer from more subtle changes, for instance feelings of hopelessness, sleep disturbances, lack of facial expression, isolation, fatigue, anger, and physical inactivity.

Pain is also categorized based on where it is generated. **Somatic pain** comes from injury to the body frame, such as to bones and muscles. **Visceral pain** comes from problems with internal organs, such as the kidneys or intestines. Because typical sensory nerves do not receive innervation from these internal organs, pain from this area is experienced differently. Symptoms of visceral pain include nausea, vomiting, and sweating. Patients may also describe the pain as originating somewhere else in the body (referred pain). A classic example is the pain in the left shoulder and arm that accompanies a heart attack.

Neuropathic pain comes from damage to nerve tissue itself. Symptoms include a tingling, burning, or stabbing pain in the area of injury. This type of pain is frequently radiating, meaning that it spreads throughout the area of the body supplied by the injured nerve. For example, nerve compression from an injured disc in the cervical spine may be experienced as pain down the arm of the affected side. Peripheral nerves commonly associated with neuropathic pain are the sciatic nerve in the legs, the trigeminal nerve in the face, and the peroneal nerves in the feet. This kind of pain does not always respond to typical analgesics, so alternative agents (such as antidepressants or anticonvulsants) that alter nerve signal transmission are used. Stress and painful stimuli can trigger damaged nerve tissue to begin firing in a cyclic manner. Patients may be able to reduce the occurrence or severity of these **pain cycles** through nonpharmacologic treatment, such as practicing relaxation techniques, avoiding of known triggers, getting good sleep and rest, and pursuing alternative therapies, like acupuncture.

Last, **sympathetically mediated pain** is associated with nerve overactivity. In this kind of pain, the patient feels pain when there is no obvious stimulus for it. **Phantom limb pain** (in which a patient feels pain in a limb that is no longer there, such as an amputated leg) is an example and a difficult problem to treat. Nerve-blocking agents are sometimes useful for sympathetic pain.

Pain has a huge impact on a patient's quality of life and overall health. It affects the patient's social, emotional, and psychological well-being in addition to causing physical symptoms. Misconceptions create many barriers to detecting and adequately treating pain. In fact, pain is often undertreated. Fear of addiction to medications and the subjective nature of pain make it a challenging condition to treat. In addition, many physicians are reluctant to prescribe adequate amounts of narcotic pain relievers to chronic pain patients for fear of professional disciplinary action. Adequate pain treatment involves a good assessment of the quality, intensity, and location of the pain, along with realistic and appropriate expectations for treatment.

Drugs for Pain

Mild pain can be managed with over-the-counter (OTC) **analgesics**, drugs that treat pain. **Moderate to severe pain**, however, requires prescription medications, many of which are narcotics. **Narcotic analgesics** are natural (e.g., codeine and morphine) or synthetic drugs that have morphine-like activity. All opiates can promote dependence, which can lead to addiction because they produce **euphoric effects** that mimic the natural endorphins that the body makes. **Endorphins** are produced in response to pain and stress in order to help the body deal with pain. Opiates, including natural endorphins, reduce anxiety and feelings of restlessness. They create feelings of well-being and are often abused for these effects. Patients can become dependent and addicted, so narcotics are controlled substances with regulations for handling and storage in the pharmacy.

To understand substance abuse and addiction, you must appreciate the effects of tolerance, dependence, and addiction. **Tolerance** in itself is not bad. It is a process whereby the body becomes less sensitive to the effects of a drug over time. That is, over days and weeks, higher and higher doses are required to produce the same therapeutic effects. Tolerance occurs with many different medications but is not always a precursor to dependence and addiction. For example, although someone using narcotic analgesics for legitimate pain may need more and more over time to achieve adequate pain control, the same is not true for opiates. In fact, the euphoric effects of opiates are not as apparent when they are used for legitimate pain. In such cases of true pain, the long-term use of opiates is not always associated with addiction.

Dependence can be both physiological (i.e., physical) and psychological (i.e., emotional). **Physiological dependence** occurs when the body becomes used to the effects of a drug over time and physically adjusts. When the drug is withdrawn, deleterious physical symptoms occur. For example, chronic use of a narcotic may lead to physical dependence and patients may become quite ill if they suddenly stop taking the drug. Physiological dependence happens with many drugs besides narcotics. For instance, rapid discontinuation of blood pressure medications causes rebound hypertension, and abruptly stopping antidepressants is associated with worsened depression. Sometimes **withdrawal symptoms** are life threatening. In any case, these symptoms are usually unpleasant for the patient, which tends to reinforce continued use of the offending drug.

Psychological dependence is related to the euphoric effects and relief that a patient feels when analgesia for legitimate pain occurs. While psychological dependence does not always lead to addiction, it can contribute. Patients who are physically or emotionally dependent on a medication may or may not need medical assistance to stop therapy when desired. Simply reducing doses slowly over time (called tapering) may avoid or minimize withdrawal symptoms.

Addiction is a compulsive behavioral disorder in which the patient becomes preoccupied with opiates or narcotics above all other drugs. The patient no longer takes the drug as instructed, displays decreased general function and ability to participate in normal life activities, and begins altering normal behavior to obtain more of the drug. Patients who are addicted may see multiple prescribers and visit many pharmacies to satisfy their need for more drug. Patients struggling with addiction will likely need counseling in addition to medical treatment. Patients are usually more successful at overcoming addiction if withdrawal symptoms are treated appropriately. For example, drugs like benzodiazepines can help with alcohol withdrawal. Methadone, a narcotic analgesic with less of a euphoric effect, can be substituted for opiates, including heroin, when addiction is present.

Fear of addiction is a major barrier to adequate pain control. When pain is not adequately controlled, patient behavior can appear to be drug-seeking and inappropriate when instead it is simply an attempt to get adequate pain relief. Pharmacists and technicians can help patients to understand the nature of the tolerance and dependence effects inherent in opiate drug use. Many times, patients believe that tolerance and dependence are addiction, so they resist appropriate therapy. Technicians can assist pharmacists to identify when psychological dependence and addiction are developing. Alerting the pharmacist to such situations will help the pharmacist to make appropriate interventions when needed and to work with prescribers when patient safety is at risk.

Acetaminophen Mild pain and fever can be relieved with **acetaminophen**. It is also used in combination with opiates for moderate to severe pain. Combining this non-narcotic analgesic with opiate drugs achieves pain relief through synergistic drug therapy: Smaller doses are needed and fewer side effects occur with this therapy than by using either agent alone (see Table 9.1). Acetaminophen works by inhibiting prostaglandin production in the CNS. It is especially good for pain associated with headache or osteoarthritis (OA), and for children experiencing pain or fever. Note that acetaminophen, unlike NSAIDs, does not have an appreciable anti-inflammatory effect.

Table 9.1 Acetaminophen and Aspirin Analgesics

Generic (Brand)	Dosage Form	Route of Administration	Common Dose
Acetaminophen (Tylenol, various, acetaminophen) Common abbreviation: APAP	Tablet, orally disintegrating tablet, chewable tablet, liquid, suspension	Oral	650 mg every 4–6 hours (max 4 g a day)
Aspirin (Bayer, Ecotrin, various, aspirin) Common abbreviation: ASA	Tablet, effervescent tablet, suppository	Oral, rectal	325–650 mg every 4–6 hours

Side Effects Common side effects of acetaminophen are few and may include stomach upset or excitation. Usually it is well tolerated.

Cautions and Considerations When taken in high doses (over 4 g a day) or used chronically at daily maximum dose levels, acetaminophen can cause liver toxicity. Intentional overdose can cause permanent liver damage or death. Patients who drink alcohol regularly should limit the total daily dose of acetaminophen to 2 g because serious liver impairment can occur. Acetaminophen should be taken in the lowest doses possible for short-term use, in order to avoid liver damage and toxicity.

Aspirin Mild to moderate pain and fever can be relieved with **aspirin**. It is especially useful for pain associated with inflammation, such as OA and menstrual cramps. It is also used in low doses for stroke and heart attack prevention (see Chapter 12), based upon its ability to make platelet cells less adherent to one another during blood clot formation (thrombogenesis). Aspirin is sometimes used in combination with opiates for moderate to severe pain. Combining this non-narcotic analgesic with opiate drugs relieves pain through synergistic drug therapy. Aspirin works by inhibiting cyclooxygenase, the enzyme that converts arachidonic acid to prostaglandins.

Side Effects Common side effects of aspirin include stomach upset; gastrointestinal irritation, erosion, and bleeding; headache; dizziness; and rash. Taking it with food can help avoid stomach upset and irritation. Signs of bleeding include blood in the urine or stool, black tarry stools, bleeding in the mouth or gums, unusual or unexplained bruising, vomiting blood (which can look like coffee grounds to some people), and nosebleeds. If such effects occur, the patient should see his or her physician. Aspirin should not be used in patients who are already at risk for bleeding, such as during surgical procedures. Patients will usually be instructed to stop taking aspirin prior to the procedure and until well after it.

Aspirin can cause or exacerbate gout. Patients with a history of gout should use other medications for pain or fever relief.

Signs of aspirin toxicity include ringing in the ears (tinnitus), dizziness, and confusion. Patients taking aspirin who experience these effects should stop taking it and contact their healthcare providers.

Cautions and Considerations Aspirin is contraindicated in patients who have asthma or are pregnant. Some patients are allergic to aspirin. You should take a thorough drug allergy history when doing prescription intake. You should inform patients that aspirin is contained in many OTC products. Patients do not always realize this.

When taken for viral infection, aspirin has been associated with **Reye's syndrome**, especially in children. Symptoms of Reye's syndrome include lethargy, confusion, disorientation, agitation, amnesia, seizures, coma, and respiratory failure. Permanent brain damage can occur. Therefore, aspirin is not recommended for use in children with fever or pain. Most pediatric aspirin products have been taken off the market.

Aspirin should not be used by patients with bleeding disorders or a history of ulcers because the risk of severe hemorrhage is too high. For this same reason, patients should not take NSAIDs along with aspirin. NSAIDs not only affect platelet activity and increase bleeding risk, they also compete for activity with aspirin and decrease its effectiveness.

NSAIDs and COX-2 Inhibitors Relief of mild to moderate pain can be achieved with **NSAIDs** and **cyclooxygenase-II (COX-2) inhibitors**. NSAIDs are also used to treat fever. They are especially useful for pain associated with inflammation, such as injuries and some forms of arthritis. Some NSAIDs are used along with opiates for moderate to severe pain. Combining a non-narcotic analgesic with opiate drugs relieves pain through synergistic drug therapy.

NSAIDs work by inhibiting cyclooxygenase I and II, the enzymes that convert arachidonic acid to prostaglandins body-wide. COX-2 inhibitors work by preferentially inhibiting cyclooxygenase II, an enzyme that produces prostaglandins as part of the inflammatory response. COX-2 inhibitors are less likely to inhibit prostaglandin production in gastric mucosa, allowing the protective effects on that tissue to continue. These two drug classes are covered in Chapter 6.

Narcotic Analgesics Relief for moderate to severe pain may require narcotic analgesics, alone or in combination with other analgesics (see Table 9.2). Most narcotic analgesics are opiate derivatives similar in action to **morphine**. Opiates work by inhibiting **mu and kappa opioid pain receptors**. Natural endorphins work at these receptors to produce analgesia and a sense of well-being. When these drugs connect with opioid receptors, pain perception and processing are decreased.

Methadone is used for severe pain relief as well as for drug abuse treatment. Methadone has opiate analgesic effects with fewer euphoric effects. Consequently, it is useful for heroin addiction. Heroin can be a difficult drug to stop using due to severe withdrawal effects and dependence. Patients are switched to methadone, and then doses are slowly tapered. Methadone reduces the patients' preoccupation with where the next "fix" will come from, allowing them to get assistance for their addiction and dependence.

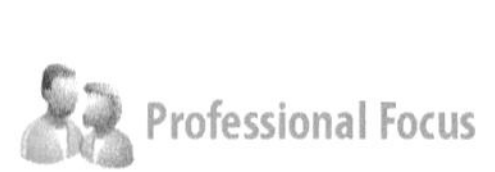

Vicodin and OxyContin are especially sought after on the street market and are targets for theft and robbery. You should be familiar with procedures to maintain safety and security in the pharmacy.

Tramadol is an **opioid analgesic** used for short-term treatment (five days or fewer) of moderate to severe pain. It is an alternative to narcotics when strong pain control is needed but the side effects of opiates are intolerable or addiction potential is high. Tramadol works by modulating serotonin and norepinephrine in addition to blocking mu-opioid receptors, so its effects differ slightly from those of other opioid analgesics. Although tolerance and dependence can occur, tramadol is not typically habit-forming, nor is it a controlled substance in every state.

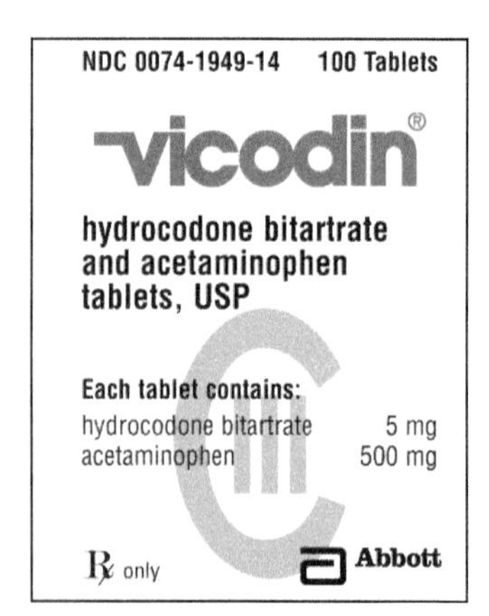

Vicodin, the most frequently dispensed drug in the United States, contains acetaminophen, which can cause liver failure if taken in large doses.

Side Effects Common side effects of narcotic analgesics include sedation, dizziness, stomach upset, fatigue, headache, and constipation. Taking these medications with food may alleviate stomach upset. Patients on high doses or taking a narcotic for longer than a few days may need to take a stool softener to help with constipation. Patients should drink plenty of fluids and maintain good fiber intake to counteract constipation effects. Less common effects include changes in blood pressure and heart rate.

Opiates can cause respiratory depression, especially at high doses. Proper monitoring for respiratory function and rate should be performed for patients who need to take large doses. This effect often worries prescribers and caregivers, especially when treating malignant pain. This type of pain often requires doses in a range that can affect respiration. Although tolerance to this effect can develop, the risks and benefits of therapy must be carefully weighed in these situations.

Some patients experience dysphoria instead of euphoria. In these patients, nausea and vomiting are common side effects. Antiemetic drug therapy may be useful when needed.

May Cause DROWSINESS
Use Caution while Driving

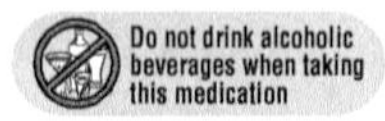

Cautions and Considerations Drowsiness and fatigue can be severe with these agents, so an auxiliary label warning patients about driving or operating machinery should be used when dispensing narcotics.

All narcotics are controlled substances. Technicians must be familiar with legal restrictions for handling and dispensing narcotics in the pharmacy. A warning label to this effect is often affixed to vials containing these medications. Pharmacy personnel must use care and sensitivity so that appropriate analgesia is provided without promoting dependence or abuse.

Because narcotics are nervous system depressants, they should not be used with alcohol because excessive sedation and respiratory depression can occur. A warning label informing patients to avoid alcohol while taking one of these agents is recommended when dispensing.

Table 9.2 Commonly Used Narcotic Analgesics

Generic (Brand)	Dosage Form	Route of Administration	Common Dose	Control Schedule
Acetaminophen + codeine (Tylenol No. 3 and No. 4)	Tablet, capsule, suspension	Oral	1–2 tablets every 3–4 hours (do not exceed 4 g acetaminophen a day)	CIII and CV
Hydrocodone + acetaminophen (Lortab, Vicodin)	Tablet, capsule, solution, elixir	Oral	1–2 tablets/capsules every 4–6 hours (do not exceed 4 g acetaminophen a day)	CIII
Hydrocodone + ibuprofen (Vicoprofen)	Tablet	Oral	1–2 tablets every 4–6 hours	CIII
Hydromorphone (Dilaudid)	Tablet, liquid, injection, suppository	Oral, IM, IV, rectal	1–4 mg every 4–6 hours	CII
Meperidine (Demerol)	Tablet, syrup, injection	Oral, IM, SC	50–150 mg every 3–4 hours	CII
Methadone (Dolophine)	Tablet, oral solution, liquid concentrate, injection	Oral, IM, IV, SC	Varies depending on dosage form and use	CII
Morphine (Duramorph, MS Contin, others)	Tablet, capsule, oral solution, suppository, injection	Oral, IM, IV, IT	Varies depending on dosage form	CII
Oxycodone (OxyContin)	Tablet, capsule, liquid, oral solution	Oral	Acute: 5 mg every 6 hours Chronic: 10–160 mg every 12 hours	CII
Oxycodone + acetaminophen (Percocet, Endocet, Tylox)	Tablet, capsule, oral solution	Oral	1–2 tablets/capsules every 4–6 hours (do not exceed 4 g acetaminophen a day)	CII
Oxycodone + aspirin (Percodan, Endodan)	Tablet	Oral	1–2 tablets every 4–6 hours	CII
Oxymorphone (Opana)	Tablet	Oral	10–20 mg every 4–6 hours	CII
Propoxyphene (Darvon)	Tablet, capsule	Oral	1–2 tablets/capsules every 4 hours	CIV
Propoxyphene + acetaminophen (Darvocet)	Tablet, capsule	Oral	1–2 tablets/capsules every 4 hours	CIV
Tramadol (Ultram)	Tablet	Oral	50–100 mg every 4–6 hours (400 mg a day max)	Rx only
Tramadol + acetaminophen (Ultracet)	Tablet	Oral	2 tablets every 4–6 hours (8 tablets a day max)	Rx only

MS Contin and OxyContin have sound-alike, look-alike names. You should double-check orders and drug selection to be sure you dispense the correct product.

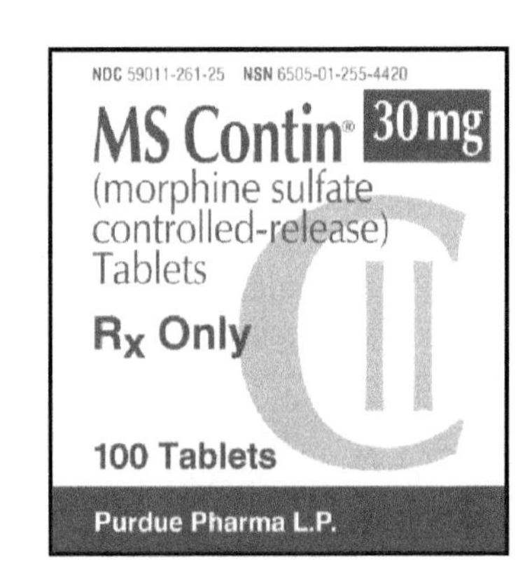

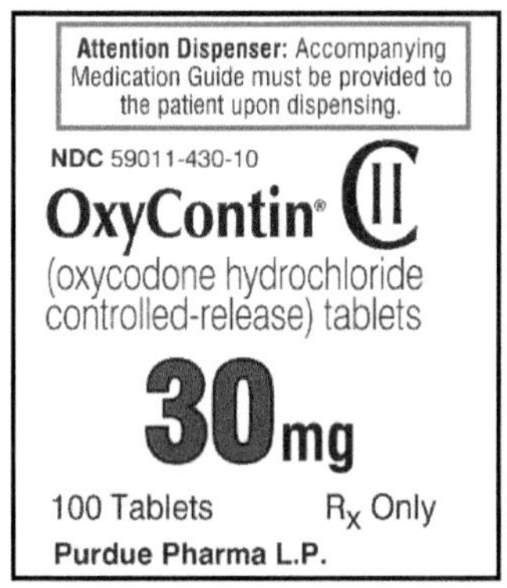

Some narcotic analgesics are intended for chronic pain use, especially when treating malignant pain. Examples include oxycodone (OxyContin) and oxymorphone (Opana). Some of these dosage forms are extended-release formulations and should not be crushed or chewed. Technicians should pay attention to labeling to identify these long-acting dosage forms and apply appropriate auxiliary warning labels as necessary.

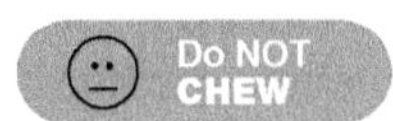

Tramadol can lower seizure threshold, so patients with seizure disorders should discuss therapy with their healthcare providers before taking this medication.

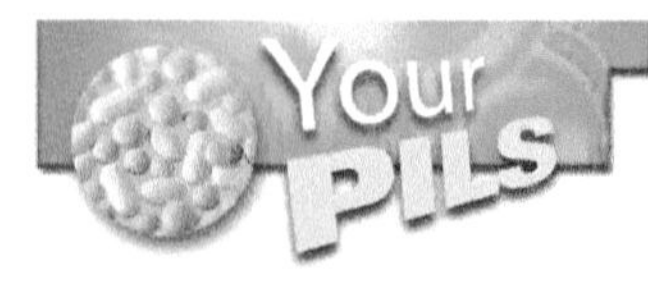

Take a few minutes to search the Internet for information and images of Vicodin and OxyContin, two popular street drugs. Whether you have a flair for the dramatic like Creators or are detail oriented like Producers, you may find the information presented informative. Of course, not everything on the Internet is correct. Next, find the Web site for the Drug Enforcement Agency (DEA) and read up on why the DEA is concerned about diversion and fraudulent prescriptions. Think about your role in preventing prescription drug abuse and diversion.

Neuropathic Pain Agents As mentioned previously, neuropathic pain does not always respond to conventional analgesics. **Gabapentin**, an anticonvulsant, and **tricyclic antidepressants**, including amitriptyline and nortriptyline, are frequently used to treat this type of pain (see Chapters 7 and 8). These agents are usually taken at bedtime on a long-term basis for spinal cord injury, sciatica, trigeminal neuralgia, and diabetic peripheral neuropathy.

Headache

Headache, a specific type and location of pain, is extremely common, affecting millions of patients in the United States each year. Headaches are caused by migraine, tension, or neuralgia, and can also be a side effect of many drugs and other conditions.

Migraine headaches are characterized by a throbbing, unilateral pain in the head that impacts normal activity of life. A migraine is not fully understood but is thought to be a vascular phenomenon caused when cerebral surface blood vessels constrict and then rapidly dilate. Serotonin, a potent vasoconstrictor and neurotransmitter, is possibly involved. Migraines are differentiated from typical headaches by the fact that the patient can also experience nausea, vomiting, and/or sensitivity to light. Increased sensitivity to sound is also common. Migraines are categorized as occurring with or without **aura**. Aura involves vision disturbances, including seeing halos, flashing lights, floating spots, or areas of darkness or blurriness. Aura is associated with the initial blood vessel constriction of migraine and usually precedes other symptoms. Aura is part of the **prodrome** (or early) phase of a migraine and is a warning for patients to seek immediate treatment. Treating migraines involves acute pain medication and abortive therapies. Preventing migraines involves avoiding known triggers including certain foods, stress, sleep deprivation, medications, and environmental irritants. The hormone fluctuations associated with menstrual cycles also trigger migraines in women. Therefore, hormonal regulation and careful timing of preventive drug therapies are employed.

Overuse of pain medication can also cause headaches. This kind of headache occurs in response to withdrawal from prolonged use of acute headache treatment medications. Signs that headaches are due to medication overuse include daily headaches, onset of pain during night or early morning, and onset of pain when preventive headache therapy becomes ineffective. **Medication overuse headache** occurs when triptans are used more than six times a month and other analgesics are used three or more times a day for three to five days a week.

Drugs for Acute Headache

Treatment for headaches caused by stress, tension, or neuralgia can include nonnarcotic or neuropathic pain medications. Migraine headache treatment is different in that it is divided into acute abortive and chronic preventive treatments. When a patient has more than two or three migraines a month, preventive drug therapy is indicated. Otherwise, abortive treatment can be kept on hand for when a migraine occurs. Abortive therapy works best when started within minutes of the first symptoms, preferably during the prodrome or aura phase.

Alternative medications include NSAIDs, ergotamine drugs, and corticosteroids. NSAIDs are covered earlier in this chapter and in Chapter 6, and oral corticosteroids are covered in Chapter 4. These drug classes are considered rescue therapy to assist in pain control when typical abortive therapies at maximum doses are not working. Ergotamines are rarely used and have many side effects and contraindications, so they are not discussed here. Antiemetic drugs are also used for the nausea and vomiting associated with migraines (Chapter 15).

Selective Serotonin Receptor Agonists (Triptans) The class of drugs known as **triptans** is the mainstay of **abortive therapy** for migraine pain. For best results, they must be used at the first sign that a migraine is starting. They begin to work in as little as fifteen minutes and last anywhere from two to several hours. Once severe throbbing pain has started, these agents are not as effective. Each of the triptans has limits on the total number of doses or total dosage that patients can take every twenty-four hours. Injectable forms are used less frequently because fast-acting oral forms have become available (see Table 9.3).

Triptans work by stimulating serotonin receptors to cause vasoconstriction. Constricting cerebral blood vessels counteracts the vasodilation that causes throbbing headache pain.

Table 9.3 Commonly Used Triptans

Generic (Brand)	Dosage Form	Route of Administration	Common Dose
Almotriptan (Axert)	Tablet	Oral	6.25–12 mg, may repeat in 2 hours (12–24 mg max a day)
Eletriptan (Relpax)	Tablet	Oral	20–40 mg, may repeat in 2 hours (80 mg max a day)
Frovatriptan (Frova)	Tablet	Oral	2.5 mg, may repeat in 2 hours (7.5 mg max a day)
Naratriptan (Amerge)	Tablet	Oral	1–2.5 mg, may repeat in 4 hours (5 mg max a day)
Rizatriptan (Maxalt)	Tablet, disintegrating tablet	Oral	5–10 mg, may repeat in 2 hours (30 mg max a day)
Sumatriptan (Imitrex)	Tablet, disintegrating tablet, nasal spray, injection	Oral, nasal, SC injection	PO: 25 mg, may repeat in 2 hours (100 mg max a day) Nasal: 1 spray, may repeat in 2 hours (40 mg max a day) SC: 6 mg, may repeat in 1 hour (12 mg max a day)
Zolmitriptan (Zomig)	Tablet, orally disintegrating tablet, nasal spray	Oral, nasal	PO: 2.5 mg, may repeat in 2 hours (10 mg max a day) Nasal: 5 mg, may repeat in 2 hours (10 mg max a day)

Side Effects Common side effects of triptans include dizziness, hot flashes, tingling, chest tightness, muscle aches, weakness, increased blood pressure, and sweating. When administered by injection, bruising sometimes occurs at the injection site. These effects are normal; if they are bothersome, alternative therapy will be needed. You should use an auxiliary warning label for dizziness when dispensing triptans.

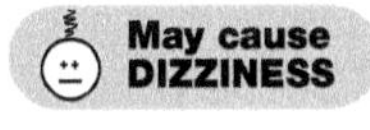

Cautions and Considerations Patients with high blood pressure, heart disease, or angina should not take triptans because these drugs can worsen these conditions. Patients taking monoamine oxidase inhibitors (MAOIs) should not use triptans because serotonin syndrome could occur. Patients on ergotamine drug therapy should not take triptans. Ergotamine therapy is saved for when triptans do not work.

Professional Focus
Many health insurance plans limit the number of tablets of triptan medication a patient can get a month. You can help patients understand these limitations and assist them in avoiding undesirable frustration when they are receiving refills.

Combination Agents Combinations of non-narcotic analgesics and **caffeine** are used to treat mild migraine headaches. Using analgesics from multiple classes attacks pain from different mechanisms, producing an advantage due to the effects of synergistic drug therapy. Caffeine is sometimes combined with other analgesics (see Table 9.4) because it improves pain control by constricting blood vessels, but to a lesser extent than do triptans.

Barbiturate products are controlled substances that are sometimes used for migraines. Only a few such products are used for acute headache pain. Butalbital is available in combinations with acetaminophen and caffeine or aspirin. It is used for tension and migraine headache pain. Butorphanol, a mixed opiate receptor agonist-antagonist, is a nasal spray useful for migraine headache pain and is also available for IM and IV administration.

Side Effects Common side effects of non-narcotic analgesics include drowsiness, dizziness, confusion, nervousness, skin rash, nausea, vomiting, heartburn, and constipation. If severe, these effects can limit therapy.

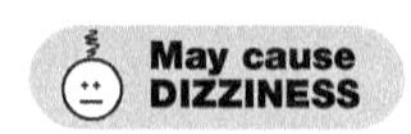

Common side effects of barbiturate-containing medications include drowsiness, dizziness, stomach upset, nasal congestion, and "hangover" feelings the following day. Therefore, these medications should be used with caution and on a limited basis only when needed.

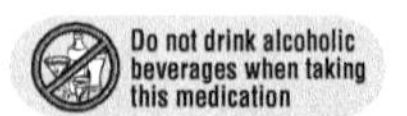

Cautions and Considerations Warning labels alerting patients to the drowsiness and dizziness effects of barbiturate and opiate medications are important. Patients should be warned not to drink alcohol while taking these medications because these effects could worsen.

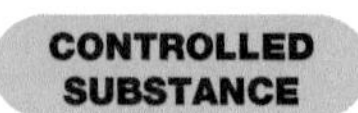

Barbiturates and opiates produce tolerance and dependence, so they may be habit forming. Appropriate auxiliary warning labels should be used to reinforce that patients need to know the risks of taking these medications. Limited and short-term use, only when needed is recommended.

Patients allergic to aspirin or NSAIDs should not take combination products with aspirin.

Table 9.4 Commonly Used Combination Products for Headache Pain

Generic (Brand)	Dosage Form	Route of Administration	Common Dose
Acetaminophen + aspirin + caffeine (Excedrin Migraine)	Tablet, caplet	Oral	Acetaminophen 500 mg Aspirin 500 mg Caffeine 130 mg
Isometheptene + dichloralphenazone + acetaminophen (Midrin)	Capsule	Oral	Isometheptene 130 mg Dichloralphenazone 200 mg Acetaminophen 650 mg
Barbiturates and Opiates			
Butalbital + acetaminophen + caffeine (Fioricet, various) CIII	Capsule, tablet, liquid	Oral	Butalbital 50 mg Acetaminophen 325–650 mg Caffeine 40 mg
Butalbital + aspirin (Fiorinal) CIII	Capsule, tablet	Oral	Butalbital 50 mg Acetaminophen 325 mg Caffeine 40 mg
Butorphanol (Stadol) CIV	Nasal spray, injection	Nasal, IM, IV	Nasal: 1 spray in 1 nostril, may repeat in 60–90 minutes IM/IV: 1–4 mg every 3-4 hours

Drugs for Headache Prevention

Preventive drug therapy is indicated when migraines affect normal life activities and occur more than twice a month. These drugs are taken daily or at regular intervals to prevent migraines from occurring as often. Migraine prevention drugs include beta blockers (see Chapter 7), antidepressants (tricyclics and serotonin reuptake inhibitors; see Chapter 8), anticonvulsants (valproic acid, topiramate, and gabapentin; see Chapter 7), calcium-channel blockers (verapamil and nimodipine; see Chapter 12), and NSAIDs (see Chapter 6). The importance of preventive therapy should be emphasized because it can greatly improve a patient's quality of life, increase productivity, and decrease time missed from work.

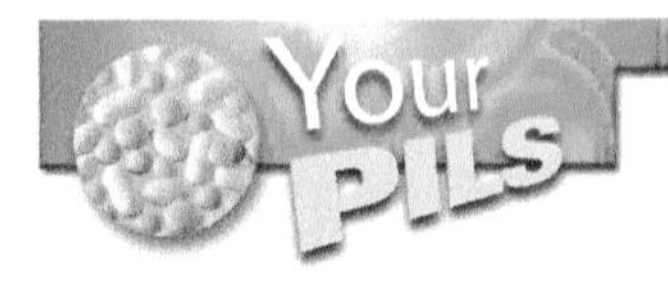

While all learners may find this exercise useful, Producers and Directors may find it matches their learning styles best. Make a set of painkiller flash cards. Use a differently colored card for each location in which you find these products (i.e., OTC aisle, prescription drug stock shelves, and locked cabinet/room for controlled substances). Assign each drug class (NSAIDs, narcotics, non-narcotics, triptans, and combination products) a different color of ink. Write the brand name on one side, and the generic name on the other side. Use your cards to quiz yourself and classmates. Keep them in your pocket as a reference for when you put away drug orders from wholesalers.

Anesthesia

Anesthesia inhibits sensation and pain during procedures such as surgery, dental work, and colonoscopy. Anesthetics are also used during obstetric and diagnostic procedures. Depending on the type of procedure, a general or local anesthetic will be used.

General anesthesia affects the entire body, and loss of consciousness occurs. Body-wide, skeletal muscle relaxes, and the patient has no memory of the event upon recovery. General anesthesia affects respiratory function and urination. Breathing slows, respiratory mucus production increases, and urination stops. Cardiac function slows, causing a decrease in blood pressure. Therefore, general anesthesia requires close monitoring of blood pressure, ventilation, pulse rate, oxygen level in the blood, and urinary output.

In contrast, **local anesthesia** affects only a select part of the body, causing loss of pain, tactile sensation, and temperature sensation. Skeletal muscle in the anesthetized area also relaxes. A person receiving local anesthesia may also lose the ability to recognize body position in that area. However, the patient does not lose consciousness and recalls everything that happened during the procedure.

For short diagnostic procedures or to enhance relaxation, pain control, and amnesia associated with surgery, **preanesthetic medications** are used. Selected benzodiazepines (see Chapter 8) and narcotic pain medications are frequently used in advance of general anesthesia. The most common preanesthetics are midazolam (Versed), diazepam (Valium), and lorazepam (Ativan), followed by fentanyl in various forms. These agents are administered systemically, so they alter consciousness and cause amnesia. They reduce patient anxiety and resistance to therapy.

General Anesthetics

General anesthetics are used for surgery and other procedures for which overall muscle relaxation is necessary to keep the patient still during manipulation. With one exception (nitrous oxide), these agents cause loss of consciousness. Nitrous oxide is used during dental procedures to relax patients and provide analgesia. General anesthetics are available in inhaled and injectable forms. Although these agents have varying lengths of effect, most act for only a few minutes. Therefore, an anesthesiologist or anesthetist administers and adjusts these medications throughout the procedure to individualize therapy and achieve proper sedation, relaxation, analgesia, and ventilation.

Inhaled anesthetics are stored in steel containers as compressed gas or liquid and then inhaled through a face mask. Most reduce blood pressure, so concomitant intravenous (IV) fluids must be given to counteract this effect. Technicians do not handle inhaled anesthetics but may prepare the IV fluids that accompany them. **Injectable anesthetics** are administered via continuous infusion. Pharmacy technicians working in surgical satellites prepare these agents (see Table 9.5 for information on commonly used general anesthetics).

Table 9.5 Commonly Used General Anesthetics

Generic (Brand)	Dosage Form	Control Schedule
Inhaled Agents		
Desflurane (Suprane)	Gas	
Enflurane (Ethrane)	Gas	
Halothane	Gas	
Isoflurane	Gas	
Nitrous oxide	Gas	
Injectable Agents		
Etomidate (Amidate)	IV	
Ketamine (Ketalar)	IV	CIII
Methohexital (Brevital)	IV	CIV
Propofol (Diprivan)	IV	
Sufentanil (Sufenta)	IV	CII
Thiopental (Pentothal)	IV	CIII

Side Effects Common side effects of anesthetics are nausea, vomiting, decreased blood pressure, and reduced renal function. Antiemetic medications are often ordered along with anesthetics to alleviate nausea. IV fluids are coadministered to counteract drops in blood pressure and reduced renal function.

Respiratory function is usually suppressed during general anesthesia. Because breathing slows and respiratory secretions increase, proper ventilation must be monitored throughout the procedure, and oxygen is sometimes given.

Cautions and Considerations General anesthesia can lower seizure threshold, so anticonvulsants may be ordered along with these agents. General anesthesia should be avoided when possible in patients with seizure disorders.

A rare but life-threatening effect of certain general anesthetics is **malignant hyperthermia**. Body temperature rises suddenly and rapidly to dangerous levels, accompanied by heart arrhythmias, difficulty breathing, and muscle rigidity. Hyperthermia is caused by a marked increase in intracellular calcium. Dantrolene, an intracellular calcium blocker, is used to treat malignant hyperthermia (see Chapter 10). One serious potential aspect of malignant hyperthermia is rhabdomyolysis. In this process, skeletal muscle is degraded, and the breakdown products can lead to acute renal failure. Pharmacy technicians are responsible for stocking and maintaining dantrolene in emergency drug kits in the surgical suite. Vials of this drug must be checked frequently for expiration date to ensure they will be effective when needed in emergency.

Local Anesthetics

When loss of sensation is desired in a defined area of the body, **local anesthetics** are used. Procedures such as dental work, stitches, and sutures may require local anesthetic action. These agents come in a variety of dosage forms to accommodate the level of anesthesia needed in the location and size of area being treated (see Table 9.6). For instance, they can be used topically for pain and burn relief, injected locally for dermatologic procedures, and injected as epidurals for obstetrical procedures (i.e., cesarean delivery).

Local anesthesia works by depressing first the nerve activity of small axons, followed by that of larger myelinated nerve fibers. Time of onset is usually within a few minutes, but length of action depends on drug choice, drug concentration, and the size of the area to which the drug is administered. **Esters** are short-acting drug molecules metabolized by local tissue fluids, whereas **amides** are longer-acting drug molecules metabolized in the liver.

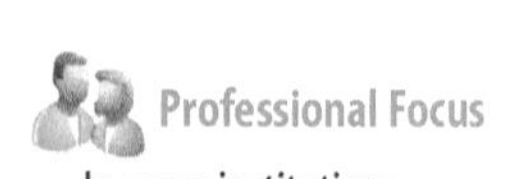

In some institutions, cocaine is used as a nasal anesthetic for sinus procedures. Cocaine is a Schedule II controlled substance and has significant restrictions for storage and use. If you work at such an institution, follow the special procedures for handling, preparing, and dispensing cocaine preparations.

Side Effects Common side effects of local anesthetics include allergic reaction, skin rash, and swelling at the application site. These are usually mild. If allergy to one chemical form (e.g., an ester) occurs, the alternate form (amide) should be used instead.

Other side effects include CNS excitation. Symptoms include anxiety, nervousness, confusion, and possibly seizure. These effects can be treated by diazepam. Sometimes these symptoms are followed by CNS depression, including sedation, loss of consciousness, and respiratory or cardiac arrest. These effects are life threatening, and patients must receive medical treatment immediately.

Occasionally, local anesthetics are absorbed into the bloodstream and cause cardiac arrhythmias. Thus, the lowest dose is administered to the smallest area possible.

Cautions and Considerations When absorbed systemically, local anesthesia can lower seizure threshold. Patients with seizure disorders should consult their prescribers before receiving any prescription-strength local anesthetics.

Table 9.6 Commonly Used Local Anesthetics

Generic (Brand)	Dosage Form	Prescription Status
Esters		
Benzocaine (Auralgan, Dermoplast, Solarcaine, Lanacane)	Cream, eardrops, gel, lozenge, ointment, spray, topical liquid	OTC
Chloroprocaine (Nesacaine)	IT	Rx
Dyclonine (Cepacol)	Topical liquid	OTC
Procaine (Novocain)	Injection, IV	Rx
Tetracaine (Pontocaine)	Injection	Rx
Amides		
Bupivacaine (Marcaine)	Injection	Rx
Levobupivacaine (Chirocaine)	Injection, IV	Rx
Lidocaine (Solarcaine)	Cream, gel, oral solution, topical spray	OTC
Lidocaine (Xylocaine)	Injection, IV	Rx
Lidocaine + prilocaine (EMLA)	Cream	Rx
Mepivacaine (Carbocaine)	Injection, IV	Rx

Analgesic and Anesthetic Antagonists

Naloxone (Narcan) is an opiate receptor antagonist that counteracts opioid pain and preanesthetic medications. It is used to reverse opiate effects in intentional and accidental overdoses. **Flumazenil** (Romazicon) is a benzodiazepine receptor antagonist used to reverse excessive sedation. It is used to speed recovery of consciousness in accidental or intentional overdose situations. It is also used in managing overdose of benzodiazepines. Both agents are usually given in the emergency or operating rooms.

Herbal and Alternative Therapies

Caffeine is a CNS stimulant used in combination with other analgesics for headache. It is also used some for fatigue and drowsiness in doses of 100–200 mg. It should not be used more than every three to four hours. It is available in tablets, capsules, and lozenges. Side effects include rapid heartbeat, palpitations, insomnia, restlessness, ringing in the ears, tremors, lightheadedness, nausea, vomiting, stomach pain, and itchy rash. Taking it with food can help with these effects, and normally doses should be decreased if such effects occur.

Capsaicin is a chemical derived from cayenne peppers. It is used as a topical treatment for pain. It has been found to be effective in diabetic neuropathy, arthritis, and headache pain. It works by exhausting the supply of substance P, a substrate in pain nerve endings in the skin. At first, burning, itching, and tingling occurs, and then analgesic effects take hold once substance P is depleted. If taken orally, inhaled, or touched to the eye, severe burning can occur. Patients should wear gloves during application and wash their hands thoroughly afterward to avoid these effects.

Feverfew is a plant product used orally for migraine pain. It is occasionally used for other pain conditions, including menstrual cramps and arthritis. It has been found to improve nausea, vomiting, and the sensitivity to light experienced during migraine. Feverfew is generally well tolerated, but side effects include heartburn, nausea, diarrhea, constipation, abdominal pain, and gas. Chewing on feverfew leaves has caused mouth ulceration. Feverfew is taken 50–100 mg daily to prevent migraine, rather than treating migraine once it has already started.

Chapter Summary

The peripheral nervous system is responsible for transmitting signals to the brain, where they are interpreted as pain. Pain is a useful biological response to harmful stimuli. It is categorized in multiple ways that help guide treatment. Acute pain is felt in response to injury to tissue and usually subsides as healing occurs. Chronic pain is a long-term condition that can cause depression in addition to the physical responses normally associated with pain. Pain is also categorized based on where it occurs. Headache pain is specifically associated with constriction and dilation in the cerebral vasculature. Treatment for migraine headache pain is categorized into abortive and preventive modalities. Triptans are the mainstay of abortive migraine treatment.

Analgesia usually starts with non-narcotic medications such as aspirin, acetaminophen, or NSAIDs. When pain is moderate or severe, narcotic medications may be necessary. These medications have side effects including drowsiness and respiratory depression and have a tendency to promote tolerance and dependence. Their euphoric effects make narcotic analgesics a target for abuse and misuse. Pharmacy technicians must be aware of special handling requirements and restrictions for these controlled substances. Natural and herbal products for pain include caffeine, capsaicin, and feverfew.

Anesthesia is the loss of sensation to touch and pain and is used for procedures such as surgery or dental work. General anesthesia involves a loss of consciousness; local anesthesia results in a loss of sensation in a specific area of the body. General anesthetics are either intravenous or inhaled, whereas local anesthetics are either topical or injected. Pharmacy technicians prepare anesthetics in the inpatient setting.

Chapter Review

For the following sets of exercises, write the exercise heading, exercise numbers, and your answers on a separate sheet of paper. Your instructor may direct you to turn in the sheet of paper or discuss your answers as a class.

REVIEW THE BASICS

Choose a, b, c, or d as the correct answer to each multiple-choice question.

1. Which of the following effects would be considered a physiological response to acute pain?
   a. decreased pulse
   b. increased blood pressure
   c. depression
   d. all of the above
2. Which of the following would be considered a response to chronic pain?
   a. depression
   b. sleep disturbances
   c. physical inactivity
   d. all of the above
3. Which of the following best describes how narcotic analgesics work?
   a. activation of mu opiate receptors
   b. blockade of mu opiate receptors
   c. activation of kappa opiate receptors
   d. blockade of kappa and mu opiate receptors
4. Which of the following drugs works best if used as soon as the first symptoms (aura) associated with a migraine appear?
   a. aspirin
   b. methohexital
   c. rizatriptan
   d. propoxyphene
5. Which of the following is a common side effect of opiate drugs?
   a. constipation
   b. drowsiness or sedation
   c. nausea/vomiting
   d. all of the above
6. Which of the following drugs interacts with opiates to cause further CNS depression?
   a. alcohol
   b. isometheptene + dichloralphenazone + acetaminophen
   c. acetaminophen
   d. all of the above
7. Which of the following is/are a CII narcotic?
   a. propoxyphene
   b. oxycodone/acetaminophen
   c. hydrocodone/acetaminophen
   d. all of the above
8. Which of the following is used topically to treat neuropathic pain?
   a. caffeine
   b. capsaicin
   c. benzocaine
   d. none of the above
9. Which of the following is an injectable anesthetic?
   a. propofol
   b. halothane
   c. naloxone
   d. benzocaine
10. Which of the following anesthetics is used for local anesthesia?
    a. methohexital
    b. desflurane
    c. lidocaine
    d. etomidate

KNOW THE DRUGS

Match each brand name drug with its corresponding generic name and most common use. Your answers should follow this example format: Generic Name: 1. a; 2. b; 3. c; etc. Most Common Use: 1. h; 2. i; 3. j; etc.

Brand Name	Generic Name	Most Common Use
1. Xylocaine	a. oxycodone	h. Migraine
2. OxyContin	b. sumatriptan	i. Mild pain
3. Ultram	c. lidocaine	j. Moderate to severe pain
4. Suprane	d. desflurane	k. General anesthesia
5. Ecotrin	e. aspirin	l. Local anesthesia
6. Axert	f. almotriptan	
7. Imitrex	g. tramadol	

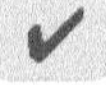

PUT IT TOGETHER

For each item, write a single term to complete the sentence, match each term with its correct description, or supply a short answer.

1. ______________ pain often requires drug therapy outside of the typical analgesics, such as an antidepressant or anticonvulsant agent.

2. ________________ is considered a mixed opiate receptor agonist-antagonist analgesic for migraine pain and is available as a nasal spray.

3. Match each of the following terms with its correct description.

   _____ Addiction

   _____ Dependence

   _____ Tolerance

   a. physiological process in which the body becomes used to drug effects and needs higher and higher doses to produce the same effect
   b. physiological process in which withdrawal symptoms will occur if the drug is discontinued
   c. compulsive psychological disorder in which a person is preoccupied with drug use

4. ________________ is a local anesthetic that is available via prescription and over the counter. What are the brand names for the prescription and OTC versions of this drug?

5. List all of the narcotic analgesics (brand names) that also contain acetaminophen.

THINK IT THROUGH

Read and think through each numbered scenario carefully and then write several sentences in reply to the question(s) presented. Question 4 requires you to do some Internet research before completing your answer(s).

1. Name three medications that are controlled substances used for migraine or headache pain. Identify their brand and generic names. How do these agents differ from other acute treatments, such as the serotonin receptor agonists? What limitations do these products have?
2. Describe how nitrous oxide differs in action and use from isoflurane, methohexital, novocaine, and benzocaine. Which of these four products is a pharmacy technician most likely to prepare?
3. Mrs. Martin comes to pick up her prescription for Darvocet and adds a bottle of Excedrin to ring up with her purchase. She has been a regular customer for years and takes Darvocet for back pain from severe osteoporosis. What should you do?

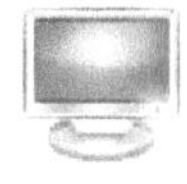

4. **On the Internet,** look up news reports on the Tylenol product recalls of 2010, 2009, and 1982. As a technician, you will be responsible for pulling recalled items from the OTC shelves and may receive inquiries from patients about this product. What was the nature of these recall efforts? What happened, and how did the company respond? What was the impact of these events?

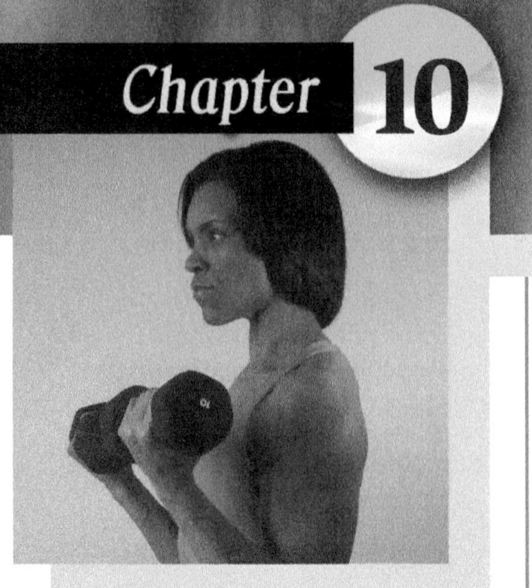

Chapter 10 The Muscular System and Drug Therapy

LEARNING OBJECTIVES

- Describe the basic anatomy and physiology of the muscular system.
- Explain the therapeutic effects of prescription medications, nonprescription medications, and alternative therapies commonly used to treat diseases of the muscular system.
- Describe the adverse effects of prescription medications, nonprescription medications, and alternative therapies commonly used to treat diseases of the muscular system.
- Identify the brand and generic names of prescription and nonprescription medications commonly used to treat diseases of the muscular system.
- State the doses, dosage forms, and routes of administration of prescription and nonprescription medications commonly used to treat diseases of the muscular system.

Interactive self-quizzes, games, audio files, and glossaries help you to learn drug names and facts.

Muscles give us the ability to move and react to the environment. Everything from running and jumping to smiling and sitting upright requires muscle tone and movement. Unfortunately, muscle injuries are also a common part of life. Trauma, neck strains, and back problems frequently necessitate prescriptions for muscle relaxants, making them some of the most commonly ordered prescriptions in the United States. Pharmacy technicians are involved in dispensing prescriptions and assisting patients with over-the-counter remedies for muscular injuries on an almost daily basis in community pharmacy.

This chapter begins with an overview of the types and functions of muscles. Knowing specific muscle location is essential to administering intramuscular (IM) drug therapy such as vaccines. Understanding drug therapies for lower back and sports injuries is important because these conditions are common. Advertising and media have popularized Botox injections for cosmetic use. However, this locally acting muscle relaxant is covered only briefly because it is rarely dispensed in the pharmacy. A few specialized muscle relaxants and neuromuscular blockers are also discussed.

Anatomy and Physiology of the Muscular System

The **muscular system** is responsible for movement, posture, and (to a great extent) body heat. It is divided into three types of muscle: skeletal, cardiac, and smooth (see Figure 10.1 for a comparison). **Skeletal muscles** are connected to bones and joints by tendons and provide voluntary movement, such as walking, clapping, and chewing. Bodybuilding and performance training in sports focus on developing and enhancing skeletal muscles.

Cardiac muscle is found only in the heart. These muscle cells are specifically designed for the pumping and squeezing action required for each heartbeat. Cardiovascular activities such as aerobics and jogging exercise the cardiac smooth muscle by raising the heart rate.

Smooth muscle can be found in the intestines and blood vessel walls. These cells are designed for **peristalsis**, a kind of movement that pushes material through tubes, such as when food progresses through the intestines or blood flows through the vasculature. These muscles are involuntarily controlled by the autonomic nervous system (see Chapter 7).

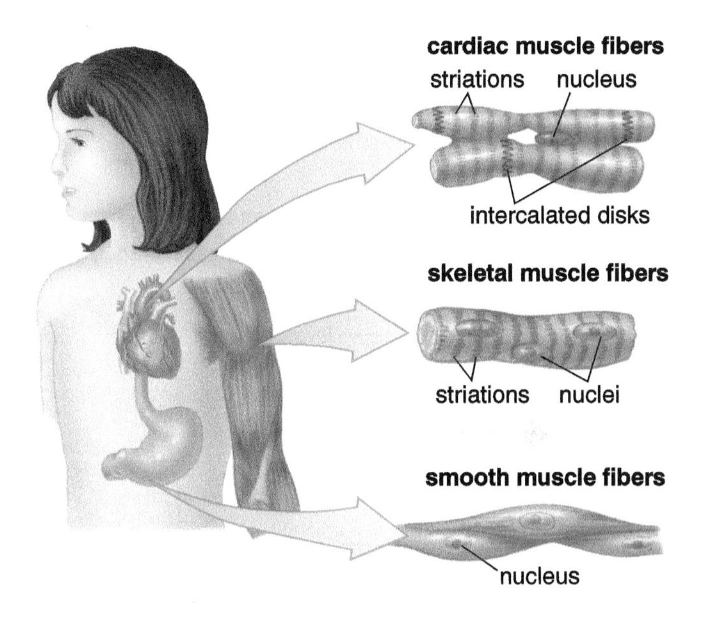

Figure 10.1
Types of Muscle Tissue
Under the microscope, both cardiac and skeletal muscles appear to have stripes called striations.

The **neuromuscular junction** (see Figure 10.2) is where nerve cells interface with muscle cells to initiate muscle contraction. **Acetylcholine (ACh)** is a neurotransmitter that is released from the nerve cell, travels across the synaptic cleft, and stimulates muscle cell receptors to cause membrane depolarization. **Depolarization** changes the balance of positive and negative electrical charges along the membrane surface and opens channels, allowing sodium (Na) to enter. **Sodium influx** causes the release of the **intracellular calcium** stores that stimulate muscle fiber contraction. **Muscle fibers** contract and shorten the muscle, which in turn pulls on attached bones and joints, creating movement. Muscle contraction stops when ACh is deactivated in the synaptic cleft by **acetylcholinesterase,** an enzyme that inactivates acetylcholine.

The muscles most relevant in the study of drug therapy are those that are commonly injured (see Figure 10.3) and those that are used for IM drug administration. **Intramuscular injections (IM injections)** are administered to adults in the **deltoid** of the upper arm and the **gluteus medius** in the buttocks. In children, injections are often given in the vastus lateralis, a muscle group in the quadriceps group of the legs. Up to 2 mL of a drug can be injected into the deltoid muscle and vastus lateralis, and up to 5 mL can be injected into the gluteus medius.

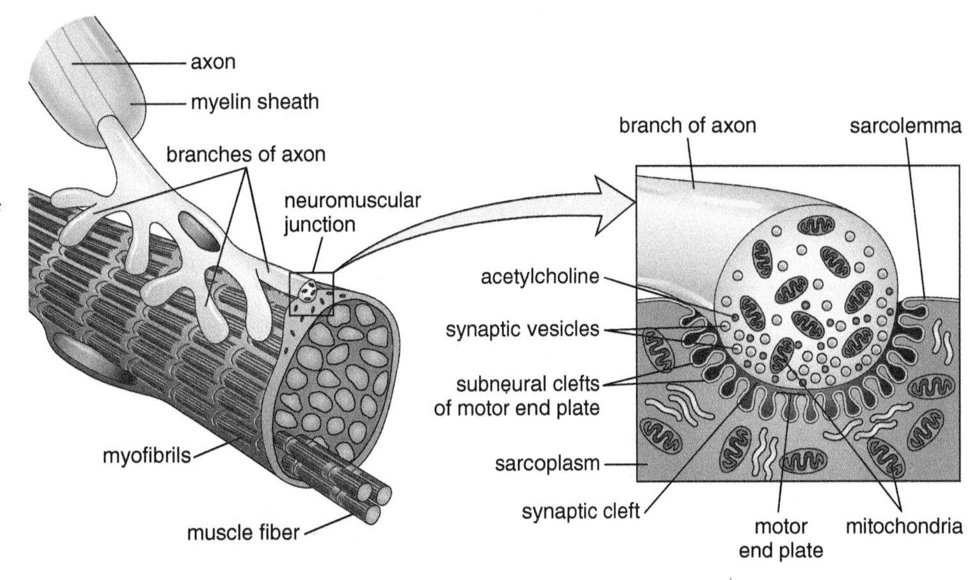

Figure 10.2
Neuromuscular Junction
The energy needed for muscle contraction comes from breaking the chemical bond that holds a phosphate functional group to adenosine triphosphate (ATP) molecules inside of muscle cells.

Figure 10.3

Anatomy of the Muscular System

Muscles commonly injured or strained tend to be those of the lower back (latissimus dorsi), head and neck (trapezius), and legs (hamstring group, quadriceps, and soleus).

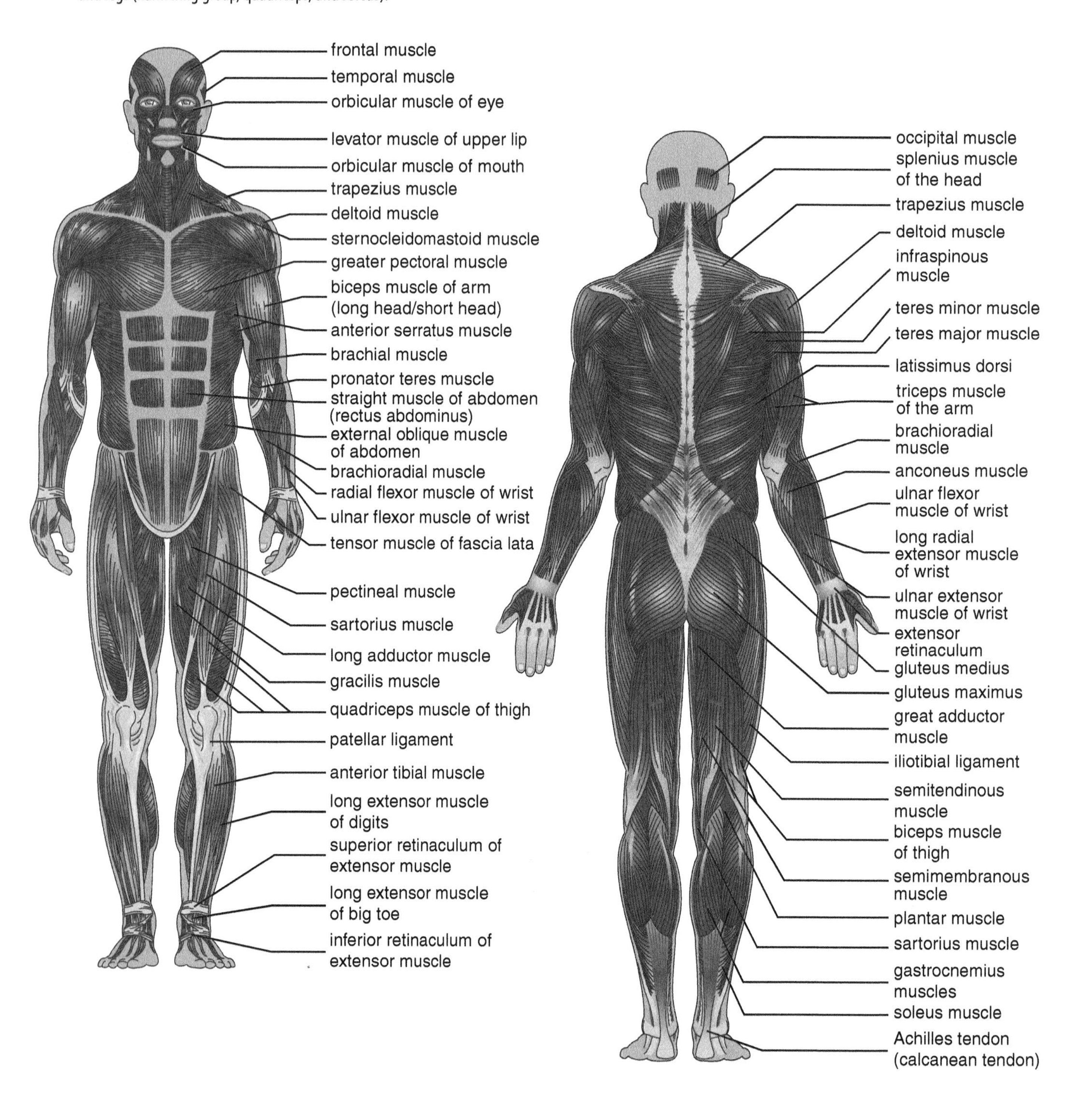

Muscle Spasm and Relaxation

Diseases and disorders of the **musculoskeletal system** are relatively uncommon. **Muscle injuries**, however, are frequently encountered at all ages. Muscle cells damaged from injury become inflamed and **spasm**, which is an involuntary contraction of muscle fibers. Until repair and healing occurs, spasms and inflammation can be quite painful. Drugs to relax muscles and dull pain can help while the healing process takes place.

Nondrug therapy for muscle relaxation includes immobilization of the affected area, physical therapy, heat and cold packs, ultrasound, and massage. Patients may be referred to physical therapists for these treatment modalities.

Muscle **spasticity** is a different condition than spasm. In spasticity, the muscles become rigid and difficult to control for coordinated movement. Spasticity can be caused by brain damage, spinal cord injury, multiple sclerosis, cerebral palsy, or malignant hyperthermia, a rare but serious side effect of anesthesia. In this condition, muscles become rigid and body heat rises to threatening levels.

Drugs for Muscle Relaxation

Drugs work in multiple ways to block and slow muscle contraction (see Figure 10.4). The most commonly used muscle relaxants block signals coming from the brain and spinal cord that control muscle contraction. These drugs are **central nervous system (CNS) depressants**. The exact mechanism or place of action within the CNS for these centrally acting drugs is unknown and probably varies among agents. All are generally sedating, which slows reflexes and relaxes muscle spasms. Some are also used as anticonvulsants and antianxiety agents due to their CNS depressive effects (see Chapters 7 and 8).

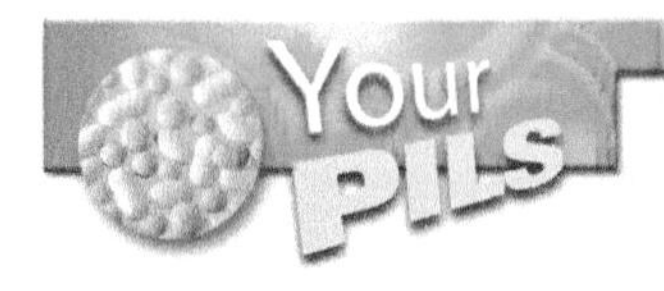

Learners who prefer interpersonal activities and fieldwork (like Enactors and Directors) when applying new concepts to real-life situations may enjoy interviewing a pharmacist about handling prescriptions for muscle relaxants. Because some agents have dependence potential, how does he or she assess prescriptions for fraud and abuse? How does the pharmacist counsel patients taking these medications? What can technicians do to help handle these prescriptions and patients appropriately and efficiently?

Centrally Acting Muscle Relaxants Muscle spasms related to acute injury are frequently treated with **centrally acting muscle relaxants,** which are primarily used for this condition. They are usually given for a defined amount of time (days to weeks) until relief and healing occur. Baclofen and tizanidine are used chronically for muscle spasticity. Centrally acting muscle relaxants are often used in conjunction with over the counter (OTC) and prescription-strength anti-inflammatory drugs such as ibuprofen to control pain and swelling associated with injuries (see Table 10.1 for descriptions of these drugs).

May Cause DROWSINESS
Use Caution while Driving

Side Effects Sedation is the most common side effect of centrally acting muscle relaxants. Patients may complain of drowsiness, dizziness, fatigue, confusion, impaired

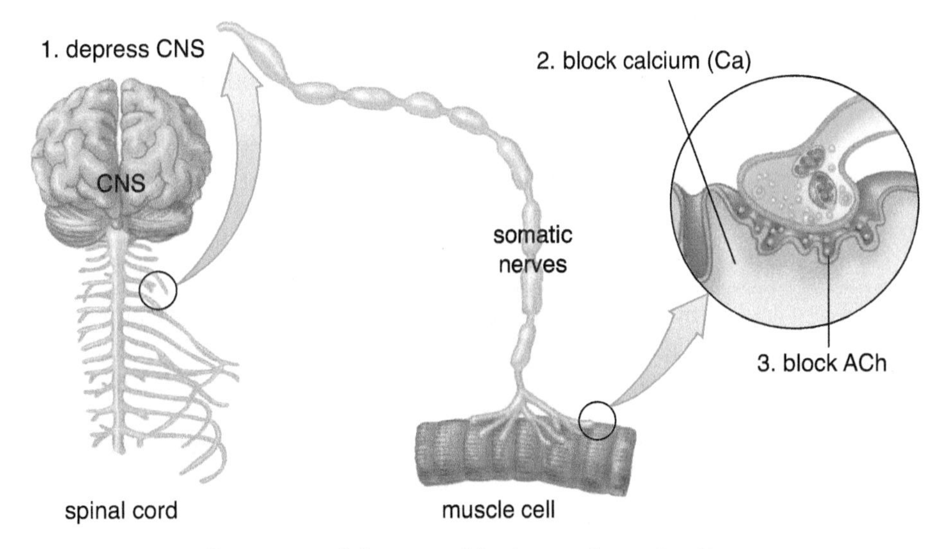

Figure 10.4
Muscle Control and Relaxation
Muscle relaxants work by slowing CNS signal conduction, inhibiting ACh at the neuromuscular junction, or preventing intracellular calcium release.

Table 10.1 Centrally Acting Muscle Relaxants

Generic (Brand)	Dosage Form	Route of Administration	Common Dose
Baclofen (Lioresal)	Tablet, oral solution, intrathecal (IT) solution	Oral, IT	PO: 20–80 mg/day in divided doses 3–4 times a day IT: 90–800 mcg/day via continuous infusion pump
Carisoprodol (Soma)	Tablet	Oral	250–350 mg 3 times a day and bedtime
Chlorzoxazone (Paraflex, Parafon Forte)	Tablet	Oral	250–750 mg 3–4 times a day
Cyclobenzaprine hydrochloride (Flexeril)	Tablet, extended-release (ER) capsule	Oral	Tablet: 5–10 mg 3 times a day ER capsules: 15–30 mg a day
Metaxalone (Skelaxin)	Tablet	Oral	800 mg 3 times a day
Methocarbamol (Robaxin)	Tablet, injectable solution	Oral, IM, IV	PO: 750–1,500 mg 3–4 times a day IM/IV: 1,000 mg (maximum infusion rate of 300 mg/min), may be repeated every 8 hours as needed
Orphenadrine citrate (Norflex)	Tablet, ER tablet, injectable solution	Oral, IM, IV	PO: 100 mg 2 times a day in morning and evening IM/IV: 60 mg, may be repeated every 12 hours as needed
Tizanidine (Zanaflex)	Tablet, capsule	Oral	4–8 mg every 6–8 hours

judgment, and altered coordination. Other side effects include headache, nausea/vomiting, dry mouth, blurred vision, and constipation. Taking these drugs with food can help to reduce nausea and vomiting. Although rare, centrally acting muscle relaxants can cause serious changes in heart function and blood pressure. Consequently, cardiac function and blood pressure should be monitored in patients with cardiovascular conditions.

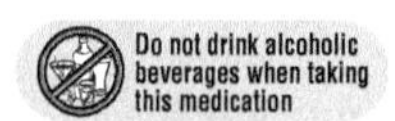

Cautions and Considerations Because these drugs cause sedation and sometimes changes in mental function, patients should be careful when driving, operating machinery, or making important decisions. Patients should not drink alcohol while taking these medications. Those taking other drugs that also cause CNS depression (such as opioids/narcotic pain drugs, antihistamines, or other controlled substances) probably should not take muscle relaxants. Patients taking antidepressants or antipsychotic medications should be monitored closely if they need to take muscle relaxants.

Centrally acting muscle relaxants interact with monoamine oxidase inhibitors (see Chapters 7 and 8) and should not be taken in conjunction with them. Patients with heart conditions, high blood pressure, or clotting disorders should either be monitored closely when taking these medications or avoid them entirely. If skin rash or yellowing of the eyes occurs, patients should be referred to their healthcare providers right away because these effects may indicate allergic reaction or liver dysfunction.

Tolerance and **dependence** can occur if these medications are taken long term. Due to euphoria-like symptoms, addiction and abuse can be an issue and must be monitored as with all controlled substances. Many of these drugs can cause hallucinations and other withdrawal symptoms if they are stopped abruptly. Instead, doses should be slowly decreased over time if the patient has been taking the medication for longer than a couple of weeks.

One particular muscle relaxant that needs heightened monitoring for abuse and addiction is carisoprodol (Soma). After absorption into the bloodstream, this drug is metabolized by the liver to meprobamate, an antianxiety medication that is a controlled substance with high risk for abuse. Consequently, patients taking carisoprodol feel some of the same euphoric effects as occur with meprobamate. Some in the pharmacy field have suggested that carisoprodol be changed to a controlled substance and be given Schedule IV status, which is true for meprobamate. This change would put limits on prescribing and dispensing, making carisoprodol more difficult to obtain. Technicians should alert the pharmacist whenever a patient receives multiple refills at once or requests frequent early refills of carisoprodol, so that proper counseling and intervention can take place.

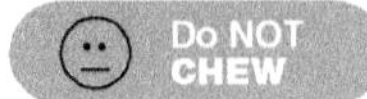

Methocarbamol can turn urine brown, black, or green, so patients should be warned of this harmless but sometimes alarming effect.

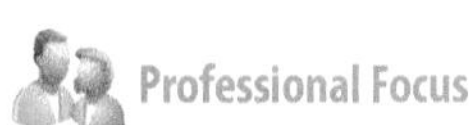

Orphenadrine should be swallowed whole, not chewed. A warning label should be used to alert patients to this important point.

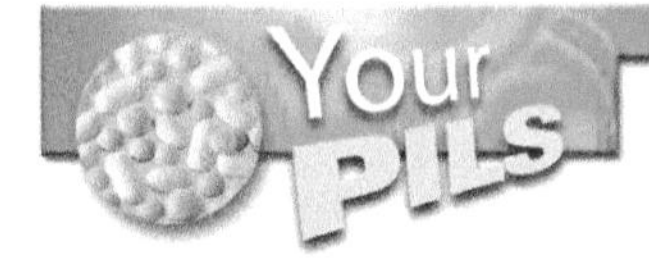

Reflective learners like Creators and Producers might find it useful to look back to Chapter 9 and compare analgesics used in combination with muscle relaxants with drugs from this chapter. Which combinations seem appropriate and which do not? Have you or a family member ever taken medication for a muscle injury? What combination was prescribed?

Professional Focus

Some muscle relaxant names look like other drug names, creating the potential for mix-ups. For example, tizanidine looks and sounds like tiagabine (generic for Gabitril), an antiseizure drug.

Locally Acting Muscle Relaxants One locally acting muscle relaxant, **botulinum toxin (Botox),** works by blocking release of ACh in the neuromuscular junction. Although botulinum toxin is approved for a few select conditions (e.g., migraine headache, spasticity, and **hyperhidrosis** [excess sweating]), the most widespread use of this drug is to reduce facial lines and wrinkles. It is administered as a subdermal injection in doses individualized to the patient. Once injected, localized muscle paralysis occurs, making small lines and wrinkles in the skin less apparent. The effect lasts for weeks to months, after which normal function and contractility return. To maintain the cosmetic effect indefinitely, repeated injections are needed. Botulinum toxin is considered a **cosmetic treatment** rarely covered by health insurance.

Side Effects Side effects from botulinum toxin are rare but can include dry mouth, headache, neck or back pain, pain/itching at the injection site, upper respiratory tract infection, fever, and flulike symptoms. Less common but more serious side effects include allergic reaction, chest pain, difficulty swallowing, difficulty breathing, and heart attack or arrhythmias. These effects are more likely at high doses and when the drug is used to treat conditions not based on cosmetic preferences. If these effects occur, patients should seek medical attention. If muscle weakness or paralysis occurs in a larger area than where administered or affects the ability to swallow, see, breathe, or otherwise move, medical attention should be obtained immediately.

Cautions and Considerations Botulinum toxin should be used carefully in patients with muscle dysfunction such as cerebral palsy, muscle spasm, or dystonia. Patients who have hyperhidrosis should avoid using deodorant for twenty-four hours prior to injection and avoid situations that cause sweating for at least thirty minutes prior to injection.

Direct Acting Muscle Relaxants One **direct acting muscle relaxant** that works by blocking the intracellular release of calcium and weakening muscle contractility is **dantrolene** (Dantrium). Dantrolene is used for muscle spasticity due to spinal cord injury or cerebral palsy. It is the drug of choice for malignant hyperthermia, an emergency situation. Injectable dantrolene is typically kept in emergency drug kits in areas where anesthesia is administered. Technicians are often responsible for stocking and monitoring these kits. Dantrolene is administered by IV injection and orally (capsule) and commonly dosed at 1–10 mg/kg.

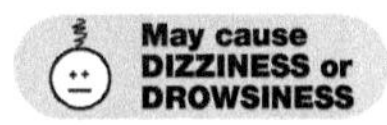

Side Effects Common side effects of dantrolene are drowsiness, dizziness, fatigue, confusion, impaired judgment, and altered coordination. If diarrhea develops, patients should consult their healthcare providers because this side effect can sometimes become severe. This drug can possibly cause photosensitivity. With long-term use, dantrolene can be toxic to the liver, so special monitoring must be performed.

Cautions and Considerations Dantrolene should be used with great caution in patients with liver disease. Women older than thirty-five tend to have more problems with liver toxicity and should be monitored closely or avoid using dantrolene altogether. Dantrolene can turn urine orange or red.

May Discolor Urine

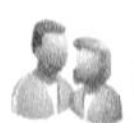

Professional Focus

Dantrolene tends to have a short shelf life, so technicians should frequently check the drug's expiration date in emergency drug kits. An emergency situation is not a good time to find out that this life-saving drug is no longer effective.

Neuromuscular Blocking Agents In all cases, **neuromuscular blockers** (see Table 10.2) cause temporary paralysis. These agents are used with anesthesia for short-term muscle relaxation during endotracheal intubation, mechanical respiration, and surgical procedures. Under no circumstance would these drugs be prescribed in the outpatient setting or for anyone not on a ventilator. Therefore, only technicians working in the inpatient setting will handle such drugs.

Neuromuscular blockers work by competitively blocking ACh receptors or inhibiting breakdown of ACh, allowing the muscle to continuously contract until fatigue and paralysis occur. Drug choice among these agents depends on the length of the procedure (a few minutes to hours) or the desired amount of time for ventilation (days or longer).

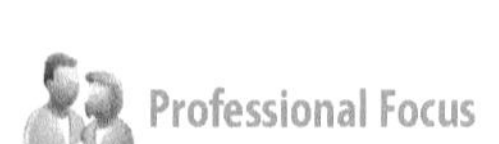

Patients have received neuromuscular blocking agents by mistake, causing death in a few circumstances. All orders for neuromuscular blockers should be double-checked to be sure they are appropriate.

Table 10.2 Neuromuscular Blocking Agents

Generic (Brand)	Dosage Form	Route of Administration
Short-Acting Agent (onset of action: immediate; duration of action: seconds to minutes)		
Succinylcholine (Anectine, Quelicin)	Injectable and IV solution	IM, IV
Intermediate-Acting Agents (onset of action: few minutes; duration of action: 30–40 minutes)		
Atracurium (Tracrium)	IV solution	IV
Cisatracurium (Nimbex)	IV solution	IV
Rocuronium (Zemuron)	IV solution	IV
Vecuronium (Norcuron)	IV powder for solution	IV
Long-Acting Agents (onset of action: few minutes; duration of action: 60–100 minutes)		
Doxacurium (Nuromax)	IV solution	IV
Mivacurium (Mivacron)	IV solution	IV
Pancuronium (Pavulon)	IV solution	IV
Pipecuronium (Arduan)	IV solution	IV

Side Effects Low blood pressure and respiratory depression are the most common side effects of neuromuscular blocking agents. Blood pressure and respiratory rate are monitored closely whenever these agents are used.

Cautions and Considerations Cardiac arrest and changes in cardiac function have occurred in patients, especially children, treated with these agents. These drugs must be dosed individually.

Pharmacy technicians should be careful to apply warning labels indicating that these drugs should be given for intubation or to ventilated patients only. Neuromuscular blockers paralyze all muscles, including those that control respiration.

Other Muscle Disorders

Rhabdomyolysis is a syndrome where muscle breakdown occurs and toxic cell contents are released into the bloodstream. This syndrome is a rare, but serious side effect of the cholesterol-lowering class of drugs called statins. Symptoms may be silent

Rhabdomyolysis is a syndrome where muscle breakdown occurs and toxic cell contents are released into the bloodstream. This syndrome is a rare, but serious side effect of the cholesterol-lowering class of drugs called statins. Symptoms may be silent but can include muscle aches and pain, red- to brown-colored urine, and muscle weakness. Laboratory tests are used to detect muscle enzymes (creatinine kinase or CK) in the blood when rhabdomyolysis is suspected. Acute renal failure is common, so patients taking statins are monitored closely for this effect. Patients taking statins should report any unexplained muscle pain or weakness to their healthcare providers.

Fibromyalgia is a chronic muscle pain condition that is not fully understood. Symptoms include musculoskeletal pain in the neck, back, shoulders, chest, arms, and legs. Patients also complain of fatigue, tingling/numbness, dizziness, and mood disturbances, including depression. Fibromyalgia is diagnosed by physical exam and the presence of specific tender points on the body. Drugs used to treat fibromyalgia include duloxetine (see Chapter 8) and pregabalin. Milnacipran (Savella) is a drug recently approved for use in fibromyalgia. It works by blocking the reuptake of norepinephrine and serotonin and is taken in doses of 100–200 mg a day. It has similar side effects and cautions to selective serotonin reuptake inhibitors and serotonin-norepinephrine reuptake inhibitors (see Chapter 8).

Myasthenia gravis is an autoimmune process that attacks and destroys ACh receptors on muscle cells in the neuromuscular junction. It is a progressive disease that begins with muscle weakness in the face and neck and eventually impairs movement in all limbs. Drugs for myasthenia gravis include neostigmine (Prostigmin) and pyridostigmine (Mestinon), agents that enhance muscle strength; and azathioprine (Imuran) and cyclophosphamide (Cytoxan), immunosuppressants that slow the progression of this disorder. Neostigmine and pyridostigmine can also be used to reverse the action of muscle relaxants in cases of overdose.

Poliomyelitis, commonly referred to as **polio**, is an infection of the nerves that control the muscular system. It is now rare in the United States because the polio vaccine has nearly eradicated it here and in most developed countries. The vaccine is not readily available in all countries, and polio remains a significant health threat in underdeveloped areas of the African, Asian, and South American continents.

Muscular dystrophy refers to a group of genetically acquired conditions causing muscle atrophy (shrinking) and wasting. Depending on the specific gene affected, muscular dystrophy can be severely debilitating and fatal. Few drugs are used to treat this condition, but many Americans can recall references to muscular dystrophy as part of the annual Jerry Lewis Muscular Dystrophy Association (MDA) Telethon held on Labor Day weekend.

Herbal and Alternative Therapies

Few herbal and natural products are used for treating muscular conditions. However, several herbal therapies taken for other problems can interact with prescription muscle relaxants. St. John's wort, valerian, and kava are examples of products taken for depression and insomnia that could intensify the CNS depression of muscle relaxants. Take notice of patients purchasing such products along with their prescription muscle relaxants. Warn them about interactions and offer to have the pharmacist counsel them appropriately.

Spinal realignment performed by a chiropractor has been found to relieve muscle pain and injury. Patients interested in **chiropractic therapy** should check with their health insurance providers for availability and coverage of this service. Many benefits packages now include it.

Chapter Summary

The muscular system is divided into skeletal, cardiac, and smooth muscle. Acetylcholine, or ACh, is a chemical transmitter that travels across the neuromuscular junction to stimulate muscle fiber contraction. Muscle contraction is also dependent on sodium influx and calcium release within the muscle cell. Muscle injury is the most common reason for using drug therapy. Centrally acting muscle relaxants are dispensed frequently for this reason. They work by suppressing the CNS, which controls muscle contraction. These drugs tend to cause sedation. Direct acting muscle relaxants are used primarily for muscle spasticity due to select conditions. They work by inhibiting intracellular calcium release. Botulinum toxin is an expensive cosmetic agent frequently administered by local injection to relax muscles in the face and reduce wrinkles. During intubation and ventilation, neuromuscular blocking agents are used to temporarily relax and paralyze muscles for specialized procedures to be completed. Special precautions should be taken with these drugs to prevent medication errors. Few herbal products are used to treat muscle spasm directly, but some products interact with muscle relaxants. Chiropractic therapy has been found to be effective in treating muscle pain and injury.

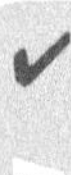

Chapter Review

For the following sets of exercises, write the exercise heading, exercise numbers, and your answers on a separate sheet of paper. Your instructor may direct you to turn in the sheet of paper or discuss your answers as a class.

REVIEW THE BASICS

Choose a, b, c, or d as the correct answer to each multiple-choice question.

1. Skeletal muscle is considered which of the following?
   a. cardiac muscle
   b. involuntary muscle
   c. voluntary muscle
   d. smooth muscle

2. On what type of muscle do commonly prescribed muscle relaxants work?
   a. cardiac
   b. skeletal
   c. smooth
   d. involuntary

3. Which of the following muscles is used most often to administer vaccines (such as the flu shot) in the pharmacy setting?
   a. trapezius
   b. deltoid
   c. gluteus maximus
   d. gluteus medius

4. Which of the following neurotransmitters causes muscles to contract by stimulating receptors on the surface of muscle cells?
   a. calcium
   b. acetylcholine
   c. acetylcholinesterase
   d. all of the above

5. Which of the following drugs is used primarily for spasticity caused by head injury or cerebral palsy?
   a. baclofen (Lioresal)
   b. cyclobenzaprine (Flexeril)
   c. carisoprodol (Soma)
   d. metaxalone (Skelaxin)

6. Although all muscle relaxants have some potential for addiction and abuse, which of the following has the greatest potential (leading some to believe it should be a controlled substance)?
   a. vecuronium
   b. cyclobenzaprine
   c. carisoprodol
   d. botulinum toxin

7. On which of the following should you put the following warning label when dispensing?

   CAUTION:
   may turn urine brown,
   black, or green

   a. Soma
   b. Skelaxin
   c. Robaxin
   d. Paraflex

8. Which of the following is a long-acting neuromuscular blocking agent?
   a. vecuronium
   b. methocarbamol
   c. pancuronium
   d. succinylcholine

9. Which of the following relaxes muscle by blocking ACh?
   a. Botox
   b. Dantrium
   c. Nimbex
   d. all of the above

10. Which of the following drugs can be given intrathecally?
    a. Zanaflex
    b. methocarbamol
    c. Flexeril
    d. baclofen

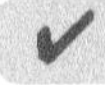

KNOW THE DRUGS

Match each brand name drug with its corresponding generic name and most common use. Your answers should follow this example format: Generic Name: 1. a; 2. b; 3. c; etc. Most Common Use: 1. h; 2. i; 3. j; etc.

Brand Name	Generic Name	Most Common Use
1. Arduan	a. dantrolene	h. muscle spasm due to injury
2. Quelicin	b. pipecuronium	i. muscle relaxation for intubation
3. Robaxin	c. carisoprodol	j. malignant hyperthermia
4. Parafon Forte	d. methocarbamol	
5. Dantrium	e. succinylcholine	
6. Flexeril	f. chlorzoxazone	
7. Soma	g. cyclobenzaprine	

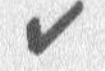

PUT IT TOGETHER

For each item, write down either a short answer or a single term to complete the sentence.

1. What cautionary label is put on all muscle relaxant prescriptions? Why?
2. Name three drugs for which you should use a warning label about administering only to ventilated patients.
3. Name two drugs that you may be asked to check in emergency drug kits in the surgical satellite or emergency room for patients who have malignant hyperthermia or need intubation.
4. ________________ should be swallowed whole, not crushed or chewed.
5. A drug mixed in ______mL or less can be injected in the deltoid or the vastus lateralis muscles, and a drug volume of ______mL or less can be injected into the gluteus medius.

THINK IT THROUGH

Read and think through each numbered scenario carefully and then write several sentences in reply to the question(s) presented. Question 4 requires you to do some Internet research before completing your answer(s).

1. You are ringing up a patient's prescription for Flexeril at the cash register when he adds a few other items to the basket. You see a bottle of Advil and some valerian among these items. What should you do?
2. You receive the following prescription in the pharmacy. What is wrong with it? What should you do?

   Soma 250 mg #40

   Sig: Take 3 tablets QID PRN
3. You receive the following prescription in the pharmacy. What is wrong with it?

   Orphenadrine (Norflex)

   Sig: 100 mg IM bolus, repeat q 12 h PRN

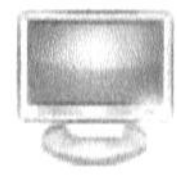

4. **On the Internet,** look up the cost, history, and additional purported side effects of Botox cosmetic. How much might a patient expect to spend on this elective treatment? Where did Botox come from, and what are the risks of using it?

Chapter 11 Drugs for Eyes, Ears, Nose, and Throat

LEARNING OBJECTIVES

- Describe the basic anatomy and physiology of the eyes, ears, nose, and throat.
- Explain the therapeutic effects of prescription medications, nonprescription medications, and alternative therapies commonly used to treat diseases of the eyes, ears, nose, and throat.
- Describe the adverse effects of prescription medications, nonprescription medications, and alternative therapies commonly used to treat diseases of the eyes, ears, nose, and throat.
- Identify the brand and generic names of prescription and nonprescription medications commonly used to treat diseases of the eyes, ears, nose, and throat.
- State the doses, dosage forms, and routes of administration of prescription and nonprescription medications commonly used to treat diseases of the eyes, ears, nose, and throat.

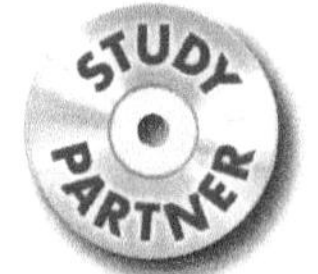

Interactive self-quizzes, games, audio files, and glossaries help you to learn drug names and facts.

Medications for the eyes, ears, nose, and throat are dispensed and purchased in pharmacies on a daily basis. The eyes and ears are unique administration sites for drug therapies, requiring special instructions for use. Patients can find these medications challenging to apply properly and may come to you with many related questions. Patients also regularly purchase cough and cold products to self-treat conditions of the nose and throat. The cough and cold section is often the largest over-the-counter (OTC) aisle. Consequently, the abundance of products and the challenges for their proper use present many difficulties. Pharmacists should assist patients in choosing these products wisely and avoiding self-treatment errors, and technicians can help patients understand which active ingredients these products contain.

After introducing the anatomy and physiology of eyes, ears, and upper respiratory tract, this chapter discusses the conditions affecting these sensory organs, including glaucoma, conjunctivitis, ear infections, ototoxicity, allergies, and the common cold. Drug classes treating eye conditions include topical beta blockers, carbonic anhydrase inhibitors, and prostaglandin agonists. Drug classes treating allergies and the common cold include antihistamines, decongestants, and cough suppressants. Last, a few natural and herbal products used for the common cold and other upper respiratory tract infections are covered.

Anatomy and Physiology of the Eyes, Ears, Nose, and Throat

The **sensory system** includes organs that produce the **five senses**: **vision**, **hearing**, **smell**, **taste**, and **touch**. Sensory organs associated with drug therapy are the eyes and ears, because they are sites of administration for medication. Many drugs used to treat eye and ear conditions are applied topically.

The **eyes** are sensory organs specially designed to sense light and produce vision. Light enters the eye through the **pupil** and is focused by the **lens** (see Figure 11.1). The lens is located just behind the pupil, the black center of the eye. The lens of the eye acts like a lens in a camera, focusing light onto the back of the eye. The **iris**, which surrounds the pupil, determines eye color. The **sclera** is the outer coating of the eyeball, commonly referred to as the white of the eye.

Sight begins with light that travels through the lens to the back of the eye, the **retina**. In the retina, photoreceptor cells detect light and color. These rod- and cone-

Figure 11.1
Anatomy of the Eye
Drugs are used to treat problems in the conjunctiva, anterior chamber, retina, and macula.

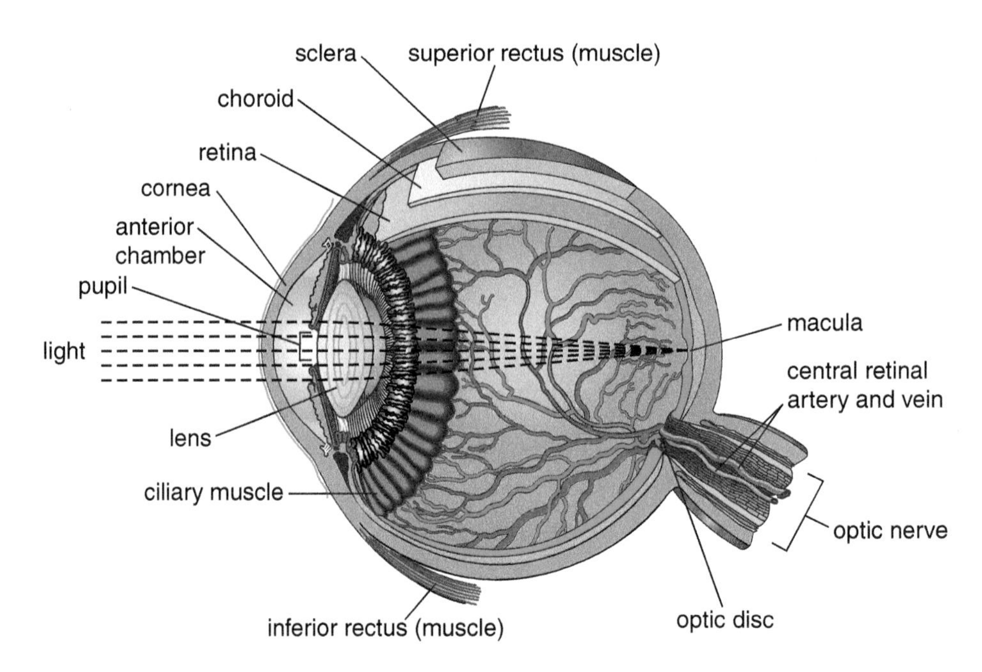

shaped sensory cells send signals via the optic nerve to the brain, where sight is ultimately perceived and interpreted (see Figure 11.2). **Rod cells** are sensitive to light in dimly lit conditions. They are responsible for night vision. Vitamin A deficiency can cause malfunctions in retinal rod cells, which then affects night vision. **Cone cells** sense color and are responsible for day vision. **Color blindness** (frequently a genetic trait that affects mostly males) is a condition in which cone cells do not differentiate colors. The most common form of color blindness is being unable to differentiate red from green. Inside the **macula** (see Figure 11.1) is the focal point (fovea centralis) on the retina where light is concentrated for vision. This part of the retina is rich in cone cells.

Other parts of the eye relevant to drug therapy include the cornea, anterior chamber, aqueous humor, ciliary muscle, and conjunctiva. The **cornea** covers the **anterior chamber**.

Figure 11.2
Anatomy of the Retina
Rod cells help animals with good night vision see in the dark.

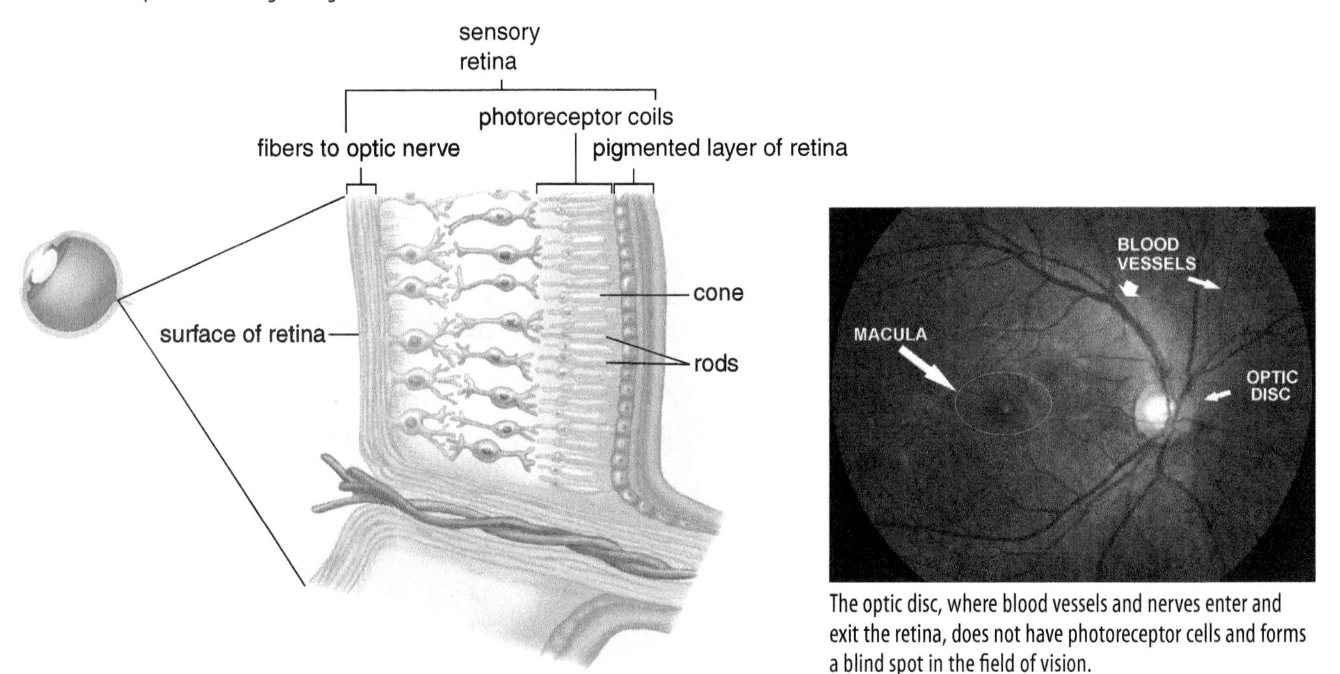

The optic disc, where blood vessels and nerves enter and exit the retina, does not have photoreceptor cells and forms a blind spot in the field of vision.

The anterior chamber holds **aqueous humor**, a fluid that lubricates and protects the lens. **Vitreous humor** is the fluid inside the eye, behind the lens. The **ciliary muscle** holds the lens in place. The **conjunctiva** forms the mucous membranes of the socket that hold the eye in place.

The **ears** are sensory organs designed to sense sound waves and produce hearing. As seen in Figure 11.3, the ear is divided into three parts: external, middle, and inner. The **external ear** captures **sound waves** and directs them through the **auditory canal** to the **tympanic membrane** (eardrum). **Cerumen** (earwax) is produced by follicles lining the auditory canal.

The eardrum separates the **middle ear** from the external ear. It vibrates in response to sound waves, causing the three bones (**malleus**, **incus,** and **stapes**) of the middle ear to move. The stapes in effect taps on the **oval window**, the entrance to the inner ear. The **eustachian tube** connects the middle ear to the throat to allow fluid to drain when atmospheric air pressure changes. The **inner ear** includes the semicircular canals and the cochlea. Fluid in the **cochlea** responds to the tapping on the oval window, producing pressure waves that flow through the spiral-shaped organ (see Figure 11.4). Sensory hairs line the surface of the cochlea in what is called the **organ of Corti**. Sound is perceived and interpreted when corresponding vibrations in these tiny hairs send signals via nerves to the brain. Damage to sensory hairs in the inner ear occurs naturally with age and exposure to loud noise. This kind of hearing loss is called **presbycusis**. The first sounds lost to perception are those produced by high-pitched sound waves.

Fluid in the **semicircular canals** maintains balance and orientation. The semicircular canals are arranged in a three-dimensional manner. Gravity pulls the fluid in these

Figure 11.3

Anatomy of the External, Middle and Inner Ear

Ear "popping" created by yawning is the characteristic sound of fluid exchange in the eustachian tube.

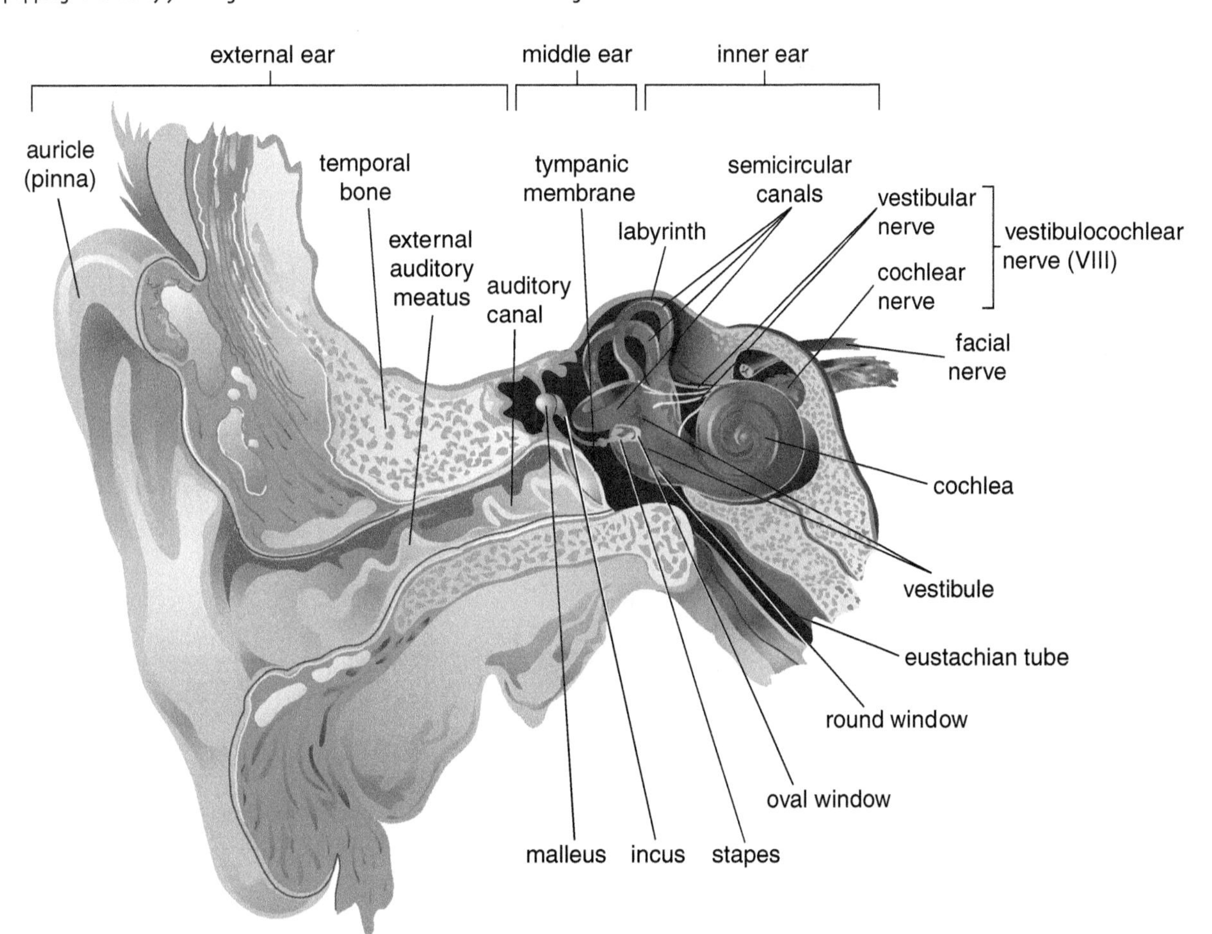

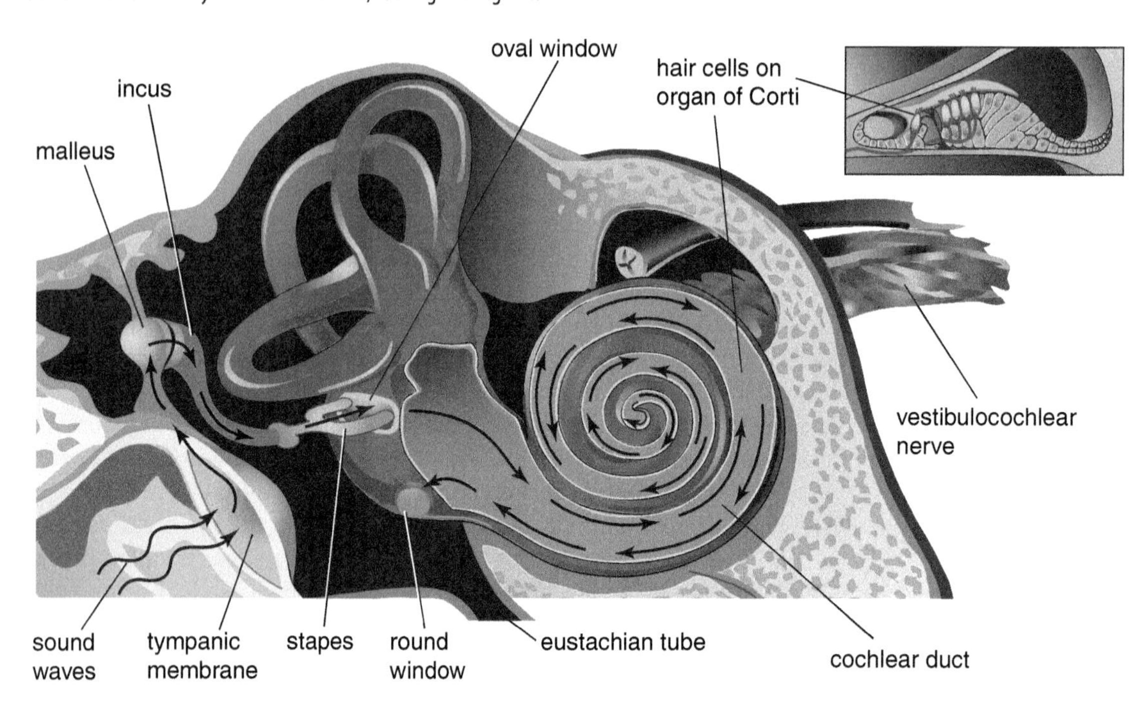

Figure 11.4
Sound Movement through the Inner Ear
Strong waves from loud noises break off tiny hairs in the cochlea, causing hearing loss.

channels downward, signaling to the **vestibular nerves** when the body is vertical, horizontal, or upside down. **Vertigo** is a condition or malfunction of these semicircular canals whereby balance is affected and dizziness is problematic.

The nose and throat are parts of the **upper respiratory tract (URT).** The URT includes **nasal passages**, **sinuses**, the back of the **throat** (where the tonsils are located), the **pharynx** (Adam's apple), and the **larynx**, or voice box (see Figure 11.5). The URT encompasses structures above the **trachea**, the opening to the lungs; the lower respiratory tract includes structures below the trachea.

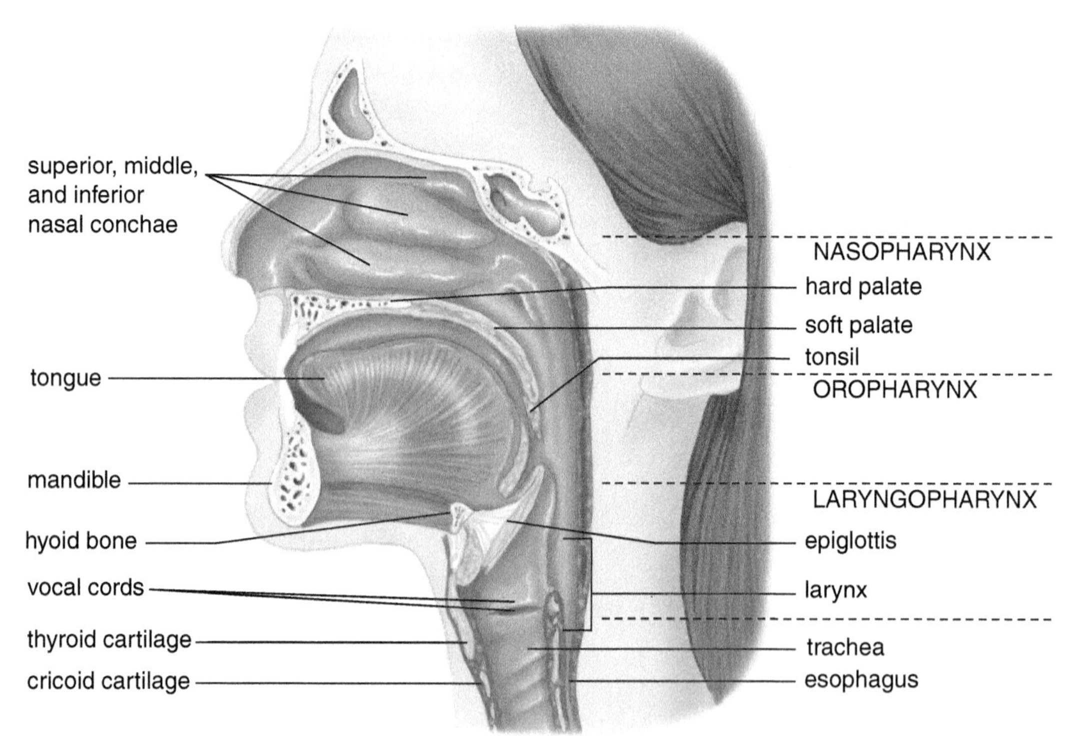

Figure 11.5
Upper Respiratory Tract
Laryngitis is inflammation of the larynx, affecting vocal cord function.

Chemoreceptors in the **nose** produce the sense of smell. The sinuses and throat are common sites for viral and bacterial infections. The common cold typically causes symptoms affecting the URT, including coughing, sinus pain, and postnasal drainage. Inflammation associated with allergies also affects URT tissues, causing congestion and runny nose (rhinitis).

Glaucoma

Glaucoma is a condition in which abnormally high **intraocular pressure** pushes on the **optic nerve** and damages it. Glaucoma can lead to blindness if it is not treated. The increased pressure comes from either overproduction of aqueous humor or blockage of its outflow from the anterior chamber (see Figure 11.6). As fluid builds up in the anterior chamber, intraocular pressure increases, and pressure is applied to the optic nerve. **Open-angle glaucoma** is a slowly progressing, chronic condition managed with medication alone. **Narrow-angle glaucoma** is an acute condition that comes on quickly and is resolved with surgery followed by drugs.

Figure 11.6

Normal Aqueous Humor Flow and Glaucoma

In open-angle glaucoma, the trabecular meshwork becomes congested, restricting the flow of aqueous humor from the anterior chamber, whereas in narrow-angle glaucoma, the canal of Schlemm is blocked completely, cutting off aqueous humor flow.

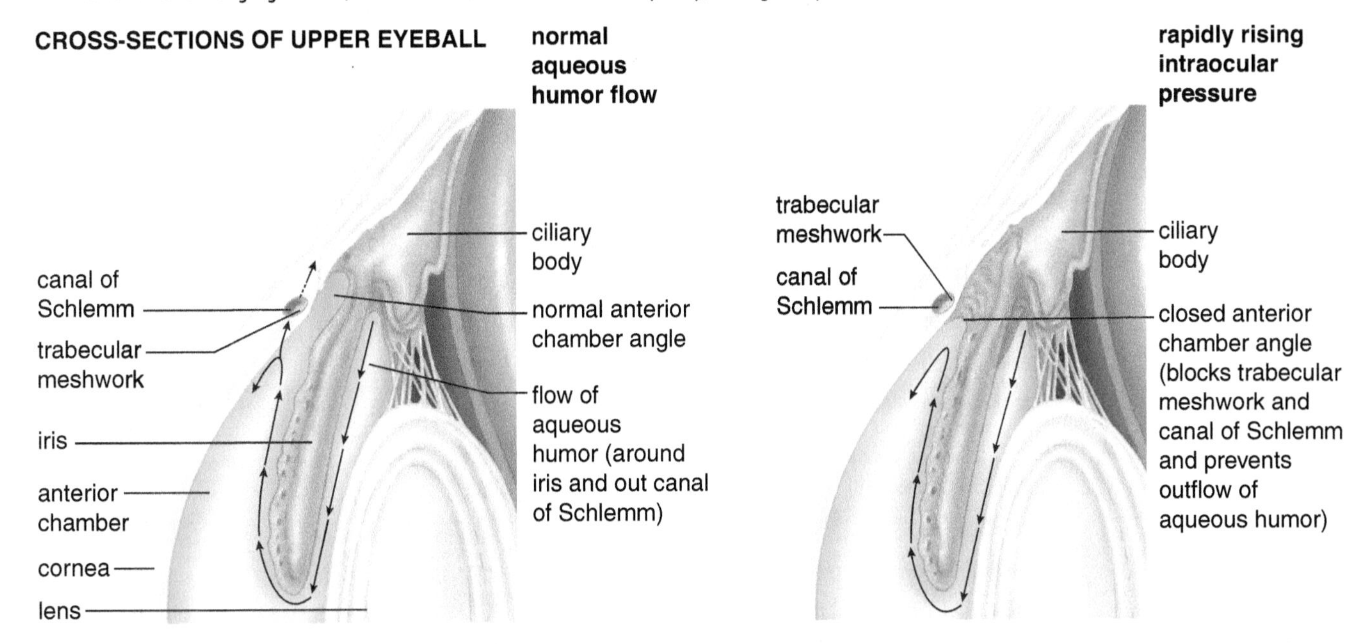

Administering Eyedrops

Most eye conditions, especially glaucoma, are treated with topical agents administered directly in the eyes. Although oral medication administration may be more convenient for most patients, the undesirable systemic effects of oral therapy can pose problems. Ophthalmic agents limit drug therapy to local effects.

Ophthalmic drops must remain sterile so as not to cause infection in the eye. Thus, the dropper bottle should be kept in a clean place. The tip of the drop applicator must not touch anything, including your fingers or the eye itself. To instill eyedrops, have the patient lie down, pull the lower eyelid downward, and gently squeeze the container to allow the required number of drops to fall into the eye (see Figure 11.7) without touching the tip of the applicator to the eye, eyelid, eyelashes, or fingers. Remove contact lenses prior to application and leave them out for at least fifteen minutes afterward.

Do not touch tip of applicator

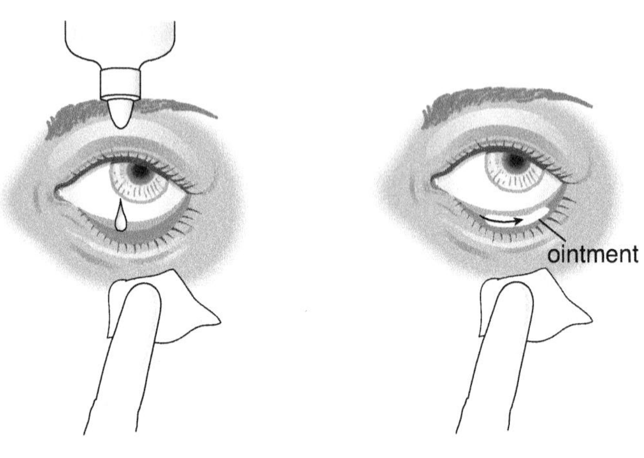

Figure 11.7
Instilling Eyedrops and Applying Eye Ointment
Eye drops are typically solutions, but a few are suspensions that should be shaken well before being used. The technique for applying eye ointment is not easy and may take some practice to do properly.

Drugs for Glaucoma Multiple drug classes are used to treat glaucoma (see Table 11.1). **Ophthalmic glaucoma agents** work by reducing aqueous humor production and, in some cases, enhancing its drainage from the anterior chamber. Miotic agents constrict the pupil slightly by contracting the ciliary muscle. This contraction enhances aqueous humor outflow. Beta blockers are first-line therapy for glaucoma and tend to be used most frequently.

Side Effects Glaucoma agents are usually well tolerated. Side effects include mild stinging, tearing, itchy eyes, and dry eyes. These effects generally improve with time.

Table 11.1 Ophthalmic Agents for Glaucoma

Generic (Brand)	Dosage Form and Route of Administration
Beta Blockers	
Betaxolol (Betoptic)	Ophthalmic solution and suspension
Carteolol (Ocupress)	Ophthalmic solution
Levobunolol (Betagan)	Ophthalmic solution
Metipranolol (OptiPranolol)	Ophthalmic solution
Timolol (Timoptic)	Ophthalmic solution
Alpha Receptor Agonists	
Apraclonidine (Iopidine)	Ophthalmic solution
Brimonidine (Alphagan P)	Ophthalmic solution
Sympathomimetics	
Dipivefrin (Propine)	Ophthalmic solution
Miotics	
Carbachol (Carbastat, Miostat)	Ophthalmic solution
Echothiophate (Phospholine Iodide)	Ophthalmic powder for reconstitution
Pilocarpine (Isopto Carpine)	Ophthalmic gel and solution
Carbonic Anhydrase Inhibitors	
Acetazolamide (Diamox)	Oral tablet and capsule
Brinzolamide (Azopt)	Ophthalmic solution
Dorzolamide (Trusopt)	Ophthalmic solution
Methazolamide (various)	Oral tablet
Prostaglandin Agonists	
Bimatoprost (Lumigan)	Ophthalmic solution
Latanoprost (Xalatan)	Ophthalmic solution
Travoprost (Travatan)	Ophthalmic solution

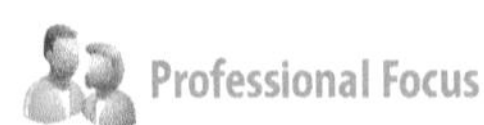

Carefully choose ophthalmic agents from the stock shelves. Be careful because otic medications come in small dropper bottles, like ophthalmic agents do. However, otic agents should never be applied in the eye—they can damage vision and cause harm to the patient.

Many glaucoma agents have the potential to cause systemic effects if enough is absorbed into the bloodstream. These effects are primarily associated with beta blockers and include slowed heartbeat, heart problems, insomnia, dizziness, vertigo, headaches, tiredness, and difficulty breathing. If any of these effects occur, patients should contact their prescribers right away. A change in drug therapy will be needed. Patients who have heart disease should discuss treatment options for glaucoma before starting to take one of these products.

Cautions and Considerations Patients with heart or thyroid problems should discuss their choices for glaucoma treatment with their prescribers before selecting and using these products. Specifically, the systemic effects of beta blockers can interfere with these conditions and the other drug therapies used to treat them.

CAUTION may change eye color

Prostaglandin agonists have a unique effect in that they cause the iris of the eye to turn brown. Patients should be informed of this effect because their eye color will likely change. For this reason, these agents are used only after others have failed.

Oral dosage forms of carbonic anhydrase medications have several drug interactions and cautions that patients and their prescribers should know about. Patients with kidney or liver problems, diabetes, gout, or asthma should talk with their healthcare providers before using a carbonic anhydrase inhibitor agent.

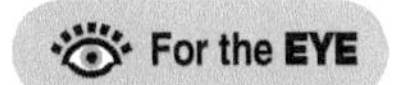

Auxiliary warning labels should also be applied to alert patients to the fact that these products are to be used in the eyes only.

Eye Infections

Common eye infections seen by pharmacy personnel include bacterial infections such as **conjunctivitis** and viral infections such as **cytomegalovirus (CMV)** and herpes. Conjunctivitis (commonly called "pink eye") is inflammation caused by bacteria in the mucous membranes surrounding the eye. Symptoms include redness of the sclera and insides of the eyelids, itching, pain, tearing, and the release of matter. Matter and exudates can be white, yellow, or green. Treatment with antibiotics is relatively easy.

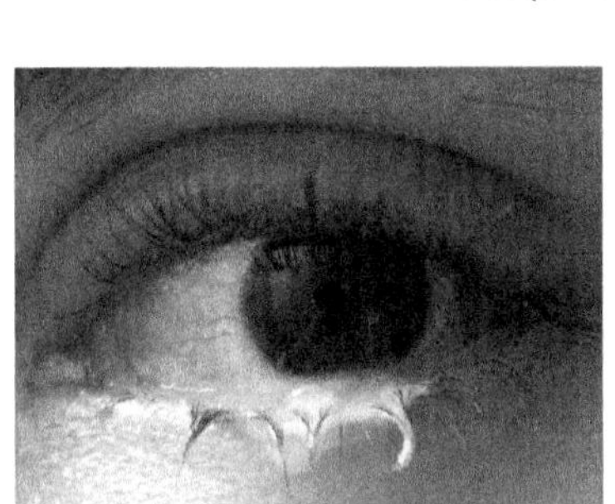

In children, conjunctivitis is often associated with prior cold and flu symptoms.

Newborns of mothers with untreated gonorrhea are at high risk for gonococcal conjunctivitis. Newborns who are suspected to be infected are often given topical ophthalmic anti-infectives for prevention and systemic antibiotics. Pregnant women should be tested for gonorrhea and treated before giving birth, if possible.

CMV is a viral infection of the inner eye that occurs almost entirely in patients with HIV or AIDS. Most people are exposed to this virus early in life but do not develop an active infection because a normally functioning immune system easily defends against it. In immunocompromised patients including those with HIV, CMV becomes an active infection that can lead to blindness. It is most common in patients at the end stages of AIDS and those who have high virus counts in the bloodstream. CMV is difficult to cure; treatment involves chronic suppression with antiviral medication to control symptoms and preserve eyesight.

Herpes zoster, the virus that causes chickenpox and shingles, and **herpes simplex**, the virus that causes cold sores, can cause various problems with the eyes and eyelids. Symptoms usually include eye pain and can also include redness, cloudiness of the cornea, tearing, decreased vision, and aversion to bright light. Serious herpetic viral infections can cause blindness. Treatment involves topical antiviral agents, which may be used in addition to systemic agents when necessary.

Administering Eye Ointment

To apply **eye ointment**, pull the lower eyelid downward and squeeze a continuous ribbon of ointment (half-inch long) along the space between the eyeball and lower lid (see Figure

11.7). Like ophthalmic drops, eye ointments must remain sterile. The applicator tip should not touch the eye or eyelid. The patient should close the eye for a few minutes to allow the ointment to liquefy. Vision may be blurry for a few minutes until the ointment dissipates. Excess ointment can be gently wiped away. If the patient wears contact lenses, the lenses should be removed and left out for at least fifteen minutes after the eye ointment is applied.

Drugs for Eye Infections Anti-infective agents for the eyes include antibiotics and antiviral medications (see Table 11.2). **Topical anti-infective** treatment for the eyes is

Table 11.2 Commonly Used Ophthalmic Anti-Infectives

Generic (Brand)	Dosage Form	Route of Administration	Common Dose
Aminoglycosides			
Gentamicin (Garamycin, Genoptic)	Solution, ointment	Ophthalmic	1–2 drops every 4 hours; half-inch ribbon 2–3 times a day
Neomycin, bacitracin, polymyxin B	Ointment	Ophthalmic	Apply small amount every 3–4 hours
Tobramycin (Tobrasol, Tobrex)	Solution, ointment	Ophthalmic	1–2 drops every 4 hours; half-inch ribbon 2–6 times a day
Macrolides			
Erythromycin	Ointment	Ophthalmic	Half-inch ribbon 2–6 times a day
Sulfonamides			
Sulfacetamide (Bleph-10, Cetamide, Sulamyd)	Solution, ointment	Ophthalmic	1–2 drops every 2–3 hours; thin ribbon 1–4 times a day and at bedtime
Trimethoprim, polymyxin B (Polytrim)	Solution	Ophthalmic	1–2 drops every 4–6 hours
Quinolones			
Ciprofloxacin (Ciloxan)	Solution, ointment	Ophthalmic	1–2 drops every 2–5 hours; half-inch ribbon 2–3 times a day
Levofloxacin (Iquix, Quixin)	Solution	Ophthalmic	1–2 drops every 2–4 hours
Ofloxacin (Ocuflox)	Solution	Ophthalmic	1–2 drops every 2–4 hours or 4 times a day
Miscellaneous Combinations			
Gentamicin, prednisolone (Pred-G)	Suspension, ointment	Ophthalmic	1 drop every 2–4 hours; half-inch ribbon 1–3 times a day
Neomycin, bacitracin, polymyxin B, hydrocortisone (Cortisporin)	Ointment	Ophthalmic	Half-inch ribbon every 3–4 hours
Neomycin, dexamethasone (NeoDecadron)	Solution	Ophthalmic	1–2 drops every 3–4 hours
Neomycin, polymyxin B, dexamethasone (Dexasporin, Maxitrol)	Suspension, ointment	Ophthalmic	1–2 drops every 3–4 hours; half-inch ribbon 3–4 times a day
Neomycin, polymyxin B, prednisolone (Poly-Pred)	Suspension	Ophthalmic	1–2 drops every 3–4 hours
Sulfacetamide, fluorometholone (FML-S)	Solution	Ophthalmic	1–3 drops every 2–3 hours
Sulfacetamide, prednisolone (Blephamide)	Solution, ointment	Ophthalmic	1–3 drops every 2–3 hours; apply 1–4 times a day
Tobramycin, dexamethasone (TobraDex)	Suspension, ointment	Ophthalmic	1–2 drops every 4 hours; apply 2–3 times a day
Antivirals			
Cidofovir (Vistide)	Solution	IV	5 mg/kg IV over an hour given every 1–2 weeks
Ganciclovir (Cytovene)	Capsule, injection	Oral, IV, intravitreal	1,000 mg orally 3 times a day; 5 mg/kg IV every 12–24 hours; 1 implant every 5–8 months
Foscarnet (Foscavir)	Solution	IV	60–120 mg/kg given every 8, 12, or 24 hours
Trifluridine (Viroptic)	Solution	Ophthalmic	1 drop every 2–4 hours
Valganciclovir (Valcyte)	Tablet	Oral	900 mg once or twice a day

chosen based on the type of infection and suspected organism. Unless the infection is systemic, topical ophthalmic agents are used.

Sometimes **ophthalmic corticosteroids** (see Table 11.3) are useful for calming inflammation caused by an infection. These agents do not help cure the infection but can reduce pain, redness, and irritation. Patients should follow instructions for using ophthalmic drops and ointments to keep the product sterile and prevent reintroducing infection into the eye.

Do not touch tip of applicator

Table 11.3 Commonly Used Ophthalmic Corticosteroids

Generic (Brand)	Dosage Form	Route of Administration	Common Dose
Dexamethasone (Dexasol, Maxidex, Ozurdex)	Solution, suspension	Ophthalmic	1–2 drops every 1–4 hours
Difluprednate (Durezol)	Emulsion	Ophthalmic	1 drop 2–4 times a day
Fluorometholone (FML, Flarex)	Suspension, ointment	Ophthalmic	1 drop 2–4 times a day; half-inch ribbon 1–3 times a day
Loteprednol (Altrex, Lotemax)	Suspension	Ophthalmic	1–2 drops 4 times a day
Prednisolone (Prednisol, Pred Mild, Econopred, Pred Forte)	Solution, suspension	Ophthalmic	2 drops 4 times a day
Rimexolone (Vexol)	Suspension	Ophthalmic	1–2 drops every 2 hours or 4 times a day
Triamcinolone (Triesence, Trivaris)	Suspension, gel	Intravitreal	1–4 mg once, then as needed

Side Effects Common side effects of topically administered anti-infectives are few, and if present they are usually mild and tolerable. Although systemic absorption is typically low with these dosage forms, systemic side effects are possible. For a discussion of side effects seen for the drug classes listed here, refer to Chapter 3.

Cautions and Considerations Anti-infectives are drugs to which many patients have allergies. Therefore, pharmacy personnel should ask each patient about allergies and document them in the patient's profile. Even topical agents such as these can cause serious allergic reactions, so updated allergy information is important for patient safety.

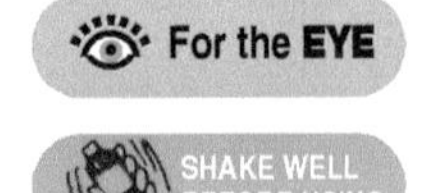

An auxiliary warning label should be used on all ophthalmic products to indicate that they are intended for use in the eyes only. Suspensions should also have a "shake well" label applied.

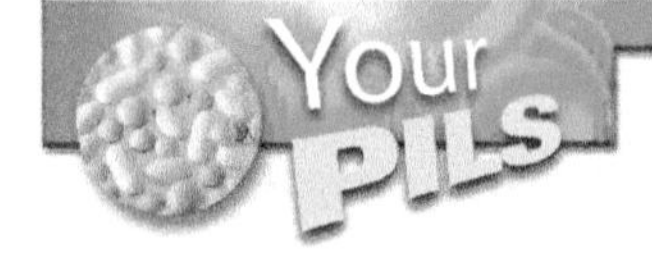

Learners who like details and reflective learning, such as Producers, may find this exercise useful for putting eye and ear antibiotics into context. Compare the drugs listed in Tables 11.2 and 11.5 to the antibiotics covered in Chapter 3. Which antibiotics are available in oral, ophthalmic, and otic dosage forms? Which drug classes from Chapter 3 are represented in this chapter? Think about ways you can keep these agents physically separated in the pharmacy as well as in your own memory.

Eye Allergies and Chronic Dry Eye

Exposure to allergens (including pollen, dust, smoke, and pollution) triggers the redness, itching, and tearing that are the symptoms of **eye allergies.** Allergies can also cause inflammations such as conjunctivitis. **Chronic dry eye** is the inability to produce sufficient tears and lubrication for the eye. It can be a side effect of some drugs with anticholinergic effects (see Chapter 7).

Drugs for Eye Allergies and Chronic Dry Eye

Drug therapy for eye allergies includes **topical antihistamines, decongestants, mast cell stabilizers**, and **nonsteroidal anti-inflammatory drugs (NSAIDs)** (see Table 11.4). These agents reduce the redness and inflammation caused by eye allergies. Ophthalmic NSAIDs are also used for the pain associated with cataract surgery.

Drug therapy for chronic dry eye starts with **normal saline** drops or **artificial tears**. If serious enough, the condition may be treated with cyclosporine, which directly reduces immune activity within the eye. This drug is available in single-use vials. Patients who choose to continue using artificial tears should separate their use of cyclosporine and artificial tears by at least fifteen minutes in order to avoid diluting cyclosporine's effects.

Side effects of these ophthalmic agents, if present, are typically mild and tolerable. Mild stinging or burning immediately after application may occur. The time to maximum effect varies, depending on the specific agent. Antihistamines and anti-inflammatory agents can take a few days for relief of symptoms to occur; cyclosporine and mast cell stabilizers can take four weeks or more for full effect. Patients should be informed of the length of these delays, so that they do not get discouraged and quit a therapy before it starts to work.

Table 11.4 Ophthalmic Agents for Allergies and Chronic Dry Eye

Generic (Brand)	Dosage Form	Dispensing Status	Route of Administration	Common Dose
Cyclosporine (Restasis)	Emulsion	Rx	Ophthalmic	1 drop twice a day
Antihistamines				
Azelastine (Optivar)	Solution	Rx	Ophthalmic	1 drop twice a day
Emedastine (Emadine)	Solution	Rx	Ophthalmic	1 drop 4 times a day
Epinastine (Elestat)	Solution	Rx	Ophthalmic	1 drop twice a day
Ketotifen (Alaway, Zaditor)	Solution	OTC, Rx	Ophthalmic	1 drop every 8–12 hours
Olopatadine (Patanol, Pataday)	Solution	Rx	Ophthalmic	1–2 drops 2 times a day
Decongestants				
Naphazoline (Clear Eyes, Naphcon, AK-Con)	Solution	OTC, Rx	Ophthalmic	1–2 drops every 3–4 hours
Oxymetazoline (Visine LR)	Solution	OTC	Ophthalmic	1–2 drops every 6 hours
Phenylephrine (Altafrin, Relief, AK-Dilate, Neofrin)	Solution	OTC, Rx	Ophthalmic	1 drop up to 3 times a day
Tetrahydrozoline (Altazine, Murine, Opti-Clear, Visine)	Solution	OTC	Ophthalmic	1–2 drops 4 times a day
Mast Cell Stabilizers				
Cromolyn sodium (Crolom)	Solution	Rx	Ophthalmic	1–2 drops 4–6 times a day
Lodoxamide (Alomide)	Solution	Rx	Ophthalmic	1–2 drops 4 times a day
Nedocromil (Alocril)	Solution	Rx	Ophthalmic	1–2 drops twice a day
Pemirolast (Alamast)	Solution	Rx	Ophthalmic	1–2 drops 4 times a day
NSAIDs				
Bromfenac (Xibrom)	Solution	Rx	Ophthalmic	1 drop twice a day
Diclofenac (Voltaren)	Solution	Rx	Ophthalmic	1–2 drops 4 times a day
Ketorolac (Acular)	Solution	Rx	Ophthalmic	1 drop 4 times a day
Nepafenac (Nevanac)	Suspension	Rx	Ophthalmic	1 drop 3 times a day

Retinopathy and Macular Degeneration

Retinopathy refers to destruction of the retina. It can be caused by a variety of conditions, and the most common is diabetes. In diabetic retinopathy, tiny blood vessels that supply the retina with blood are damaged, allowing minute hemorrhaging to occur. Diabetic retinopathy is a leading cause of blindness in the United States, but it can be prevented through proper treatment and control of blood glucose levels. If retinopathy is detected early, laser treatments can keep vision loss at bay. Pharmacists and technicians can help by reminding patients with diabetes that annual eye exams are important for preserving eyesight.

Macular degeneration is generally associated with increasing age and is a painless condition that can go undetected until vision is significantly affected. The macula is responsible for central vision. Central vision is used for reading, driving, and focusing on others' faces. When the breakdown of tissue in this area occurs slowly with age, the condition is referred to as **dry macular degeneration**. Changes in sight include blurry vision and requiring more light to read. **Wet macular degeneration**, in which tissue breakdown occurs rapidly from fast blood vessel growth and rupture, is not associated with age. Vision changes are quick to develop and make straight lines appear wavy.

Ear Infections

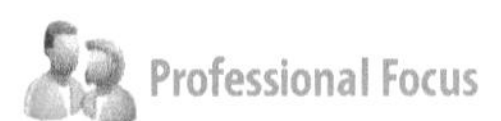

Pharmacy personnel should keep inventories of ophthalmic and otic products separate to prevent medication errors. Take care when putting new stock away to be sure the eye- and eardrop bottles are stored in a way that prevents dispensing errors. Double-check the labeling on the bottle every time you choose an eye- or eardrop from the shelf.

External ear infection (**otitis externa**) is an infection of the ear canal and involves bacteria or fungi that thrive in moist environments such as that found in earwax. Regular swimmers have the highest propensity to develop external ear infections. **Middle ear infection** (**otitis media**) is most common in children. Because the eustachian tube is more horizontal than vertical in children as compared with adults, fluid from the middle ear does not drain well in children, allowing bacteria and viruses to flourish. Most middle ear infections are viral in nature and clear on their own or develop after a viral respiratory tract infection in which mucus and fluid build up and provide a growing medium for bacteria. Symptoms of an ear infection include ear pain, jaw pain, sinus pain, itching, and fever. Pain is often dramatic enough to cause patients (or their parents) to seek medical attention. Primary care prescribers attempt to be judicious when prescribing antibiotics for ear infections so as to reduce antibiotic resistance.

Administering Eardrops

Eardrops are topical medications effective only for certain infections, such as otitis externa. If an infection is in the middle or inner ear, medication applied to the external ear will not reach the intended site of action. Systemic absorption of otic preparations usually is not possible. Oral drug therapy is necessary for middle ear infections, unless the eardrum has ruptured or ear tubes have been surgically placed, creating an opening through which the medication can enter. Inner ear infections require oral therapy.

To receive eardrops, the patient should lie down with the affected ear pointing upward. In children younger than three years old, pull the earlobe gently down and back. In older children and adults, pull the earlobe up and out. This manipulation creates the best angle for administration (see Figure 11.8). Then gently squeeze the dropper bottle to apply the required number of drops into the ear canal.

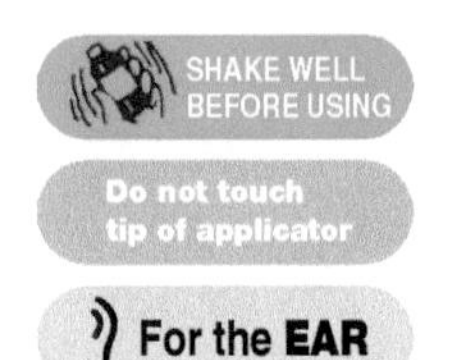

Eardrops are more likely than ophthalmic agents to come in suspensions as well as solutions. Proper shaking instructions should be given. Patients who have tubes in their ears should use suspensions only. Pharmacy technicians should ask patients about ear tubes when filling new prescriptions for otic preparations. Also, patients with ear tubes should keep otic preparations sterile so as not to cause infection. The dropper tip should be kept clean and should not touch anything, including the ear or fingers.

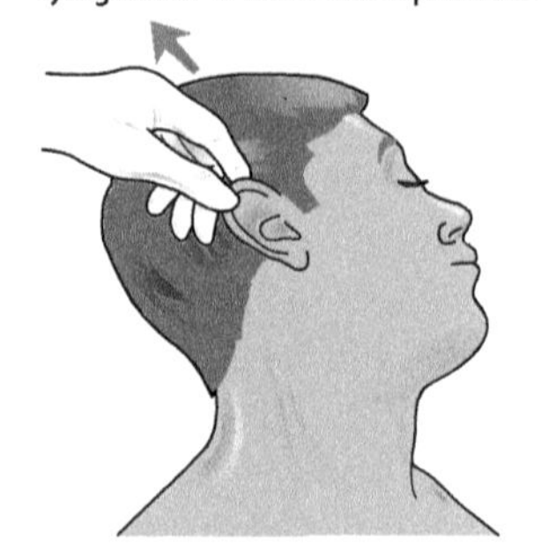
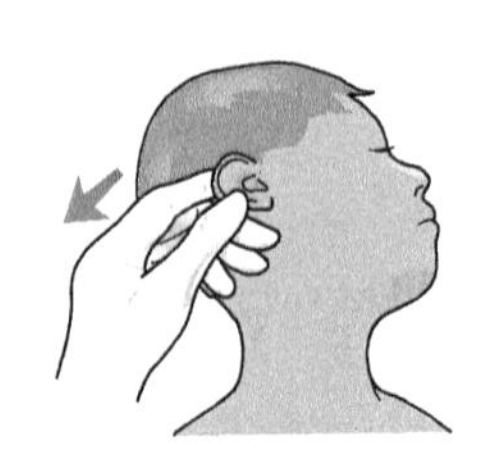

Figure 11.8
Applying Otic Drops
In children older than age 3 and adults, pull the ear up and out. For children under age 3 , pull it down and back. The patient should remain lying down to allow the liquid to travel down and coat the ear canal.

Some physicians prescribe ophthalmic products to be used in the ear. Although it is appropriate to use ophthalmic drops in the ear, in contrast, it is quite painful to use otic drops in the eyes. A warning label to this effect should be applied to prescriptions for eardrops.

Drugs for Ear Infections Bacterial infections of the external ear and cases of middle ear infection in which the tympanic membrane has ruptured or ear tubes are present are treated with **otic antibiotic preparations** (see Table 11.5). **Drying agents** are used for treatment or prevention of external ear infections, especially for patients prone to such infections, such as swimmers. Treatment for swimmer's ear may be on a short-term basis for active infection or a regular (even daily) basis to prevent potential infection. **Earwax removers** are used for patients with cerumen impaction. When cerumen builds up, hearing can become impaired and infection can follow. Earwax removers first loosen and dissolve cerumen, after which irrigation with warm water flushes it out. Topical otic analgesics are used for patients with severe ear pain associated with infection. These products work by temporarily numbing the ear canal (see Table 11.6).

The few side effects of otic agents are rarely (if ever) experienced. And although systemic absorption is rarely seen with otic agents, allergic reactions are still possible.

Table 11.5 Commonly Used Otic Antibiotics

Generic (Brand)	Dosage Form	Route of Administration	Common Dose
Aminoglycosides			
Gentamicin (Garamycin Otic)	Solution	Otic	3–4 drops 3 times a day
Quinolones			
Ciprofloxacin (Cetraxal)	Solution	Otic	1 single-use container twice a day
Ofloxacin (Floxin Otic)	Solution	Otic	10 drops a day
Combinations			
Ciprofloxacin, dexamethasone (Ciprodex)	Solution	Otic	3–4 drops 2–4 times a day
Ciprofloxacin, hydrocortisone (Cipro HC)	Solution	Otic	3 drops twice a day
Neomycin, polymyxin B, hydrocortisone (Cortisporin, Otosporin, AntibiOtic)	Solution	Otic	3–4 drops 2–4 times a day

Table 11.6 Miscellaneous Otic Products

Generic (Brand)	Dosage Form	Route of Administration	Common Dose
Drying Agents			
Acetic acid (various)	Solution	Otic	5–10 drops 2–4 times a day
Boric acid (Dri-Ear Otic)	Solution	Otic	2–3 drops after swimming or showering
Isopropyl alcohol, glycerin (Dri-Ear)	Solution	Otic	4–5 drops in each ear
Earwax Removers			
Carbamide peroxide (Debrox)	Solution	Otic	5–10 drops twice a day
Analgesics			
Antipyrine, benzocaine (Auralgan)	Solution	Otic	Instill a few drops in ear and place cotton pad every 1–2 hours as needed

Pharmacy technicians should be sure to update allergy information for patients, especially when filling a prescription for an antibiotic.

Ototoxicity

Ototoxicity is damage to the ear as a result of chemical or drug exposure. Some drugs, such as aminoglycosides, can cause hearing loss, although the loss is usually temporary if caught early. Symptoms can begin as ringing in the ears (tinnitus) and progress to noticeable hearing loss. Several drugs can cause ototoxicity (see Table 11.7).

Table 11.7 Drugs that Can Cause Ototoxicity

Aminoglycosides
Aspirin and salicylates
Benzodiazepines
Calcium-channel blockers
Cisplatin and some chemotherapy agents
Erythromycin and macrolides
Furosemide
Neomycin
NSAIDs
Quinine
Some antiviral agents used in HIV
Tricyclic antidepressants
Valproic acid

Rhinitis, Seasonal Allergies, and Colds

Conditions of the URT commonly include **rhinitis** (runny nose), **sinus congestion**, **pharyngitis** (sore throat), **laryngitis** (loss of voice), and **epistaxis** (nose bleeding). Runny nose and nasal congestion are frequently caused by seasonal allergies or the common cold. When associated with allergies, symptoms such as watery, itchy eyes; sneezing; runny nose; and sinus congestion tend to occur in relation to a specific trigger. Common allergens that trigger such symptoms include dust, pollen, pet dander, and cigarette smoke. Cells in the respiratory tract release histamine and other inflammatory mediators in response to allergen exposure. **Histamine** dilates arterioles, allowing blood contents to leak into the local area. This process facilitates the movement of white blood cells, which fight disease and foreign allergens, to the affected area. It also causes swelling, mucus production, and soreness. Treatment of allergies includes avoidance of allergens, use of anti-inflammatory medication, and obtaining symptomatic relief with antihistamines and decongestants.

Cold viruses can elicit a similar response. The common cold has no cure because there are too many virus strains that quickly mutate. Treatment for a cold centers around symptom relief. While the disease runs its course, antihistamines, decongestants, cough suppressants, and mucolytics can be used to relieve runny nose, stuffy nose, coughing, and chest congestion.

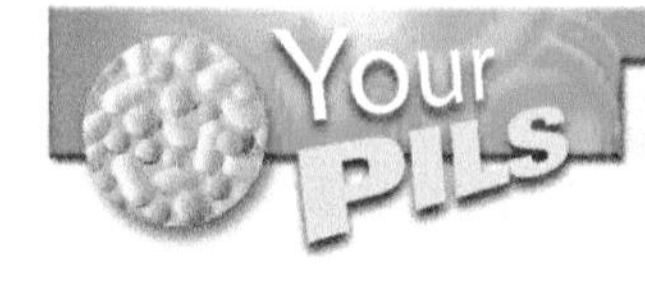

Before you go through this section on cough and cold products, take a look in your medicine cabinet. What medications do you use when you have a stuffy or runny nose? What cough medicine works best for you? Enactors and Directors appreciate hands-on learning activities that apply new information to real life. Make a list of the active ingredients in the products you use, and think about how they work as you learn about their mechanism of action, side effects, and other details.

Drugs for Rhinitis, Seasonal Allergies, and Colds

Treatment for rhinitis and nasal allergies includes many of the same drugs that treat common cold symptoms, including antihistamines, decongestants, and cough remedies. Antihistamines and nasal corticosteroids are used to treat symptoms including runny nose, watery/itchy eyes, and sneezing, whether the symptoms are caused by allergies or infection. Decongestants may be used for allergies that are severe enough to cause nasal congestion. They are used more frequently when a cold produces symptoms of stuffy nose and sinus pain.

Many cough and cold products contain various combinations of antihistamines, decongestants, cough suppressants, and expectorants. These products also contain analgesics such as acetaminophen or ibuprofen. Patients sometimes do not realize which active ingredients they are receiving when taking a combination product. This confusion can lead to duplicate therapy and overdose if a patient takes more than one product. This confusion also leads to unnecessary treatment when a patient takes a combination product for multiple symptoms when all he or she really needs is just one active ingredient for one or two specific symptoms. Pharmacy technicians can play an important role in educating patients about the contents of cough and cold preparations.

Antihistamines This drug class is used for symptomatic relief of excess nasal secretions, itching, sneezing, and coughing. **Antihistamines** are also used to relieve the itching and redness resulting from allergic reactions (such as hives and rashes). These drugs cause sedation, which is useful for mild insomnia and relaxation prior to anesthesia or other anxiety-producing procedures. In fact, the active ingredient in most OTC sleep aids is an antihistamine. First-generation antihistamines tend to cause the most sedation. Second-generation antihistamines do not cross the blood-brain barrier as readily; therefore, they cause less sedation. Antihistamines have also been used for motion sickness and Parkinson's disease.

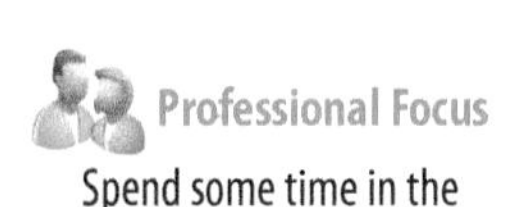

Spend some time in the cough and cold aisle of the OTC section. Familiarize yourself with the active ingredients of products that patients purchase most often. Become the expert on the specific symptoms each brand treats.

Antihistamines work by blocking **histamine (H_1) receptors**, which reduces capillary dilation and leakage. Doses for each agent vary widely based on patient age, dosage form, and reason for use (see Table 11.8). Product packaging should be consulted whenever possible to verify proper dosing for the age of the patient being treated.

Side Effects The most common side effects of antihistamines are drowsiness (first-generation), dry mouth, and urinary retention. Patients who take other medications that also cause drowsiness should take care with antihistamines because sedation could be excessive. For this same reason, patients should avoid drinking alcohol while taking antihistamines. Patients who have urination problems, including patients with prostate enlargement, should not use antihistamines because they can make urination even more difficult.

In some children, antihistamines have a paradoxical effect, causing excitation rather than drowsiness. Parents should be aware of this potential side effect.

Cautions and Considerations Patients who have high blood pressure or heart problems should talk with their prescribers before taking antihistamines. Antihistamines should not be given to infants or mothers who are breast-feeding. Patients with glaucoma or who are using monoamine oxidase inhibitors should not take antihistamines.

Table 11.8 Commonly Used Antihistamines

Generic (Brand)	Dosage Form	Route of Administration	Common Dose
First Generation			
Chlorpheniramine (Chlor-Trimeton)	Tablet, capsule, syrup, suspension	Oral	Varies by age
Clemastine (Tavist)	Tablet, syrup	Oral	Varies by age and use
Diphenhydramine (Benadryl)	Tablet, capsule, oral strip, liquid, elixir, syrup, suspension, injection	Oral, IM, IV	Varies depending on age, dosage form, and use
Second Generation			
Cetirizine (Zyrtec)	Tablet, syrup	Oral	Varies by age and use
Desloratadine (Clarinex)	Tablet, syrup	Oral	Varies by age
Fexofenadine (Allegra)	Tablet, suspension	Oral	Varies by age
Loratadine (Claritin)	Tablet, syrup	Oral	Varies by age

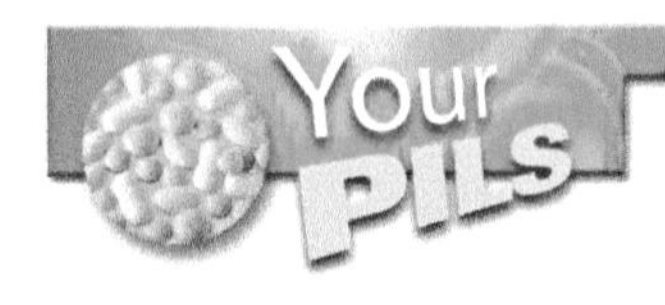

If you currently work in a pharmacy and are a reflective learner, as are Creators and Producers, try this activity. Sit down at the end of your shift and write down all brand name cough and cold products you saw that day. Try to recall the generic drug names and symptoms treated for each product you write down.

Decongestants This class of drugs is used for the sinus congestion and pain caused by common colds, infections, or allergies. They reduce sinus tissue swelling and allow for better drainage. **Decongestants** (see Table 11.9) work by stimulating adrenergic receptors in nasal passages, which constricts blood vessels and reduces swelling.

Doses for each agent vary widely based on patient age, dosage form, and reason for use. Product packaging should be consulted whenever possible to verify proper dosing for the age of the patient being treated.

Side Effects Common side effects of decongestants include headache, dizziness, lightheadedness, insomnia, nervousness, and nausea. These effects are usually mild, but if they persist or are severe, the patient should contact a healthcare provider. Topical preparations can cause sneezing and nasal irritation.

Potentially serious effects include increased blood pressure and fast or irregular heartbeat. Patients with high blood pressure or heart problems should not use decongestants unless they talk with their prescribers first.

Cautions and Considerations When used topically, decongestants can cause rebound swelling and congestion if used for longer than three days. As a result, patients using decongestant nasal sprays for longer than a few days at a time may have worsened congestion when they stop using them. This rebound swelling lasts a few days and then subsides. Rebound congestion can make stopping decongestant use difficult, because symptoms will seem to have returned and worsened. Patients may find themselves using such a product longer than is truly needed.

Some decongestants, including **pseudoephedrine**, are available over the counter but are restricted. These drugs can be used illegally as precursor substances in preparing methamphetamine (crystal meth), a highly addictive and illegal drug. Consequently, most state and federal laws have limits on the quantities of these drugs that can be purchased. Usually patients must be at least eighteen years old, provide proof of age, and sign specific records at the time of purchase. To protect themselves as well as patients, pharmacy technicians must be familiar with these laws and the procedures for the handling and sale of these products at their worksites.

Table 11.9 Commonly Used Decongestants

Generic (Brand)	Dosage Form	Route of Administration	Common Dose
Phenylephrine (Sudafed PE, Pedia Care, Neo-Synephrine, Triaminic)	Tablet, oral liquid, chewable tablet, oral strip, nasal spray	Oral, nasal	Varies by age and dosage form
Pseudoephedrine (Sudafed, Simply Stuffy, Dimetapp, Drixoral, others)	Tablet, capsule, oral liquid, syrup, drops, suspension	Oral	Varies by age and dosage form

Cough Suppressants and Expectorants When coughing is excessive and nonproductive (dry, hacking), **cough suppressants** are used. These agents depress the cough reflex in the cough center of the medulla in the brain. Dextromethorphan is a relative of the codeine molecule that does not have the pain-relieving or addictive properties of opiates. Hydrocodone and codeine are opiates that treat pain at higher doses.

Expectorants are used when a cough is productive (wet, mucus-producing). They are also called mucolytic agents. Mucolytics work by liquefying respiratory secretions to allow them to be cleared easily.

Doses for each agent vary widely based on patient age, dosage form, and reason for use (see Table 11.10). Product packaging should be consulted whenever possible to verify appropriate dosing for the age of the patient.

Table 11.10 Commonly Used Cough Medications

Generic (Brand)	Dosage Form	Route of Administration	Common Dose
Suppressants			
Codeine phosphate (many)	Tablet, capsule, syrup	Oral	Varies by product and dosage form
Dextromethorphan (Robitussin, Sucrets DM, Triaminic, Vicks 44, PediaCare, others)	Capsule, lozenge, oral strip, liquid, syrup, suspension, solution, freezer pop	Oral	Varies by age and dosage form
Hydrocodone (many)	Tablet, liquid	Oral	Varies by product and dosage form
Expectorant/Mucolytic			
Guaifenesin (Robitussin, Mucinex, others)	Tablet, granules, syrup, liquid	Oral	Varies by age and dosage form

May Cause DROWSINESS
Use Caution while Driving
Do not drink alcoholic beverages when taking this medication

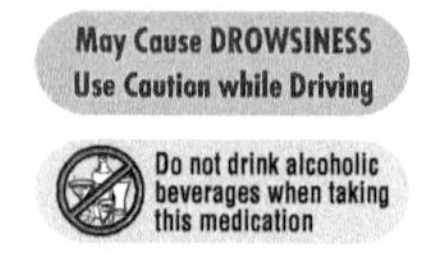

Side Effects Common side effects of cough suppressants include drowsiness, dizziness, and stomach upset. Patients should see how these agents affect them before driving. They should also avoid alcohol or other drugs that cause drowsiness while taking cough suppressants. Additive effects can cause excessive drowsiness and dangerously slow breathing.

Side effects of guaifenesin are rare and mild when they occur. Side effects could include stomach upset and headache.

Cautions and Considerations Codeine-derivative cough suppressants may be available over the counter but are restricted. Many states limit the quantities of these drugs that can be purchased at once. The pharmacist must dispense these medications. To protect themselves as well as patients, pharmacy technicians must be familiar with these laws and the procedures for handling and sale of these products at their worksites.

Nasal Corticosteroids Nasal allergy symptoms localized to the URT (i.e., nasal passages) are often treated with **topical nasal corticosteroids** (see Table 11.11). Using these agents during seasons when allergies are most likely reduces inflammation and allergy symptoms.

These products are administered intranasally and the patient should be in the upright position with the head tilted slightly forward. Gently insert the sprayer tip into the nostril and depress the applicator to deliver a metered dose. Patients should breathe through the nose gently and slowly when depressing the sprayer. The patient does not

Table 11.11 Commonly Used Nasal Corticosteroids

Generic (Brand)	Dosage Form	Route of Administration	Common Dose
Beclomethasone (Beconase AQ)	Spray	Nasal	1–2 inhalations in each nostril twice a day
Budesonide (Rhinocort Aqua)	Spray	Nasal	2–4 sprays each nostril once a day
Ciclesonide (Omnaris)	Spray	Nasal	2 sprays each nostril once a day
Flunisolide (AeroBID)	Spray	Nasal	1–2 sprays each nostril 2–3 times a day
Fluticasone (Flonase, Veramyst)	Spray	Nasal	2 sprays each nostril once a day
Mometasone (Nasonex)	Spray	Nasal	1–2 sprays each nostril once a day
Triamcinolone (Nasacort AQ)	Spray	Nasal	1–2 sprays each nostril once a day

need to breathe in quickly or forcefully. The patient also does not need to hold his or her breath. The site of action is in the nose, not deep in the sinuses or lungs.

Side Effects Common side effects of nasal allergy products include cough, sore throat, headache, and runny nose. Typically, these effects are mild and tolerable. Nosebleeds can also occur, especially in children. Patients who experience nosebleeds while taking one of these agents should speak with their healthcare providers.

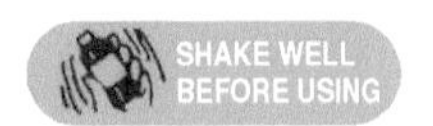

Cautions and Considerations For proper dosing, patients should shake these products well before administration. An auxiliary warning label should be used to remind patients to shake the container prior to using it.

The spray application bottle should be primed when new and when it has not been used for a while. Priming means that the patient should pump the sprayer a few times until an even amount of spray exits the applicator.

Herbal and Alternative Therapies

Echinacea, **zinc**, and **vitamin C** are natural or herbal products that patients often take to boost immune function and fight off cold and flu viruses. Cold and flu viruses are the most common causes of symptoms involving the ears, nose, and throat. Although some success with these products has been seen, standardized regimens have not been proven in the scientific literature. Echinacea or zinc, if used, must be started at the first sign of infection to have any significant effect on the severity or length of symptoms. Vitamin C is best taken as a preventive agent during the cold and flu season. For further discussion of these agents, see Chapter 3 on anti-infective agents.

Vitamin A is essential for photoreceptor cell growth and regeneration. Deficiency in vitamin A can cause night blindness. Vitamins A (**beta carotene**), C, E, and zinc may slow disease progression of age-related macular degeneration. Ocuvite is a brand-name combination product made especially for this use. It is taken in doses of two tablets each morning and evening with food. This combination of vitamins does not cure or prevent macular degeneration. Patients who smoke or have a high risk of certain types of cancer may not be good candidates for therapy with this product. Patients should talk with their healthcare providers before starting to take any vitamin products to treat eye conditions.

Chapter Summary

Eye conditions include glaucoma, infections, retinopathy, and macular degeneration. The most common eye conditions for which drug therapy is used are glaucoma, bacterial infections, and viral infections. Topical beta blockers, alpha agonists, sympathomimetics, miotics, carbonic anhydrase inhibitors, and prostaglandin agonists are given as ophthalmic drops for glaucoma. Numerous antibiotics and antiviral medications are administered as eyedrops and ointments. Eyedrops must be kept sterile, so the applicator tip should not touch anything. Applying eye ointments requires a technique that can take practice to learn and perform well.

Eardrops are used most often for external ear infections but can be used for inner ear infections in some cases. Applying eardrops to young children (under age 3) requires one to pull the ear down and back; administering eardrops to older children and adults requires pulling the ear up and out. Eyedrops can be used in the ears, but eardrops should not be used in the eyes. Technicians should take care to accurately choose eye and ear products from the shelves when dispensing.

Conditions of the nose and throat URT for which drug therapy is used include cold and flu viral infections. Symptoms such as runny nose (rhinitis), sinus congestion, and cough frequently accompany URT infections. Antihistamines, decongestants, cough suppressants, and expectorants are used to combat symptoms of colds and respiratory tract infections, but they do not cure the infections. Natural and herbal products used for ear, nose, and throat conditions include vitamin A, vitamin C, echinacea, and zinc.

✔ Chapter Review

For the following sets of exercises, write the exercise heading, exercise numbers, and your answers on a separate sheet of paper. Your instructor may direct you to turn in the sheet of paper or discuss your answers as a class.

REVIEW THE BASICS

Choose a, b, c, or d as the correct answer to each multiple-choice question.

1. Which part of the eye is responsible for central, focused eyesight in the daytime?
   a. conjunctiva
   b. macula
   c. incus and stapes
   d. retina

2. Which part of the ear is a tube that allows fluid to drain from the middle ear to the throat?
   a. anterior chamber
   b. eustachian
   c. larynx
   d. semicircular canals

3. Which of the following drug classes are used topically *and* orally for eye allergies and sinus stuffiness?
   a. beta blockers
   b. expectorants
   c. carbonic anhydrase inhibitors
   d. decongestants

4. Which of the following is an otic agent used for the ear pain associated with otitis media?
   a. Auralgan
   b. Patanol
   c. Tobrex
   d. Vistide

5. Someone with heart problems or high blood pressure should not take which of the following drug classes?
   a. decongestants
   b. otic antibiotics
   c. ophthalmic corticosteroids
   d. all of the above

6. Which of the following drugs is available in an oral dosage form used for glaucoma?
   a. Azopt
   b. Diamox
   c. Timoptic
   d. Travoprost

7. Which of the following drugs can change the color of a patient's eyes?
   a. bimatoprost
   b. carbamide peroxide
   c. cyclosporine
   d. levofloxacin

8. Which of the following drugs is used for cough and comes as an oral liquid and a tablet?
   a. clemastine
   b. dextromethorphan
   c. guaifenesin
   d. pseudoephedrine

9. Which of the following can cause rebound sinus congestion if used longer than three days?
   a. Benadryl
   b. Neo-Synephrine
   c. Nasonex
   d. Mucinex

10. Which of the following has a usual dosage amount of ten drops a day?
    a. bromfenac
    b. ofloxacin
    c. ketotifen
    d. latanoprost

KNOW THE DRUGS

Match each brand name drug with its corresponding generic name and most common use. Your answers should follow this example format: Generic Name: 1. a; 2. b; 3. c; etc. Most Common Use: 1. h; 2. i; 3. j; etc.

Brand Name	Generic Name	Most Common Use
1. Nasonex	a. cetirizine	h. glaucoma
2. Zyrtec	b. betaxolol	i. eye allergies
3. Alomide	c. fexofenadine	j. antihistamine
4. Ocupress	d. carteolol	k. nasal corticosteroid
5. Azopt	e. mometasone	
6. Betoptic	f. brinzolamide	
7. Allegra	g. lodoxamide	

PUT IT TOGETHER

For each item, write down a short answer, indicate true or false, or provide a single term to complete the sentence.

1. What do Claritin and Patanol have in common? How do they differ?
2. Name two auxiliary warning labels you should put on all ophthalmic medications.
3. True or False: Ophthalmic drops can be given in the ear.
4. ______________ keep you from coughing, whereas ______________ help to liquefy mucus, allowing you to cough it out more easily.
5. Vitamin _____ helps photoreceptor cells to grow and regenerate, which is helpful for night vision and preventing macular degeneration.
6. ______________-generation antihistamines tend to cause less drowsiness as a side effect.
7. Name two drug classes that can cause ototoxicity.

THINK IT THROUGH

Read and think through each numbered scenario carefully and then write several sentences in reply to the question(s) presented. Question 4 requires you to do some Internet research before completing your answer(s).

1. Explain how to administer eardrops to a toddler versus to an adult. What do you do differently?
2. Mr. Collins comes to the counter to purchase Sudafed. As you proceed with the proper procedures for the sale of this drug precursor item, he mentions he would like to have his blood pressure taken. He says he just saw his doctor, who recommended he check his blood pressure regularly. He does not have a home blood pressure monitor and doesn't feel he can trust the electronic blood pressure machine in the pharmacy. What should you do?
3. A patient approaches you in the OTC aisle to ask about cough and cold products. He says that he has been taking Benadryl for seasonal allergies, but it makes him too drowsy at work. He wants to know which cold medicine would help his runny nose, sneezing, and watery eyes without making him feel so tired. What should you do?

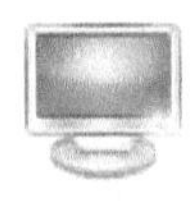

4. **On the Internet,** look up an alternative brand name and use for bimatoprost. Research the available similar products on the market. What do they contain and how are they used? To where should you refer patients asking about such products?

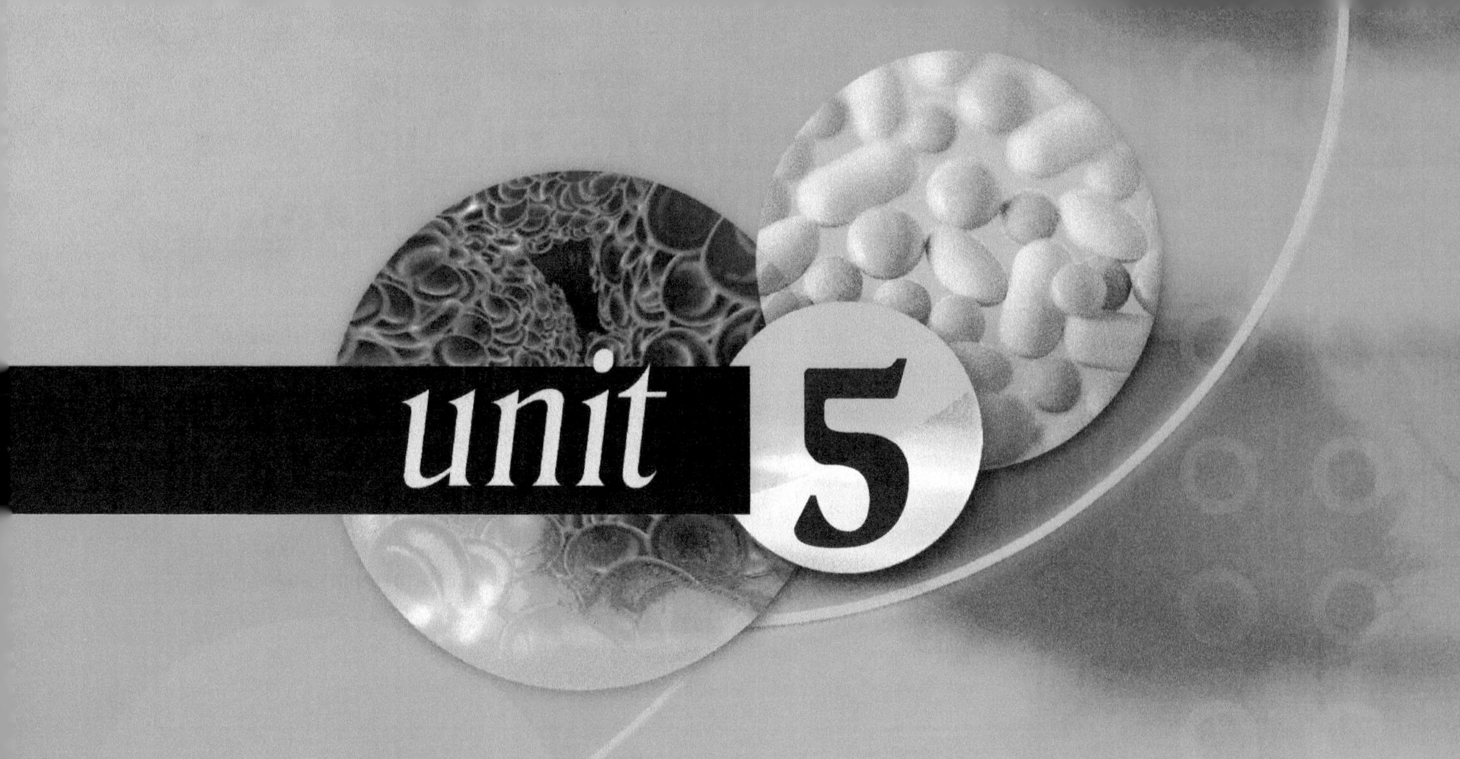

unit 5

Drugs for the Cardiovascular and Respiratory Systems

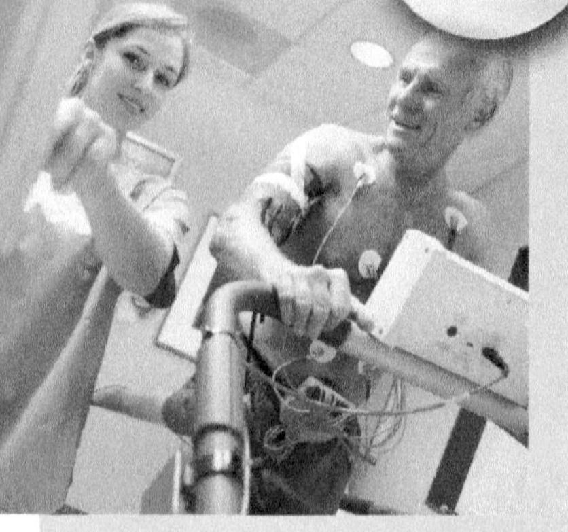

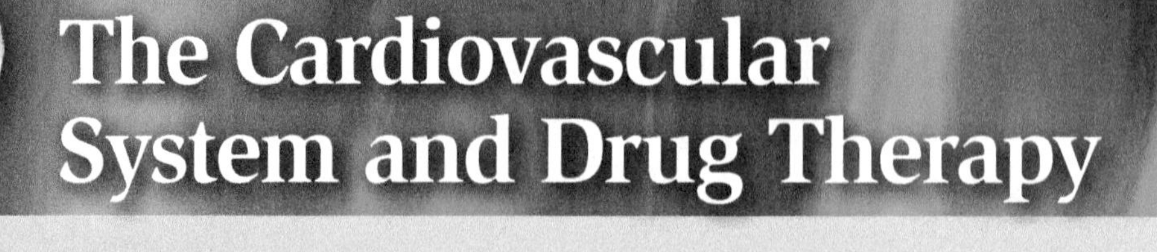

Chapter 12 The Cardiovascular System and Drug Therapy

- Describe the basic anatomy and physiology of the cardiovascular system.
- Explain the therapeutic effects of prescription medications, nonprescription medications, and alternative therapies commonly used to treat diseases of the cardiovascular system.
- Describe the adverse effects of prescription medications, nonprescription medications, and alternative therapies commonly used to treat diseases of the cardiovascular system.
- Identify the brand and generic names of prescription and nonprescription medications commonly used to treat diseases of the cardiovascular system.
- State the doses, dosage forms, and routes of administration for prescription and nonprescription medications commonly used to treat diseases of the cardiovascular system.

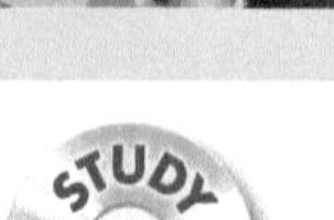

Interactive self-quizzes, games, audio files, and glossaries help you to learn drug names and facts.

Because **heart disease**, more formally known as **cardiovascular disease**, is the leading cause of death in the United States, many healthcare resources are devoted to it. Unfortunately, it seems that everyone knows someone who has had a heart attack. But cardiovascular disease is more than heart attacks. It also includes hypertension (high blood pressure), arrhythmia, angina, and heart failure. The drugs used to prevent and treat cardiovascular disease represent a large number of the total prescriptions dispensed nationally. In fact, most pharmacy technicians will encounter high blood pressure medications on a daily basis. Be aware that the number of medications used for the **cardiovascular system** is large, and learning them can be a daunting task. Nonetheless, the frequency with which pharmacy technicians prepare and dispense such agents makes familiarity with these drugs imperative.

This chapter describes the function of the heart and blood vessels and then outlines the most common conditions (listed above) affecting the cardiovascular system. The drug classes used most frequently for these conditions include beta blockers, angiotensin-converting enzyme (ACE) inhibitors, calcium-channel blockers, antiarrhythmic agents, digoxin, and nitroglycerin. Last, this chapter also covers hyperlipidemia, because this condition contributes to cardiovascular disease.

Anatomy and Physiology of the Cardiovascular System

The cardiovascular system, which includes the heart and blood vessels, circulates blood throughout the body, bringing needed oxygen and nutrients to tissues and carrying away carbon dioxide and toxic by-products. Without a properly functioning cardiovascular system, life is not sustainable. The heart pumps blood out to the body through **arteries,** which carry blood away from the heart, and receives blood back from the tissues via **veins** (see Figure 12.1). In the **capillaries,** which are tiny blood vessels, critical fluids, gases, and nutrients are exchanged between the blood and body tissues. The heart also pumps blood through the lungs, where the blood is replenished with **oxygen** and releases **carbon dioxide**, which is then exhaled.

The heart is made of specialized **cardiac muscle** fibers that make up the heart's four chambers: the right and left **atria** and the right and left **ventricles**. Figure 12.2 shows the functional anatomy of the heart. The atria receive the blood that is brought to the heart, and the ventricles push blood out, either to the lungs or to other body tissues.

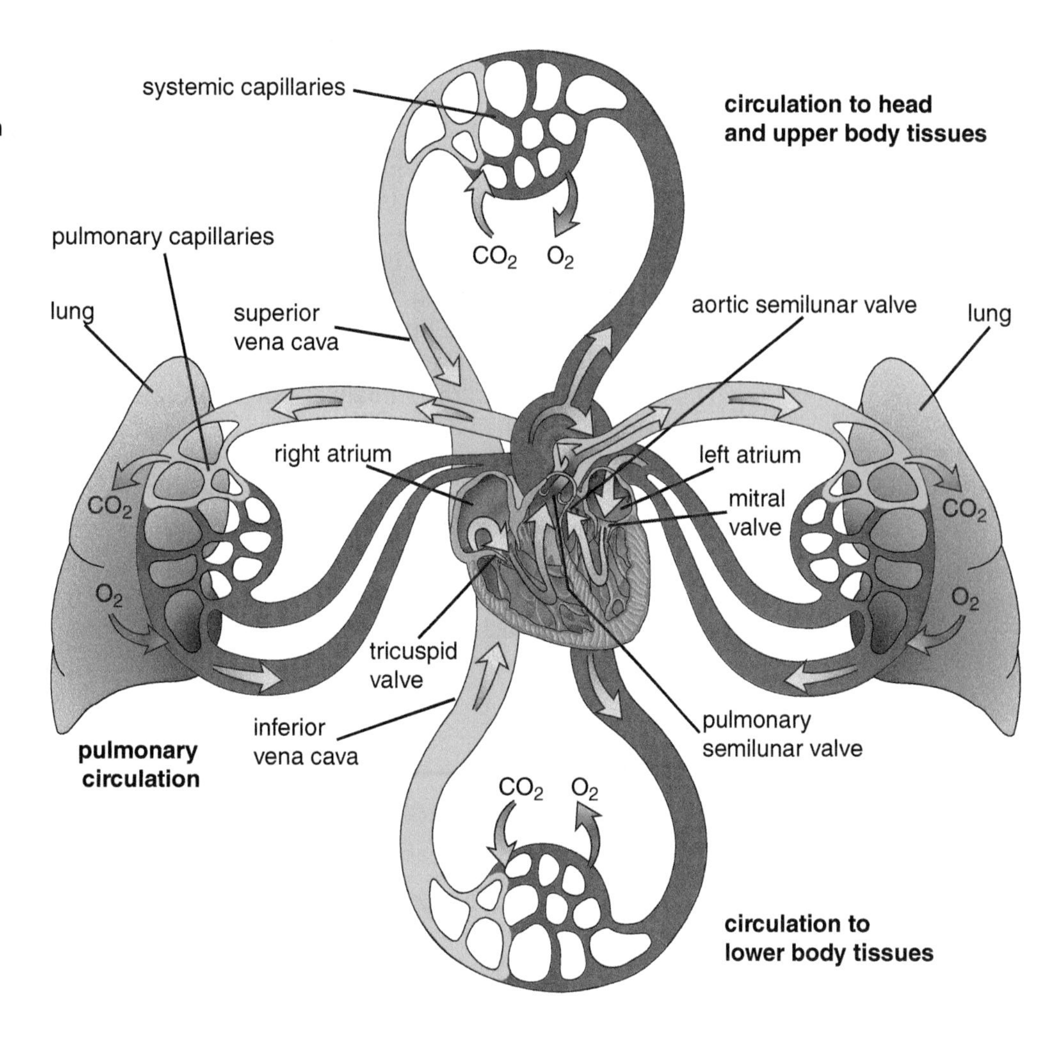

Figure 12.1
Blood Flow through the Circulatory System
Oxygenated blood is depicted in red, whereas blood returning from the body, in need of oxygen, is shown in blue.

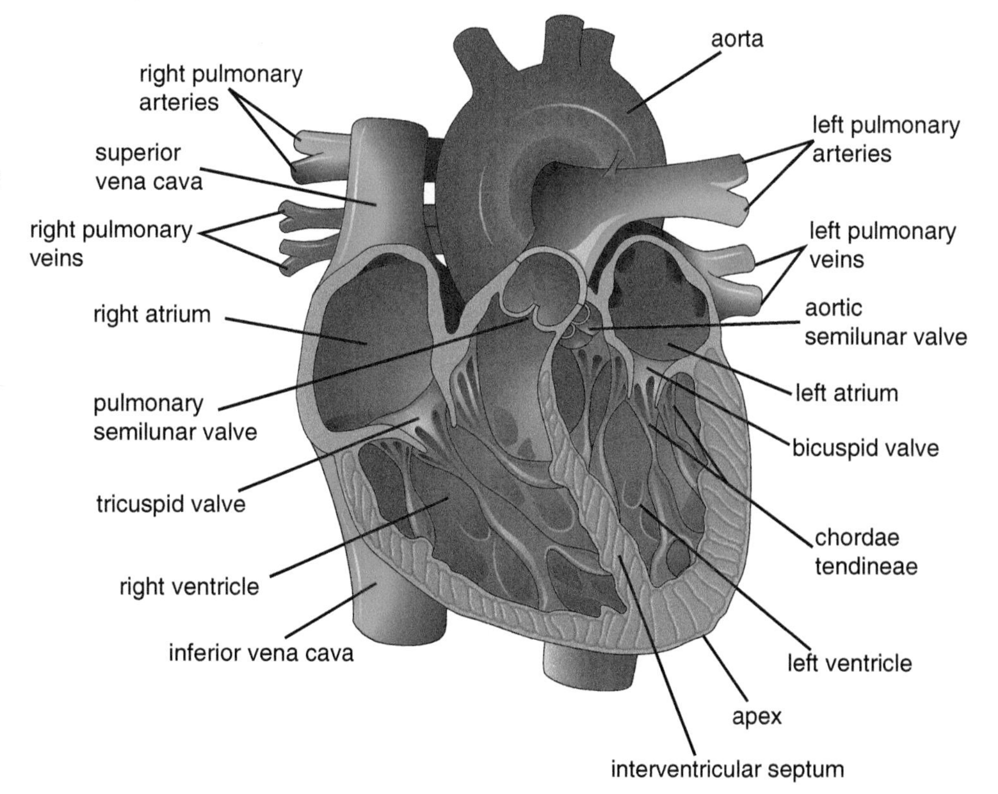

Figure 12.2
Anatomy of the Heart
Blood is prevented from flowing backward within the heart by the one-way valves between the atria and ventricles. These valves snap shut in a coordinated, two-step process that creates an audible sound—the distinctive "lub-dub" of a heartbeat.

Systole refers to the time period during which the heart is contracting and actively pumping blood. **Diastole** refers to the time period when heart muscle relaxes, allowing blood to passively flow in and fill up the heart chambers. Cardiac muscle contraction in the atria and ventricles is coordinated by special conduction fibers that carry electrical signals through the heart tissue (see Figure 12.3). These electrical signals control muscle contraction (systole) and relaxation (diastole) by depolarizing and repolarizing the surface of cardiac muscle cells. In effect, a wave of positive-to-negative electrical charges passes from cell to cell, causing them to contract in sequence. Potassium, sodium, and calcium ions, all positively charged, cross the cell membrane through tiny channels and create the waves of positive and negative charge.

The heartbeat starts in the **sinoatrial (SA) node**, a bundle of conduction fibers in the right atrium and often called the heart's natural pacemaker. The electrical signal is carried through the atria and at the same time down to the **atrioventricular (AV) node**. After a delay, the signal travels through the **bundle of His**. At this point, the signal branches into the **Purkinje fibers**, which stretch into the ventricles to contract the lower—and largest—part of the heart. The signal travels down to the apex of the heart first, and then back up to the ventricular myocardium. The typical rate at which the SA node fires to initiate each heartbeat is seventy to eighty times per minute. **Heart rate**

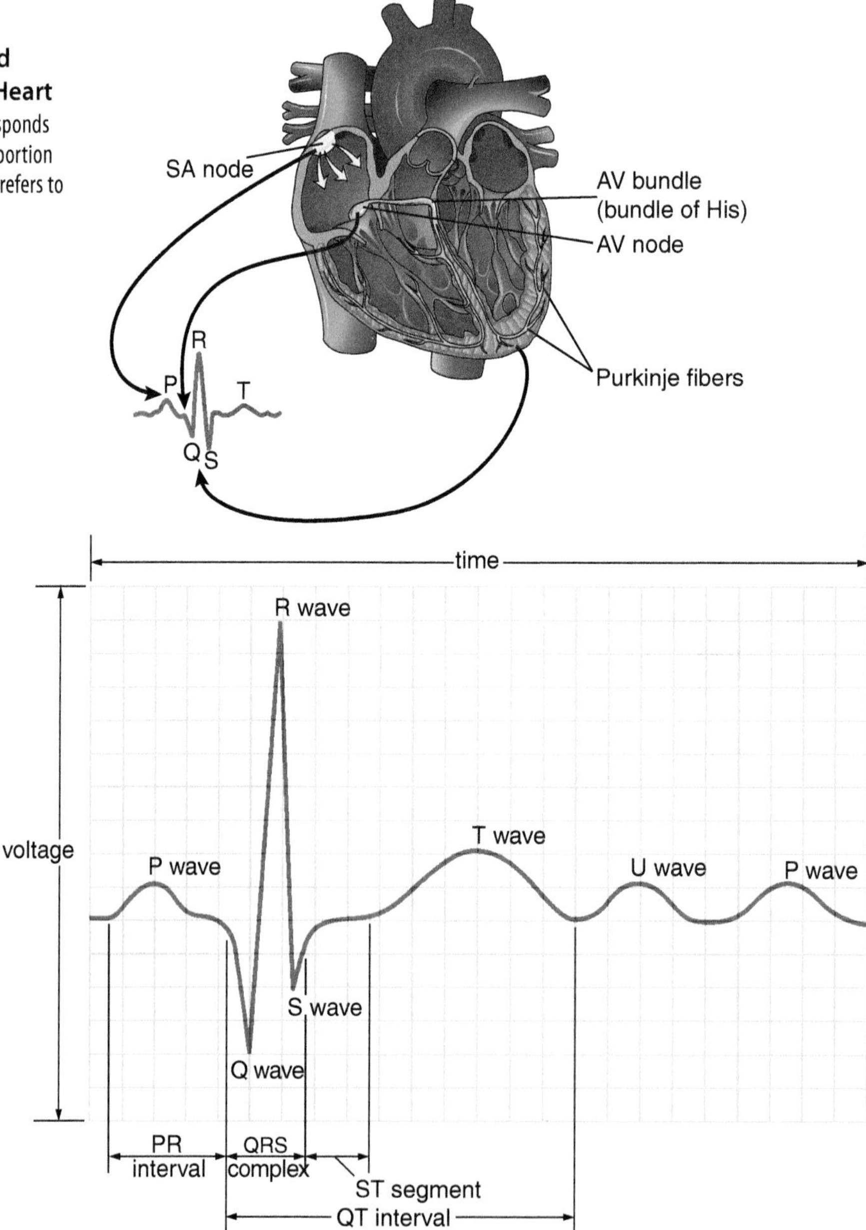

Figure 12.3
Electrocardiogram (ECG or EKG) and Electrical Conduction through the Heart
Each section of the ECG wave is labeled and corresponds to action in a particular part of the heart. The PR portion corresponds to atrial function and the QT interval refers to ventricular function.

(HR) is reported in **beats per minute (BPM)** and is measured by taking a person's **pulse**. Easy places to feel a pulse are at the carotid artery in the neck or at the radial pulse on the thumb side of the wrist.

The electrical signal flowing through the heart is measured with an **electrocardiogram (ECG or EKG)** machine. This machine translates these signals into a wave line that is drawn onto paper or displayed on a screen (see Figure 12.3). Cardiologists look for abnormalities in the shape or size of these waves to diagnose heart dysfunction.

Blood pressure, the force of blood that fills the circulatory system, is maintained by complex feedback mechanisms. Figure 12.4 shows the variety of mechanisms that work together to properly balance blood pressure. In simple terms, blood pressure is a function of:

- **Capacitance**—how much blood is held in the system
- **Peripheral vascular resistance (PVR)**—how constricted or relaxed the blood vessels are
- **Cardiac output (CO)**—the force and volume of blood coming from the heart
- **Renin–angiotensin system**—a feedback mechanism that is regulated by the kidneys and balances fluid volume and vessel constriction

If blood vessels are constricted, causing increased PVR, the heart has to work harder to maintain the same CO to keep blood pressure stable. Therefore, constriction or dilation of blood vessels will raise or lower blood pressure, respectively. High blood pressure is often caused by elevated PVR. Stress on the heart from high blood pressure may cause cardiac disease. High blood pressure also affects vital organs and can eventually result in kidney failure and stroke. Sympathetic nerves in the autonomic nervous system (see Chapter 7) regulate this multifaceted system. Alterations in any one of these compensatory checks and balances can cause hypertension (see following page). Losing large amounts of blood lowers blood pressure to dangerous levels. If blood pressure falls low enough, the patient may go into **shock,** a condition during which vital organs are not perfused with blood and begin to die.

Measuring Blood Pressure

Blood pressure is measured with an instrument called a sphygmomanometer and a cuff that is wrapped around a patient's arm and inflated to apply pressure. The cuff briefly cuts off blood flow through the brachial artery in the upper arm. Air is slowly released

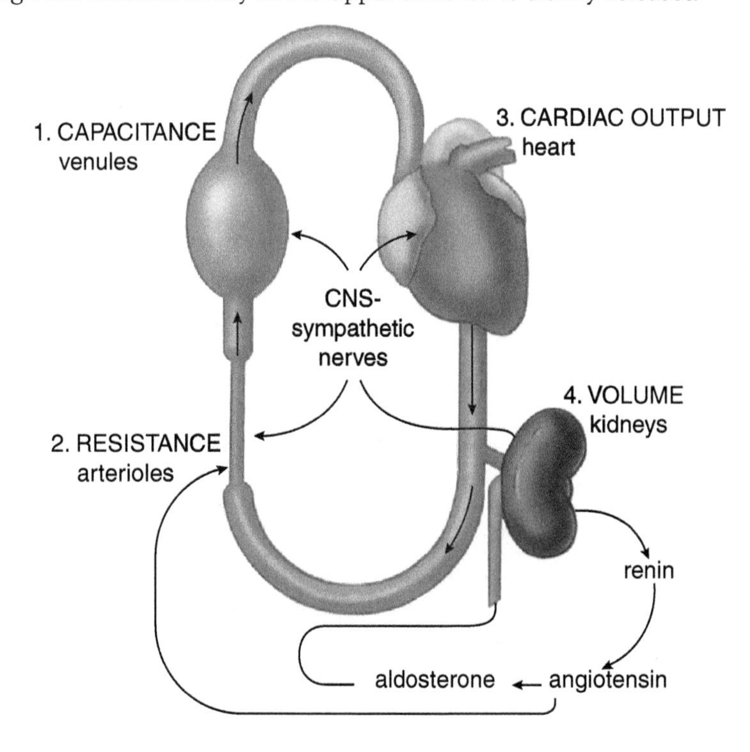

Figure 12.4
Maintaining Blood Pressure
Blood and fluid volume, one of four factors that control blood pressure, is maintained by the kidneys and renin-angiotensin system.

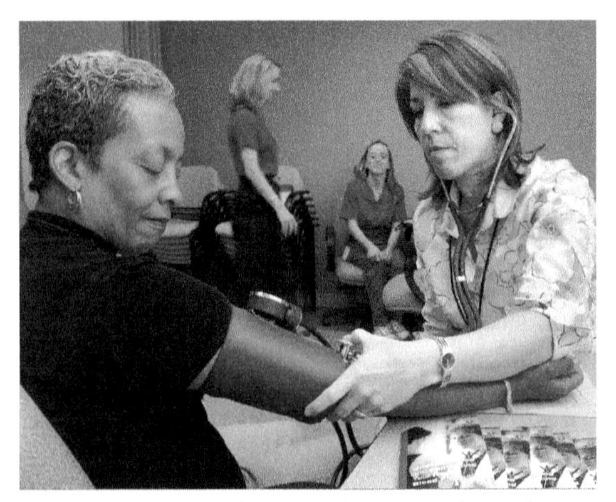

Many people, including pharmacy technicians, can be taught to measure blood pressure and, with practice, become skilled enough to perform it accurately on patients.

from the cuff, lowering the pressure to a point at which the blood begins flowing (with turbulence, however) through the artery again. This turbulent blood flow is audible through a stethoscope placed over the brachial artery. When blood starts flowing again, the first or upper number reported in a blood pressure result is taken. This number is called the systolic reading or the systolic blood pressure (SBP). The diastolic reading or the diastolic blood pressure (DBP), the lower number in a blood pressure result, is taken at the point at which the cuff is loose enough that blood freely flows without turbulence through the artery. At this turbulence-free point, the pulsing sound heard through the stethoscope fades away and becomes silent. Therefore, when taking a reading, you listen first for the start of the sound (and note the systolic reading or SBP) and second for when the sound goes away (and note the diastolic reading or DBP). Ideal blood pressure is considered to be 120/80 mm Hg or lower, but this number can be affected by recent stress, physical activity, caffeine intake, nicotine use, and various medical conditions.

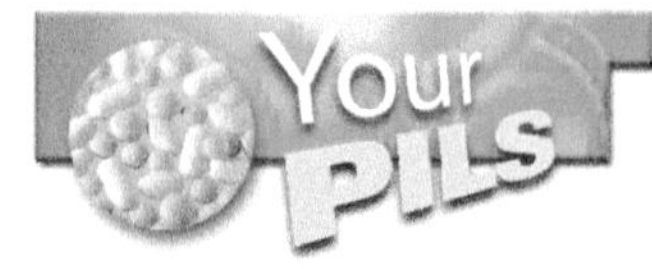

Learners who prefer visual images and abstract thought, like Creators do, may find it helpful to superimpose a list of drugs and their dosage forms onto Figure 12.4. Under each of the four primary compensatory mechanisms for maintaining blood pressure, list the drugs that affect each one. To complete this list, think about a drug's mechanism of action.

Hypertension

High blood pressure, or **hypertension**, is a silent killer that affects more than 50 million people in the United States. Patients cannot immediately feel the effects of hypertension, but damage to vital organs such as the heart, kidneys, eyes, and brain occurs when pressure is high for long periods of time. Elevation in either systolic or diastolic blood pressure or both is considered hypertension. If blood pressure is especially high (greater than 180/110 mm Hg), urgent medical attention is needed. At that pressure, capillaries might burst and cause immediate stroke and blindness. Factors that contribute to high blood pressure include smoking, diabetes, kidney disease, age, family history, and gender. High blood pressure usually develops over time, so a staging system has been implemented to guide diagnosis and treatment (see Table 12.1).

Table 12.1 Classification of Blood Pressure from The Seventh Report of the Joint National Committee on Prevention, Detection, Evaluations and Treatment of High Blood Pressure (JNC 7) (Adaptation)

JNC 7 Blood Pressure Category	SBP (mm Hg)	and/or	DBP (mm Hg)
Normal	< 120	and	< 80
Prehypertension (for patients with risk factors for heart disease including diabetes, hypertension begins at ≥ 130/85)	120–139	or	80–89
Hypertension	≥140	or	≥90
Stage 1	140–159	or	90–99
Stage 2	≥ 160	or	≥ 100
Hypertensive Emergency	≥ 180	or	≥ 110

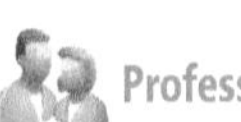

Professional Focus

Measuring blood pressure at home is now recommended for all patients who have hypertension. Become the expert on home blood pressure monitors in your pharmacy. Find out the difference between machines that measure at the arm versus those that measure at the wrist. Which machines are most reliable, easy to use, and cost-effective?

As more pharmacies implement specialized services to monitor blood pressure for patients, you may find yourself measuring blood pressure or helping pharmacists do so. Consequently, you should be familiar with what the numbers mean, because patients will ask you about them. Keep in mind, however, that a single elevated reading is not sufficient to diagnose hypertension. Encourage patients to have their blood pressure checked by their healthcare providers if readings are abnormal. Healthy lifestyle modifications, such as weight loss and regular exercise, are used in all stages; drug therapy usually starts at Stage 1. Patients with other medical conditions that affect the heart (such as diabetes, kidney disease, or a previous heart attack) will be treated with drug therapy even at the prehypertension stage.

Drugs for Hypertension

Because hypertension is a progressive condition that often worsens over time, patients may find themselves taking multiple medications to get their blood pressure under control. Goals for systolic and diastolic blood pressure are lower than in earlier decades, so care providers are more aggressive about treating hypertension than they used to be. Stepped therapy (as shown in Figure 12.5) is typically followed.

Blood pressure medications alter, over the long run, the compensatory systems that control blood pressure. Abruptly stopping therapy can cause an immediate rebound in blood pressure, putting a patient at risk for a hypertensive emergency. Therefore, technicians should use auxiliary labels that instruct patients not to stop taking their prescription without first discussing it with their healthcare providers.

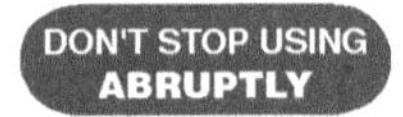

Angiotensin-Converting Enzyme (ACE) Inhibitors

This class of drugs is used for a variety of cardiac conditions: hypertension, angina, heart attack, heart failure, and kidney disease (see Table 12.2). Patients with diabetes may be prescribed **ACE inhibitors** to protect the kidneys from long-term damage. ACE inhibitors are said to be renal protective and are used even when blood pressure is not elevated. Consequently, you cannot assume that all patients with diabetes who take ACE inhibitors have hypertension.

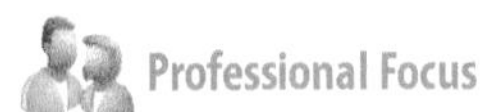

Professional Focus

All generic drug names for ACE inhibitors end with –pril.

ACE inhibitors regulate blood pressure through the renin–angiotensin system. **Renin,** an enzyme produced by the kidneys, is converted to **angiotensin I** in the bloodstream. Angiotensin I is, in turn, converted to **angiotensin II** by **angiotensin-converting enzyme (ACE).** Angiotensin II is a potent vasoconstrictor; blocking its production usually allows blood vessels to relax, which lowers vascular resistance and overall blood pressure.

Figure 12.5
Stepped Therapy for High Blood Pressure
Drug therapy for hypertension starts with one drug (most often a thiazide diuretic), and then other agents are added one by one, based on a patient's co-morbid conditions.

step 1. modify lifestyle:
- reduce salt (sodium) intake
- lose weight
- increase physical activity
- reduce alcohol consumption
- reduce stress
- quit smoking

step 2. start drug therapy with one drug:
- diuretic
- beta blocker
- ACE inhibitor
- angiotensin II receptor blocker (ARB)
- calcium channel blocker

step 3. add diuretic if first drug (step 2) was not one

step 4. add other agents (one by one) of differing mechanisms of action

Table 12.2 Common ACE Inhibitors

Generic (Brand)	Dosage Form	Route of Administration	Common Dose
Benazepril (Lotensin)	Tablet	Oral	5–40 mg a day
Captopril (Capoten)	Tablet	Oral	25–100 mg a day
Enalapril (Vasotec, Enalaprilat)	Tablet, injectable solution	Oral, IV	PO: 5–20 mg a day IV: 1.25 mg every 6 h infused over 5 min
Fosinopril (Monopril)	Tablet	Oral	10–40 mg a day
Lisinopril (Prinivil, Zestril)	Tablet	Oral	5–40 mg a day
Quinapril (Accupril)	Tablet	Oral	10–80 mg a day
Ramipril (Altace)	Tablet, capsule	Oral	2.5–20 mg a day

Side Effects Common side effects of ACE inhibitors include headache, dizziness, fatigue, mild diarrhea, and dry hacking cough. Dizziness occurs most frequently in patients taking ACE inhibitors for heart failure. Cough is a frequent but odd side effect that patients often do not associate with their blood pressure medicine. The cough is caused by a buildup of a substance called bradykinin in the respiratory tract and is an unintended effect of ACE inhibitors. Pharmacists and technicians can help identify those patients with this annoying but harmless side effect. Unfortunately, if a patient experiences a cough with one ACE inhibitor, the others will likely produce the same effect. The cough will resolve when the ACE inhibitor is discontinued.

Angioedema is a rare but serious side effect of ACE inhibitors. It is an allergic-like reaction wherein swelling of the tongue and face are severe enough to threaten breathing. If patients report slurred speech, difficulty swallowing, or enlarged tongue, medical help should be sought immediately.

Cautions and Considerations In rare instances, **hypotension**, or low blood pressure, can occur. For ACE inhibitors, hypotension can happen dramatically, sometimes on the first dose. Careful monitoring is necessary when a patient starts taking an ACE inhibitor. In some cases, the first dose may be given in the doctor's office, so the patient's blood pressure can be monitored for drastic drops.

Elevated potassium levels (hyperkalemia) is another rare but serious effect. It tends to occur when patients are also taking potassium-sparing diuretics. Periodic blood tests for potassium levels will be conducted. Patients who take diuretics along with an ACE inhibitor should be warned against taking potassium supplements.

Pregnant patients should not take ACE inhibitors because these agents can cause severe birth defects. Patients with a kidney condition called bilateral renal artery stenosis also should not take ACE inhibitors because the kidneys could shut down. Patients with other types of kidney problems can still take ACE inhibitors, but doses are adjusted downward.

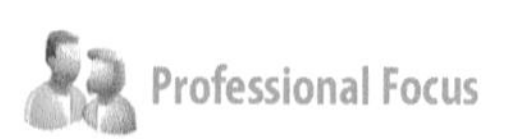

All generic drug names in the class of angiotensin II receptor blockers end with -sartan.

Angiotensin II Receptor Blockers (ARBs) Like ACE inhibitors, **angiotensin receptor blockers (ARBs)** are used for hypertension and heart failure. They are often used as an alternative choice when a patient cannot tolerate ACE inhibitors. Some ARBs can also be used for renal protective effects in patients with diabetes (see Table 12.3).

ARBs work by binding to the same receptors to which angiotensin II binds. Instead of stimulating vasoconstriction, as angiotensin II does, ARBs block these receptors, preventing constriction and causing blood vessels to relax, which lowers blood pressure. ARBs do not cause bradykinin buildup like ACE inhibitors do, so coughing is not a typical side effect.

Side Effects Common side effects of ARBs include headache, dizziness, fatigue, and mild diarrhea. Dizziness occurs most frequently in patients who also have heart failure. Patients taking ARBs may also have more respiratory tract infections, but the reason for

Table 12.3 Common ARBs

Generic (Brand)	Dosage Form	Route of Administration	Common Dose
Candesartan (Atacand)	Tablet	Oral	8–32 mg once or twice a day
Eprosartan (Teveten)	Tablet	Oral	400–800 mg a day
Irbesartan (Avapro)	Tablet	Oral	150 mg a day
Losartan (Cozaar)	Tablet	Oral	25–100 mg a day
Olmesartan (Benicar)	Tablet	Oral	20–40 mg a day
Telmisartan (Micardis)	Tablet	Oral	20–80 mg a day
Valsartan (Diovan)	Tablet, capsule	Oral	80–320 mg a day

this side effect is unknown. Finally, patients also taking diuretics may experience hypotension. Patients should be careful about getting up too quickly from a sitting or lying position until they know how these drugs affect them. A drop in blood pressure upon sitting or standing is called orthostatic hypertension. Dizziness, fainting, and falling down may be signs of hypotension. Patients with kidney or liver impairment may need special dosing and monitoring if they are to take these medications.

Calcium-Channel Blockers This drug class is used regularly to treat hypertension, heart failure, and arrhythmias. Due to adverse effects, **calcium-channel blockers** (see Table 12.4) are not usually the first therapeutic choice for high blood pressure. They can be useful when a patient has more than one cardiovascular condition, necessitating drug therapy.

Calcium-channel blockers decrease blood pressure by preventing calcium from entering into smooth muscle cells in arterial walls. When calcium cannot enter as usual, smooth muscle cells relax to open up blood vessels and lower blood pressure.

Side Effects Common side effects of calcium-channel blockers include headache, dizziness, fatigue, constipation, nausea, heartburn, and flushing. In most cases, these effects are mild. If patients cannot tolerate these effects, they should be referred to their physicians for a change of medication.

Cautions and Considerations Some calcium-channel blockers cause fluid retention (edema) and heart palpitations. To balance the beneficial with the negative effects on the heart, this class of drugs is chosen and monitored carefully.

Some calcium-channel blockers come in extended-release dosage forms that need to be taken just once a day. These products should be swallowed whole, not crushed or

Table 12.4 Common Calcium-Channel Blockers

Generic (Brand)	Dosage Form	Route of Administration	Common Dose
Amlodipine (Norvasc)	Tablet	Oral	5–10 mg a day
Diltiazem (Cardizem, Dilacor)	Tablet, capsule, powder for injection	Oral, IV	PO: 180–240 mg a day IV: 20–25 mg infused over 2 minutes or 5–10 mg/h continuous infusion × 24 h
Felodipine (Plendil)	Tablet	Oral	2.5–10 mg a day
Isradipine (DynaCirc)	Tablet, capsule	Oral	5–20 mg a day
Nicardipine (Cardene)	Capsule, injectable solution	Oral, IV	PO: 20–40 mg three times a day IV: 0.5–2.2 mg/h continuous infusion
Nifedipine (Procardia, Adalat)	Tablet, capsule	Oral	30–120 mg a day
Verapamil (Calan, Isoptin, Verelan)	Tablet, capsule, injection	Oral, IV	PO: 240–320 mg a day IV: 5–10 mg infused over 2–3 min

chewed, which would ruin the release mechanism and might result in drastically lowered blood pressure because the entire large dose would be released at once.

Patients should be warned that some of the extended-release dosage forms (such as the oral form of verapamil) work by releasing the drug from a capsule or tablet (called a ghost tablet) that will appear in their stool. Patients should not be alarmed—the drug has already been released while in their digestive system.

Diuretics As a cornerstone of hypertension treatment, **diuretics** have been on the market for years. Diuretics are either the first or second choice when trying to get a patient's blood pressure under control. These drugs work by helping the kidneys eliminate sodium and fluid from the body, which decreases blood volume and lowers blood pressure. These drugs are covered in Chapter 19 in greater detail.

Alpha and Beta Blockers For many patients, drug therapy for hypertension begins with a **beta blocker** (see Figure 12.5). As explained in Chapter 7, alpha and beta blockers are adrenergic inhibitors that block certain adrenaline receptor types found in the body. **Alpha blockers** are especially useful for men with both high blood pressure and benign prostatic hyperplasia. Beta blockers are a mainstay of treatment for high blood pressure for many patients. They have beneficial effects on the heart, especially after a heart attack. These drugs have been on the market for years, and most are inexpensive and available generically. Alpha and beta blockers (adrenergic inhibitors) are covered in Chapter 7 in greater detail.

Cardiac Arrhythmias

Normal heart rhythm is called **sinus rhythm** because it originates from the sinus node, or pacemaker, which is located in the left atrium (see Figure 12.3). Any deviation from sinus rhythm is considered **arrhythmia**. Such deviations could be changes in the rate at which the heart beats or alterations in electrical conductivity through the heart. **Tachycardia** refers to increased heart rate, and **bradycardia** is decreased heart rate. Other terms, such as **flutter** and **fibrillation**, refer to changes in the way certain parts of the heart beat out of sync with each other. Flutter occurs when select portions (the atria, for example) are slightly out of sync with the rest of the heart. It is not necessarily life threatening. In contrast, fibrillation can be life threatening and occurs when large portions of the heart beat out of sequence. In ventricular fibrillation, no blood flows through the heart and electronic defibrillation to the chest is necessary to shock the heart components back into sequence. ECG readings are used to observe heart function and diagnose arrhythmias (see Figure 12.6). Symptoms of cardiac arrhythmias include palpitations, syncope (fainting), lightheadedness, weakness, sweating, chest pain, and pallor (skin paleness).

Figure 12.6
Abnormal Heart Rhythms
A straight flat-line on the ECG means there is no heartbeat, signaling the point of death.

Arrhythmia	Beats per Minute	Electrocardiogram
tachycardia	150–250	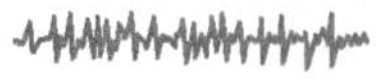
bradycardia	<60	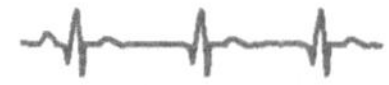
atrial flutter	200–350	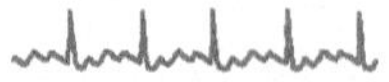
atrial fibrillation	>350	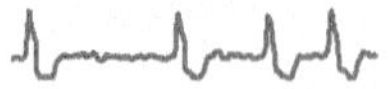
premature atrial contraction	variable	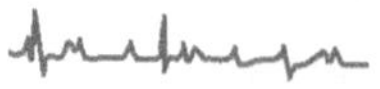
premature ventricular contraction	variable	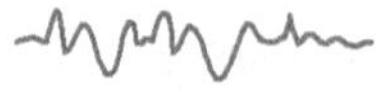
ventricular fibrillation	variable	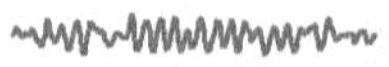
absence of rhythm	0	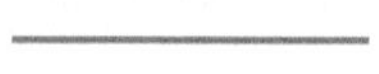

Drugs for Cardiac Arrhythmias

Treatment for arrhythmias attempts to restore normal sinus rhythm by changing the heart rate and conductivity. Antiarrhythmic drugs are categorized into classes by their mechanisms of action. These categories include other drug classes that have effects on heart rhythm. Such medications are chosen and dosed individually, based on desired patient results. Drug interactions can alter the effectiveness of these drugs (see Table 12.5), so you should heed all interaction warnings on the computer when filling these prescriptions.

Class I (Membrane-Stabilizing Agents) The large group of drugs known as **membrane-stabilizing agents** (class I) includes a combination of medications from a few different drug classes that all happen to block sodium channels in cardiac muscle cells. By slowing the influx of sodium, a positively charged ion, the cell membrane becomes more stable and less able to depolarize. Thus, the electrical charge must be stronger to stimulate the cardiac muscle cells to contract and make the heart beat. This effect regulates heart rhythm because it decreases the incidence of abnormal beats.

Table 12.5 Antiarrhythmic Agents

Generic (Brand)	Dosage Form	Significant Drug Interactions	Common Side Effects	Special Notes
Class I (Membrane-Stabilizing Agents)				
Disopyramide (Norpace)	Capsule	Clarithromycin, erythromycin, fluoroquinolones	Hypotension, anticholinergic effects*, headache, gas, muscle aches/pains	Only used for life-threatening ventricular arrhythmias. Avoid use in patients with heart failure as can reduce heart rate too much.
Flecainide (Tambocor)	Tablet	Cisapride, ritonavir	Dizziness, shortness of breath, headache, nausea, fatigue, palpitations, chest pain tremor, angina	Only used for life-threatening ventricular arrhythmias. Avoid use in patients with heart failure as can reduce heart rate too much.
Lidocaine (Xylocaine)	IV	Anticonvulsants	Bradycardia, hypotension, dizziness, drowsiness, blurred vision, confusion	Only used for life-threatening ventricular arrhythmias. Often used to treat acute heart attack.
Mexiletine (Mexitil)	Capsule	Cimetidine, caffeine, theophylline, rifampin	Palpitations, chest pain, dizziness, tremor, nervousness, insomnia, nausea, vomiting, blurred vision, headache, shortness of breath	Only used for ventricular arrhythmias. Can cause leukopenia (low white blood cells) and agranulocytosis, a severe blood condition.
Procainamide (Procanbid)	Tablet, capsule, IV	Amiodarone, antiarrhythmics, cimetidine, ranitidine, fluoroquinolones, thioridazine, ziprasidone	Anorexia, nausea, vomiting, diarrhea, lupus-like syndrome	Only used for atrial arrhythmias. Can cause heart failure in patients with ventricular dysfunction. Can cause leukopenia (low white blood cells) and agranulocytosis, a severe blood condition.
Propafenone (Rythmol)	Tablet, capsule	Cimetidine, ritonavir, SSRI antidepressants, digoxin, theophylline	New arrhythmias, dizziness, nausea, vomiting	Only used for life-threatening arrhythmias.
Quinidine (Quinidine Gluconate, Quinidine Sulfate)	Tablet, IV	Amiodarone, antacids, cimetidine	Hypotension, anticholinergic effects*, headache, tinnitus, confusion, nausea	Gluconate, polyglyconate, and sulfate salts of quinidine contain varying amounts of active drug and thus are not interchangeable. Can cause thrombocytopenia, a life-threatening condition of low platelet production.
Class II (Beta Blockers)				
Acebutolol (Sectral)	Capsule	Reserpine	Dizziness, fatigue, headache, diarrhea, indigestion, nausea, gas	
Esmolol (Brevibloc)	IV	NSAIDs, calcium-channel blockers, theophylline	Hypotension	

continued

Table 12.5 Antiarrhythmic Agents, *continued*

Generic (Brand)	Dosage Form	Significant Drug Interactions	Common Side Effects	Special Notes
Propranolol (Inderal)	Tablet, capsule, oral liquid, IV	Antacids, cimetidine, SSRI antidepressants, fluoroquinolones, ritonavir, phenytoin, haloperidol, fluconazole, zolmitriptan, rizatriptan, theophylline	Hypotension, dizziness, fatigue, lupus-like syndrome	
Sotalol (Betapace)	Tablet, IV	Antiarrhythmics, calcium-channel blockers, reserpine, antacids, fluoroquinolones, thioridazine, ziprasidone	New arrhythmias, bradycardia, chest pain, nausea, vomiting, fatigue, shortness of breath	Only used for life-threatening arrhythmias. Should not be used in patients with asthma.
Class III (Potassium-Channel Blockers)				
Amiodarone (Cordarone)	Tablet, IV	Azole antifungals, cimetidine, fentanyl, fluoroquinolones, loratadine, macrolide antibiotics, statin antihyperlipidemics, other antiarrhythmics	Fatigue, tremor, photosensitivity, anorexia, constipation, nausea, vomiting, blurred vision	Takes days to months for full effect. Must use glass bottle for IV solution. Can cause fatal toxicities to lungs, liver, and heart—used with caution.
Dofetilide (Tikosyn)	Capsule	Verapamil, cimetidine, trimethoprim, ketoconazole	New arrhythmias, headache, chest pain, dizziness, shortness of breath, nausea	Used in cardioversion procedures to restore normal rhythm.
Class IV (Calcium-Channel Blockers)				
Diltiazem (Cardizem, Dilacor)	Tablet, capsule, IV	Cimetidine, benzodiazepines, carbamazepine, rifampin	Hypotension, bradycardia, nausea, constipation, headache, dizziness, fatigue	Only used for atrial arrhythmia.
Verapamil (Calan, Covera, Isoptin, Verelan)	Tablet, capsule, IV	Cimetidine, carbamazepine, alcohol, grapefruit juice, amiodarone, macrolide antibiotics	Hypotension, bradycardia, nausea, constipation, headache, dizziness, fatigue, indigestion, increased infections	Only used for atrial arrhythmia.

*Anticholinergic effects = blurred vision, dry mouth, constipation, and reduced urination

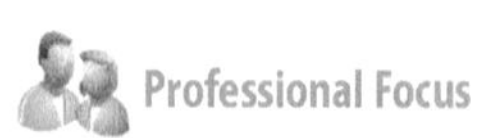

An amusing way to remember beta blockers by name is to note that all generic drug names in this class end with -lol ("laugh out loud").

Class II (Beta Blockers) Certain (but not all) **beta blockers** inhibit beta-one receptors on the heart (class II). They are used for arrhythmia because they inhibit sympathetic nervous system activity on the heart. Normally, sympathetic stimulation makes the heart beat harder and faster. By blocking this stimulation, conduction is slowed through the AV node. This effect slows the rate and force of heartbeats just enough to reduce arrhythmia (for more details on beta blockers, see Chapter 7).

Class III (Potassium-Channel Blockers) Another class of agents, **potassium-channel blockers** (class III), blocks potassium channels in cardiac muscle cells. Like class I antiarrhythmic agents, these drugs work by slowing the influx of a positively charged ion (i.e., potassium), which makes the cell membrane more stable and less able to depolarize. The electrical charge must thus be stronger to make the heart beat. This effect regulates heart rhythm because it decreases the incidence of abnormal beats.

Class IV (Calcium-Channel Blockers) Two **calcium-channel blockers** (class IV), diltiazem and verapamil, are used frequently for atrial fibrillation, a common but non-fatal heart arrhythmia. These agents block calcium, another cation, from entering cardiac muscle cells. This effect dilates cardiac arteries, providing better oxygen supply. The heart rate slows because the heart works more efficiently.

Digoxin This drug is not included in Table 12.5 because, although it is considered an antiarrhythmic drug, it is in a class by itself. **Digoxin** is especially useful for atrial fibrillation and flutter. It is not often used for other arrhythmias. Digoxin works by inhibiting sodium-potassium ATPase, an enzyme that regulates the influx of these ions in cardiac muscle cells. Digoxin alters SA node conductivity, conduction velocity through the heart, and rest time between beats. Digoxin also increases the force and velocity of muscle contraction, making the heart pump more efficiently.

Side Effects Digoxin has a narrow therapeutic window. In other words, the amount needed to produce the desired effect is not much lower than the amount that causes toxicity. Side effects are not common when doses are maintained within the therapeutic range (see Table 12.6 for drug interaction cautions). Patients must get regular lab work done to monitor effects and adjust doses accordingly. Patients also should not change between the brand and generic drugs because even small differences in tablet strength between manufacturers can affect blood concentrations. When toxicity occurs, patients should seek medical attention right away. Symptoms of digoxin toxicity are visual disturbances: (seeing yellow or green halos around objects), headache, dizziness, confusion, nausea, and vomiting. If a patient taking digoxin complains of these symptoms, a technician should refer the patient to the pharmacist and help to get medical attention. Other side effects include gynecomastia (breast enlargement), anorexia, mental disturbances (anxiety, depression, delirium, hallucination), and heart block (extremely slow heartbeat). If these effects occur, the patient should discuss them with his or her prescriber.

Table 12.6 Digoxin

Generic (Brand)	Dosage Form	Significant Drug Interactions
Digoxin (Lanoxin)	Tablet, elixir, IV	IV calcium, succinylcholine, thyroid hormones (use with caution with beta blockers, calcium-channel blockers, beta agonists, diuretics)

Angina and Heart Attack

Angina pectoris, or simply angina, is chest pain caused by inadequate blood flow to a portion of the heart (i.e., **myocardial ischemia**). Ischemia usually occurs as a result of a blockage in the coronary arteries that supply the heart itself with blood (see Figure 12.7). When one or more of these arteries become significantly blocked (usually by 70% or more), tissue damage in that area of the heart ensues, causing a heart attack. In angina, tissue damage is not extensive enough to be considered a heart attack but does cause recurring chest pain episodes.

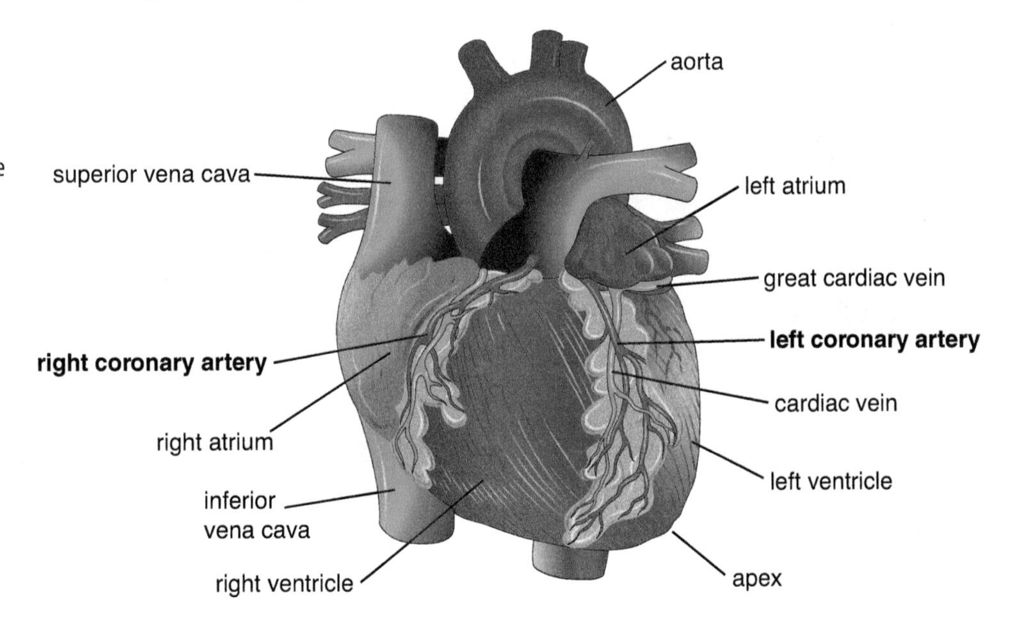

Figure 12.7
Coronary Arteries
Cardiac bypass surgery takes a vein from the leg and inserts it on the heart as a bypass around a blockage in a coronary artery.

Stable angina refers to a predictable pattern of chest pain and tightness that happens in response to specific triggers, such as exercise, physical pain, emotional stress, exposure to cold, or smoking. **Unstable angina** is chest pain and tightness that occurs with increasing frequency and less predictability. It occurs with less exertion or may be brought on by factors other than physical activity or stress. Unstable angina can be a warning that a heart attack is impending. **Variant angina** is another type of chest pain that involves spasm of the coronary blood vessels, rather than blockage.

When heart muscle is deprived of oxygen long enough, muscle cells die (infarct) causing a **heart attack (myocardial infarction, MI)**. If blockage in the coronary arteries is extensive, **cardiac catheterization** (a procedure to reopen blocked arteries) or **coronary bypass surgery** is performed. In bypass surgery, a vessel from the leg is used to create an arterial bypass around a blockage in a coronary artery, thus restoring blood flow to previously blocked off heart tissue. **Stents**, supportive structures made of metal wire mesh, are also placed surgically to keep coronary arteries open. If tissue damage becomes permanent, electrical conductivity in that part of the heart is affected, increasing the likelihood of permanent arrhythmia.

Drugs that dilate and relax blood vessels, allowing better blood flow to the heart and decreasing the amount of vascular resistance that the heart must push against, are used to treat and control angina attacks. Symptoms of heart attack include:

- tightness, heaviness, or squeezing in chest
- chest, neck, or jaw pain
- chest pain that radiates down the left arm
- indigestion or nausea
- a sense of impending doom
- weakness or fatigue
- sweating

Drugs for Angina and Heart Attack

Treatment for angina is twofold: providing immediate relief of chest pain and preventing it entirely. The ischemia and coronary artery blockage that cause angina can progress to a heart attack. Therefore, the goal of drug therapy is to dilate blood vessels to reduce the demand for and increase the delivery of oxygen to myocardial tissue and prevent ischemia from approaching the level of infarction.

During a heart attack, a multitude of drugs is used to open blocked arteries, control blood pressure, and regulate heart rhythm. Heart attack is an emergency; pharmacy technicians do not dispense many of the drugs that would be used during an attack. In some institutions, pharmacists may assist with codes, the emergency procedures to care for a patient in cardiac arrest, but this is not universal. Therefore, specific drug therapies used in the emergency room during treatment of a heart attack are not covered here in depth. Drugs used to break up the blood clots and open the clogged coronary arteries that cause a heart attack are covered in Chapter 13.

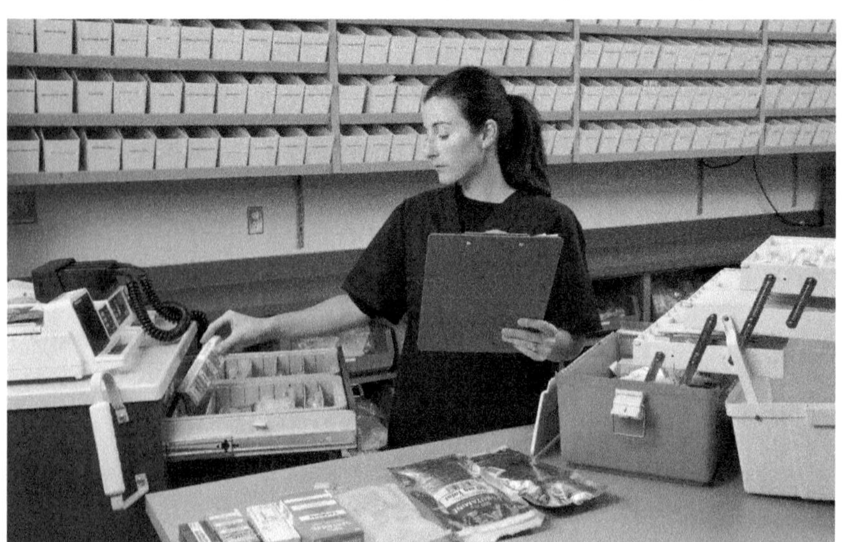

Emergency drug kits are often kept as part of a crash cart, a portable unit containing all equipment needed to aid in cardiac arrest.

Pharmacy technicians who work in an inpatient setting may be involved in stocking **emergency room drug kits** and **crash carts** for the floors. Making sure that these supply stations are stocked with appropriate drugs that are not expired is an important task and should not be taken lightly: Their readiness can mean the difference between life and death. Drug expiration dates must be checked to ensure that all agents will work when needed. Many of these drugs are injectable vasopressors (see Table 12.7). Vasopressors produce vasoconstriction and a rise in blood pressure to restore cardiovascular system function during and after cardiac arrest and shock situations. You should refer to your institution's protocol for specific medications kept in emergency drug kits.

Table 12.7 Drugs Commonly Stocked in Emergency Crash Carts

Generic (Brand)	Common Use
Atropine	Cardio stimulant used to restore heart rate and blood pressure after sudden drop.
Bretylium (Bretylol)	Antiarrhythmic used in ventricular fibrillation and acute arrhythmia.
Calcium chloride	Electrolyte solution used to restore balance after cardio resuscitation.
Dantrolene (Dantrium)	Muscle relaxant used for malignant hyperthermia.
Dextrose Solution ($D_{50}W$)	Sugar solution used to restore blood glucose levels in severe hypoglycemic episodes.
Diazepam (Valium)	Benzodiazepine used for seizures, anxiety, and alcohol withdrawal.
Diphenhydramine (Benadryl)	Antihistamine used for allergic reactions.
Dobutamine	Antiarrhythmic used in ventricular fibrillation and acute arrhythmia.
Dopamine in D_5W	Vasopressor used to correct hemodynamic balance in shock.
Epinephrine	Vasopressor used in allergic reactions, asthma attacks, and cardiac arrest.
Flumazenil (Romazicon)	Benzodiazepine blocker used for excessive sedation from anesthesia or drug overdose.
Furosemide (Lasix)	Diuretic used for severe edema and fluid retention in heart and kidney failure.
Hetastarch (Hespan)	Plasma expander used to restore fluid volume in circulatory system in times of sudden, severe loss.
Isoproterenol (Isuprel)	Vasopressor used for heart block.
Lidocaine (Xylocaine)	Antiarrhythmic used in ventricular fibrillation and acute arrhythmia.
Magnesium sulfate	Electrolyte solution used as antiarrhythmic drug and for tetany.
Midazolam (Versed)	Benzodiazepine used for anxiety as preanesthetic prior to immediate surgical procedures.
Naloxone (Narcan)	Opiate blocker used for excessive sedation from anesthesia or drug overdose.
Nitroglycerin	Vasodilator used to relieve chest pain due to angina or heart attack.
Procainamide	Antiarrhythmic used in ventricular fibrillation and acute arrhythmia.
Sodium bicarbonate	Alkalinizing agent used for metabolic acidosis due to cardiac arrest or shock.
Verapamil	Vasodilator used to relieve chest pain due to angina or heart attack.

Vasodilators Used to relax smooth muscle and dilate blood vessels, **vasodilators** are specifically helpful for dilating the coronary arteries. Such dilation allows greater oxygen and nutrient supply to reach cardiac muscle tissue, which relieves chest pain and ischemia (low blood supply). The most frequently used vasodilators are **nitrates**.

Nitrates come in immediate-release products used for an angina attack and in long-acting dosage forms to prevent frequent angina attacks (see Table 12.8). The short-acting forms (nitroglycerin forms) are all designed to produce rapid absorption after one dose. The most common dosage forms used to abort an anginal episode are sublingual tablets and sprays. Patients should keep their nitroglycerin with them at all times and use it when they experience chest pain. Long-acting forms are used on a scheduled daily basis

Table 12.8 Nitrates for Angina

Short-Acting Nitrates

Nitroglycerin
(Nitro-Bid)—ointment
(Nitrogard)—buccal tablet
(Nitrolingual)—sublingual spray
(Nitrostat)—sublingual tablet

Long-Acting Nitrates

Isosorbide
Isosorbide dinitrate (Isordil)—tablet
Isosorbide mononitrate (Ismo)—tablet

Nitroglycerin
(Nitro-Dur)—transdermal patch

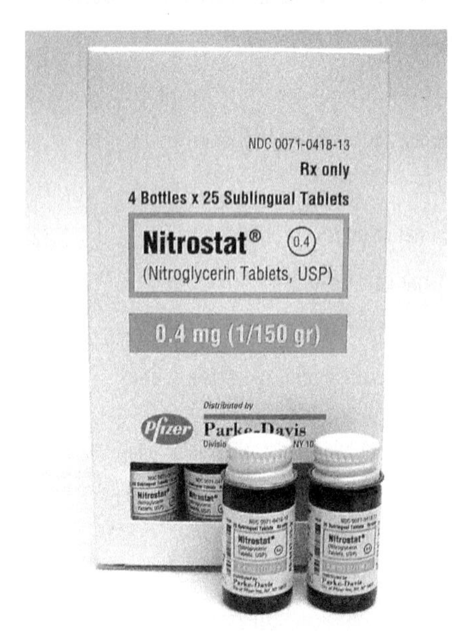

Standard labeling does not fit on a nitroglycerin bottle, which is quite small and meant to be kept in a patient's pocket.

to prevent angina attacks from occurring. Patients should take these forms once a day and allow for at least an eight-hour time span during which they are drug-free.

Side Effects The most common side effects of nitrates are headache, dizziness, blurred vision, flushing, increased heart rate, hypotension, and agitation. Some of these effects can intensify if the drug is taken with alcohol, hypertension drugs, and other drugs that cause vasodilation.

Cautions and Considerations Erectile dysfunction drugs (e.g., Viagra, Levitra, and Cialis) should not be taken if someone also takes nitrates. These agents cause vasodilation too, and additive effects between these drug classes could lower blood pressure to dangerous levels.

Because short-acting forms are designed for immediate absorption, sublingual and buccal tablets should not be swallowed. Instead, they are placed in the mouth and allowed to dissolve. Long-acting oral forms are swallowed and should be taken on an empty stomach with a full glass of water.

If patients do not get relief from chest pain within fifteen minutes of taking a short-acting nitroglycerin, they can repeat one dose, and they should then call 911 for emergency care. If this second dose is needed, a patient could be experiencing a heart attack and should be medically evaluated immediately.

Sublingual nitroglycerin tablets must be kept in their original amber-colored container and protected from light, heat, and moisture. These tablets lose their effectiveness easily in warm and moist conditions. Once the bottle is opened, they are only good for six months, so even if they have not been used, the patient should throw them away and get a new bottle if it has been opened for that long.

Tolerance to the beneficial effects of nitrates is a concern. Tolerance occurs after constant exposure to the drug, resulting in reduced effectiveness of the medication for the patient. Therefore, a drug-free period of approximately eight hours a day (usually overnight) is necessary. For example, the transdermal nitrate patch should be removed before bedtime and left off overnight. A new patch should be applied in the morning.

Other Drugs for Angina ACE inhibitors, calcium-channel blockers, and beta blockers are all used to treat angina and heart attack. In some cases, these agents are used during the acute heart attack itself, but usually they are used after one has occurred. These drugs have shown beneficial effects on heart tissue that has already experienced ischemia. They increase oxygen supply to cardiac tissue and increase pumping efficiency. They can reduce stress on a heart that has suffered an infarction.

Heart Failure

Over time, high blood pressure and coronary artery blockage can cause the heart to be overworked, which can result in enlargement and weakening. The heart is then no longer able to pump sufficiently to supply the body with oxygenated blood. **Heart failure** is characterized by weakness, fatigue, severe fluid retention, and difficulty breathing due to pulmonary edema (fluid accumulation in the lungs). Eventually, vital organs such as the heart, brain, kidneys, and liver shut down due to lack of blood supply, which explains why half of patients die within five years of experiencing heart failure. Hypertension and coronary artery disease are the primary causes of heart failure; other factors, including alcoholism, liver disease, kidney disease, valvular heart disease, anemia, and even drug therapy, can contribute to this condition.

Drugs for Heart Failure

Drug therapies for heart failure have already been covered in this chapter in sections on hypertension and arrhythmias. In heart failure, just about any of the drugs already covered in this chapter may be used, depending on the situation. Many of these drugs help to regulate heart rhythm, and some help the heart to pump more efficiently. In most cases, the difference between using these drugs for heart failure and using them for other cardiovascular conditions, such as hypertension or angina, centers on dosing amounts and frequencies. Loop diuretics (see Chapter 20) are also used frequently in heart failure to eliminate extra body fluid so that the heart does not have to work so hard.

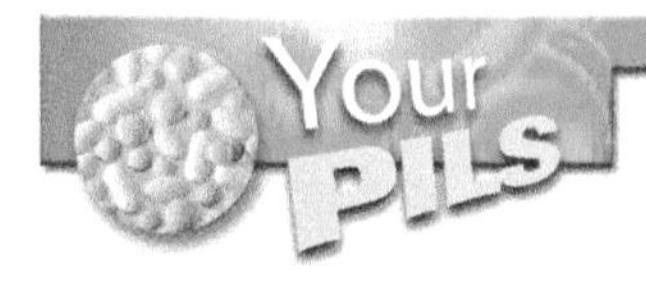

Try this exercise if you like working with details as do Producers. On a piece of paper, write "high blood pressure," "arrhythmia," "angina," "heart failure," and "high cholesterol" across the top. Under each condition column, list the drug classes used to treat it. Remember, some classes will be listed under multiple conditions. For each drug class, list as many generic drug names as you can remember. Write the brand name next to each generic drug name. Try to do this exercise from memory first, and then refer to the text for answers. Put a star next to the drugs that need a warning label "take with food." Underline the drugs that expire six months after being opened. Circle those needing a warning label about avoiding drinking grapefruit juice. Last, draw a box around the drugs that are usually stocked in a crash cart or emergency room drug kit.

Hyperlipidemia

Hyperlipidemia is a condition of elevated cholesterol, phospholipids, and/or triglycerides in the blood and leads to cardiovascular disease and coronary artery blockage. **Cholesterol** itself is both made within the body and ingested with foods. Cholesterol is used to build cell membranes and form hormones. Eating foods high in fat and cholesterol can raise a person's blood cholesterol above normal levels. However, many people with hyperlipidemia also make too much cholesterol in their livers. In some individuals, a genetic factor causes high cholesterol that cannot be overcome by diet and exercise. An accumulation of cholesterol in the bloodstream leads to blockage of and dysfunction in blood vessel walls. Blockages cause angina and heart attacks.

In the bloodstream, cholesterol is packaged into multiple types of molecules: lipoproteins and triglycerides. **Low-density lipoproteins (LDL)** are the worst type of cholesterol and contribute to artery blockages. **High-density lipoproteins (HDL)** are the good kind and help to break up plaques and blockages in blood vessels. **Triglycerides**, another kind of lipid molecule, contribute to atherosclerosis (blocking and hardening of artery walls due to fat buildup). Hyperlipidemia exists when LDL cholesterol or triglycerides are elevated in the blood (see listing at left for abnormal levels). Often, hyperlipidemia coexists with low HDL cholesterol. Treatment begins with reducing fat and cholesterol in the diet, but if this is unsuccessful, drug therapy is started.

Abnormal Blood Lipid Levels

Total cholesterol > 200 mg/dL
LDL > 160 mg/dL
HDL < 45 mg/dL
Triglycerides > 150 mg/dL

Drugs for Hyperlipidemia

Lowering cholesterol (lipid) levels in the blood has been found to significantly reduce the risk of heart attack. Once someone has had one heart attack, the risk for subsequent heart attacks rises dramatically. Drugs for hyperlipidemia are used either to prevent a first heart attack (primary prevention) or to prevent subsequent attacks after an MI (secondary prevention).

Many pharmacies now offer fingerstick testing for blood cholesterol. This testing is conducted to screen for high cholesterol or to monitor drug therapy for hyperlipidemia. Pharmacy technicians may be asked to assist with ordering supplies and operating the

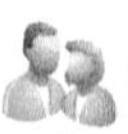
Professional Focus

You should be aware that the cassettes for cholesterol testing machines can be costly (over $10 each) and must be kept in the refrigerator. Plan ahead for appropriate storage of cassettes, and be sure to take them out far enough in advance because they must be warmed to room temperature before use.

machine that runs these tests. Special technique is needed to perform this test accurately, so proper training is recommended for anyone performing it. Universal precautions against blood-borne pathogens and proper disposal of biohazardous waste must be followed.

HMG-CoA Reductase Inhibitors (Statins) The drug class of **HMG-CoA reductase inhibitors** lowers LDL cholesterol primarily and can have beneficial effects on other lipids as well (see Table 12.9). They are usually the first-line choice of therapy for hyperlipidemia. **Statins** reduce the amount of cholesterol made in the body by blocking an enzyme, **HMG-CoA reductase**, which is required for cholesterol production.

Side Effects Most side effects of statins are mild and tolerable. However, they can cause upset stomach and diarrhea, so patients may take them with food if needed. Muscle aches and weakness can also occur. Muscle breakdown (rhabdomyolysis) is a rare but serious side effect. Severe rhabdomyolysis may cause permanent kidney failure. Patients should report any muscle aches or weakness to their healthcare providers to determine whether the symptom is simply due to muscle weakness or to true muscle breakdown. Occasionally, statins cause liver toxicity, so patients should get blood tests periodically.

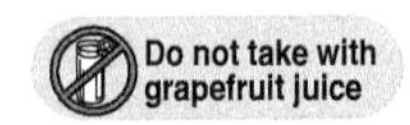

Cautions and Considerations HMG-CoA reductase inhibitors work best when taken at night. They should not be taken during pregnancy or by patients planning to get pregnant. Grapefruit juice alters the activity of statins, so patients should avoid drinking it when taking these medications. Several other drugs also interact with these medications, so technicians should heed all computer alerts that come up when filling a statin drug prescription.

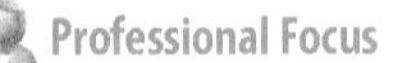
Professional Focus

Because only a few statin drugs are available in generic form, many insurance plans offer preferred pricing and co-pays on generics to encourage cost saving. You may receive prescription claim rejections based on this practice. Suggesting a generic statin can save patients money.

Table 12.9 Common Antihyperlipidemic Drugs

Generic (Brand)	Dosage Form	Route of Administration	Common Dose
Statins			
Atorvastatin (Lipitor)	Tablet	Oral	10–20 mg a day
Fluvastatin (Lescol)	Tablet	Oral	20–80 mg a day
Lovastatin (Mevacor)	Tablet	Oral	20–80 mg a day
Pravastatin (Pravachol)	Tablet	Oral	40–80 mg a day
Rosuvastatin (Crestor)	Tablet	Oral	5–40 mg a day
Simvastatin (Zocor)	Tablet	Oral	10–80 mg a day
Fibrates			
Fenofibrate (TriCor, Lofibra, Triglide, Antara)	Tablet, capsule	Oral	130–200 mg a day
Gemfibrozil (Lopid)	Tablet	Oral	600 mg twice a day, before morning and evening meals
Miscellaneous			
Ezetimibe (Zetia)	Tablet	Oral	10 mg a day
Ezetimibe + simvastatin (Vytorin)	Tablet	Oral	10 mg + 10 mg to 10 mg + 80 mg a day

Fibrates One class of drugs used daily to lower high cholesterol, especially elevated triglycerides, is **fibrates**. These drugs are also used as an alternative to statins when statins cannot be tolerated. Fibrate drugs, also called fibric acid derivatives, lower LDL cholesterol but are best at lowering triglycerides and increasing HDL cholesterol. The exact mechanism of action is not well understood.

Common side effects of fibrates include upset stomach, diarrhea, indigestion, and abdominal cramps. These effects improve over time and can be diminished by taking the medication with food. Patients with gallbladder problems probably should not take fibrates, nor should they be taken in combination with statins because rhabdomyolysis can occur.

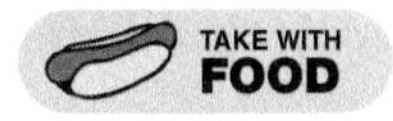

Ezetimibe The drug known as **ezetimibe** inhibits cholesterol absorption from the gastrointestinal tract. It works on all forms of cholesterol but may not significantly reduce lipid levels when large reductions are needed. Side effects, such as abdominal cramps and diarrhea, are usually mild, making this drug quite tolerable.

Niacin Vitamin B_3 (nicotinic acid) is also known as **niacin**. This dietary supplement is available over the counter as well as via prescription (see Table 12.10). Niacin reduces triglycerides and LDL cholesterol while raising HDL cholesterol. Its main side effect is vasodilation in the face and neck, which causes flushing (reddening) and itching. This effect can be quite uncomfortable and is a barrier for some patients. The flushing effect can be reduced by taking an aspirin thirty minutes prior to the niacin dose. Sometimes taking niacin before bedtime will ensure that flushing, if it occurs, happens while sleeping and may go unnoticed. The prescription dosage forms are formulated specifically to release the drug slowly to reduce this side effect.

Table 12.10 Niacin Products

Generic (Brand)	Dosage Form	Prescription Status	Common Dose
Various products	Tablet, capsule	OTC	1 g–2 g, 2–3 times a day
Niacin (Niacor)	Tablet	Rx	250–750 mg a day
Niacin (Niaspan)	Tablet	Rx	250–750 mg at bedtime
Niacin (Slo-Niacin)	Tablet	OTC	250–750 mg a day

Herbal and Alternative Therapies

Omega 3 fatty acids are polyunsaturated fatty acids (also called **DHA** and **EPA**) available in a variety of fish oil products. Patients can get DHA and EPA from eating fish or taking fish oil supplements. Fish oil is used frequently to treat high cholesterol, hypertension, and coronary artery disease. Although not as effective as other prescription drugs for high triglycerides, fish oil supplements or increased dietary intake of fish has been found to lower triglycerides significantly. A variety of fish oil products are available; Lovaza (465 mg EPA and 375 mg DHA) is approved by the Food and Drug Administration to treat hypertriglyceridemia. Consuming 1 g of fish oil a day or eating fish (3 ounces) twice a week has been found to prevent cardiovascular disease.

Plant sterol esters have been found to significantly lower LDL cholesterol and can be helpful adjuncts to diet and drug therapy for hyperlipidemia. **Beta-sitosterol** is a plant sterol similar in chemical structure to cholesterol. It is used in several food products (nutraceuticals), such as margarine and juice, for cardiovascular disease. It is taken 800 mg to 6 g a day in divided doses with or in meals. It should not be taken with ezetimibe (Zetia), because this drug blocks sitosterol absorption and renders the dose ineffective.

Alpha tocopherol (vitamin E) supplements are used for a variety of conditions, such as cardiovascular disease, cancer, and diabetic neuropathy. The effectiveness of vitamin E for these uses has not been proven; even so, many take this antioxidant for better health. A total daily dose of 400 IU has been found to be safe and possibly effective for selected conditions, whereas higher doses can cause side effects and are associated with poor outcomes. More information on vitamin E can be found in Chapter 16.

Garlic contains organosulfur compounds that have antihyperlipidemic, antihypertensive, and antifungal effects. A variety of garlic products and supplements is available and has been found to be possibly effective in treating atherosclerosis, high blood pressure, some cancers, and skin fungal infections. The garlic product must contain **allicin**, the odorous, active ingredient produced upon crushing garlic cloves. Doses of 600–1,200 mg a day, divided into three doses, have been used in clinical trials. One clove of fresh garlic a day has also been used. Patients taking warfarin, saquinavir (an HIV drug), or NNRTIs (other HIV drugs) should not take garlic.

Chapter Summary

Cardiovascular disease is a frequent diagnosis in the United States and encompasses multiple conditions for which drugs are used. The most common conditions are hypertension, arrhythmia, angina, heart attack, and heart failure. Hyperlipidemia contributes to cardiovascular disease. In fact, drugs used to treat high cholesterol are on the list of the top fifty drugs dispensed.

ACE inhibitors, beta blockers, and calcium-channel blockers are used in almost all of these cardiovascular conditions. Consequently, they can be challenging to learn and remember. Other classes covered are ARBs for hypertension, nitrates for angina, and antihyperlipidemic agents (statins and fibrates). The drugs used for heart arrhythmias are divided into four classes, all of which have complications to keep in mind. Some have serious side effects and toxicities. Beta blockers and calcium-channel blockers are also used for arrhythmia. Last, a variety of dietary supplements are used for cardiovascular disease. Niacin, for which both OTC and prescription products are available, is prescribed frequently for high cholesterol.

Chapter Review

For the following sets of exercises, write the exercise heading, exercise numbers, and your answers on a separate sheet of paper. Your instructor may direct you to turn in the sheet of paper or discuss your answers as a class.

REVIEW THE BASICS

Choose a, b, c, or d as the correct answer to each multiple-choice question.

1. Which part of the heart pumps blood out to the rest of the body?
   a. right atrium
   b. left atrium
   c. tricuspid valve
   d. left ventricle

2. Which of the following heart rates would be considered bradycardia?
   a. > 100 BPM
   b. 70–80 BPM
   c. < 60 BPM
   d. none of the above

3. The heart's natural pacemaker is the:
   a. AV node
   b. SA node
   c. SV node
   d. VA node

4. Which of the following is the number in a blood pressure reading that represents the pressure when the heart is at rest?
   a. systolic
   b. diastolic
   c. ventricular
   d. hypotensive

5. Which of the following is considered a healthy cholesterol result?
   a. total cholesterol 210 mg/dL
   b. LDL 100 mg/dL
   c. HDL 30 mg/dL
   d. triglycerides 301 mg/dL

6. Which of the following drugs is a vasodilator used during acute angina attack?
   a. propranolol
   b. nifedipine
   c. nitroglycerin
   d. niacin

7. Which of the following is a form of vitamin B_3 used for hyperlipidemia?
   a. niacin
   b. fish oil
   c. alpha tocopherol
   d. allicin

8. Which of the following drug classes produces antihypertensive effects via the renin-angiotensin system?
   a. calcium-channel blockers
   b. vasodilators
   c. ACE inhibitors
   d. beta blockers

9. Seeing yellow or green halos around objects is a signal of toxicity for which of the following drugs?
   a. losartan
   b. diltiazem
   c. digoxin
   d. gemfibrozil

10. Which of the following medications can cause flushing?
    a. lisinopril
    b. candesartan
    c. nifedipine
    d. niacin

KNOW THE DRUGS

Match each brand name drug with its corresponding generic name and most common use. Your answers should follow this example format: Generic Name: 1. a; 2. b; 3. c; etc. Most Common Use: 1. k; 2.l; 3.m; etc.

Brand Name	Generic Name	Most Common Use
1. Zestril	a. isosorbide dinitrate	k. hypertension
2. Procardia	b. simvastatin	l. angina
3. TriCor	c. lisinopril	m. arrhythmia
4. Atacand	d. ramipril	n. hyperlipidemia
5. Zocor	e. fenofibrate	
6. Isordil	f. rosuvastatin	
7. Altace	g. disopyramide	
8. Cardene	h. nifedipine	
9. Norpace	i. candesartan	
10. Crestor	j. nicardipine	

PUT IT TOGETHER

For each item, write down either a single term to complete the sentence or a short answer.

1. HMG-CoA reductase inhibitors end with the suffix ________________.
2. Angiotensin II receptor antagonists end with the suffix ____________________.
3. Beta blockers tend to end with the suffix ________________.
4. ACE inhibitors end with the suffix ________.
5. What medication must be kept in the original container and protected from light and moisture to remain effective?
6. Name two drugs for which you should use the warning label "take with food" to avoid stomach upset and diarrhea.

THINK IT THROUGH

Read and think through each numbered scenario carefully and then write several sentences in reply to the question(s) presented. Question 4 requires you to do some Internet research before completing your answer(s).

1. Mr. Carlson brings the following new prescription to the pharmacy. As you are entering this prescription into the computer, you notice he also has scripts for Prinivil, Nitrostat, and metformin. What concern does this raise? What will you do about it?

Cialis 10 mg	#5	Sig: Take one tablet as desired for sexual activity

2. You are stocking the OTC shelves when a customer stops you to ask where to find the cough syrup. He tells you he has a nagging cough that just will not go away. After you show him where the cough and cold products are, you ring him up at the register. He asks you to add his prescription refill for Lotensin to his purchase. What should you do?
3. Mrs. Nelson comes to the counter to ask you where she could find some niacin. She states that her physician told her to start taking it for her cholesterol. What other OTC product should you recommend she purchase along with her niacin? If she complains of cost or the complexity of this dual-therapy option, what else can you do?

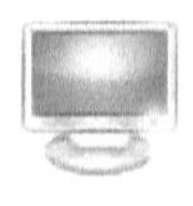

4. **On the Internet,** look up a couple of sources for lists of the most commonly prescribed or dispensed drugs in the United States. Look at how many of the top 100 medications are drugs for cardiovascular disease. Make a list of these drugs (brand and generic names) and their classes. Use your list as a guide for remembering these important drugs, which you will see every day in the pharmacy.

Chapter 13 The Blood and Drug Therapy

LEARNING OBJECTIVES

- Describe the basic anatomy and physiology of the blood and the hematologic system.
- Explain the therapeutic effects of prescription medications, nonprescription medications, and alternative therapies commonly used to treat diseases of the blood and the hematologic system.
- Describe the adverse effects of prescription medications, nonprescription medications, and alternative therapies commonly used to treat diseases of the blood and the hematologic system.
- Identify the brand and generic names of prescription and nonprescription medications commonly used to treat diseases of the blood and the hematologic system.
- State the doses, dosage forms, and routes of administration for prescription and nonprescription medications commonly used to treat diseases of the blood and the hematologic system.

Interactive self-quizzes, games, audio files, and glossaries help you to learn drug names and facts.

The blood is a vital organ, carrying needed nutrients and oxygen to cells and tissues of the body. Without constant blood flow to essential organs including the brain, heart, lungs, and kidneys, life is not possible. To work properly, the blood must adequately perfuse body tissues, contain functional blood cells able to do their various jobs, and clot when injury or bleeding occurs. The blood is a hematologic system that makes a variety of blood cells and sustains life by circulating needed oxygen and other nutrients. This chapter describes the components of the hematologic system that makes the blood and supports its physiological functions. You will also learn about the coagulation cascade, the process by which blood forms clots. When clots form unnecessarily and cut off blood flow, the results are stroke, heart attack, and pulmonary embolism (clot in the lungs). Stroke, clotting disorders, and hemophilia are covered, as well as iron deficiency and pernicious anemia.

Some of the medications for these conditions are inexpensive and used extensively, whereas others are rarely used and quite costly. In this chapter, anticoagulants such as warfarin (a top 100 drug) are discussed. Like all of the medications for blood disorders, warfarin has special considerations for side effects and drug interactions. As the reports of medication errors with heparin have proven, attention to detail is imperative when dealing with these medications. Errors with these lifesaving therapies can have dire consequences. Pharmacy technicians must appreciate the sensitive nature of these agents and understand their special considerations in order to ensure patient safety.

Anatomy and Physiology of the Blood

The **blood** serves several functions besides supplying the cells of the body with oxygen and nutrients. It also carries the hormones and enzymes that control bodily functions and helps regulate body temperature. The blood is made up of cells suspended in liquid plasma. Blood **plasma** contains water, **protein** (albumin and immunoglobulins), and various dissolved substances. Drug molecules are carried by the blood either as dissolved substances in the plasma or when bound to proteins such as **albumin**.

Three types of cells are found in the blood including **red blood cells (RBCs)**, **white blood cells (WBCs)**, and **platelets** (see Figure 13.1). **Erythrocytes** (RBCs) contain the iron and **hemoglobin** to which oxygen and carbon dioxide bind during transport. **Iron**,

Figure 13.1
Components of the Blood
RBCs give blood its characteristic red color.

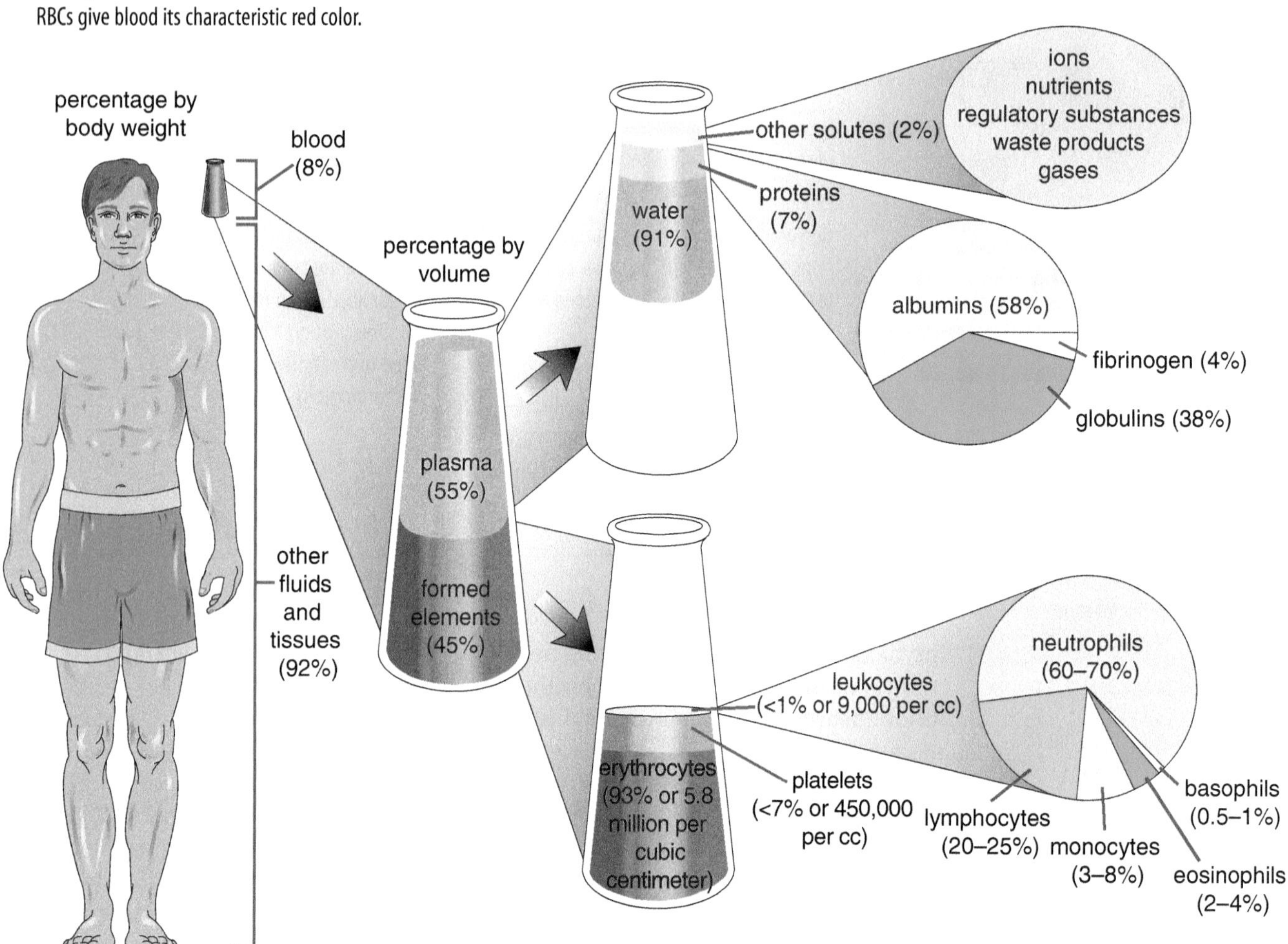

folate, and **vitamin B$_{12}$** are all necessary nutrients used in forming RBCs. They help hemoglobin bring oxygen to cells. **Erythropoiesis** is the process whereby new RBCs are made in the bone marrow and released into the bloodstream. This process is stimulated by erythropoietin, a substance made by the kidneys.

Leukocytes (WBCs) in the blood are responsible for fighting disease as a central component of the immune system. The function of WBCs is discussed in Chapter 3.

Platelets (**thrombocytes**) are another type of blood cell. They help the blood to clot during injury or bleeding by clumping together and adhering to surrounding tissue.

The **coagulation cascade** is the process by which blood clots form. The cascade involves a complicated series of reactions that attract **thrombin** and **fibrin**, coagulation proteins that facilitate the growth of a functional blood clot (see Figure 13.2). The combination of platelet activity, the coagulation cascade, and reactions involving natural anticoagulants (TPA and proteins C and S) produces the body's ability to build and break down clots. The two pathways of the cascade, which stimulate blood clotting, are the **extrinsic** and **intrinsic**. An abnormality in a single step of either pathway can affect coagulation and produce too much or too little clotting. These pathways converge with the use of **clotting factor** X, thrombin, and fibrin (see Figure 13.3). If a problem occurs with this common pathway, clotting is severely affected.

When clotting is unable to slow bleeding, blood loss can be life threatening and may require transfusion. Blood typing allows donor blood to be matched to a recipient for transfusion. Blood type is determined by specific antigen proteins on the surface of RBCs. If the blood that is given to a patient possesses different surface antigens than are

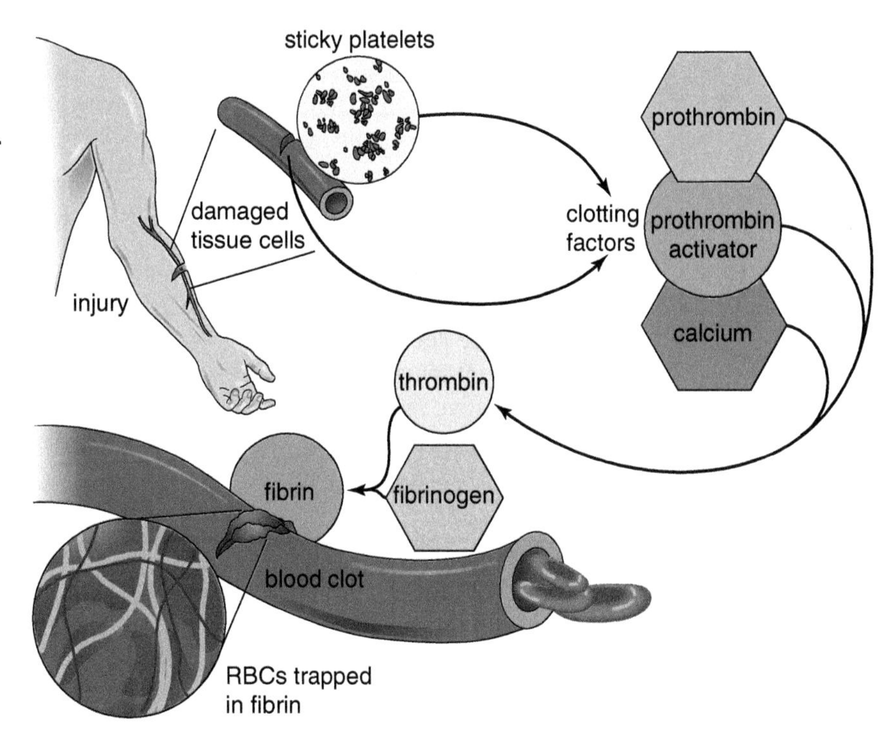

Figure 13.2
Forming Blood Clots
Tissue damage triggers platelets to accumulate and activates clotting factors to start coagulation.

Figure 13.3
Coagulation Cascade
When one pathway malfunctions, usually the other pathway compensates.

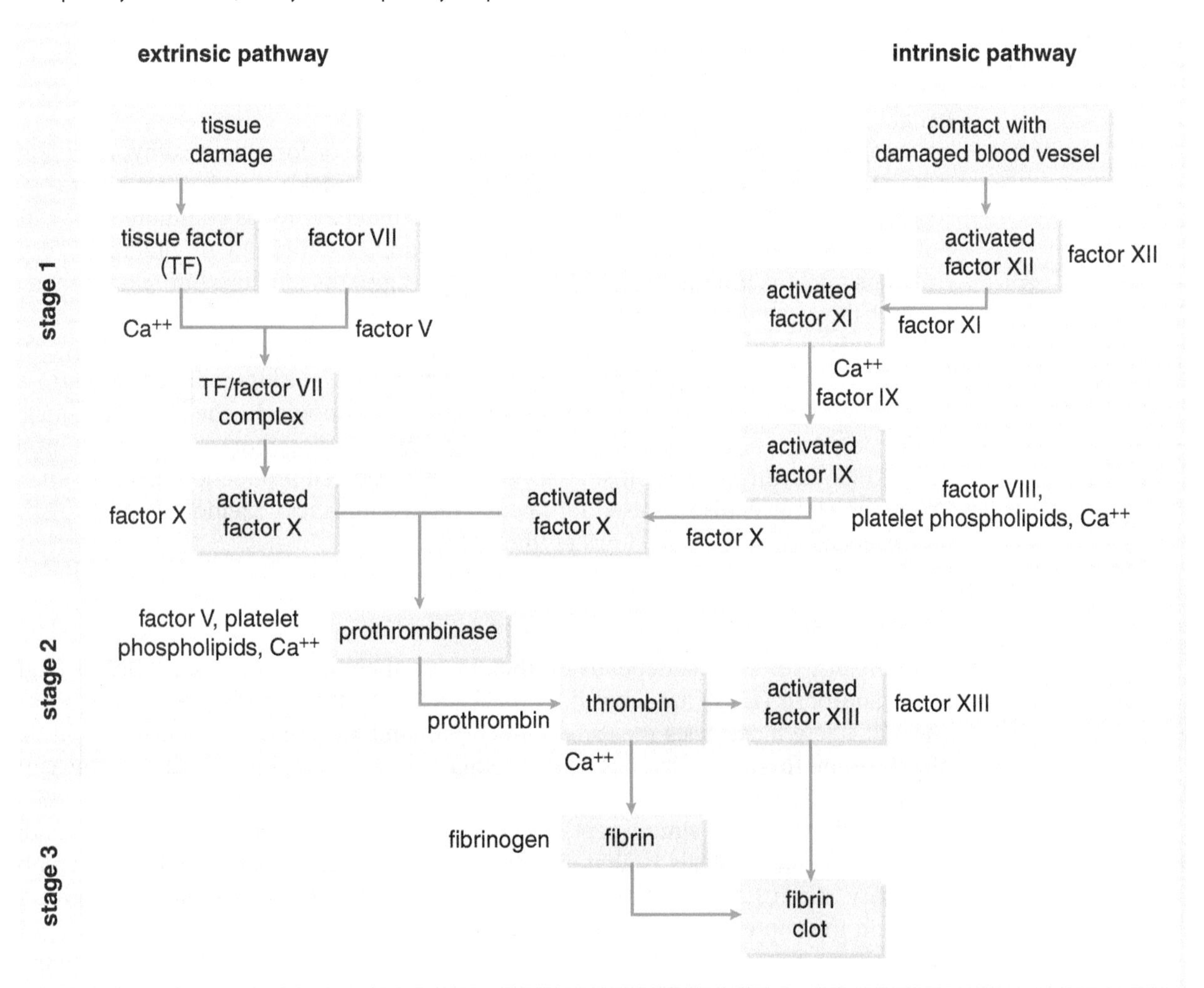

present in the patient's own blood, antibodies form and cause RBCs to clump together. **Blood types** are categorized as A, B, AB, and O, such that AB has both kinds of antigens, and O has none. Blood type O is considered the universal donor, because it does not introduce new antigens to a recipient. Blood type AB is considered the universal recipient, because it already contains any antigens the donor blood could bring.

Rh factor is another marker molecule on RBCs for which blood is typed for transfusion. If a patient is Rh positive, he or she has the marker. The presence of this marker and the antibodies made against it are most important during pregnancy. If the mother is Rh negative and the fetus is Rh positive, the mother's blood will form antibodies against the baby's RBCs. These antibodies can build up over a pregnancy and jeopardize the survival of the current fetus and also significantly impact subsequent pregnancies. Mothers who are Rh negative receive an immune globulin injection (RhoGAM) that inhibits the production of these antibodies and protects the fetus in any future pregnancy.

Anemia

Anemia is a lack of normal, healthy RBCs containing functional hemoglobin in the blood. Symptoms depend on the type of anemia present. Some signs of recent-onset anemia may include rapid heartbeat, lightheadedness, and breathlessness. Chronic anemia may cause fatigue, weakness, headache, vertigo, faintness, sensitivity to cold, pallor, and loss of skin tone.

Many causes of anemia exist, but most can be categorized into one of three types: that caused by rapid destruction of RBCs, by blood loss, or by inadequate production of RBCs. **Hemolytic anemia**, defined by the excessive destruction of RBCs, can be caused by infection or even drug therapy. Blood loss usually requires blood transfusion for treatment. However, the inadequate production of RBCs is the most common cause of anemia. It is found in up to half of the patients admitted to an inpatient setting and is usually related to nutrition.

Iron, folate, and vitamin B_{12} are essential nutrients for forming healthy, abundant RBCs. **Iron-deficiency anemia** can happen relatively quickly, but it takes several months to replenish iron stores in the body. **Folate deficiency** is common among alcoholics, because they tend not to get proper nutrition. A deficiency in vitamin B_{12} is called **pernicious anemia**. It takes from weeks to months to occur but takes only days or weeks to replenish.

Chronic kidney disease can also cause anemia. The kidneys produce erythropoietin, the substance that stimulates bone marrow to make RBCs. Kidney disease reduces the kidneys' ability to make erythropoietin, and thus erythropoiesis, the process of making RBCs, slows down. In this kind of anemia, simply providing more iron will not produce more RBCs. Erythropoietin must be given to get blood cell production going again. Erythropoietin may also be used for anemia related to cancer chemotherapy, which damages bone marrow and slows erythropoiesis.

Drugs for Anemia

Drug therapy for anemia depends on the type of anemia present. **Hemoglobin (Hgb)** and **hematocrit (HCT)** are laboratory markers for the blood tests used to diagnose anemia. These blood tests measure hemoglobin and oxygen-carrying capacity in the blood. When these numbers are low, anemia is suspected. Other diagnostic measures and iron studies are used to determine the cause(s) of the anemia. If nutrient deficiency is the cause(s), simply replacing the appropriate missing nutrient corrects the anemia. If **hematopoiesis** is altered, administration of erythropoietin therapy will be necessary. For instance, patients with chronic renal failure do not make enough erythropoietin to support adequate hematopoiesis. They are given exogenous erythropoietin to treat their anemia. Sometimes multiple causes contribute to anemia, making drug treatment more complicated.

Iron and Other Supplements Iron, folate, and vitamin B_{12} (**cyanocobalamin**) are used as supplements for the anemia that is caused by nutrient deficiency (see Table 13.1). Iron is used alone for iron-deficiency anemia or in combination with hematopoietic agents for anemia associated with chronic kidney disease. **Iron supplementation** can take up to six months to replenish iron stores and produce normal RBCs with adequate hemoglobin content.

Table 13.1 Commonly Used Supplements for Anemia

Generic (Brand)	Dosage Form	Route of Administration	Common Dose
Cyanocobalamin (vitamin B_{12})	Tablet, injection, intranasal gel	Oral, IM, SC injection, intranasal	PO: 1,000 mcg/day Injection: 100–1,000 mcg for 5 days, then weekly for 1 month, then monthly Intranasal: 500 mcg once a week for 5–10 days followed by injections
Ferrous gluconate (Fergon)	Tablet	Oral	100–200 mg elemental iron a day in divided doses
Ferrous gluconate complex (Ferrlecit)	Injection	IV	Test dose first 1 g in divided doses
Ferrous sulfate (Feosol)	Tablet, capsule, oral drops, elixir syrup	Oral	100–200 mg elemental iron a day in divided doses
Folic acid	Tablet, injection	Oral, IM, IV, SC injection	Pregnancy: 0.4–0.8 mg a day Deficiency: 1–5 mg a day
Iron dextran (INFeD, Dexferrum)	Injection	IM, IV	25–100 mg a day
Iron sucrose (Venofer)	Injection	IV	20–100 mg a day

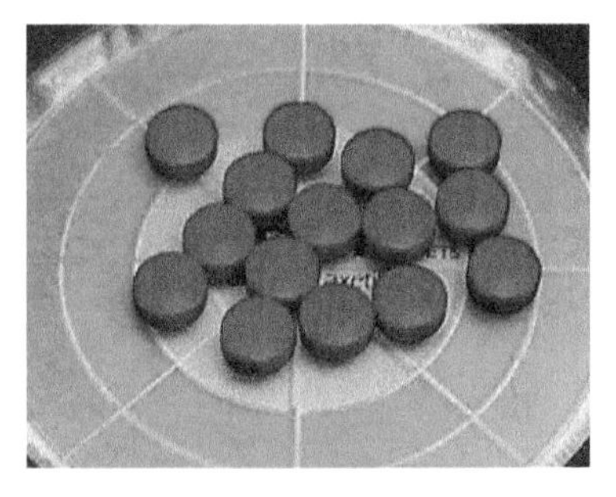

The shiny enteric coating on iron tablets makes the pills resemble candy, which leads to a potential poisoning hazard for children.

Folic acid is used in low doses for prenatal supplementation to support fetal brain and spinal development. In fact, it is a recommended supplement for all women who are pregnant or planning to become pregnant. Folic acid in higher doses is used for anemia due to alcoholism, because folic acid is frequently found to be deficient in these patients.

Vitamin B_{12} is used for pernicious anemia and to prevent neuropathy and certain types of dementia. Vitamin B_{12} builds and protects nerve tissue. Unlike the length of time needed for iron replacement, replenishing a deficiency of vitamin B_{12} takes only days to weeks.

May Discolor Urine

Side Effects Common side effects of iron supplementation include constipation, stomach upset, urine discoloration, and dark stools. Constipation can be relieved by drinking plenty of fluid, incorporating fiber into the diet, and taking a stool softener if needed. Most oral dosage forms are enteric coated to help with stomach upset, but if nausea occurs, taking iron with food may help. Technicians should use an auxiliary warning label to alert patients to the potential for urine discoloration.

Common side effects of vitamin B_{12} are itching, diarrhea, headache, and anxiety. These effects are usually mild and may improve over time.

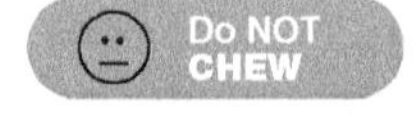

Cautions and Considerations Oral iron supplements are enteric coated and should not be crushed or chewed.

Most oral iron supplements are available over the counter, making them cost-effective and easily accessible. However, they can pose a poison risk to children. Iron overdose in children can be fatal, and doses do not have to be extremely large to cause significant problems. Patients should be instructed to keep iron supplements in child-proof packaging and out of reach of children.

Iron supplements should not be taken with antacids or other acid-reducing medications, because absorption of iron will be decreased. Iron supplements are sometimes given with vitamin C because it increases iron absorption. Iron supplements should not

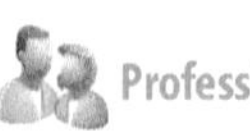

Professional Focus

Iron doses are based on the amount of elemental iron the product contains. The elemental iron content is different for various salts (e.g., gluconate, sulfate). You can help patients to select a product that will deliver the correct dose of elemental iron. Advise patients to stick with one product once they have started treatment.

be taken with tetracycline or fluoroquinolones, because iron binds to these antibiotics and reduces their effectiveness at fighting infection.

Iron dextran has been associated with severe allergic reactions; therefore, a test dose must be given first. Other intravenous (IV) forms of iron do not tend to cause this same allergic reaction, so they are used more often.

Hematopoietic Agents Two **hematopoietic agents**, **erythropoietin** and **darbepoetin**, are used to treat anemia associated with chronic kidney disease. They are sometimes used when cancer chemotherapy causes bone marrow suppression and affects blood cell production. These products should always be used in combination with iron supplements because they will deplete iron stores as RBC production increases. These agents (see Table 13.2) work by supplementing the body's normal production of erythropoietin, which stimulates blood cell production in the bone marrow. Full onset of the agents' effects can take a few weeks.

Side Effects Common side effects of erythropoietin and darbepoetin include headache, fatigue, fever, muscle/joint pain, swelling, diarrhea, nausea, and vomiting. These agents can also cause high blood pressure, clotting, and rapid heartbeat. Therefore, careful monitoring of blood pressure and cardiac function is necessary. Patients with uncontrolled high blood pressure may not be good candidates for hematopoietic therapy. Patients with a history of seizures need to inform their prescribers and pharmacists before using one of these agents.

Cautions and Considerations Laboratory tests used to monitor hematopoietic therapy include complete blood count (CBC), Hgb, and HCT. In some settings, technicians may help pharmacists retrieve these results. When monitoring erythropoietin and darbepoetin therapy, Hgb levels should not exceed 12 g/dL because increased cardiac and clotting problems can occur.

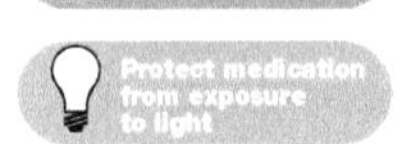

Erythropoietin and darbepoetin products should be refrigerated and cannot be shaken during preparation. They should not be diluted. Some erythropoietin products have a limited shelf life and must be discarded after twenty-one days if not used. Darbepoetin should be protected from light.

Table 13.2 Commonly Used Hematopoietic Agents

Generic (Brand)	Dosage Form	Route of Administration	Common Dose
Darbepoetin (Aranesp)	Injection	IV, SC injection	100 mcg every week or 200 mcg every 2 weeks
Erythropoietin or epoetin alpha (Epogen, Procrit)	Injection	IV, SC injection	40,000 units every week or 150 units/kg 3 times a week

Stroke

A common cause of death and disability around the world, **stroke** (**cerebrovascular accident** or **CVA**) is an interruption in oxygen supply to the brain. The brain is an oxygen-rich organ and requires a constant supply of oxygenated blood to remain alive and functional. When oxygen cannot reach parts of the brain, it takes only minutes to lose consciousness and for tissue damage to occur. The brain is incapable of regeneration, so cell death is permanently disabling.

The two types of stroke are ischemic and hemorrhagic. **Ischemic stroke** results from an obstruction of blood flow: A blood clot or cholesterol plaque occludes a blood vessel that supplies brain tissue. If the block in blood flow is brief and causes only temporary dysfunction, it is called a **transient ischemic attack (TIA)**. TIA is often a precursor and forewarning of stroke. Risk factors for ischemic stroke include high cholesterol, cardiac arrhythmia, coronary artery disease, prosthetic heart valve, diabetes, hypercoagulable states, obesity, and physical inactivity. These conditions increase the likelihood of blood clots forming and traveling to the brain.

Hemorrhagic stroke is a rupture in a blood vessel that supplies an area of the brain. Blood spills out of the ruptured vessel and then cannot reach the part of the brain that the vessel serves. Risk factors for hemorrhagic stroke are high blood pressure, cigarette smoking, and excessive alcohol intake. In these conditions, tiny vessels in the brain become weakened and form an **aneurysm**, a thin-walled protrusion in an artery wall that can easily burst. Other risk factors for any kind of stroke include diabetes, increased age, male gender, genetic predisposition, and prior stroke.

Because brain cell death is irreversible, most drug therapy for stroke is aimed at prevention rather than treatment after the fact. However, it is difficult to accurately predict risk for stroke. Many times, anticoagulation therapy starts only after someone has had a stroke or a TIA. Thrombolytic (fibrinolytic) therapies can be used to break up an ischemic clot if it caused a massive stroke. However, there is a limited window of opportunity from the time of the onset of symptoms to when thrombolytic therapy would no longer be effective. Proper diagnosis of the type of stroke and timing is necessary. Consequently, anticoagulation and antiplatelet therapies are used more often to prevent stroke rather than to break up a clot once it has already caused a stroke. Sometimes patients who do not have a history of stroke but who do have multiple risk factors, such as diabetes and high cholesterol, will be prescribed low-dose aspirin therapy to reduce the risk of stroke and heart attack. Anticoagulants, antiplatelet drugs, and thrombolytic therapies are described later in this chapter.

Clotting Disorders

A class of diseases known as **clotting disorders** involves both **hypercoagulation** (over-production of blood clots) and **hemophilia** (inability to produce blood clots). Many causes for clotting disorders exist, and most involve genetics in some way. For instance, patients with hemophilia usually lack the genes that control the ability to produce specific clotting factors in the coagulation cascade. Type A hemophilia is the inability to produce factor VIII, and Type B hemophilia is a deficiency in factor IX. Both types are rather rare. Other, more common clotting disorders include deficiencies in Von Willebrand factor, protein C, protein S, and factor V Leiden. Because many clotting factors are made in the liver, liver disease also affects coagulation.

In many cases, however, specific causes for coagulation abnormalities are not apparent. In **deep-vein thrombosis (DVT)**, a clot forms in an extremity such as the lower leg or calf. In **pulmonary embolism (PE)**, a clot forms in the lungs. These clotting problems are the results of hypercoagulation (excess clotting). Physical inactivity has been found to increase risk of DVT as blood pools in the legs and then forms clots. Many patients in the inpatient setting who are immobile due to sickness will receive preventive anticoagulation therapy. Risk factors for DVT include age over forty years, estrogen therapy (such as birth control pills) with smoking, obesity, surgery, trauma, prolonged immobility, hip replacement, and varicose veins.

Other conditions that can create a hypercoagulable state are pregnancy, severe infection, liver disease, and cancer. The greatest concern other than relieving pain and local tissue injury associated with an unwanted clot is that a piece of the clot (called an embolus) can dislodge and travel to the heart, brain, or lungs. Occlusion of small vessels in one of these organs is a life-threatening emergency. Therefore, treatment for DVT and PE will usually last for at least three to six months to prevent emboli as the body dissolves a clot.

Drugs for Stroke and Clotting Disorders

Prevention and treatment of unwanted clots, whether the cause is stroke or a clotting disorder, employs anticoagulants, antiplatelet agents, and thrombolytics. Patients on such therapies will be monitored regularly with specific laboratory tests.

- **Partial thromboplastin time (PTT)** measures the function of the intrinsic and common pathways of the coagulation cascade. This marker monitors heparin therapy.
- **Prothrombin time (PT)** measures the function of the extrinsic and common pathways of the coagulation cascade. It can vary, so reference ranges produced by the local laboratory must be used to interpret this test. This measure monitors warfarin therapy.
- **International normalized ratio (INR)** gives a reference for coagulation involving the extrinsic and common pathways of the coagulation cascade. It standardizes the PT to remove variability. This marker monitors warfarin therapy.

Some pharmacies use fingerstick technology to measure INR for patients. Pharmacist-run anticoagulation clinics monitor patients and adjust drug therapies by protocol with prescribers. Pharmacy technicians may help pharmacists by gathering these lab test results or administering the fingerstick.

Anticoagulant Agents Blood clots that have already formed can be treated with a choice of **anticoagulant agents**. These agents do not necessarily break down a clot that has already formed, but they halt growth and keep emboli from forming as the body reabsorbs the clot on its own.

Treatment usually starts with IV **heparin** to keep the clot from growing. Later, therapy is often switched from heparin to a **low molecular weight heparin (LMWH)** product that can be given via self-injection, which facilitates discharge from the hospital. Next, oral **warfarin** therapy can begin. But because warfarin is used for long-term anticoagulation and requires five or more days for onset of effect, it cannot initially be used alone when treating an acute clot. Instead, it must be overlapped by at least five days with either heparin or an LMWH. This dual therapy may continue longer as doses of warfarin are adjusted to achieve the desired therapeutic range. When there is no immediate need to treat an acute clot, warfarin is given alone as a preventive therapy and doses adjusted to achieve the desired results.

Heparin is used for immediate, short-term IV anticoagulation treatment of blood clots or in pregnancy when other anticoagulants are contraindicated. It is also used as a flushing agent to keep IV lines open and used subcutaneously for prevention in patients at high risk for developing clots. Heparin works by inhibiting clotting factors in the coagulation cascade and inactivating thrombin and factor Xa. It also affects the platelets' ability to clump together. Heparin does not affect an existing clot but prevents emboli from forming while the body slowly dissolves and absorbs a clot. Heparin is the only anticoagulant used during pregnancy because it does not cross the placental barrier.

LMWHs work similarly to heparin, but they affect factor Xa more than they affect thrombin. LMWHs can be injected subcutaneously and have a longer half-life than heparin does. LMWHs are more convenient to use because they can be given once or twice a day as self-injections rather than via continuous infusion (see Table 13.3). LMWHs are used as a bridge therapy from IV heparin to oral warfarin.

When patients cannot tolerate heparin or LMWHs, alternatives are available. **Fondaparinux** works by selectively inhibiting factor Xa in the coagulation cascade. It is injected subcutaneously once a day. **Direct thrombin inhibitors** work by inhibiting thrombin directly. Direct thrombin inhibitors are all given as continuous infusions, as is heparin.

Conditions for which warfarin is used include heart valve disease, artificial heart valve placement, prior stroke, atrial fibrillation, DVT, PE, heart attack, and other heart conditions in which clot formation in the heart is a concern. Warfarin works by inhibiting the production of vitamin K–dependent clotting factors in the liver. Warfarin is adjusted to each patient individually, so frequent laboratory testing is necessary. Pharmacists and technicians should emphasize patient compliance with monitoring visits and laboratory tests to ensure patient safety.

Table 13.3 Anticoagulants

Generic (Brand)	Dosage Form	Route of Administration	Common Dose
Fondaparinux (Arixtra)	Injection	SC injection	2.5 mg once a day
Heparin or unfractionated heparin (UFH)	Injection	Continuous IV infusion, SC injection	IV: doses individualized but often in thousands of units per infusion SC: 3,000–5,000 units every 8–12 hours
Warfarin (Coumadin)	Tablet, injection	Oral, IV	2–10 mg a day (doses are individualized)
Direct Thrombin Inhibitors			
Argatroban (Acova)	Injection	Continuous IV infusion	Doses individualized but often given as 2 mcg/kg a minute
Bivalirudin (Angiomax)	Injection	Continuous IV infusion	Doses individualized but often given as 1.75 mg/kg an hour
Lepirudin (Refludan)	Injection	Continuous IV infusion	Doses individualized but often given as 0.15 mg/kg an hour
Low Molecular Weight Heparins			
Dalteparin (Fragmin)	Injection	SC injection	200 units/kg a day given in doses twice a day
Enoxaparin (Lovenox)	Injection	SC injection	1–1.5 mg/kg a day given in doses once or twice a day
Tinzaparin (Innohep)	Injection	SC injection	175 units/kg a day given once a day

Professional Focus

In some institutions, pharmacy technicians take patient education and self-injection teaching materials to patients' rooms when orders for LMWH are received. They advise patients to review the materials and to expect the pharmacist or nurse to come by later to explain the use of this new medication. You can offer encouragement to patients, noting that this medication will help them go home sooner and is only a temporary treatment until the warfarin begins to work.

Side Effects Common side effects of heparin include bruising, bleeding due to excessive anticoagulation, and thrombocytopenia (low platelet count). Heparin-induced thrombocytopenia (HIT) is a rare but serious side effect that can be life threatening. It can only be fully detected by laboratory tests but often is preceded by skin rash. Patients should report any signs of bleeding or skin rashes to their prescribers right away.

Common side effects of LMWHs include bruising, bleeding due to excessive anticoagulation, fever, pain at the injection site, and thrombocytopenia. Patients who have had HIT should not take LMWHs. Patients should report any signs of bleeding or skin rashes to their prescribers right away.

Common side effects of fondaparinux include nausea, fever, anemia, bleeding due to excessive anticoagulation, and thrombocytopenia. Patients should report any signs of bleeding to their prescribers and follow instructions regarding laboratory tests.

Common side effects of direct thrombin inhibitors include nausea, headache, back pain, and bleeding due to excessive anticoagulation. Patients should report any signs of bleeding to their prescribers and follow instructions regarding laboratory tests.

The most common side effects of warfarin include bleeding due to excessive anticoagulation, hair loss, skin lesions, and purple/blue toe syndrome (in which clots form in the toe, causing tissue death and even gangrene if not treated). Signs of bleeding include blood in the urine or stool, black tarry stools, bleeding in the mouth or gums, unusual or unexplained bruising, vomiting blood (or material that resembles coffee grounds), and nosebleeds. If any of these or other side effects occur, patients should see their prescribers. Pharmacists and technicians should help patients understand the urgency of such effects and help them seek medical care.

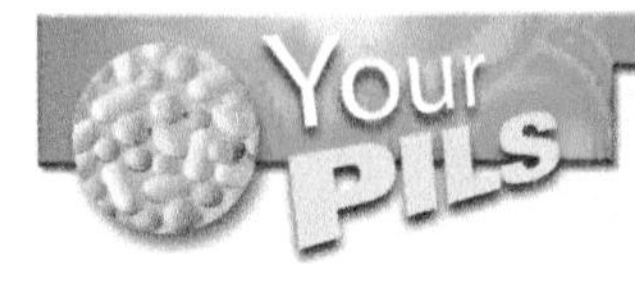

Opportunistic learners, like Enactors, may find looking through their own medicine cabinets a useful way to become familiar with warfarin drug interactions. Using a reputable drug information resource, look up the drugs you have at home and determine which ones interact with warfarin. Be aware that many patients on warfarin have these same drugs in their medicine cabinets. The next time a patient purchases one of these products along with a warfarin refill, you can point out the potential for problems.

Cautions and Considerations Heparin should not be injected intramuscularly because severe bruising can occur.

LMWHs, fondaparinux, and direct thrombin inhibitors require dose adjustment in patients with impaired renal function and are contraindicated in some cases of severe kidney problems. Patients should inform their prescribers and pharmacists if they know they have kidney disease.

Table 13.4 Drugs that Interact with Warfarin

Carbamazepine	Metronidazole
Cimetidine	Phenytoin
Fenofibrate	Rifampin
Fluconazole	Rosuvastatin
Fluoxetine	Simvastatin
Fluvastatin	Sulfamethoxazole
Gemfibrozil	Tamoxifen
Levothyroxine	Voriconazole
Lovastatin	

Warfarin is highly protein-bound and metabolized through the liver, so it interacts with many OTC and prescription drugs. The **drug interactions with warfarin** are too numerous to list here, but some of the most common prescription drugs that interact with warfarin are listed in Table 13.4. Aspirin and NSAIDs affect clotting by changing platelet action, so they should not be taken with warfarin.

Interactions that affect warfarin activity can be serious. A decrease in effectiveness can cause unwanted clots; an increase in effectiveness can cause bleeding. Either way, the results of these interactions can be life threatening. Patients should tell their prescribers and pharmacists about all medications they take so interactions can be detected. You can help by obtaining a thorough medication history upon prescription intake.

Professional Focus

Look up specific foods that are high in vitamin K. Put a list of these foods into an information leaflet that you can give to patients picking up prescriptions for warfarin. Remind them that they can eat these foods but that they should not dramatically vary the amount of them that they would normally eat.

Warfarin is also affected by certain foods. Because it inhibits vitamin K–dependent clotting factors, changes in the amount of vitamin K a patient ingests can affect warfarin activity. Pharmacists should educate patients, especially those just starting warfarin therapy, about food and drug interactions. Foods high in vitamin K (such as leafy green vegetables) do not have to be totally avoided, but patients should not vary the amount of these foods that they normally eat. Warfarin doses are adjusted according to each patient's typical daily food intake. Pharmacy technicians can reinforce these teaching points with patients as they dispense refills.

Alcohol increases warfarin's effects. Patients taking anticoagulant drugs should not drink excessive amounts of alcohol or bleeding could occur. Modest alcohol intake, one to two drinks a day, does not affect anticoagulant drug therapy.

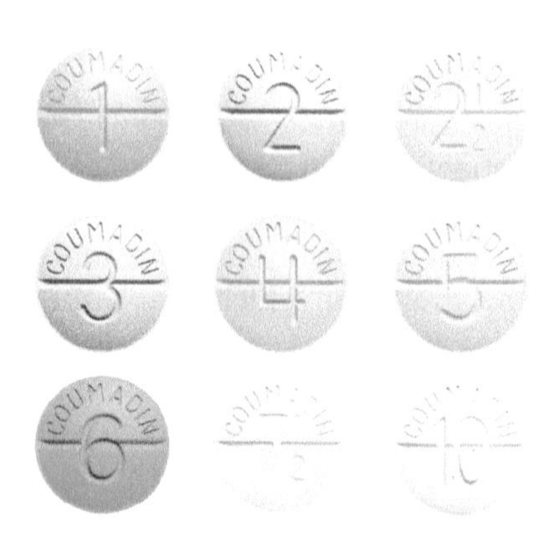

For patient safety reasons, all companies that make warfarin use the same color-coding that corresponds with tablet strength. You should become familiar with the tablet colors for the strengths dispensed most often in your pharmacy.

Warfarin therapy requires frequent laboratory tests and close monitoring. Compliance is essential for successful anticoagulation therapy. Doses should be taken at the same time each day. Missed doses should be taken as soon as the patient remembers but should not overlap with subsequent doses. Missed doses should be reported to the prescriber or pharmacist adjusting doses.

Because anticoagulants are used frequently, especially in the inpatient setting, technicians encounter them daily. Slight changes in doses can have large effects on patient health and safety. These agents do not leave much room for error, and under- or overdosing can have life-threatening consequences. Anticoagulants are considered high-risk medications for potential mistakes. Both pharmacists and technicians should never assume doses are correctly written as ordered. Use appropriate references to look up doses, double-check all calculations during mixing and preparation, and be sure proper labeling is used to avoid medication errors.

Anticoagulation Antagonists One class of drugs used to treat coagulation problems is **anticoagulation antagonists** (see Table 13.5). **Vitamin K** is used in the body to make clotting factors II, VII, IX, and X

Table 13.5 Anticoagulation Antagonists

Generic (Brand)	Dosage Form	Route of Administration	Common Dose
Phytonadione or vitamin K (Mephyton)	Tablet, injection	Oral, IM, IV, SC injection	1–10 mg a dose
Protamine	Injection	IV	Based on degree of heparin reversal desired

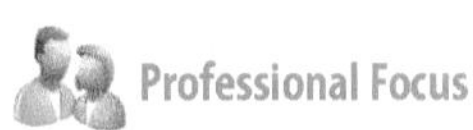
Professional Focus

Oral vitamin K tablets are not the same as potassium supplements—although these supplements are abbreviated in prescription orders and on labels as "K." It is crucial that you take extra care to ensure that vitamin K is not mixed up with K-Dur and K-Tab, which are potassium supplements. A dispensing error between these products could be fatal.

in the coagulation cascade as well as proteins C and S. It is used to reverse warfarin effects when signs of bleeding are present. If the INR lab results are elevated but signs of bleeding are not present, the patient may simply be instructed to skip a dose or two of warfarin. The pharmacist and prescriber should handle these decisions and adjustments in direct conjunction with the patient. If bleeding is severe, the patient will be given fresh whole blood with clotting factors to stop blood loss.

Protamine is used to reverse heparin effects. It works by combining with heparin to form a complex that is no longer able to exert coagulation effects. It is used when hemorrhage or high risk of hemorrhage is present.

Side Effects Common side effects of vitamin K include flushing, changes in taste sensation, dizziness, sweating, rapid pulse, and difficulty breathing. Pain at the injection site can also happen. Vitamin K should be administered under direct supervision to monitor for these effects and signs of anaphylaxis (severe allergic reaction).

Cautions and Considerations Vitamin K should be used subcutaneously whenever possible; when IM or IV administration is unavoidable, it must be given very slowly (no faster than 1 mg a minute). Fatalities have occurred with more rapid administration of vitamin K. Also, vitamin K should be mixed in preservative-free normal saline or dextrose 5% in water (D_5W).

Antiplatelet Agents These medications are used to decrease the risk of stroke, DVT, and clotting associated with cardiovascular blockage. **Antiplatelet agents** are usually used once a patient has had a stroke, DVT, or heart attack in order to prevent further clotting events. **Low-dose aspirin** (81 mg to 325 mg a day) is used to prevent clots associated with stroke and heart attack (see Table 13.6). This dose of aspirin has antiplatelet effects but may not alleviate pain or fever. Aspirin can be used during a heart attack to keep clots from completely occluding blood vessels in the heart. Other uses for aspirin along with a full discussion of side effects and special considerations are covered in Chapter 9.

Side Effects Common side effects of aspirin, clopidogrel, and ticlopidine include bleeding due to excessive anticoagulation, stomach upset, headache, dizziness, and rash. Signs of bleeding include blood in the urine or stool, black tarry stools, bleeding in the mouth or gums, unusual or unexplained bruising, vomiting blood (or material that resembles coffee grounds), and nosebleeds. If any of these effects occur, the patient should see his or her prescriber. These agents should not be used in patients who are already at risk for bleeding, such as those about to have surgical procedures. Usually patients will be instructed to stop taking these drugs prior to the procedure.

Cautions and Considerations Antiplatelet and anticoagulant agents should not be used by patients with bleeding disorders or a history of ulcers because their risk of severe hemorrhage is too high. For this same reason, patients should not take NSAIDs along with antiplatelet or anticoagulation therapy. NSAIDs can affect platelet activity and increase bleeding risk.

Table 13.6 Commonly Used Antiplatelet Agents

Generic (Brand)	Dosage Form	Route of Administration	Common Dose
Aspirin	Tablet, chewable tablet, effervescent tablet, suppository	Oral, rectal	81–325 mg a day
Clopidogrel (Plavix)	Tablet	Oral	75 mg a day
Dipyridamole (Persantine)	Tablet, injection	Oral, IV	PO: 75–100 mg 3–4 times a day IV: Doses individualized by weight
Pentoxifylline (Trental)	Tablet	Oral	400 mg 3 times a day
Ticlopidine (Ticlid)	Tablet	Oral	250 mg twice a day with food

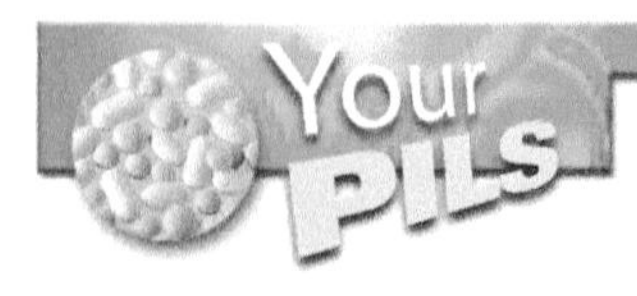

All learners can benefit from putting the drug therapies they handle into the context of patient care. Anticoagulant and antiplatelet drugs (see Tables 13.3 and 13.6) are used to maintain a patient's INR within in a specific range. Look up the goal ranges for patients taking anticoagulation therapy for DVT treatment, atrial fibrillation, and prosthetic heart valve. The goal of therapy is to elevate INR just enough to prevent clot formation but not overshoot and cause bleeding.

Clopidogrel and ticlopidine can cause thrombocytopenia (low platelets) and neutropenia (low WBCs). CBC is used to monitor for drops in platelet or WBC counts. Liver function tests are usually tracked as well.

TAKE WITH FOOD

Antiplatelet agents work best when taken with food. An auxiliary warning label to this effect is recommended when dispensing these medications.

Thrombolytic Agents When immediate return of blood flow is crucial, these agents are used to dissolve clots that have formed (see Table 13.7). Use of **thrombolytic agents** is limited to select situations, including massive myocardial infarction, stroke, and PE. These agents can yield dramatic life-saving results but must be administered within hours to days of the event to be effective.

Thrombolytic medications work through a variety of mechanisms, all of which break up clots that have already formed. Many work by dissolving fibrin. Unlike the other medications discussed earlier in this chapter that prevent formation or further growth of clots, these drugs, in contrast, dissolve and shrink blood clots. However, their cost and potential serious side effects must be weighed along with their benefits.

Table 13.7 Commonly Used Thrombolytic Agents

Generic (Brand)	Dosage Form	Route of Administration	Common Dose
Alteplase (TPA, Activase)	Powder for injection	IV	0.09–0.75 mg/kg over 30–60 minutes
Anistreplase (Eminase)	Injection	IV	30 units over 2–5 minutes
Reteplase (Retavase)	Injection	IV	10 units over 2 minutes
Streptokinase (Streptase, Kabikinase)	Powder for injection	IV	Doses individualized but often given in thousands to millions of units per infusion
Tenecteplase (TNKase)	Powder for injection	IV	Depends on patient weight
Urokinase (Abbokinase)	Powder for injection	IV	4,400–6,000 units/kg an hour

Side Effects Common side effects of thrombolytic medications include bleeding, bruising, slow heart rate, decreased blood pressure, arrhythmias, fever, and allergic reactions. These agents are administered in the inpatient setting, so these effects are monitored closely. Risk of severe bleeding is high, so use of these agents is limited to life-threatening situations.

Cautions and Considerations Tenecteplase should not be shaken during reconstitution. It should be mixed with sterile water only, not dextrose solution, and allowed to sit for a few minutes. Reteplase must be refrigerated and protected from light.

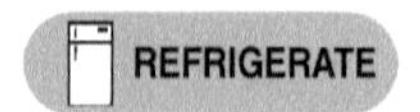

Hemophilia Agents Drugs for hemophilia replace specific missing clotting factors in patients with this condition. Replacing missing factor(s) allows the coagulation cascade to function and restores normal coagulation. These injectable **hemophilia agents** include factors VIIa, VIII, IX, and Von Willebrand factor. You will not prepare or dispense many of these products unless you work in a specialty pharmacy. These agents are quite expensive and thus closely monitored by prescribers and by patients' insurance providers. Few pharmacies stock them. Prevention of major bleeding events in patients with hemophilia is important for sustaining life as well as keeping costs of healthcare down. One hospitalization for a hemophilia-related bleeding event can cost millions of dollars.

Herbal and Alternative Therapies

Other than iron, folate, and vitamin B_{12} supplements, few herbal or natural products are used to treat blood disorders. **Vitamin C** is sometimes prescribed along with iron supplements to boost absorption. No other OTC products are available for coagulation and clotting disorders. Frequently, however, patients take herbal products that interact with drugs discussed in this chapter. For instance, anticoagulants (warfarin) and antiplatelet agents (aspirin and ticlopidine) interact with numerous herbal products, including cranberry juice, *dong quai*, feverfew, ginger, garlic, ginkgo biloba, green tea, St. John's wort, and vitamin E.

Pharmacy technicians can help patients and pharmacists detect these drug interactions by making sure they take thorough medication histories of all patients on anticoagulants, antiplatelet drugs, and other medications mentioned in this chapter. By asking about herbal and natural products specifically, you can remind patients to inform their healthcare providers when they take these products. Entering these medications into the patient's profile is an important step in checking for drug interactions.

Chapter Summary

The blood contains plasma and three main types of blood cells: RBCs, WBCs, and platelets. RBCs contain hemoglobin, which carries oxygen to the body's tissues. Iron, folate, and vitamin B_{12} are essential building blocks of hemoglobin and RBCs. Anemia is a reduction in the amount of healthy RBCs containing functional hemoglobin. It can be caused by a deficiency in these nutrients or a reduction in hematopoiesis, the process whereby RBCs are produced. Drug therapy for anemia includes iron, folic acid, and vitamin B_{12} supplementation as well as hematopoietic agents such as epoetin alpha and darbepoetin.

Platelet activity and the coagulation cascade regulate the blood's ability to form clots. When the blood cannot clot, dangerous bleeding can occur. Hemophilia, a life-threatening bleeding condition, is a genetic disorder in which certain clotting factors are absent or deficient. Missing clotting factors are administered to prevent bleeding. These therapies are quite expensive and dispensed by specialty pharmacies only.

When the blood forms unwanted clots, blood flow can be cut off to vital organs, including the brain, heart, and lungs. Clots cause stroke, heart attack, PE, and DVT. Anticoagulants and antiplatelet drug therapies are used frequently to prevent and treat such clots. These drugs have many drug interactions and side effects that must be monitored closely. Thrombolytic drugs can be used in certain situations to break down clots that have formed. They are also expensive and not without risk.

Chapter Review

For the following sets of exercises, write the exercise heading, exercise numbers, and your answers on a separate sheet of paper. Your instructor may direct you to turn in the sheet of paper or discuss your answers as a class.

REVIEW THE BASICS

Choose a, b, c, or d as the correct answer to each multiple-choice question.

1. Which of the following blood components is primarily responsible for the transport of oxygen to the cells of the body?
   a. plasma
   b. RBCs
   c. WBCs
   d. platelets

2. Which of the following contain(s) protein, such as albumin, to which drug molecules bind?
   a. plasma
   b. RBCs
   c. WBCs
   d. platelets

3. Which of the following drugs works by preventing platelets from clumping together and forming blood clots?
   a. iron
   b. aspirin
   c. heparin
   d. alteplase

4. Which of the following drugs stimulates RBC production to treat anemia?
   a. ticlopidine
   b. vitamin K
   c. darbepoetin
   d. fondaparinux

5. Eating more green leafy vegetables than usual while taking which of the following drugs could cause an unwanted blood clot?
   a. vitamin B_{12}
   b. warfarin
   c. clopidogrel
   d. enoxaparin

6. Which of the following drugs is *not* available in an oral dosage form?
   a. folic acid
   b. heparin
   c. vitamin K
   d. cyanocobalamin

7. Hemophilia is caused by which of the following?
   a. lack of platelets
   b. lack of clotting factors
   c. iron deficiency
   d. all of the above

8. Anemia is caused by which of the following?
   a. folate deficiency
   b. RBC destruction
   c. blood loss
   d. all of the above

9. Which of the following drugs is a thrombolytic (fibrinolytic) agent?
   a. pentoxifylline
   b. tenecteplase
   c. erythropoietin
   d. lepirudin

10. Which of the following is dosed in thousands of units per infusion?
    a. iron sucrose
    b. heparin
    c. vitamin K
    d. dalteparin

KNOW THE DRUGS

Match each brand name drug with its corresponding generic name and most common use. Your answers should follow this example format: Generic Name: 1. a; 2. b; 3. c; etc. Most Common Use: 1. g; 2. h; 3. i; etc.

Brand Name	Generic Name	Most Common Use
1. Venofer	a. vitamin K	g. anemia
2. Procrit	b. iron sucrose	h. stroke prevention
3. Fergon	c. enoxaparin	i. reversal of overanticoagulation
4. Activase	d. alteplase	j. deep-vein thrombosis
5. Mephyton	e. epoetin alpha	k. fibrinolysis
6. Lovenox	f. ferrous gluconate	

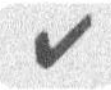

PUT IT TOGETHER

For each item, write down either a single term to complete the sentence or a short answer.

1. ________________ require use of an auxiliary warning label warning patients of urine discoloration.
2. List the anticoagulation antagonists and then list the primary drug that each antagonist is used against in cases of overdose or toxicity risk.
3. Oral ______________ products should not be crushed or chewed.
4. List three natural or herbal products that interact with warfarin.
5. What laboratory tests are used to detect, diagnose, and monitor anemia?
6. ________________ can be measured with a fingerstick test in pharmacist-run anticoagulation clinics.

THINK IT THROUGH

Read and think through each numbered scenario carefully and then write several sentences in reply to the question(s) presented. Question 4 requires you to do some Internet research before completing your answer(s).

1. You work at a retail pharmacy in a grocery store. A patient asks you to ring up a couple of other items along with her refill for warfarin. She adds a bottle of Tums, a bag of lettuce, and salad dressing. What interaction should you alert the patient to in this situation? What should you do?
2. A pharmacist you work with gets a call from the floor with an order for bridge therapy for a patient on heparin. The pharmacist instructs you to get the typical order ready and send it to the floor. What drugs are part of anticoagulation bridge therapy? What additional information do you need to fill this request?
3. Mr. Martin comes to pick up his prescriptions for his diabetes, high cholesterol, and high blood pressure. He says his doctor told him to start taking baby aspirin every day. He asks you why he can't just take an adult aspirin instead. What should you tell him?

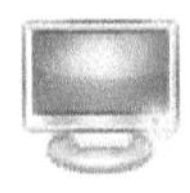

4. **On the Internet,** look up some reports of medication errors that have occurred with heparin. The Institute for Safe Medication Practices (ISMP) has many resources available on its Web site for preventing such errors. Which drugs from this chapter are on the High-Alert Medication List? Heparin is dosed in units; look to see how this should be written in medication orders to prevent errors (see the ISMP's Error-Prone Abbreviation List). Think about ways you could avoid errors when working with heparin and other anticoagulants.

Chapter 14 The Respiratory System and Drug Therapy

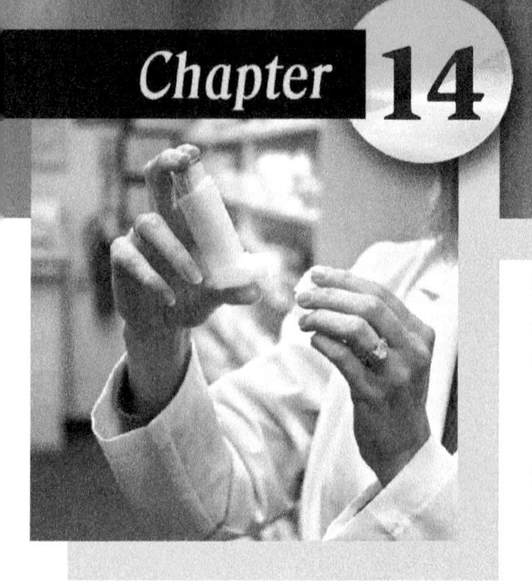

LEARNING OBJECTIVES

- Describe the basic anatomy and physiology of the respiratory system.
- Explain the therapeutic effects of the prescription medications, nonprescription medications, and alternative therapies commonly used to treat diseases and disorders of the respiratory system.
- Describe the adverse effects of the prescription medications, nonprescription medications, and alternative therapies commonly used to treat diseases and disorders of the respiratory system.
- Identify the brand and generic names of the prescription and nonprescription medications commonly used to treat diseases and disorders of the respiratory system.
- State the common doses, dosage forms, and routes of administration of the prescription and nonprescription medications commonly used to treat diseases and disorders of the respiratory system.

STUDY PARTNER

Interactive self-quizzes, games, audio files, and glossaries help you to learn drug names and facts.

Diseases and conditions of the respiratory tract range from the common cold and seasonal allergies to asthma and tuberculosis. If you are involved in healthcare, you will encounter some sort of respiratory disease on a regular basis. Drug therapies for respiratory problems are dispensed daily, and pharmacy technicians see them frequently. In fact, the success of these drug therapies is highly dependent on patient adherence to prescribed regimens. When you are familiar with the proper use of these medications, you can help the pharmacist emphasize to patients just how important adherence to treatment is and also help identify when problems arise.

For the purposes of this text, the upper and lower respiratory tracts are discussed in separate chapters. This chapter covers the normal physiology of the lower respiratory system, followed by an explanation of the conditions that most often affect it. Such conditions include asthma, chronic obstructive pulmonary disease (COPD), and pneumonia. The chapter then briefly touches on tuberculosis and cystic fibrosis treatments. Last, it addresses smoking cessation. Conditions affecting the upper respiratory tract, such as seasonal allergies and colds, are covered in Chapter 11 in the discussion of medications for the eyes, ears, nose, and throat.

Anatomy and Physiology of the Respiratory System

The respiratory tract is divided into the upper and lower regions. The **upper respiratory tract** includes the nasal passages, sinuses, and the throat area where the **epiglottis** and **larynx** (voice box) are located (see Figure 14.1). The **lower respiratory tract** includes the **bronchi**, **bronchioles**, **lungs**, and **alveoli**. Different diseases and conditions tend to affect the upper and lower respiratory tracts, so different drug therapies may be used for each.

When a person breathes, air is pulled into and pushed out of the lungs. This mechanical process facilitates bringing oxygen into the lungs and releasing carbon dioxide. In the lungs, small air sacs called alveoli fill with air and allow for **gas exchange** with the blood. The surface area of the alveoli is extremely large, and respiratory tissue is well supplied with blood vessels, allowing gases such as oxygen and carbon dioxide to move easily into and out of the bloodstream.

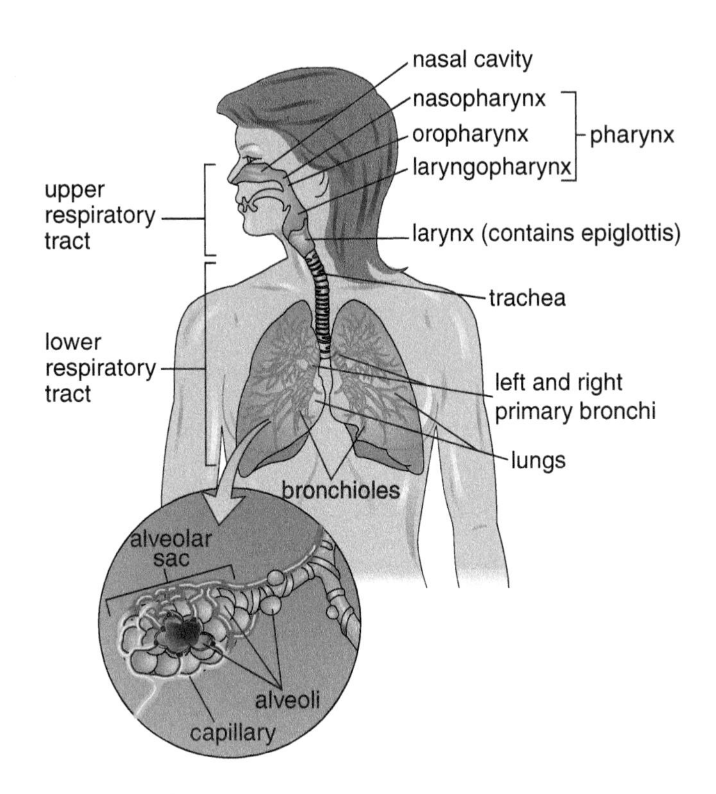

Figure 14.1
Upper and Lower Respiratory Tracts
The epiglottis, a flap of tissue that covers the tracheal opening to the lungs when you swallow, is in effect the dividing line between the upper and lower respiratory tracts.

Inside the alveoli, oxygen moves into the blood, and carbon dioxide, a by-product of cellular function, leaves the blood. This gas-exchange process (see Figure 14.2) provides needed oxygen to the cells of the body to supply energy and to fuel cellular respiration. This process also helps maintain the acid/base balance in the blood. As a result, blood pH is kept within safe limits.

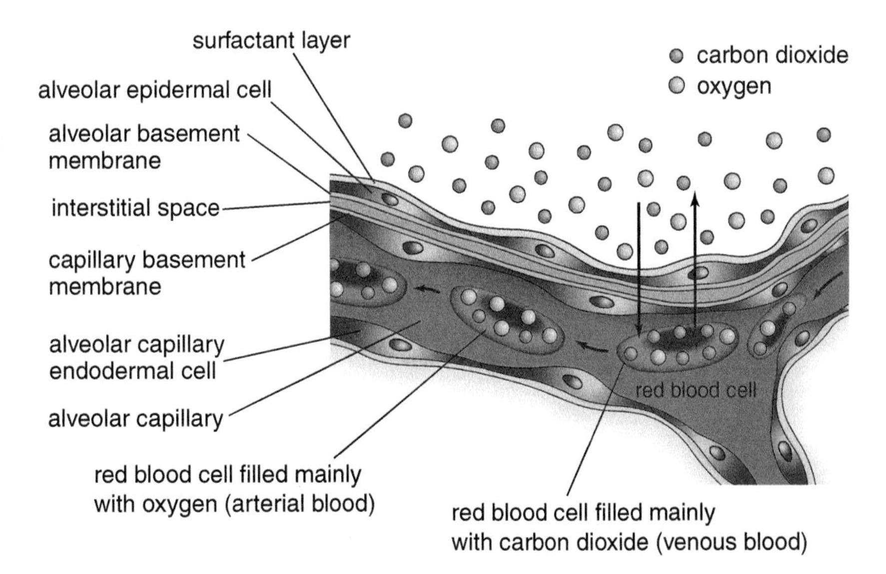

Figure 14.2
Gas-Exchange Process
Oxygen picked up in the lungs is carried by red blood cells to all the cells of the body, while carbon dioxide is brought back to the lungs to be expelled during exhalation.

Asthma

Asthma affects over 22 million people in the United States. Six million of these people are children. The number of people living with asthma in the United States has increased in the past twenty years. In fact, each year asthma accounts for thousands of emergency room visits, hospitalizations, and even deaths. The primary goal of treatment is to reduce acute and chronic troublesome symptoms, prevent exacerbations, and minimize hospitalizations or visits to the emergency room. Other goals of treatment are for asthmatics to be as physically active as they would like, and to sleep without interruption from asthmatic symptoms.

Asthma is an inflammatory disorder of the airways and causes coughing, wheezing, breathlessness, and chest tightness. Bronchioles constrict, mucus production increases, and lung tissue swells (see Figure 14.3), making normal breathing difficult. This condition is **chronic**, meaning that it is not curable. However, asthma is a reversible lung disease in that it can improve or be controlled if a patient uses appropriate medications. If the patient regularly takes anti-inflammatory medication, lung function may return to normal.

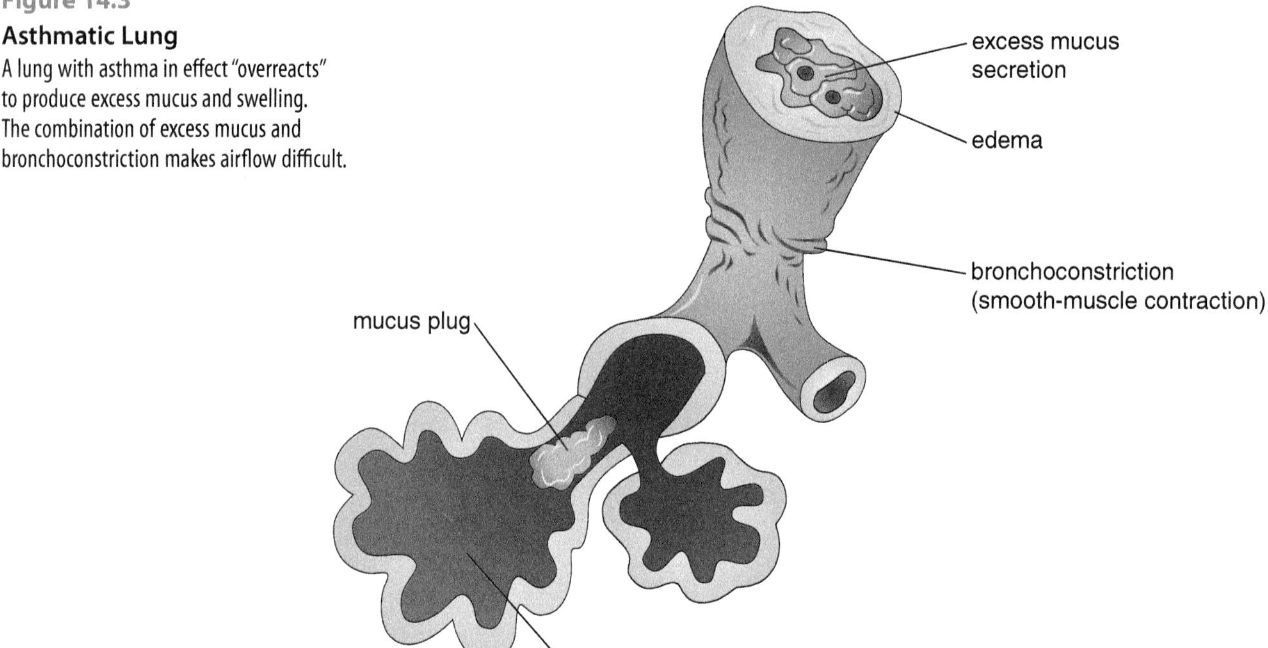

Figure 14.3

Asthmatic Lung

A lung with asthma in effect "overreacts" to produce excess mucus and swelling. The combination of excess mucus and bronchoconstriction makes airflow difficult.

Asthma is also episodic, meaning that times of poor airflow and difficulty breathing alternate with times of normal function. Acute difficulty breathing, known as an **asthma attack**, is characterized by hyperreactivity of the airways and **bronchospasm,** usually in response to allergens or irritants. Common triggers include smoke, dust, exercise, pet dander, cold weather, and colds or flu. Other potential triggers can include medications, anxiety, laughing, and certain foods. Immediately after exposure to a trigger, mast cells in the lung tissue release histamine and other chemical mediators that cause bronchospasm and increased mucus production.

An asthma attack not only produces anxiety for the patient, it can be life threatening when severe. Over time, continued release of histamine, bradykinins, prostaglandins, and leukotrienes causes tissues to inflame and airways to constrict, and can result in permanent lung tissue damage. Fortunately, in many cases, breathing symptoms and

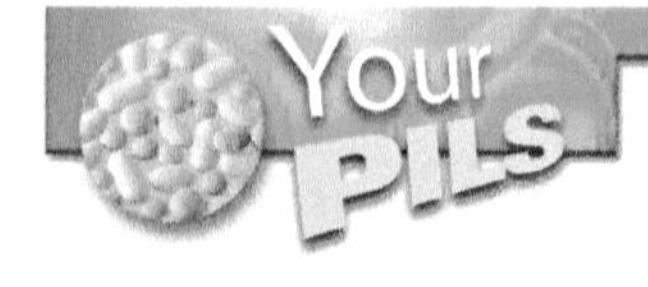

To see what it's like to have an asthma attack, try this exercise. Creators who have a flair for the dramatic or Directors who like hands-on creativity may particularly like this exercise. Run in place for a few minutes until your breathing rate is increased. Now, put a straw in your mouth and try to breathe exclusively through it. You will feel how difficult it is to get enough air to satisfy your need for oxygen and hopefully appreciate the anxiety that patients go through during an asthma attack.

airway constriction can be controlled with proper treatment. Without treatment, lung function can steadily decline.

Asthma is categorized into levels of severity (intermittent, mild, moderate, and severe), based on how patients' symptoms affect their ability to sleep at night, continue normal daily activities, and breathe freely. Objective **pulmonary function tests** can be done to assess asthma severity. In addition, if a patient is waking up at night more than twice a month or using relief medication such as an inhaler more than twice a week, asthma is considered "not controlled." Patients should understand that if their asthma is not controlled, they should seek medical treatment and be sure to adhere to prescribed medication schedules. Drug therapy for asthma includes long-term treatment to prevent exacerbations as well as rescue treatment to help once symptoms have begun. Many patients need more than simple rescue therapies. Long-term, steady treatment can improve overall lung function, reduce exacerbations, and decrease the need for short-term relief therapies.

One way patients can monitor their lung function at home is to use a peak flow meter (see photo, below). This small, portable device is sold in most pharmacies and measures the strength of airflow exiting the lungs. The patient takes a deep breath and then blows into the device as fast and as forcefully as possible. The indicator moves in response to airflow, and a number is generated. Although this device is not diagnostic, it can provide a crude assessment of lung function if patients use it regularly and chart the results daily. The chart helps patients see if their lung function is declining over time. In such cases, patients can work with their healthcare providers to prevent worsening lung function before the trend leads to a bigger problem and asthma attacks intensify. As a pharmacy technician, you might suggest that patients using multiple inhalers for asthma also use a peak flow meter regularly. The pharmacist can offer instruction for proper use.

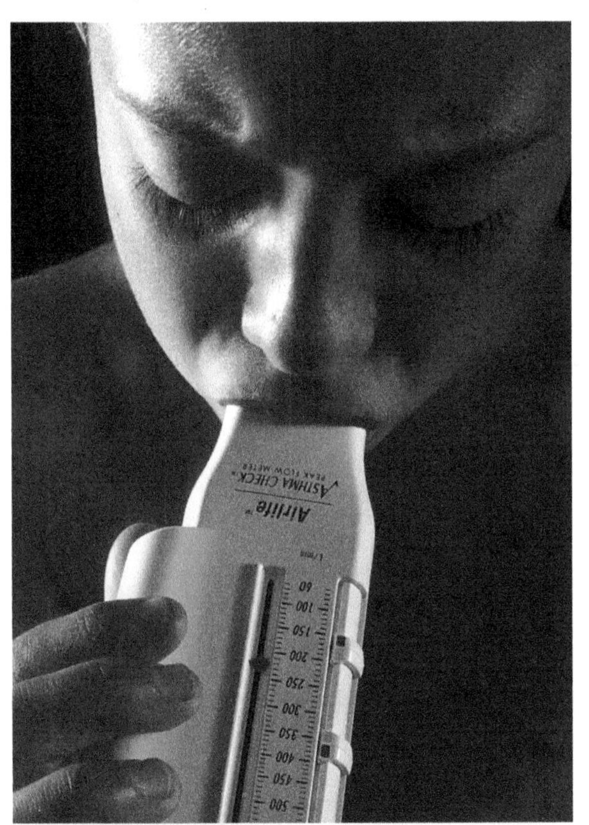

A peak flow meter is a valuable tool for asthma patients to measure lung function and manage symptoms.

Drugs for Asthma

Drug therapy for asthma has two components: **rescue inhalers** for quick relief during an asthma attack and **long-term anti-inflammatory agents** (inhaled corticosteroids) leukotriene inhibitors and mast cell inhibitors, to improve **bronchoconstriction** and prevent attacks. Sometimes, patients rely too heavily on rescue inhalers, which provide immediate improvement in breathing. However, pharmacy technicians can help patients remain adherent to anti-inflammatory treatment so that long-term asthma control improves.

The goal of asthma treatment is to improve breathing so that patients do not wheeze and cough as much and are able to sleep better at night, go to work and school every day, and participate in desired activities including exercise. Asthma management is a step-wise process that generally begins with inhalers and proceeds to oral therapies. Typically, short-acting beta agonists (with or without an inhaled corticosteroid) are the first treatment and then other agents such as leukotriene inhibitors or mast cell inhibitors are added for more severe cases. Health professionals also recommend that patients with asthma get a flu shot every year.

Metered dose inhalers (MDIs) are used most often to deliver beta agonist agents and inhaled corticosteroids. You should be aware that inhaler technology is changing to remove propellants that can be harmful to the atmosphere. Improved inhalers are labeled with the letters "HFA,"

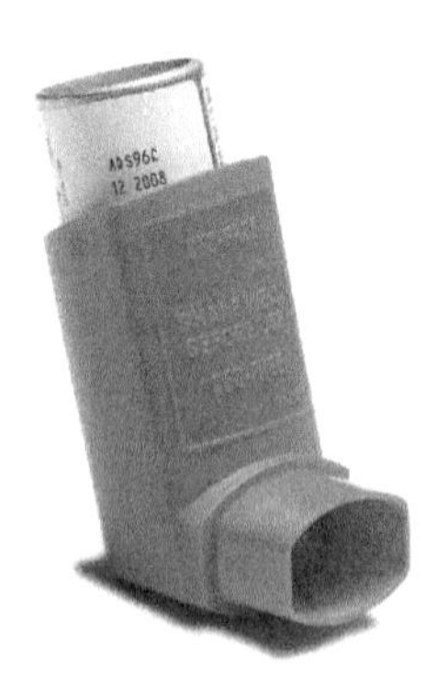

MDIs spray a controlled amount of medication through the opening when the canister is pressed downward.

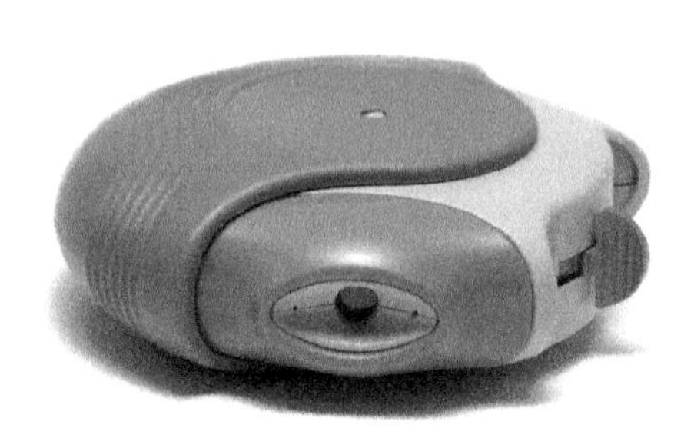

Dry powder inhalers look like a discus and are actuated by breathing in deeply at the opening instead of pressing with the fingers.

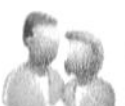

Professional Focus

Nebulizer solutions come as single-dose vials in multipack boxes. You can teach patients how to open the vials, put the solution into the compartment below the mask, run the treatment until all of the solution is gone, and clean the tubing and accessory equipment.

which stands for hydrofluoroalkane. In most cases, healthcare providers recommend that patients use a **spacer** along with MDIs to improve drug delivery to the lungs. A spacer suspends the medication mist in the air for a few seconds, allowing patients more time to coordinate the two required actions: breathing in and activating the inhaler.

Some inhalers contain plain dry powder that patients pull into their lungs when they breathe in quickly and forcefully at the inhaler opening. Such **dry powder inhalers** can be easily identified because they are often shaped like a discus (see photo above).

Young children or elderly patients who find it difficult to use an inhaler or who cannot breathe in forcefully enough to use a dry powder inhaler will need to have nebulizer treatments. A **nebulizer machine** (see photo below) sends a stream of air through the drug solution, creating a fine mist that patients inhale by breathing normally through a mask for 10–15 minutes.

Short-Acting Beta Agonists Used via inhalation for short-term relief of breathing symptoms related to asthma, and sometimes COPD (covered later in this chapter), **short-acting beta agonists** (see Table 14.1) are prescribed for adults and children. The medication is supplied as a hand-held MDI and as a nebulizer solution. Short-acting beta agonists work by stimulating beta-2 receptors in the lungs and by producing smooth muscle relaxation in the bronchioles, which open airways. Because their effects last only a few hours, these agents may need to be used multiple times a day. Although oral dosage forms are available, most patients use these agents by inhaling them into the lungs.

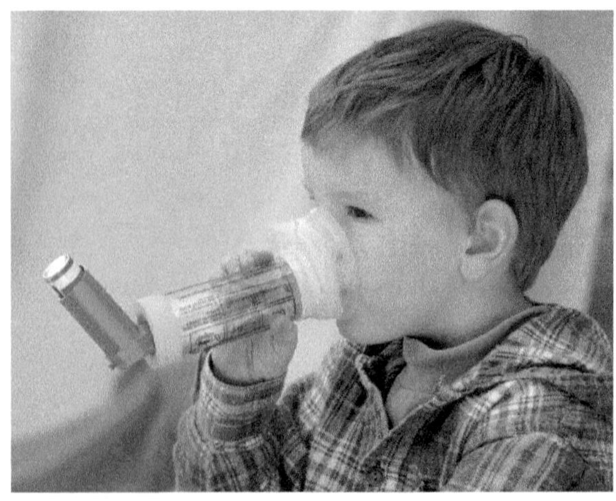

If a spacer is added to an MDI, the medication is more likely to penetrate deeper into the lung tissue than if the MDI is used alone.

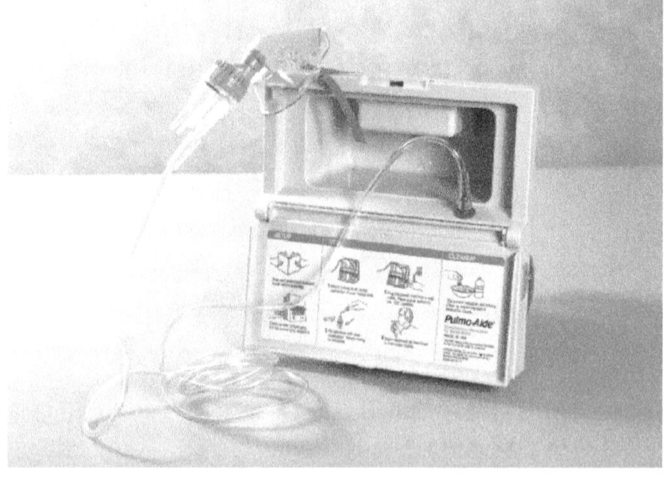

Nebulizer machines usually have clear tubing, a compartment to hold solution from single-dose vials, and an adjustable mask strap.

Table 14.1 Common Short-Acting Beta Agonists

Generic (Brand)	Dosage Form	Route of Administration	Common Dose
Albuterol (Proventil, Ventolin, AccuNeb)	Tablet, syrup, aerosol (MDI), nebulizer solution	Oral, inhalation	PO: 2–4 mg 3–4 times a day MDI: 1–2 puffs 3–4 times a day Inhalation: 2.5 mg 3–4 times a day via nebulizer
Levalbuterol (Xopenex)	Aerosol (MDI), nebulizer solution	Inhalation	MDI: 2 puffs every 4–6 hours Inhalation: 0.31–0.63 mg 3 times a day via nebulizer
Metaproterenol (Alupent)	Tablet, syrup	Oral	PO: 10–20 mg 3–4 times a day
Pirbuterol (Maxair)	Aerosol (MDI)	Inhalation	MDI: 2 puffs (400 mcg) every 4–6 hours

Side Effects Common side effects of short-acting beta agonists include dizziness, nervousness, heartburn, nausea, and tremors. They also cause cardiac effects including increased blood pressure and heart palpitations. Patients with high blood pressure or heart problems should discuss these beta agonists with their physicians before using them.

Cautions and Considerations Short-acting beta agonists interact with digoxin and beta blockers, both of which are frequently used by people with heart disease. Short-acting beta agonists can cause digoxin levels to rise, resulting in increased toxicity. Beta blockers inhibit the effect of these beta agonist drugs. Short-acting beta agonists and beta blockers should not be used together; if they must be, physicians must carefully adjust the doses.

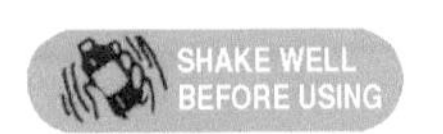

MDIs should be shaken before each use. Pharmacists should teach patients how to use their inhalers properly with each new prescription and periodically for refills.

Inhaled Corticosteroids Used for long-term treatment and control of moderate to severe asthma, **corticosteroids** are produced in oral and inhaled forms (see Table 14.2). Systemic side effects of oral corticosteroids are problematic (see Chapter 4). An advantage of inhaled corticosteroids is that there is less systemic absorption and fewer side effects than are seen with oral parenteral steroids. In severe exacerbations of asthma or COPD, an oral corticosteroid may be needed initially to gain control. Be aware that oral agents are used for short-term therapy only.

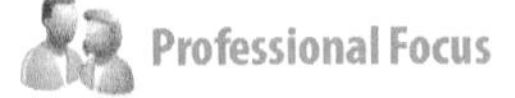

Check medication histories for corticosteroid inhaler prescriptions that were filled only once or twice and then dropped. These patients may be candidates for intervention and education. Patients often stop using inhaled corticosteroids prematurely because they do not receive noticeable relief early on.

However, if a patient must use a short-acting beta agonist inhaler more than twice a week, an **inhaled corticosteroid** is indicated. These inhaled agents can be used long term and are also sometimes used for COPD. Inhaled corticosteroids work by decreasing the inflammation that contributes to bronchoconstriction and excess mucus production. To be effective, they must be used on a regular basis rather than only when an asthma attack occurs. The purpose of these agents is to prevent frequent asthma attacks from occurring, not to treat one after it has started.

In healthcare, inhalation is the preferred route of corticosteroid administration. Topical administration directly to lung tissue produces desired effects with few systemic side effects. Pharmacy technicians can help improve patient safety by monitoring for proper inhaler use and checking refill frequency when refilling these prescriptions. If you identify potential problems, alert the pharmacist. Patients getting refills more or less frequently than prescribed may simply be confusing a corticosteroid inhaler with their beta agonist rescue inhaler. Technicians should also remind patients on checkout which inhaler is their rescue inhaler, for use only during an attack, and which is their long-term inhaler, for daily use.

Side Effects Common side effects of inhaled corticosteroids include dry mouth, headache, sore throat, hoarseness, coughing, and oral fungal infection (oral thrush). Oral thrush appears as a visible white coating on the inside of the mouth and tongue. Washing out the mouth after each inhalation decreases the incidence of oral thrush significantly and may decrease throat irritation. Using a spacer can also reduce dry mouth, sore throat, and hoarseness.

Table 14.2 Common Inhaled Corticosteroids

Generic (Brand)	Dosage Form	Common Dose
Beclomethasone (QVAR)	Aerosol (MDI)	40–160 mcg twice a day
Budesonide (Pulmicort)	Powder for inhalation, suspension for inhalation	200–800 mcg twice a day
Flunisolide (AeroBid)	Aerosol (MDI)	80–160 mcg twice a day
Fluticasone (Flovent)	Aerosol (MDI)	88–440 mcg twice a day
Mometasone (Asmanex)	Powder for inhalation	110–440 mcg 1–2 times a day
Triamcinolone (Azmacort)	Aerosol (MDI)	1–2 puffs 3–4 times a day
Combinations		
Budesonide/formoterol (Symbicort)	Aerosol (MDI)	2 inhalations twice a day
Fluticasone/salmeterol (Advair)	Aerosol (MDI), powder for inhalation	100 mcg/50 mcg to 500 mcg/50 mcg twice a day

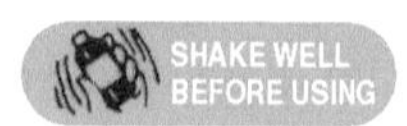

Cautions and Considerations MDIs should be shaken before each use. Dry powder inhalers should not be shaken prior to use. Instructions should be carefully followed to puncture the powder packet or capsule and then place the device in the mouth before breathing in forcefully. Pharmacists should teach patients how to use their inhalers properly with each new prescription and periodically for refills.

Leukotriene Inhibitors Used for long-term control of moderate to severe asthma as well as for allergic rhinitis, **leukotriene inhibitors** (see Table 14.3) are often prescribed when short-acting beta agonists and inhaled corticosteroids are not providing adequate control of breathing symptoms. **Leukotrienes** are inflammation mediators that cause mucus secretion and bronchoconstriction. Zileuton inhibits the enzyme involved in leukotriene synthesis, and zafirlukast and montelukast are leukotriene receptor blockers. Depending on the agent, some leukotriene inhibitors are limited to specific ages of children. For instance, montelukast is not typically used in children younger than age twelve, whereas zafirlukast can be used in children as young as age five.

Table 14.3 Common Leukotriene Inhibitors

Generic (Brand)	Dosage Form	Route of Administration	Common Dose
Montelukast (Singulair)	Chewable tablet, granules	Oral	4–5 mg once a day
Zafirlukast (Accolate)	Tablet	Oral	10–20 mg twice a day
Zileuton (Zyflo)	Tablet	Oral	600 mg twice a day

Side Effects The most common side effects of leukotriene inhibitors include nausea, sore throat, and sinusitis. Less common effects include diarrhea, stomach pain, and rash. These effects tend to be mild in nature; if they become bothersome, patients should talk with their healthcare providers.

Cautions and Considerations Leukotriene inhibitors can cause liver toxicity. Patients with liver problems should not use leukotriene inhibitors. Patients taking them will need periodic liver tests to monitor for this potentially serious side effect and should be encouraged to closely follow instructions on getting regular lab tests.

Other Asthma Agents If asthma is severe and difficult to control with other agents alone, **mast cell stabilizers** and **xanthine agents** are older therapies that may be added to a patient's regimen. Mast cell stabilizers include cromolyn and nedocromil. They are inhaled and work by blocking mast cell activity. Mast cells contribute to the overreactive inflammatory process in asthma.

Xanthine agents include theophylline and aminophylline. These older agents are taken orally and are similar in chemical structure to caffeine. They are direct bronchodilators that can also be used to treat COPD. Currently these agents tend not to be used, in part due to their side effects, which include anxiety, headache, insomnia, dizziness, tremors, heart palpitations, and increased urination. Blood levels may be read periodically to monitor xanthine therapy. Certain drugs (e.g., erythromycin) may elevate a patient's blood level.

Omalizumab is a recombinant DNA-derived humanized monoclonal antibody that selectively binds to human immunoglobulin E (IgE). It is used in patients with asthma over age twelve that is not controlled by inhaled steroids.

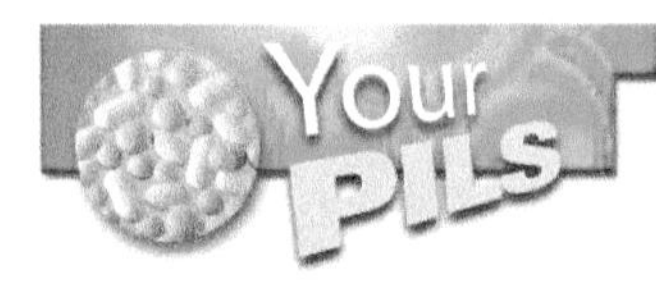

If you like working by yourself, like Producers do, you might enjoy making a list or chart of all of the inhaler medications for asthma and COPD. See if you can find a picture of each inhaler online (manufacturers' Web sites are often good sources) and place them on a chart. Then, for each inhaler, list the brand name, generic name, drug class, use (such as "asthma rescue inhaler" or "COPD long-term therapy," etc.), and the method of delivery (i.e., MDI or dry powder inhaler). Simply making this chart can be a learning experience, and you will have also produced a useful reference for memorizing the inhalers and locating them in the pharmacy.

Chronic Obstructive Pulmonary Disease (COPD)

COPD is the fourth leading cause of chronic disease and death in the United States. It is a chronic and progressive condition in which airflow is limited by an abnormal inflammatory response. Unlike asthma, COPD is not reversible, for lung function does not significantly improve on administration of a bronchodilator. In fact, COPD is a disease that progressively worsens, even with treatment.

On the positive side, COPD is largely preventable. Although some patients are genetically predisposed to getting COPD, studies show that 85% of people with COPD are smokers. Most patients have a history of smoking or exposure to pollution or occupational hazards prior to getting it. Repeated respiratory infections can also contribute to a COPD diagnosis.

COPD has two sets of symptoms: **chronic bronchitis** and **emphysema**. Chronic bronchitis is defined as a persistent cough that produces sputum lasting at least 3 months out of the year for at least 2 consecutive years. It is caused by overgrowth of mucus glands and airway narrowing in the lungs. Patients with this condition are sometimes referred to as "blue bloaters" because they may have blue lips due to lack of oxygen, and they are often overweight.

Emphysema occurs when alveolar walls are damaged or destroyed, causing enlargement of the air spaces deep within the lungs. Having fewer alveoli walls reduces the surface area available within the lungs for gas exchange. Therefore, patients use labored, fast breathing to improve oxygen exchange. These patients are sometimes referred to as "pink puffers" because, although they usually do not have blue lips, they appear to puff quickly as they breathe. Patients can have a mixture of chronic bronchitis and emphysema symptoms, depending on their condition.

Drugs for COPD

Drug therapy for COPD does not prevent progression of the disease; it simply relieves symptoms. COPD treatment can improve quality of life and allow patients to exercise or be physically active without getting out of breath. Most agents for COPD act on the bronchoconstriction that occurs as the condition gets worse. In the most severe states, patients may need oxygen to help them breathe. Oxygen is not a prescription item that pharmacy technicians typically dispense, unless the pharmacy distributes durable medical equipment. COPD patients carry portable oxygen packs or pull oxygen tanks on wheels with them. A tube called a nasal cannula delivers the gas just under their nose. Healthcare professionals recommend that patients with COPD get a flu shot every year.

Anticholinergics Used as first-line treatment for bronchoconstriction from COPD, **anticholinergic agents** (see Table 14.4) work by inhibiting acetylcholine, a neurotransmitter that stimulates smooth muscle in the lungs to constrict. Nasal spray formulations are used for rhinitis and seasonal allergies (see Chapter 11). Anticholinergics are used when long-term **bronchodilation** is needed. The purpose of these agents is to prevent frequent COPD exacerbations from occurring, not to treat acute breathing problems after they begin. These agents improve quality of life and can reduce the need for hospitalizations.

Table 14.4 Common Anticholinergic Agents

Generic (Brand)	Dosage Form	Route of Administration	Common Dose
Ipratropium (Atrovent)	Aerosol (MDI), nebulizer solution, nasal spray	Inhalation, intranasal	MDI: 2 puffs 4 times a day Nebulizer: 500 mcg 3–4 times a day Nasal spray: 2 sprays per nostril 3–5 times a day
Ipratropium/albuterol (Combivent, DuoNeb)	Aerosol (MDI), nebulizer solution	Inhalation	MDI: 2 puffs 4 times a day Nebulizer: 3 mL treatment 4 times a day
Tiotropium (Spiriva)	Powder for inhalation	Inhalation	Inhale contents of 1 capsule a day

Side Effects The most common side effects of anticholinergics are dry mouth, nervousness, dizziness, headache, cough, nausea, bitter taste, nasal dryness, upper respiratory tract infection, and nosebleeds. Patients who have glaucoma or urination problems, such as prostate enlargement, should not use anticholinergics because they can make these conditions worse.

Cautions and Considerations Patients allergic to peanuts or soy should not use anticholinergic agents. The drug itself is not the problem, but rather, the inhaler technology uses substances similar to peanut proteins, which can trigger peanut allergies.

Ipratropium inhalers require priming before first use. **Priming** the inhaler involves holding the inhaler away from the body and pushing the canister against the mouthpiece so the medicine sprays into the air. When starting to use a new canister, priming may take up to seven sprays. In cases where the inhaler has not been used for more than 24 hours, patients should prime the inhaler twice.

Tiotropium capsules are used only with an inhaler device, not swallowed. Patients should take care to follow instructions for properly puncturing the capsule and inhaling the powder using the inhaler device. Pharmacy technicians can check with patients when refills are requested, ensuring that patients are using proper technique and pointing out any problems they identify to the pharmacist for in-depth teaching.

Long-Acting Beta Agonists Used for both COPD and asthma, **long-acting beta agonists** (see Table 14.5) work in a way that is similar to the action of short-acting beta agonists (covered earlier in this chapter). They simply do not have to be administered as many times a day. Used more frequently for COPD, the long-acting agents can also be used for severe asthma, when bronchodilator therapy is needed multiple times a day, on a regular basis.

Table 14.5 Common Long-Acting Beta Agonists

Generic (Brand)	Dosage Form	Route of Administration	Common Dose
Formoterol (Foradil, Perforomist)	Powder capsule for inhalation, nebulizer solution	Inhalation	12 mcg every 12 hours
Salmeterol (Serevent Discus)	Powder for inhalation	Inhalation	1 inhalation twice a day

Side Effects As is true for short-acting beta agonists, common side effects for long-acting beta agonists include dizziness, heartburn, nausea, and tremors. Long-acting beta agonists can cause cardiac effects including increased blood pressure and heart palpitations. Patients with high blood pressure or heart problems should discuss these beta agonists with their physicians before using them.

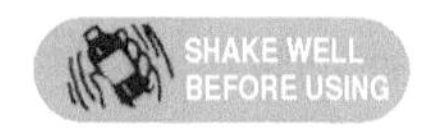

Cautions and Considerations Warnings and drug interactions for long-acting beta agonists are similar to those for short-acting agonists. Patients should not take them with beta blockers or digoxin. Importantly, MDIs need to be shaken before each use to distributed the drug evenly and ensure proper, equal doses.

Pneumonia and Tuberculosis (TB)

Pneumonia is a lower respiratory tract infection caused by bacterial, viral, or fungal pathogens. Pneumonia can be acquired from the general community or from exposure to pathogens during hospitalization. If one gets pneumonia while hospitalized or living in a long-term care facility, it is called **nosocomial pneumonia**. Nosocomial pneumonia is severe and difficult to treat because it is usually caused by more virulent pathogens. Patients in the inpatient setting encounter such pathogens because they are in close proximity to other sick patients who harbor these infections. Patients who get pneumonia from exposure outside of an inpatient facility have **community-acquired pneumonia (CAP)**.

Tuberculosis (TB) is an infectious disease caused by a mycobacterium that infects the lungs. TB causes tubercles to form in the lungs. It is quite difficult to kill. TB used to be called "consumption" and has been around for centuries. Many U.S. residents remember that TB regularly claimed lives prior to the 1960s. Once drug therapy for TB became available, people thought that TB was completely eradicated from the United States. Unfortunately, TB is on the rise now that drug-resistant strains have emerged and immunodeficiency conditions are more prevalent.

Healthcare professionals who work in inpatient or long-term care settings are usually required to get annual skin tests **(PPD skin test)** to check for exposure to TB. In a PPD skin test, an injection is placed just under the skin and then checked again 48–72 hours later for **induration** (i.e., inflammation and swelling). On testing positive for TB exposure, a person receives a chest x-ray and other tests to see if drug therapy is needed. Not everyone exposed will develop the full disease with active organisms. Symptoms of active disease include night sweats, weight loss, coughing blood, chest pain, and fatigue.

In the inpatient setting, those entering the room of a patient having TB must put on a gown, mask, and gloves prior to entry and remove those items on exiting to protect against transmission. Special respirator masks are sometimes worn over the face. You will notice signs on the door and in areas outside these hospital rooms warning people to wear appropriate garb and use universal precautions when entering.

Drugs for Pneumonia

Drug therapy for pneumonia will not be covered here in great detail because most agents are covered in Chapter 3 on infectious diseases. Prescribers must determine if a patient has CAP or nosocomial pneumonia before they can choose appropriate therapy. However, because determining the disease type takes time, a two-step treatment process is typically followed.

First, the patient is treated according to **empirical therapy**, a therapy that is applied based on common knowledge of the pathogens typically causing certain types of pneumonia. This initial drug therapy is prescribed according to the patient's symptoms, general medical history, and where the exposure is suspected to have occurred. These facts give clues to the likely pathogen so the empirical therapy can be started immediately. An antibiotic that covers a broad range of pathogens will be chosen first to increase the chances that the appropriate one is being treated.

While the first therapy is in process, a second process, called narrowing treatment, begins. Lab tests and cultures are taken to determine exactly what bacteria or fungus is present in the lungs. The patient and care providers must then wait, because results will take a couple of days to get back. Pharmacy technicians may be asked to retrieve these results when they become available. Drug therapy is then changed, if necessary, to cover the found pathogen. Bronchodilators and corticosteroids may also be administered to assist breathing, if it is labored.

Drugs for TB

Because drugs for TB are often specialized and not dispensed regularly in all settings, they are covered only briefly here (see Table 14.6). Technicians working in settings where TB is seen regularly, such as hospitals and long-term care facilities, should refer to additional texts for further detail.

One reason for the reemergence of TB is the high rate of nonadherence to drug therapy for the disease. The course of therapy for a typical infection is 7–14 days, but the course of therapy for TB is 6 months or longer. For many patients, adhering to therapy for that long is challenging, and many do not complete the entire course. Instead, they stop taking the TB medications once they begin to feel better. However, stopping therapy too soon allows the bacteria to regain a foothold and grow even stronger. Incomplete therapy only promotes the emergence of **drug-resistant TB**. Unfortunately, we now have some strains of TB that current drugs cannot eradicate.

Another reason patients find it hard to complete TB therapy is the side effects. For instance, isoniazid can cause liver toxicity. Kanamycin and streptomycin are aminoglycosides, so they can cause kidney damage and hearing loss. Rifampin causes flulike symptoms such as fever, chills, and a general feeling of illness. Ethambutol can cause changes in vision, which should be reported to the physician.

In addition to presenting side effects, most of these drugs must be taken on an empty stomach to ensure proper absorption. Patients do not always follow this requirement and take the doses inconsistently. Consequently, each of these agents can be difficult to take for the entire course of therapy. Patients can lose motivation before therapy is complete.

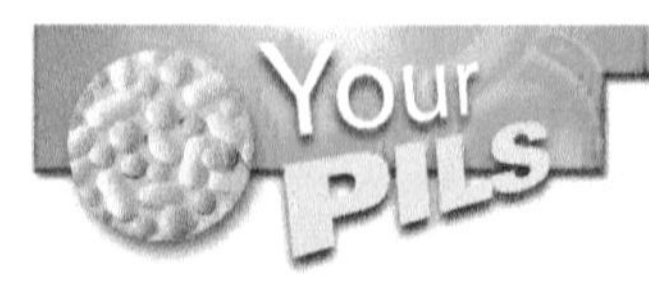

If you like to learn through discussion with others, like Enactors and Creators do, try this exercise to put a "face" on TB. Use the library and Internet to identify some historical figures (authors, politicians, world leaders, etc.) who died from "consumption." Also think about how TB is depicted in movies and theater. Then get together with a few other students to discuss your findings. Which historical figures were victims of TB? Which of your findings surprised you? Why?

Table 14.6 Common TB Drugs

Generic (Brand)	Dosage Form	Length of Therapy	Common Dose
Cycloserine (Seromycin)	Capsule	18–24 months	500 mg–1 g a day
Ethambutol (Myambutol)	Tablet	6–9 months	15 mg/kg/day daily
Isoniazid (INH)	Tablet, syrup, injection	6–24 months	5 mg/kg/day or 15 mg/kg/day 2–3 times a week
Kanamycin (Kantrex)	IM, IV	Up to 12 months	11–13 mg/kg/day daily
Pyrazinamide	Tablet	6–9 months	15–30 mg/kg/day daily
Rifampin (Rifadin)	Capsule, injection	6–9 months	10 mg/kg/day daily
Streptomycin	IM injection only	Up to 12 months	15 mg/kg/day daily or 25–30 mg/kg/day twice a day

Cystic Fibrosis

Cystic fibrosis (CF) is a genetic disease that affects exocrine glands and their ability to transport chloride across cell membranes. This abnormal chloride transport results in thick, sticky mucus production in the lungs, gastrointestinal (GI) system, and pancreas. Sweat glands and reproductive organs are also affected. However, most hospitalizations and deaths from CF occur due to pulmonary problems. The mucus accumulating in the lungs clogs airways, and infections easily take hold. In the GI system, mucus accumulation causes intestinal obstructions and affects nutrient absorption. General pancreatic function is also reduced. Therefore, treatment of CF must address nutritional needs and include pancreatic enzyme supplementation in addition to addressing respiratory complications. CF is a fatal disease from which most patients die before early to middle adulthood.

Drugs for CF

Because drugs for CF are specialized and not dispensed regularly in all settings, they are covered only briefly here. Respiratory therapy for CF includes **percussion** (non-drug treatment), antibiotics, and mucolytics (medications that liquefy and promote expulsion of thick mucus from the lungs). Percussion is a tapping, pounding movement performed on the back and chest to break up and help expectorate mucus from the lungs. Nebulizer therapy with bronchodilators, hypertonic saline, acetylcysteine, and other specialized medications is often used in conjunction with percussion to help clear airways. Several antibiotics and antifungal drugs are used to combat the bacteria and fungus that take root in the respiratory mucus secretions. Theophylline can also be used, but CF patients have vastly different pharmacokinetic profiles than do healthy patients. Special dosing and monitoring is needed.

Because the GI system and pancreas are also affected, physicians often prescribe special vitamins and **pancreatic enzyme supplements** for CF patients. These supplements help prevent ductal obstructions and steatorrhea (fatty, foul-smelling diarrhea caused by fatty foods not being absorbed). They improve growth and life expectancy for children with CF. The number of pancreatic enzyme supplements is large, so covering them here is prohibitive. However, they all contain varying amounts of **lipase, protease,** and **amylase**. Pancreatic dysfunction also contributes to malabsorption, especially for fat-soluble vitamins. Therefore, you will see many patients with CF on supplements containing vitamins A, D, E, and K. You may be more likely to encounter these oral agents in pediatric specialty centers and the outpatient setting.

Smoking Cessation

Cigarette smoking is the leading cause of preventable death. It contributes to heart disease, COPD, stroke, and many malignancies in addition to lung cancer. Because the nicotine in cigarettes is addictive, smoking can be a difficult lifestyle habit to quit. Symptoms of nicotine withdrawal include:

- anxiety
- decreased blood pressure and heart rate
- depression
- drowsiness
- headache
- increased appetite and weight gain
- insomnia
- irritability, frustration, and restlessness

Drugs for Smoking Cessation

Prescription and OTC medications can reduce nicotine withdrawal symptoms for patients trying to quit smoking. In combination with **smoking cessation** programs and social support, these medications (see Table 14.7) can help patients quit smoking successfully. Long-term cessation success is more likely when a patient uses these products along with a formal smoking cessation program rather than attempting to quit alone. Drug therapy for smoking cessation includes nicotine supplements, antidepressants, or a **nicotine blocker.**

Nicotine supplements are used to reduce absorbed nicotine slowly over time, thereby reducing many withdrawal symptoms. They are available OTC in several forms. Gradually reducing the dose helps patients get used to a smoke-free lifestyle. Gum forms work best for users of smokeless tobacco products. These forms are chewed briefly and then "parked" in the cheek until the craving for nicotine returns. Inhaled forms mimic the use and effects of smoking while eliminating the harmful toxins from inhaling smoke.

Bupropion, an antidepressant, is used to combat the mood changes and emotional instability associated with smoking cessation. It can also reduce cravings for nicotine. It is available only by prescription.

Varenicline blocks nicotine from binding to pleasure receptors and reduces withdrawal symptoms. It makes smoking less desirable and reduces weight gain. It must be started one week prior to the desired quit date. Varenicline is taken for 12 weeks and is used in conjunction with a formal smoking cessation program for best results. It is available only by prescription.

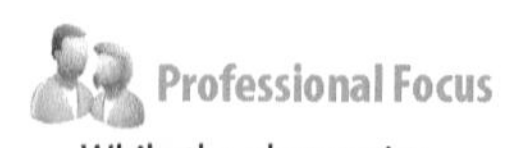

While the pharmacist should provide full counseling to patients starting on smoking cessation products, you can encourage patients by emphasizing the benefits of quitting smoking: saving money, protecting the health of family at home, healthier babies (for pregnant patients), improved stamina, better smelling breath, and better overall health.

Table 14.7 Common Smoking Cessation Products

Generic (Brand)	Dosage Form	Route of Administration	Common Dose
Bupropion (Wellbutrin, Zyban)	Tablet	Oral	150 mg twice a day
Nicotine (Commit, NicoDerm, Nicorette, Nicotrol)	Gum, inhaler, patch, spray	Buccal, inhalation, transdermal, nasal	Varies, depending on product and patient
Varenicline (Chantix)	Tablet	Oral	1 mg twice a day

Side Effects Side effects of nicotine products include those consistent with excess nicotine. These effects include abdominal pain, confusion, diarrhea, dizziness, headache, hearing loss, hypersalivation, nausea, sweating, vision changes, vomiting, and weakness. Removing or discontinuing the medication will alleviate or eliminate these effects. Inhaled dosage forms can cause mouth irritation, coughing, runny nose, headache, and indigestion. If side effects are bothersome, patients should switch to another dosage form.

Side effects of bupropion include drowsiness, dizziness, blurred vision, and insomnia. To reduce these effects, patients should avoid drinking alcohol while taking this medication and take the dose in the morning.

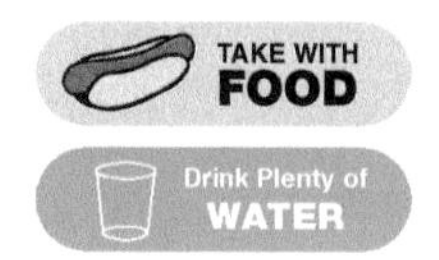

Side effects of varenicline include nausea and unusual dreams. Patients should take varenicline with food and a full glass of water to decrease nausea. In rare cases, patients have experienced serious mental status changes and events.

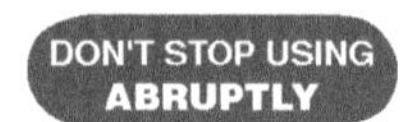

Cautions and Considerations As with starting on any antidepressant therapy, patients using bupropion should talk with their healthcare providers if they notice symptoms of depression or suicidal ideation. The FDA-approved labeling for varenicline and bupropion includes a boxed-in warning that alerts users of serious mental-health events. Patients should be observed for agitation, hostility, depression, and changes in behavior. Patients with suicidal ideation should stop taking varenicline immediately and talk with their healthcare providers. When stopping therapy with bupropion, however, doses must be decreased slowly over time to avoid a rebound of depressive symptoms. Patients should not stop taking bupropion abruptly.

Herbal and Alternative Therapies

Echinacea, zinc, and **vitamin C** are herbal and supplement products that patients often take to boost immune function and fight off cold and flu viruses that can progress to pneumonia. With varying success, these products have been found to reduce the severity and length of symptoms of the common cold or flu. Although some success with these products has been seen, standardized regimens have not been proven in the scientific literature. Little is known about their true clinical effects on lower respiratory tract infections such as pneumonia. If echinacea or zinc is used, it must be started at the first sign of infection to have any significant effects on the severity or length of symptoms. Vitamin C is best taken as a preventive agent during cold and flu season. For further discussion of these agents, see Chapter 3 on anti-infective agents.

Chapter Summary

Respiratory diseases and conditions are common in pharmacy and the healthcare setting. Hospitalizations for asthma, COPD, and pneumonia are common every year. Numerous patients depend on drug therapy to breathe well. Inhaled therapies are delivered via MDIs, dry powder inhalers, and nebulizer machines. Short-acting beta agonists dilate and open airways when immediate relief is needed, whereas inhaled corticosteroids reduce inflammation and improve breathing in asthma over the long term. Even though COPD gets progressively worse, drug therapy can help improve symptoms and quality of life. Unfortunately, too many patients still misunderstand how to use inhalers to better control their condition. Inhalers are not easy to use, and TB agents must be taken for over six months to be successful. Smoking cessation is something most people must attempt multiple times before succeeding. Although many barriers to respiratory therapies exist, pharmacists and technicians can provide a valuable service to patients by educating and supporting them.

Chapter Review

For the following sets of exercises, write the exercise heading, exercise numbers, and your answers on a separate sheet of paper. Your instructor may direct you to turn in the sheet of paper or discuss your answers as a class.

REVIEW THE BASICS

Choose a, b, c, or d as the correct answer to each multiple-choice question.

1. Which of the following is the location for oxygen exchange between air in the lungs and the blood?
   a. alveoli
   b. bronchioles
   c. bronchi
   d. sinus cavity
2. Which of the following is an oral agent used to treat asthma?
   a. varenicline
   b. rifampin
   c. Advair
   d. Singulair
3. Which of the following delivers liquid drug solution via inhaled mist generated by a machine?
   a. MDI
   b. dry powder inhaler
   c. nebulizer
   d. percussion
4. Which of the following drugs does not have bronchodilation effects?
   a. Xopenex
   b. Singulair
   c. Spiriva
   d. Serevent Discus
5. Common side effects of inhaled corticosteroids include which of the following?
   a. nervousness
   b. oral thrush
   c. nausea
   d. unusual dreams
6. Which of the following inhalers should a patient use for quick relief from an asthma attack?
   a. Atrovent
   b. Flovent
   c. Asmanex
   d. Proventil
7. Which of the following medications must be inhaled on a regular basis to have a significant long-term effect on asthma symptoms?
   a. Combivent
   b. Pulmicort
   c. Maxair
   d. montelukast
8. Which of the following TB agents has the advantage of being one of the shortest duration therapies but which can also make patients feel like they have the flu?
   a. isoniazid
   b. rifampin
   c. ethambutol
   d. cycloserine
9. Which of the following manifests effects on the respiratory system but is in fact a genetic disease that affects exocrine glands and their ability to transport chloride across cell membranes?
   a. COPD
   b. pneumonia
   c. TB
   d. CF
10. Which of the following is a smoking cessation agent that contains nicotine and is available OTC?
    a. Commit
    b. Wellbutrin
    c. Zyban
    d. Chantix

KNOW THE DRUGS

Match each brand name drug with its corresponding generic name and most common use. Your answers should follow this example format: Generic Name: 1. a; 2. b; 3. c; etc. Most Common Use: 1. i; 2. j; 3. k; etc.

Brand Name	Generic Name	Most Common Use
1 Singulair	a. pirbuterol	i. asthma
2. Maxair	b. varenicline	j. COPD
3. Advair	c. montelukast	k. TB
4. INH	d. fluticasone/salmeterol	l. smoking cessation
5. Chantix	e. tiotropium	
6. Spiriva	f. albuterol	
7. Proventil	g. isoniazid	
8. Serevent Discus	h. salmeterol	

PUT IT TOGETHER

For each item, write down either a single term to complete the sentence or a short answer.

1. ________________ are used as needed every 4–6 hours, whereas ________________ are used twice a day for bronchodilation effects.
2. Name the three pancreatic enzymes contained in supplements used to treat the GI complications of CF.
3. How long must a patient with TB take drug therapy to eradicate the disease?
4. Most patients with asthma need to use two inhalers: an inhaled corticosteroid (regularly) and a short-acting beta agonist (as needed). Some patients who need both may use only one inhaler that combines these active drugs. Name at least two brand and generic names for these drug products.
5. How many times a day are inhaled corticosteroids typically used? Which one is the exception to this rule? How often is it taken?
6. Name the most prominent (and preventable) risk factor for developing COPD.

THINK IT THROUGH

Read and think through each numbered scenario carefully and then write several sentences in reply to the question(s) presented. Question 4 requires you to do some Internet research before completing your answer(s).

1. Mr. Anderson has asthma and comes to pick up a refill of his albuterol inhaler. You see in his profile that he also uses Flovent. As you check him out at the register, he complains that his voice has been hoarse lately. He sings in the church choir and is getting frustrated with the changes in his voice. He is also using his albuterol more often. What should you do in this situation? What might help Mr. Anderson?

2. A new customer requests Nicoderm patches. As you get them out for him, he says he has heard of prescription pills you can take to help quit smoking. He asks you what they are. What should you do?

3. While working in the inpatient pharmacy, you receive an order for "albuterol nebs" with instructions that say "use 1–2 puffs 4 times a day as needed." What is wrong with this order and what should you do?

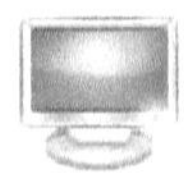

4. **On the Internet**, look up some reputable sources of patient information on asthma control and drug treatment. Many patients with asthma are children. See what resources you can find for parents of children with asthma as well as patient education materials aimed at children. Parents of children with asthma often need information and support in working with their children's schools to ensure that proper medication administration is provided. Print some information pieces that would be useful to keep in the pharmacy for parents of patients with asthma. Where did you find good patient information about the special issues that children with asthma might encounter?

unit 6

Drugs for the Digestive and Endocrine Systems

Chapter 15 The Gastrointestinal System and Drug Therapy

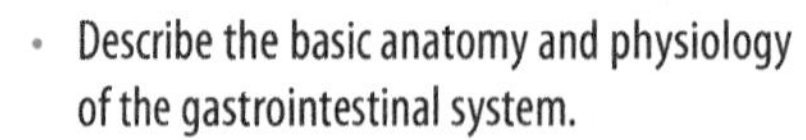

LEARNING OBJECTIVES

- Describe the basic anatomy and physiology of the gastrointestinal system.
- Explain the therapeutic effects of prescription medications, nonprescription medications, and alternative therapies commonly used to treat common problems of the gastrointestinal system.
- Describe the adverse effects of prescription medications, nonprescription medications, and alternative therapies commonly used to treat common problems of the gastrointestinal system.
- Identify the brand and generic names of prescription and nonprescription medications commonly used to treat common problems of the gastrointestinal system.
- State the doses, dosage forms, and routes of administration for prescription and nonprescription medications commonly used to treat common problems of the gastrointestinal system.

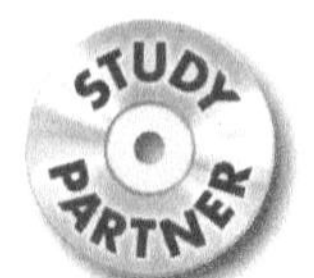

Interactive self-quizzes, games, audio files, and glossaries help you to learn drug names and facts.

Nausea, vomiting, diarrhea, constipation, and heartburn are common gastrointestinal (GI) complaints that everyone deals with at some time in life. Every day, patients visit pharmacies, clinics, and hospitals for GI problems. No matter the practice setting, young and old alike are frequently the victims of GI diseases. In fact, parents of sick children are a major group of customers looking for GI medications in the pharmacy. Acute problems in this system are treated in an institutional setting every day. Pharmacy technicians, regardless of work setting, play a central role in dispensing GI medications and are team members that help patients with GI problems.

This chapter describes the GI system and the most common prescription medications, nonprescription medications, and alternative therapies used to treat the most common problems affecting the GI system. Treatment of diarrhea, constipation, gastroesophageal reflux disease, peptic ulcer disease, and nausea and vomiting are discussed. Both over-the-counter (OTC) and prescription medications are used to treat these conditions. Herbal and alternative products such as probiotics, a growing segment of the nutraceutical market, are explained as well.

Anatomy and Physiology of the Gastrointestinal System

The **GI system** is where the body processes food and liquids. This includes **digestion** (breakdown of large food molecules to smaller ones) and **absorption** (uptake of essential nutrients into the bloodstream). The GI system is composed of the **GI** or **alimentary tract** and a number of supportive organs. The alimentary tract includes the **mouth**, **esophagus**, **stomach**, **intestines**, **colon**, and **rectum** (see Figure 15.1).

When food is swallowed, smooth muscle along the walls of the esophagus propels it into the stomach and then through the small and large intestines. This process of coordinated muscle contraction, called **peristalsis**, keeps food particles moving through the **GI tract**. Moving food through the intestines is also referred to as **GI motility**. The parasympathetic nervous system controls GI motility (see Chapter 7). Increased GI motility can result in **diarrhea**, whereas decreased GI motility can result in **constipation**.

Once food reaches the stomach, acid and enzyme secretions digest large particles and proteins in ingested food. **Gastrin**, a hormone that stimulates acid secretion, is released when the walls of the stomach stretch in response to food. **Parietal cells**,

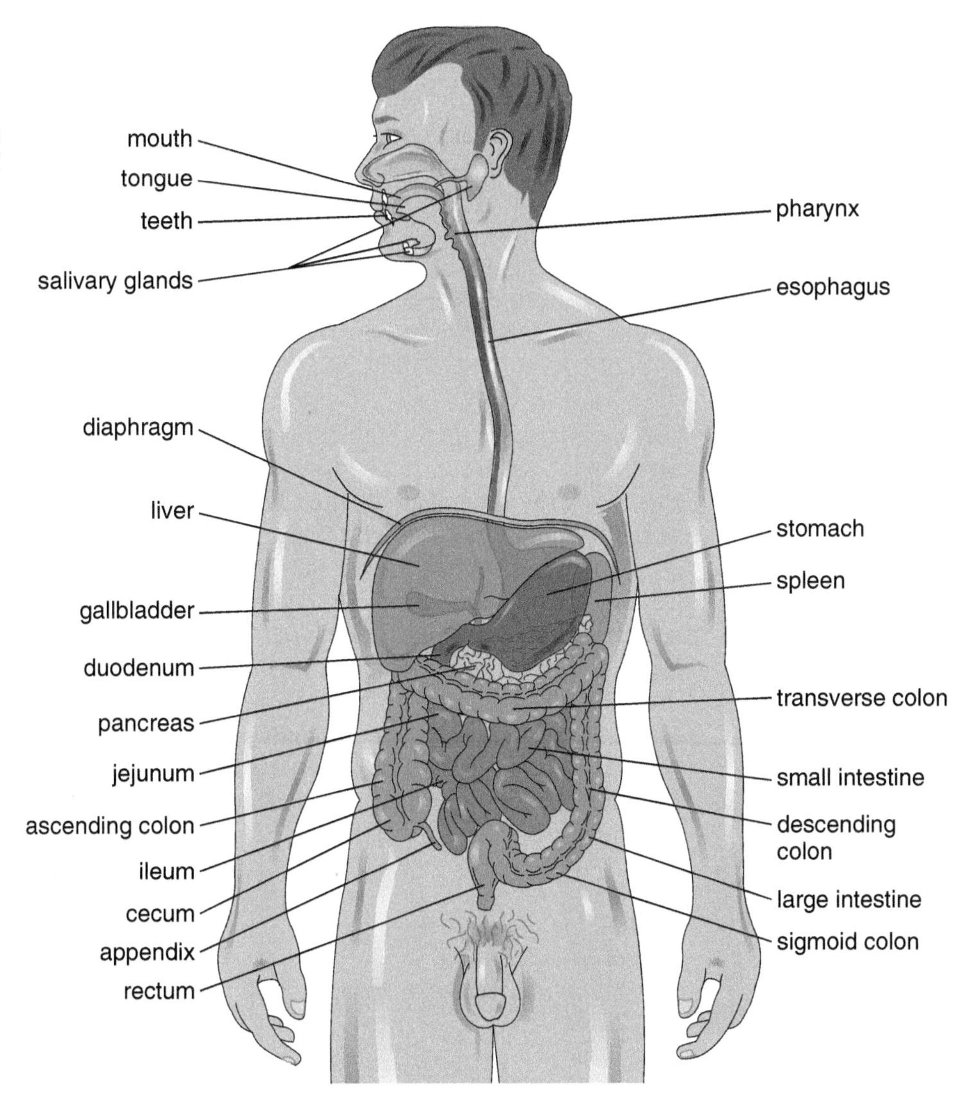

Figure 15.1
Diagram of GI Tract
The mouth, esophagus, and stomach are part of the upper GI system, and the intestines, colon, and rectum are part of the lower GI system.

which line the walls of the stomach, are responsible for producing acid from specialized structures known as **proton pumps**. Gastrin stimulates **histamine** release, which increases the number of active proton pumps.

Acidity in the GI system is measured by **pH**, a scale that indicates the amount of acid present. Normally, the pH of the stomach is approximately 1 to 2 (very acidic). Most tissues of the body would not tolerate these acidic conditions, but cells lining the stomach walls are protected by a layer of mucus. In addition to helping digest food particles, the low pH of the stomach is protective because it kills a majority of the bacteria that are ingested. Furthermore, low pH is critical for absorption of certain drugs that dissociate poorly in a neutral or basic environment.

When food particles leave the stomach, they enter the **small intestine**. This is where most digestion and nutrient absorption takes place. The small intestine has an enormous surface area, which allows for maximal nutrient absorption. A large percentage of drugs administered orally are absorbed in the small intestine.

Remaining food particles proceed to the **large intestine**. The large intestine, also known as the colon, has four distinct segments: **ascending, transverse, descending,** and **sigmoid colon**. Normally, the GI tract is very efficient, absorbing all carbohydrates, fats, and proteins that are consumed. Only nonabsorbable substances, such as fiber and bacteria, remain as waste material. This waste material, or **stool**, exits the body through the rectum and **anus** via **bowel movement** or **defecation**. Because proteins, fats, and carbohydrates have already been absorbed into the bloodstream through the small intestine, the large intestine absorbs additional salt and water, bringing the stool to the proper consistency for elimination.

Other components of the GI system include the **salivary glands, gallbladder, pancreas,** and **liver**. These organs release secretions that aid in digestion of food and absorption of nutrients. **Saliva** provides lubrication for food, making swallowing easier, and contains enzymes that begin the process of digesting sugars. The gallbladder is a holding area where **bile** is stored until it is required. Bile is produced by the liver and facilitates absorption of fat and cholesterol from the small intestine. The pancreas produces many enzymes that help digest carbohydrates, protein, and fats (see Figure 15.2). The pancreas is also important because it releases secretions that neutralize the acid from the stomach.

In addition to making bile, the liver is the major organ for **drug metabolism**. After being absorbed from the small intestine, molecules travel in the blood via the **portal vein** directly to the liver. The liver removes and metabolizes harmful substances before they reach the general circulation. Before orally administered drugs enter the circulation, they must pass through the liver. The liver metabolizes drugs before they reach their target in the body; this is called the **first-pass effect** (see Figure 15.3).

To regulate the speed at which food particles move through the GI tract, the body uses **sphincters**. These sphincters, muscle rings wrapped around the GI tract, are important because they prevent food and other digested substances from moving in the wrong direction. For example, a very important sphincter called the **lower esophageal sphincter** is located between the esophagus and stomach. This sphincter relaxes to let chewed-up food pass into the stomach, then closes to prevent the acidic contents of the stomach from traveling back up into the esophagus. Without the lower esophageal sphincter, acid travels up into the esophagus, causing pain and tissue damage.

Figure 15.2
Pancreas
Without neutralization by pancreatic secretions, acid from the stomach would damage the small intestine.

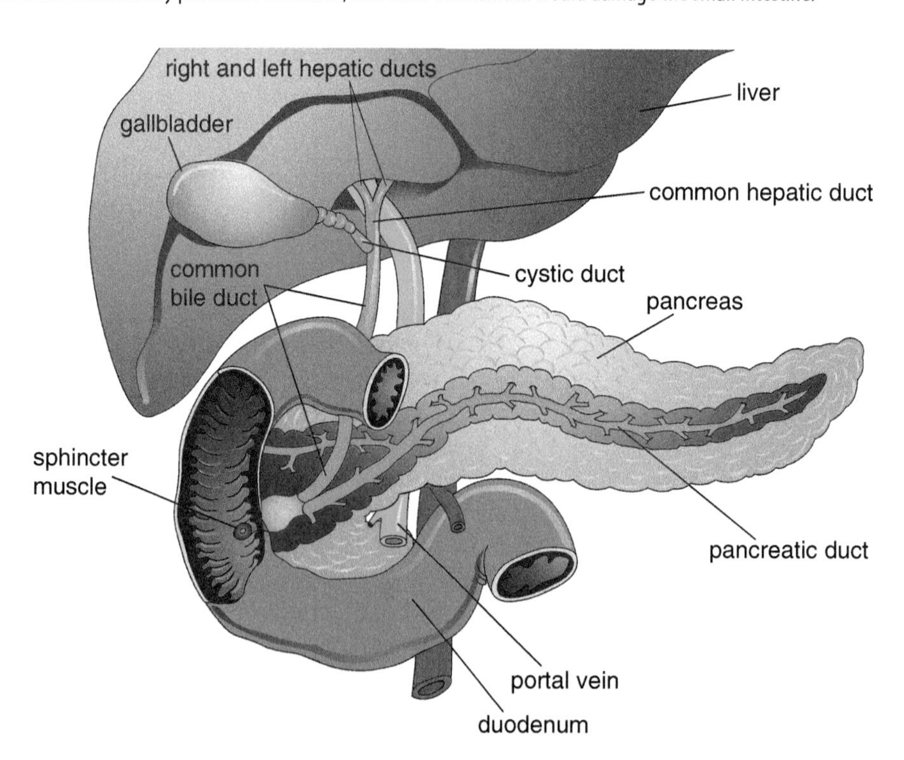

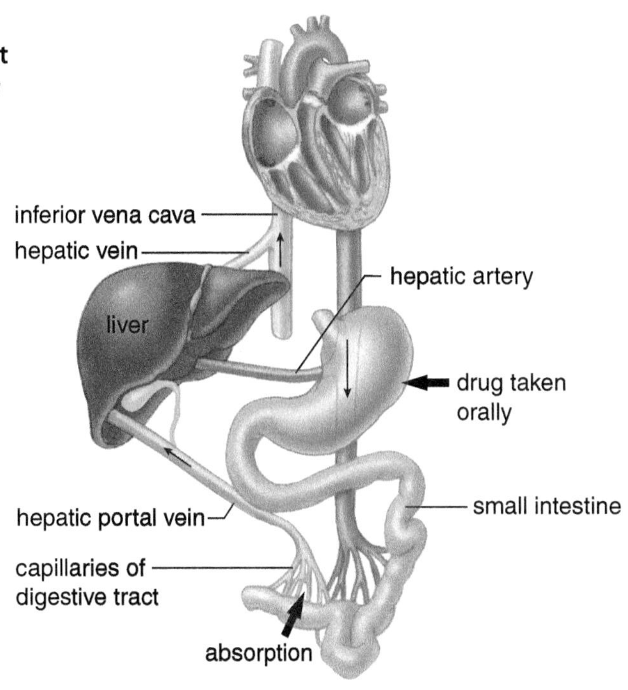

Figure 15.3
Liver Function and First-Pass Effect
Alternatives to oral administration are necessary for drugs that will lose their efficacy if they undergo the first-pass effect.

Diarrhea

Diarrhea is defined as excessive, soft, or watery stools. Excessive stool can mean large stool volume or larger number of bowel movements than normal. In diarrhea, increased GI motility leads to frequent bowel movements. Acute diarrhea is a common condition that can be caused by infections such as **traveler's diarrhea**, **food poisoning,** as well as drugs (see Table 15.1). Infectious causes of diarrhea include bacterial infections such as **salmonella** and ***Escherichia coli (E. coli)***, protozoal infections such as giardia or viral infections such as **Norwalk** and **rotavirus**. Drugs used to treat infections are covered in Chapter 3. Chronic diarrhea is less common and can be caused by irritable bowel syndrome, ulcerative colitis, or Crohn's disease.

Table 15.1 Drugs that Can Cause Diarrhea

Angiotensin-converting enzyme inhibitors	Magnesium-containing laxatives or antacids
Antibiotics	Nonsteroidal anti-inflammatory drugs
Digoxin	Proton pump inhibitors
H_2 receptor antagonists	

Drugs for Diarrhea

Professional Focus
Familiarize yourself with hydration products such as Pedialyte (in liquid and frozen ice pop forms) available in your pharmacy, so you can easily refer patients to them when needed. Hydration is key to treating diarrhea.

Antidiarrheal medications slow the transit of food through the GI tract or decrease secretions into it, which reduces stool volume and makes stool less watery. Diarrhea is a symptom of a disease, not a disease itself. Therefore, antidiarrheal medications do not treat the underlying cause of the diarrhea, but only help reduce diarrhea symptoms. Some types of diarrhea are caused by an infection. If this is the case, the patient may receive an antibiotic in addition to an antidiarrheal medication. Antibiotics used to treat infectious diarrhea are discussed in Chapter 3. Patients with diarrhea lose a large amount of water, so fluid or electrolyte replacement may be needed along with antidiarrheal medications (see Chapter 20). Technicians should refer patients with severe diarrhea to the pharmacist for proper assessment.

Opiate Derivatives Acute diarrhea can be treated on a short-term basis with medications derived from opiates. These medications are similar to narcotic analgesics in that they too are derivatives of opium (see Chapter 9). Unlike the powerful pain medicines, however, these **opiate derivatives** are poorly absorbed and do not reach the brain in high concentrations. Instead of affecting the central nervous system, they work by inhibiting peristalsis and slowing the progression of food through the GI tract. They also reduce the liquid content of stool. They are taken only when needed for short-term relief of diarrhea. **Loperamide** is available over the counter, and **diphenoxylate** with atropine is a controlled substance (Schedule V). Table 15.2 lists opiate derivatives and other commonly used antidiarrheal drugs.

Although these agents can potentially be used in children, they are usually avoided in that population. Patients seeking an opiate derivative for an infant or a young child (a child less than two years old) should first talk with the pharmacists or their healthcare providers. These medications take about six to eight hours to work.

Side Effects Loperamide can cause dizziness and constipation, even when used correctly. Diphenoxylate has very few side effects, but some patients may experience dizziness and drowsiness. However, blurred vision, dry mouth, and difficulty urinating are potential side effects of atropine. Patients can minimize these effects by not exceeding the recommended daily dose. If high doses are taken, respiratory depression is possible. Children are more likely to experience adverse events than adults.

Cautions and Considerations Loperamide is available over the counter, whereas diphenoxylate is scheduled (C-V) due to potential for abuse. Unlike loperamide, diphenoxylate can enter the brain and cause euphoria. Atropine is added to diphenoxylate to discourage misuse, because it has undesirable side effects including blurred vision, urinary retention, and dry mouth. Still, pharmacies must follow state laws regarding controlled substance dispensing. In some states, special restrictions apply to the purchase of these products, and all sales are documented in a logbook.

Opiate derivatives are not appropriate for all types of diarrhea. If fever or bloody stool is present, the patient should consult a doctor. Additionally, if diarrhea continues for forty-eight hours after use of an opiate derivative, the patient needs further evaluation by a medical professional.

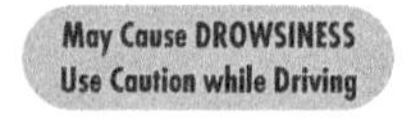

Because opiate derivatives may cause dizziness and drowsiness, patients should be reminded that activities such as driving may not be safe while taking these medications. Caution patients to take careful note of the effects of these medicines before attempting such activities. Technicians should place an auxiliary label on these prescriptions reminding them of this effect.

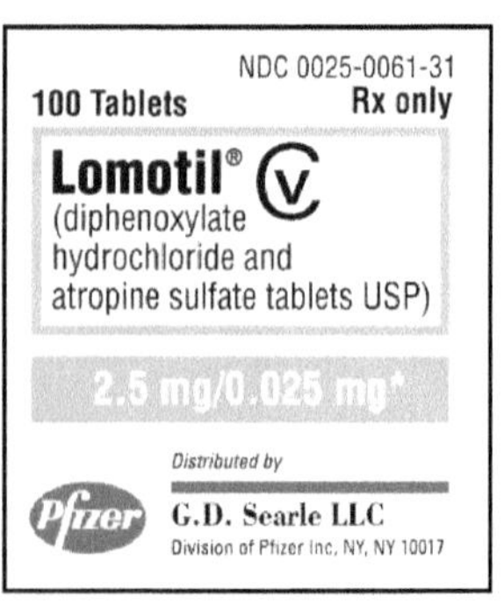

Lomotil should be stored behind the counter, because it is a controlled substance.

Bismuth Subsalicylate Acute diarrhea can be treated with **bismuth subsalicylate**. It works by an antisecretory action, making stools less watery. Bismuth subsalicylate also has anti-inflammatory and antibacterial effects, making it beneficial in treating ***Helicobacter pylori (H. pylori)*** infection and traveler's diarrhea. This product may be used in small children, but specialized doses may be required. It takes approximately twenty-four hours to work and is available over the counter.

Table 15.2 Commonly Used Antidiarrheal Drugs

Generic (Brand)	Dosage Form	Route of Administration	Common Dose
Opiate Derivatives			
Diphenoxylate and atropine (Lomotil)	Tablet, solution	Oral	5 mg four times a day (max 20 mg/day)
Loperamide (Imodium)	Tablet, capsule, solution	Oral	4 mg, then 2 mg after each loose stool (max 16 mg/day)
Bismuth Subsalicylate			
Bismuth subsalicylate (Pepto-Bismol, Kaopectate)	Chewable tablet, oral suspension	Oral	534 mg every 0.5–1 hour. Maximum 8 doses daily (4,192 mg)

Side Effects Bismuth subsalicylate may cause constipation, nausea, vomiting, and darkening of tongue and/or stools. Taking bismuth subsalicylate with food and plenty of water may relieve nausea symptoms. Although rare, neurotoxic symptoms such as tinnitus (ringing in the ears), confusion, and weakness are also potential side effects. To avoid these more serious side effects, patients should not take excessive doses of bismuth subsalicylate.

Cautions and Considerations Patients with aspirin hypersensitivity should avoid products containing bismuth subsalicylate because such products may trigger an allergic-like reaction.

Patients should be warned that their tongue and stools may darken while taking this medication. These changes are harmless and temporary.

You should inform patients to stop taking bismuth subsalicylate if they experience confusion, dizziness, or vision changes. Additionally, patients should consult their pharmacists or physicians and report these problems.

Bismuth subsalicylate may decrease the effectiveness of tetracycline antibiotics, so patients should not take them simultaneously. Additionally, these products may enhance the anticoagulant effects of warfarin, increasing a patient's risk of bleeding. Patients should tell their physicians or pharmacists about all prescription and nonprescription products they are taking to avoid or limit these potential drug interactions. Patients with renal failure or gout should consult their physicians before using bismuth subsalicylate.

Patients should consult their pharmacists or physicians before giving this product to children. Children and adolescents are at risk of a condition known as Reye's syndrome, a potentially life-threatening disorder caused by salicylate use for viral infections.

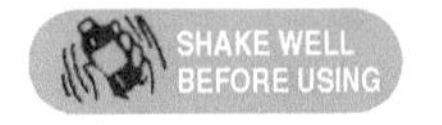

Oral suspensions must be shaken well before ingestion to ensure adequate mixing and proper dosing.

Constipation

Constipation is the opposite of diarrhea. It is characterized by infrequent bowel movements, small stool size, hard stools, or the feeling of incomplete bowel evacuation. Most people pass at least three stools a week, so fewer stools could constitute constipation. However, diagnosis depends on the individual patient. Many episodes of constipation are related to a diet low in fiber or fluid intake. Constipation can also be caused by certain foods or drugs (see Table 15.3). Although many drugs have the potential to cause diarrhea or constipation, the ones most associated with constipation include pain medicines such as opiates and antacids. Stress may also exacerbate constipation, whereas light exercise promotes GI motility.

Drugs for Constipation

Dietary modification and lifestyle changes should accompany pharmacologic treatment of constipation. Adequate dietary intake of fiber (including fruits, vegetables, and cereals) and regular exercise (even light walking) regulates GI motility. Patients with repeat bouts of constipation should drink plenty of fluids, eat adequate fiber, and exercise regularly.

Drugs that relieve constipation are known as **laxatives**. Typically, laxatives are used only as needed on a short-term basis. Electrolyte abnormalities may occur if laxatives

Table 15.3 Drugs that Can Cause Constipation

Antiemetics	Iron
Antihistamines	Nonsteroidal anti-inflammatory drugs
Calcium- and aluminum-containing laxatives or antacids	Opiates (morphine, hydrocodone, oxycodone, etc.)
Calcium-channel blockers	Tricyclic antidepressants
Diuretics	

are used too frequently. If patients are using laxatives on a regular basis, they should consult their physicians for a full evaluation.

In addition to oral dosage forms, many laxatives are available as **suppositories** or **enemas**. These dosage forms are used for rapid treatment of moderate to serious constipation. Rectal suppositories take fifteen to sixty minutes to work. They are useful for hospitalized patients who are unable to swallow. Before inserting a rectal suppository, the patient can squat or lie on his or her side with one leg straight and the other bent. The patient should remove the wrapping from the suppository and insert the pointed end first (see Figure 15.4). It needs to be inserted far enough into the rectum so that it does not slip out. Afterward, the patient should wash his or her hands.

An enema is a liquid solution that is delivered directly into the rectum. Enemas are used to rapidly clear out the bowels prior to surgery or diagnostic procedures such as a colonoscopy or barium enema. They also can remove excessive fecal matter that is blocking the GI tract. To use an enema, the patient should lie down. The enema tip is inserted into the rectum, and the liquid is allowed to drain into the rectum via gravity or by squeezing the bottle. The patient should hold the enema liquid in the rectum for a period of time (two to sixty minutes, depending on the product) and then defecate normally.

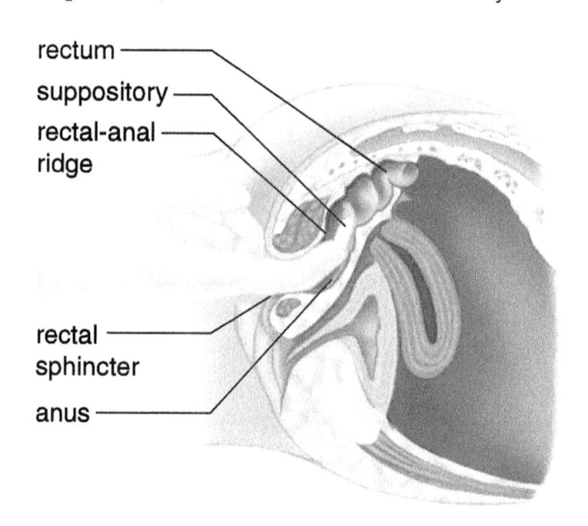

Figure 15.4
Suppository Insertion
Surprisingly, some patients may not understand that you must remove the foil wrapping before inserting a suppository.

Bulk-Forming Laxatives Mild constipation can be treated with **bulk-forming laxatives**. As with dietary fiber, bulk-forming agents are poorly absorbed and remain in the GI tract, drawing water and other electrolytes into the GI system. Increased volume in the GI tract triggers peristalsis and facilitates bowel movements. In general, these agents take between one and three days to work. Bulk-forming laxatives work best for preventing constipation rather than as acute treatment. Patients with repeated problems with constipation may consider using a bulk-forming laxative on a daily basis to remain regular. Bulk-forming laxatives may also have beneficial effects in patients who have diabetes or high cholesterol, because they absorb fat and reduce glucose. Bulk-forming laxatives are available over the counter. Table 15.4 contains information on commonly use laxatives.

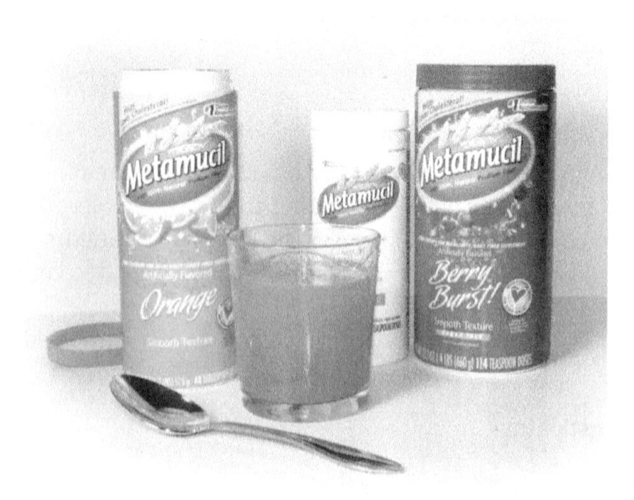

Patients dissolve powder dosage forms of bulk-forming laxatives in water or juice and then drink the solution.

Cautions and Considerations Although rare, obstruction of the esophagus or bowels is possible with bulk-forming laxatives. To avoid obstruction, patients should take bulk-forming laxatives with a full glass of liquid (at least eight ounces). Patients with intestinal stenosis should not take bulk-forming laxatives.

Table 15.4 Commonly Used Laxatives

Generic (Brand)	Dosage Form	Route of Administration	Common Dose
Bulk-Forming Laxatives			
Methylcellulose (Citrucel, Unifiber, Maltsupex)	Tablet, powder	Oral	See individual product, used 3–4 times a day
Polycarbophil (Equalactin, Konsyl Fiber, Fiber-Lax, FiberCon)	Chewable tablet, tablet	Oral	2 tablets 1–4 times a day
Psyllium (many brand names, including Metamucil, Fiberall, Genfiber, and Konsyl)	Capsule, powder to mix and form solution, wafer	Oral	Varies with product
Wheat dextrin (Benefiber)	Chewable tablet, caplet, powder	Oral	3.5 g three times a day
Stool Softeners			
Docusate sodium, calcium, and potassium (many brands, including Colace)	Capsule, solution, syrup, tablet, enema	Oral, rectal	50–500 mg a day divided between 1–4 doses
Stimulants			
Bisacodyl (many brands)	Tablet, solution, suppository, enema	Oral, rectal	Adult: 5–15 mg once a day or one 10 mg suppository Pediatric: 5–10 mg once a day orally or rectally
Senna (many brands, including Ex-Lax, Fletcher's)	Tablet, chewable tablet, solution, syrup	Oral	Adult: 15 mg once a day Pediatric: 3.75–8.6 mg daily; 5–30 mL liquid 1–2 times a day

Because they increase GI motility, bulk-forming laxatives can affect drug absorption. The small intestine is an important site of absorption for orally taken drugs. Decreasing GI transit time can decrease drug absorption. Patients should separate doses of bulk-forming laxatives from other medications by at least two hours to ensure that other drugs are absorbed properly.

Stool Softeners For patients who are at risk of becoming constipated, **emollient laxatives** (another term for **stool softeners**) are used. They are not as effective for treatment of acute constipation as they are for helping reduce or prevent constipation when it is likely to occur. Stool softeners are typically taken on a regular, daily basis. They work by increasing water and electrolyte secretions in the GI tract, which makes stool softer and easier to pass.

Side Effects Although well tolerated, side effects of stool softeners can include throat irritation, abdominal pain, diarrhea, and intestinal obstruction. Drinking plenty of fluids on a daily basis can reduce these effects.

Cautions and Considerations The syrup dosage form has a bitter taste. Taking these products with eight ounces of milk or juice can mask the bad taste. Drinking plenty of fluids while taking stool softeners enhances their effect. As with many laxatives, excessive or long-term use may lead to electrolyte imbalance. Patients should inform their physicians if constipation or abdominal pain occurs while taking a stool softener.

Stimulant Laxatives Acute constipation can be treated with **stimulant laxatives**. They work by stimulating parasympathetic neurons that control bowel muscles, enhancing peristalsis and GI motility. To avoid electrolyte imbalances, they are taken only when needed on a short-term basis. Stimulant laxatives are commonly used to treat opiate-induced constipation.

Side Effects Common side effects of stimulant laxatives include mild abdominal pain, nausea, vomiting, and rectal burning. Patients should take these agents at bedtime to avoid side effects. Serious electrolyte abnormalities are very rare but can occur with chronic use. For this reason, long-term use is not recommended.

Cautions and Considerations Patients should take bisacodyl with a full glass of water on an empty stomach to achieve the best effect. Dairy products and antacids can decrease the effects of bisacodyl, so patients should not ingest these substances simultaneously. Senna should not be taken if a patient has intestinal obstruction, Crohn's disease, or abdominal pain, or is pregnant.

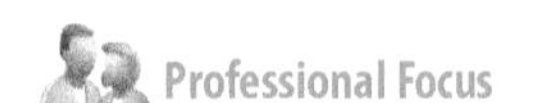

Professional Focus

Bowel prep solutions do not taste good, but patients must drink a large volume relatively quickly. Tell patients that refrigerating bowel prep solution prior to drinking it can reduce the bad taste and may make it easier to drink quickly.

Bowel Prep (Osmotic) Laxatives

Evacuating the bowels prior to surgery or a diagnostic procedure requires quick-acting, powerful laxatives. Bowel evacuation may also be necessary for clearing poisons or parasitic worms from the GI tract and for treating bowel impaction from severe constipation. **Bowel prep laxatives** work by drawing water and electrolytes into the GI tract. They prepare the bowel for examination by completely cleaning it out.

Magnesium citrate and sodium phosphate are available over the counter in oral and rectal dosage forms. Polyethylene glycol is available over the counter (MiraLAX) and by prescription (GlycoLax) as a powder for a solution that you drink. MiraLAX can be used for occasional constipation, whereas GlycoLax is usually used the day before a bowel procedure. These agents take only a few hours to work if taken orally, or less than an hour if used rectally. Therefore, patients should use these products at home where a toilet is readily accessible.

Side Effects Common side effects of bowel prep laxatives include abdominal pain, diarrhea, and electrolyte loss or imbalance. Polyethylene glycol electrolyte solution has higher rates of side effects than other fast-acting laxatives and can also cause anal irritation, bloating, and nausea and vomiting. Although bothersome, these effects are brief and improve within a few hours of using the product.

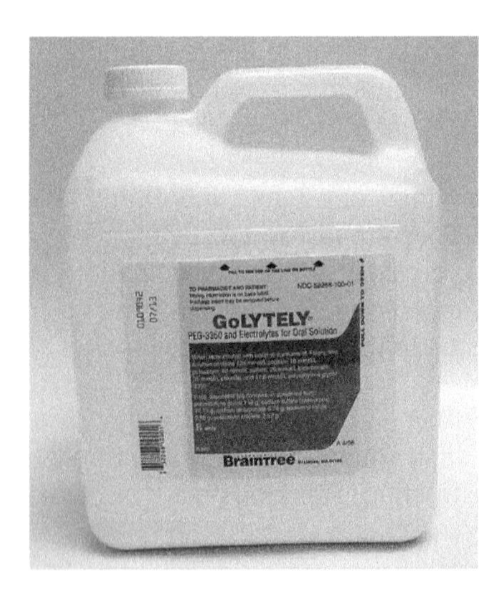

Patients who are taking bowel prep laxatives should fill the four-liter container with water and drink an eight-ounce glass of the laxative solution every ten minutes until the entire container is empty.

Cautions and Considerations Products containing magnesium or sodium should be used with caution in patients with congestive heart failure due to potential accumulation of these ions. Use with caution in patients with kidney problems and children less than two years old. To avoid significant electrolyte loss, these laxatives should only be used occasionally. If a patient is using one of these products on a regular basis, he or she should consult a physician for a full evaluation.

Miscellaneous Laxatives

A few other laxative agents bear mentioning because you will see them used in select cases. **Milk of magnesia** is used frequently over the counter and in the long-term care setting for mild constipation. It is available as a liquid and as chewable tablets. **Glycerin suppositories** are used in children with occasional constipation. **Lactulose** is an oral solution used for patients with ammonia toxicity and delirium in end-stage liver failure. It pulls ammonia from the bloodstream into the GI

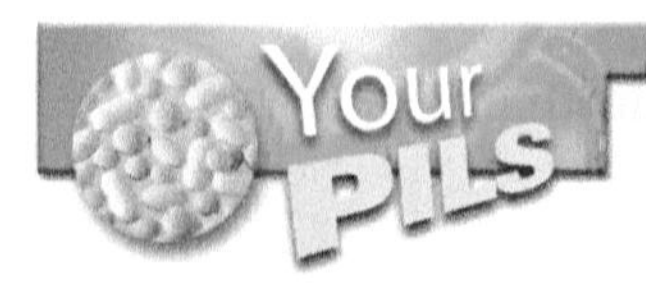

Learners who like fieldwork and live laboratory exercises, like Enactors and Directors, may find a trip to the pharmacy useful. Check out the laxatives available over the counter. Can you find the OTC bowel prep products? What brand names of bisacodyl and senna can you find? Seeing these products in person may help you remember them and recall where to find them when patients inquire.

tract and stimulates diarrhea to quickly eliminate it. Technicians working in the inpatient setting are more likely to handle lactulose, because patients with delirium and end-stage liver disease are commonly hospitalized.

Heartburn and Ulcers

Gastroesophageal reflux disease (GERD), the medical term for **heartburn,** is a common complaint for which patients seek medication. It is estimated that 10% of people in the United States get heartburn every week. Heartburn is characterized by a burning or sensation of warmth starting in the gut or chest that may radiate to the neck. In GERD, the lower esophageal sphincter allows stomach contents to move up into the esophagus, where acidic juices cause tissue damage and pain. GERD is most likely caused by a faulty lower esophageal sphincter that does not close properly (see Figure 15.5). Spicy or fatty foods, caffeine, smoking, and drinking alcohol decrease the closing pressure of this lower esophageal sphincter (see Table 15.5). Large meals and obesity increase pressure in the stomach and force its contents up to the esophagus. Weight loss, elevating the head of the bed at night, not eating before bedtime, remaining upright after a meal, reducing meal size, and decreasing alcohol and tobacco use can relieve GERD symptoms.

GERD not only produces bothersome symptoms for patients, but also, over time, causes permanent changes in the tissue lining of the esophagus. When chronically exposed to acid, the cells of the esophageal lining change. These changes have been linked to narrowing of the esophagus (esophageal stricture) and esophageal cancer, so repeated bouts of GERD indicate a condition the patient should not ignore. Long-term treatment involves reducing the acidity of the stomach contents to limit damage to the esophagus.

Ulcers occur when the protective lining of the GI tract is worn away and bleeding occurs. Ulcers are sores or patches of dead tissue along the walls of the GI tract. A bacterial parasite, *H. pylori*, is the most common culprit that causes **peptic ulcer**

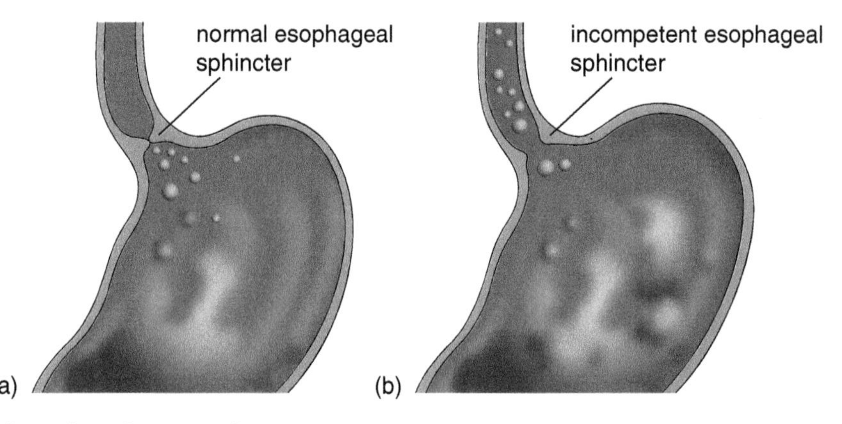

Figure 15.5
Lower Esophageal Sphincter Function
GERD is common during pregnancy, because as the growing fetus requires more room, the uterus expands and pushes upward on the stomach.

Table 15.5 Foods and Medications that May Worsen GERD

Foods	Medications
Chocolate	Alcohol
Coffee or soda	Alendronate
Fatty foods	Anticholinergics
Garlic	Aspirin
Onions	Barbiturates
Orange juice	Caffeine
Peppermint and spearmint	Dopamine
Spicy foods	Iron
	Nicotine (from smoking)
	Nitrates
	Nonsteroidal anti-inflammatory drugs
	Tetracycline

disease (PUD), or ulcers in the stomach. *H. pylori* is a spiral-shaped, gram-negative organism that attaches to the lining of the stomach. It releases toxic chemicals that damage the stomach lining, leading to ulcer formation. Additionally, *H. pylori* elicits an immune response whereby activated immune cells damage neighboring cells in the stomach and small intestine in the process of killing bacteria. **Duodenal ulcers** occur in the portion of the small intestine just below the stomach. These ulcers are caused by hyperacidity, not usually by *H. pylori*.

Stress ulcers occur in critically ill patients who are bedridden. The exact mechanism by which they form is not well understood, but it is thought that serious illness, stress, and trauma lead to a decrease in the protective mucous layer of the stomach and an increase in acid secretion in the stomach. Patients in intensive care settings are routinely given medicines that reduce stomach acid to prevent stress ulcers.

Nonsteroidal anti-inflammatory drugs (NSAIDs) (e.g., ibuprofen) and **aspirin** can cause ulcers. These acidic drugs irritate and erode GI tissue. More important, they inhibit production of prostaglandins. Prostaglandins produce inflammation and pain throughout most of the body, but in the stomach they protect the lining from acid secretion. Prolonged use of aspirin or NSAIDs removes the protective effects of prostaglandins in the stomach and can result in GI ulceration. When ulceration erodes into a blood vessel, a **GI bleed** can occur. GI bleeds may be asymptomatic for many patients and are particularly dangerous for elderly patients or those who are critically ill. Patients on long-term NSAID, aspirin, and anticoagulation therapy are at high risk for ulcers and life-threatening bleeding.

Drugs for GERD and PUD

Although the underlying problems of GERD and GI ulcers relate to damage in the GI tract from stomach acid, most treatments for these conditions do not directly fix this problem. **Antacids, proton pump inhibitors (PPIs),** and **H_2 blockers** relieve symptoms of GERD by decreasing acid production in the stomach. This means that stomach contents may still regurgitate into the esophagus or reach an ulcer in the stomach or intestines, but less damage will occur because the stomach juices are less acidic.

Antacids

Mild to moderate GERD can be treated with antacids. Antacids contain special ions that react with hydrogen ions in the stomach and neutralize acid. They only work for a few hours, so it may be necessary to take these medications after every meal. Antacids are available over the counter. See Table 15.6 for information on antacids.

Side Effects Common side effects of antacids include constipation, diarrhea, stomach pain, nausea, and vomiting. These effects are generally mild. Calcium- and aluminum-containing antacids tend to cause constipation, whereas magnesium-containing antacids tend to cause diarrhea.

Cautions and Considerations Antacids provide short-term relief for patients with heartburn. Patients requiring repeated or constant use of antacids should see their prescribers and discuss other treatment options. Continuous use of calcium-containing

Table 15.6 Commonly Used Antacids

Generic (Brand)	Dosage Form	Route of Administration	Common Dose
Aluminum hydroxide (ALternaGEL, Gaviscon)	Chewable tablet, liquid	Oral	Doses vary depending on product, dosage form, and indication for use. Refer to product packaging for proper dosing instructions.
Aluminum hydroxide with magnesium hydroxide (Maalox, Mylanta)	Liquid	Oral	
Calcium carbonate (Tums, Maalox)	Chewable tablet	Oral	
Calcium carbonate with magnesium hydroxide (Mylanta, Rolaids)	Gelcap, liquid, tablet	Oral	

antacids can cause acid hypersecretion, particularly when the medicine is discontinued, so long-term use of calcium products should be discouraged.

Antacids bind to several other oral drugs, decreasing their absorption. Antibiotics such as tetracyclines, quinolones, and isoniazid should not be given at the same time as antacids for this reason. Other interacting medications include iron supplements containing ferrous sulfate and the sulfonylureas (treatment for diabetes). Antacids should be taken more than two hours before or after the other medication.

Antacids must be used with caution in patients with renal failure because aluminum and magnesium can accumulate in the blood. Patients should let the pharmacy know if they have kidney failure, and you should enter this information into the patient profile.

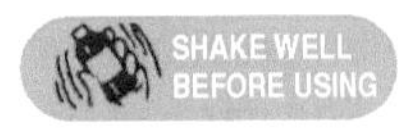

Antacid suspensions need to be shaken well before use to ensure adequate mixing of contents and proper dosing.

Proton Pump Inhibitors (PPIs) GERD, PUD, and *H. pylori* infection can all be treated with PPIs, which work by binding to proton pumps in the stomach lining, rendering them inactive. When fewer proton pumps are functioning in the stomach, less acid is produced. PPIs are long-acting agents, with effects lasting approximately twenty-four hours. Patients with chronic GERD problems take PPIs on a daily basis to continually suppress stomach acid production. Because PPIs are most effective when taken on an empty stomach, patients should take them one hour before the first meal of the day. Omeprazole and lansoprazole are available over the counter, whereas other PPIs are only available by prescription.

Infants can have GERD in the first weeks or months of life and are prescribed liquid forms of PPIs. The pharmacy specially compounds these products. Pharmacy technicians should pay particular attention to appropriate concentrations and doses to avoid harmful medication errors when compounding pediatric products.

Some PPI medications are available for intravenous (IV) use, and these may be given to patients who are critically ill in the hospital and at risk for stress ulcers.

Patients with gastric tubes are also prescribed PPIs. Although medications are often crushed and given through the gastric tube into the stomach, many PPI products are delayed-release or produced as capsules that cannot be crushed. You should alert the pharmacist about any orders for PPIs in patients with a gastric tube. Liquid dosage forms can be given via gastric tube, but tablet and capsule forms cannot. Table 15.7 has more information on common PPIs.

Side Effects PPIs are very well tolerated. Rarely, patients may experience headache, nausea, vomiting, and diarrhea. If these side effects become bothersome, patients should consult their physicians. PPIs have been associated with increased risk for developing certain infections, such as respiratory tract infections. The significance of this association is not clear.

Table 15.7 Commonly Used PPIs

Generic (Brand)	Dosage Form	Route of Administration	Common Dose	Dispensing Status
Esomeprazole (Nexium)	Capsule, granules, powder for reconstitution, tablet	Oral, IV	Adult: 20–40 mg once a day Pediatric: 10–20 mg once a day	Rx only
Lansoprazole (Prevacid)	Capsule, tablet, powder for suspension	Oral, IV	Adult: 15–30 mg once a day Pediatric: 15–30 mg once a day	OTC and Rx
Omeprazole (Prilosec)	Capsule, tablet	Oral	Adult: 20–40 mg once a day Pediatric: 5–20 mg once a day	OTC and Rx
Pantoprazole (Protonix)	Powder for reconstitution, tablet, granules for suspension	Oral, IV	Adult: 40 mg once a day (oral) Pediatric (≥ 5 years old): 20–40 mg once a day	Rx only
Rabeprazole (AcipHex)	Tablet	Oral	Adult: 20 mg once a day	Rx only

Cautions and Considerations It is important that patients know that delayed-release capsules or tablets cannot be crushed or chewed. Lansoprazole is available as orally disintegrating tablets that are placed on the tongue and allowed to dissolve. The dissolved particles must be swallowed without chewing.

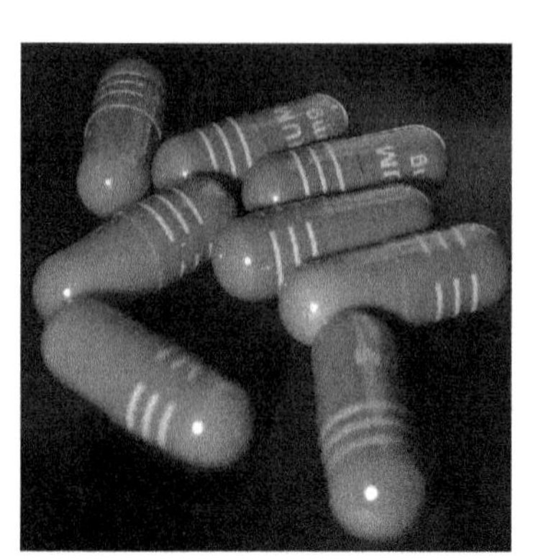

You can see why Nexium capsules are advertised as the "purple pill."

PPIs may decrease the absorption of drugs that need an acidic environment to dissolve. Both digoxin (for heart failure) and ketoconazole (an antifungal drug) are acid-soluble drugs that may not work if used simultaneously with PPIs. Because PPIs have long-lasting effects on stomach acidity, alternatives to PPIs should be sought for patients taking digoxin and ketoconazole.

In addition to decreasing the absorption of some drugs, PPIs seem to decrease the effectiveness of clopidogrel (Plavix) by an unknown mechanism. Clopidogrel is an antiplatelet drug (see Chapter 13) used following cardiac surgeries to help prevent heart attack and stroke. The magnitude and importance of this interaction is currently unclear and is still being studied.

OTC omeprazole should only be used for fourteen days. If symptoms have not resolved after two weeks, patients should consult their physicians.

H_2 Blockers As with the PPIs, GERD and PUD can be treated with H_2 blockers. They work by blocking type 2 histamine receptors in the stomach, which decreases proton pump activity and limits acid secretion. They work for approximately eight hours. They can be taken daily or on an as-needed basis (see Table 15.8). They are all available over the counter. In the inpatient setting, IV dosage forms may be useful for critically ill patients at risk for stress ulcers.

Side Effects H_2 blockers are well-tolerated medicines. However, patients may experience headache, diarrhea, and dizziness occasionally. Rarely, these medications may cause temporary confusion. If this occurs, patients should discontinue treatment and contact their physicians or pharmacists. H_2 blockers have been associated with increased risk for developing certain infections, such as respiratory tract infections. The significance of this association is not clear.

Cautions and Considerations Cimetidine interacts with several other drug therapies. For example, it increases the levels of theophylline, warfarin, phenytoin, nifedipine, and propranolol in the bloodstream. Therefore, patients taking these other medications should talk with their pharmacists before taking cimetidine. Other H_2 blockers do not interact with these medications, so patients can be switched to one of them if drug interactions are a concern. Because cimetidine is available over the counter, neither the pharmacist nor the prescriber may be aware of when an interaction occurs in a patient. You can improve patient care and safety by alerting the pharmacist when you encounter a patient purchasing cimetidine who also takes other medications.

Table 15.8 Commonly Used H_2 Blockers

Generic (Brand)	Dosage Form	Route of Administration	Common Dose	Dispensing Status
Cimetidine (Tagamet)	Solution, solution for injection, tablet	Oral, IV	Adult: 400–1,200 mg a day orally or IV (divided 2–4 times a day) Pediatric: weight-based	OTC and Rx
Famotidine (Pepcid)	Gelcap, premixed infusion, solution for injection, tablet	Oral, IV	Adult: 20 mg twice a day, orally or IV Pediatric: weight-based	OTC and Rx
Nizatidine (Axid)	Capsule, solution, tablet	Oral	Adult: 150 mg twice a day Pediatric: weight-based	OTC and Rx
Ranitidine (Zantac)	Solution for injection, premixed infusion, capsule, syrup, tablet	Oral, IV	Adult: 150 mg twice a day, orally or 50 mg every 6–8 hours IV Pediatric: weight-based	OTC and Rx

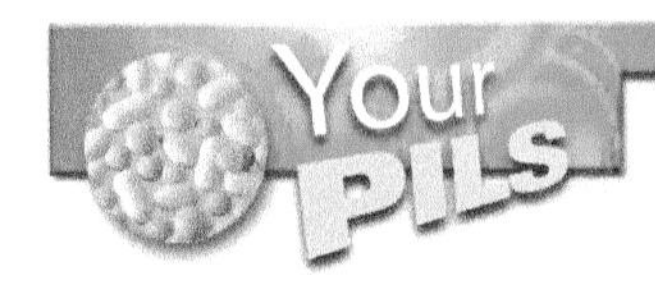

If you like to learn in a hands-on way, like Enactors do, take a look through your medicine cabinet at home. Pull out all medications for treating heartburn. What are the active ingredients in each product? Think about when and why you choose to use them. What is the difference in dose between OTC and prescription GERD medications? Talk with your family about proper use of these products. Seeing, handling, and talking about these medications will give them relevance and cement their names and uses in your memory.

H_2 blockers decrease the absorption of drugs that require an acidic environment to dissolve. Both digoxin (for heart failure) and ketoconazole (an antifungal) are acid-soluble drugs that may not be effective if used simultaneously with H_2 blockers. Because H_2 blockers have long-lasting effects on stomach acidity, alternatives should be sought for patients taking digoxin and ketoconazole.

Patients with hepatitis should not take ranitidine. Although rare, reports of liver failure and death in patients with hepatitis taking ranitidine have occurred.

Sucralfate This drug is no longer commonly prescribed. However, you may encounter it in compounded products for infants with GERD. **Sucralfate** coats the walls of the stomach and small intestine, forming a protective barrier against stomach acid. It must be taken four times a day. For best results, sucralfate should be taken on an empty stomach one hour before or two hours after a meal.

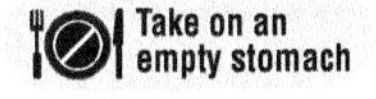

Because sucralfate is not absorbed systemically, it causes very few side effects. Constipation, diarrhea, headache, GI discomfort, and indigestion are possible. Sucralfate interacts with many other medications because it forms a barrier along the lining of the stomach, preventing absorption. Patients should avoid taking sucralfate simultaneously with other medications, particularly quinolone antibiotics, antifungals, phosphate supplements, and levothyroxine. Sucralfate suspensions must be shaken well before use to ensure adequate mixing of contents.

Regimens for *H. Pylori* If a patient with PUD is *H. pylori* positive (+), a multidrug regimen is prescribed (see Table 15.9). These drug combinations treat the ulcer, reduce symptoms, and kill *H. pylori* in the GI tract at the same time. All regimens consist of a PPI or H_2 blocker to heal the ulcer and antibiotics to destroy the bacteria. Combination products are also available. Helidac and Pylera contain bismuth subsalicylate, metronidazole, and tetracycline. Prevpac contains lansoprazole, amoxicillin, and clarithromycin.

Table 15.9 Commonly Used Regimens for *H. pylori* Eradication

PPI	Plus Antibiotic	Plus Antibiotic	
Esomeprazole (Nexium) Lansoprazole (Prevacid) Omeprazole (Prilosec) Pantoprazole (Protonix) Rabeprazole (AcipHex) (all are taken once a day)	Clarithromycin 500 mg twice a day	Amoxicillin 1 g twice a day or metronidazole 500 mg twice a day	
PPI or H_2 blocker	**Plus Antibiotic**	**Plus Antibiotic**	**Plus Antacid**
PPI listed above or Cimetidine (Tagamet) Famotidine (Pepcid) Nizatidine (Axid) Ranitidine (Zantac) (all are taken twice a day)	Metronidazole 250–500 four times a day	Tetracycline 500 mg four times a day, or amoxicillin 500 mg four times a day, or clarithromycin 250–500 mg four times a day	Bismuth subsalicylate (Pepto-Bismol) 525 mg four times a day

Nausea and Vomiting

Nausea and vomiting are related symptoms caused by a variety of diseases and conditions. Intestinal infections such as traveler's diarrhea are a common cause of nausea and vomiting. **Morning sickness** is nausea and vomiting in the first weeks of pregnancy. It is related to hormonal changes. **Motion sickness** is nausea and vomiting following movement (e.g., on a roller coaster or boat ride). It is related to vestibular responses in the inner ear that affect the sense of balance. Anesthesia used during surgery is also associated with nausea and vomiting.

Nausea is the feeling of the need to vomit. **Vomiting** is the expulsion of stomach contents out of the mouth. It involves coordinated muscle contractions along the upper GI tract **(reverse peristalsis)**. Vomiting is a defense mechanism to protect the body from harmful substances that have been consumed. All drugs are foreign substances to the body and have the potential to trigger stomach irritation, nausea, and vomiting. However, medications most commonly associated with nausea and vomiting are cancer chemotherapy and radiation treatments (see Table 15.10).

The impulse to vomit or feeling of nausea begins in the brain (see Figure 15.6). The **chemoreceptor trigger zone (CTZ)** and **vomiting center** in the medulla receive input from the cerebral cortex, hypothalamus, GI tract, and blood-borne stimuli (e.g., bacteria) to cause nausea and vomiting. For instance, when a harmful substance is detected in the stomach or normal balance is thrown off in the inner ear, the vomiting center signals the nausea sensation and stimulates vomiting.

Table 15.10 Treatments that Can Cause Nausea and Vomiting

Antibiotics	Opiates (morphine, hydrocodone, oxycodone, etc.)
Antiseizure medications (phenytoin, carbamazepine, levetiracetam, etc.)	Radiation therapy
Chemotherapy agents	Theophylline
Digoxin	

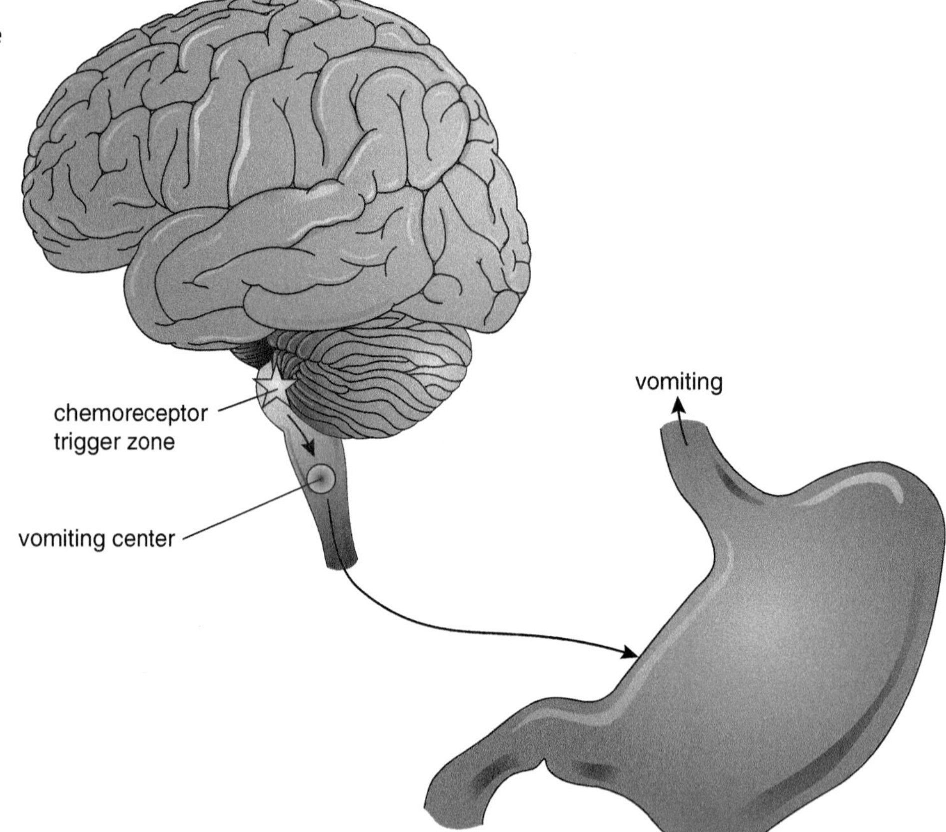

Figure 15.6
Chemoreceptor Trigger Zone (CTZ) and Vomiting Center
Blocking receptors for serotonin, dopamine, histamine, and substance P in the CTZ can relieve symptoms of nausea and vomiting.

Drugs for Nausea and Vomiting

The act of vomiting is also known as **emesis**. Therefore, drugs used to prevent vomiting are called **antiemetics**. Treatment depends on the cause and severity of the nausea and vomiting. For nausea and vomiting due to heartburn, antacids and H_2 blockers can be used. For mild nausea and vomiting related to motion sickness, OTC anticholinergic agents can be used. For moderate to severe nausea and vomiting, more potent antiemetics are needed. These medications are prescribed in clinics and hospitals for nausea and vomiting associated with severe dehydration, chemotherapy, and anesthesia following surgical procedures. Sometimes these potent agents are used in combination with oral corticosteroids (see Chapter 4).

Anticholinergic Antiemetics In general, **anticholinergic antiemetics** are similar in chemical structure to antihistamines. They are used as antiemetics for mild motion sickness. They work by blocking histamine and acetylcholine, two neurotransmitters in the CTZ and vomiting center. See Table 15.11 for more information.

Table 15.11 Anticholinergic Antiemetic Agents

Generic (Brand)	Dosage Form	Route of Administration	Common Dose
Dimenhydrinate (Dramamine)	Tablet, liquid, injection	Oral, IM, IV	Varies by age and use, usually taken 1 hour prior to when motion sickness is expected and once a day thereafter (when needed)
Hydroxyzine (Atarax, Vistaril)	Tablet, capsule, syrup, suspension, injection	Oral, IM	Varies by age and use, usually taken 1–2 hours prior to when motion sickness is expected and once a day thereafter (when needed)
Meclizine (Bonine)	Tablet, capsule	Oral	Varies by age and use, usually taken 1 hour prior to when motion sickness is expected and once a day thereafter (when needed)
Scopolamine (Transderm Scop, Scopace)	Tablet, transdermal patch	Oral, transdermal	0.4–1 mg, usually taken 1 hour prior to when motion sickness is expected

May Cause DROWSINESS
Use Caution while Driving

Side Effects Common side effects of anticholinergic antiemetics are drowsiness, dry mouth, and urinary retention. Patients who take other medications that also cause drowsiness should be careful because sedation could be excessive. Patients should avoid drinking alcohol and take care when driving until they know how the medication affects them. Patients who have prostate enlargement should not use anticholinergic antiemetics because they can make urination even more difficult.

In some children, antihistamines have a paradoxical effect, where excitation occurs rather than drowsiness. Parents should be aware of the potential for this side effect.

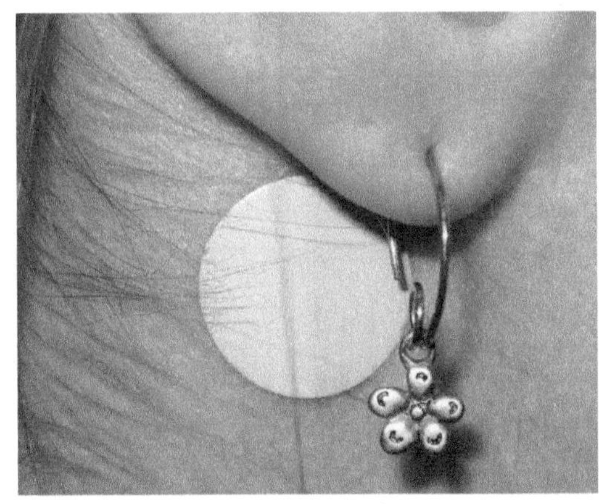
Many people use the scopolamine patch to prevent motion sickness while on boat or airplane rides.

Cautions and Considerations Patients who have high blood pressure or heart problems should talk with their prescribers before taking anticholinergic antiemetics. These agents should not be given to infants or mothers who are breast-feeding. Patients with glaucoma or who are using monoamine oxidase inhibitors (MAOIs) should not take these agents.

General Antiemetics A handful of agents make up the majority of prescription orders for antiemetics, especially in the inpatient setting. **Metoclopramide** works by increasing GI motility, which allows food to pass quickly through the stomach, preventing vomiting. **Promethazine** blocks histamine (H_1) receptors.

Phenothiazines are potent antiemetic drugs that work by blocking dopamine. They are first-generation antipsychotics when used in higher doses. Technicians working in an inpatient setting will likely dispense phenothiazines daily because they are frequently ordered in that setting.

These medications are available in many different dosage forms (see Table 15.12), an important feature because patients with nausea and vomiting may not be able to swallow a pill or oral solution. Patients can receive an IM shot, an IV injection, or rectal suppository to relieve symptoms.

Table 15.12 Commonly Used General Antiemetics

Generic (Brand)	Dosage Form	Route of Administration	Common Dose
Metoclopramide (Reglan)	Tablet, syrup, injection	Oral, IM, IV	10–20 mg 3–4 times a day
Promethazine (Phenergan, others)	Tablet, liquid, solution for injection, suppository	Oral, IM, IV, rectal	12.5–25 mg 4–6 times a day
Phenothiazines			
Chlorpromazine (Thorazine)	Tablet, liquid, solution for injection	Oral, IM, IV	10–25 mg orally or 25–50 mg IM or IV every 4–6 hours
Prochlorperazine (Compazine)	Tablet, liquid, solution for injection, suppository	Oral, IM, IV, rectal	5–10 mg 3–4 times a day orally. 2.5–10 mg IM or IV 3–4 times a day

Side Effects Common side effects of general antiemetics include drowsiness and sedation, which most patients experience. Movement disorders (called extrapyramidal symptoms [EPS] or EPS side effects), tardive dyskinesia and dystonia, are also possible with phenothiazines, particularly at high doses. EPS effects include uncontrollable movements of the eyes, face, and limbs that may become permanent. Patients, especially the elderly, have to be closely monitored for the appearance of EPS. If any symptoms of EPS appear, patients should stop taking the antiemetic. Benadryl may be used to treat dystonia.

May Cause
DROWSINESS
Do not drink alcoholic beverages when taking this medication

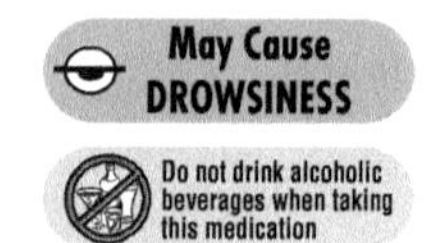

Cautions and Considerations The sedative effects of these medications may make it difficult for patients to drive or accomplish other activities. Alcohol may make the sedation worse. Auxiliary warning labels to these effects should be placed on these products when dispensed, especially in the outpatient setting.

Patients with liver problems cannot eliminate these agents from the bloodstream properly, increasing the risk for EPS. Patients should inform their prescribers if they have liver problems so that this risk can be assessed and other therapy chosen if necessary.

Serotonin Type 3 (5-HT3) Receptor Antagonists These agents are potent antiemetics used to prevent and treat severe nausea and vomiting associated with chemotherapeutic medicines, radiation treatment, or anesthesia. This class of drugs works by blocking serotonin type 3 (5-HT3) receptors in the brain and GI tract. Blocking these receptors stops nausea signals traveling from the brain to the stomach. These powerful antiemetics are prescription-only products (see Table 15.13) that technicians in the inpatient and oncology specialty clinics will encounter.

Table 15.13 Commonly Used 5-HT3 Receptor Antagonists

Generic (Brand)	Dosage Form	Route of Administration	Common Dose
Dolasetron (Anzemet)	Solution for injection, tablet	Oral, IV	100 mg orally or 12.5 mg IV
Granisetron (Granisol, Kytril, Sancuso)	Solution for injection, tablet, transdermal patch	Oral, transdermal, IV	1–2 mg
Ondansetron (Zofran)	Premixed infusion bag, solution for injection, tablet, orally disintegrating tablet	Oral, IM, IV	8–24 mg orally or 4–12 mg IM, IV
Palonosetron (Aloxi)	Solution for injection	IV	0.075–0.25 mg IV

Side Effects Common side effects of 5-HT3 receptor blockers include headache, fatigue, constipation, drowsiness, and muscle weakness. Although extremely rare, serious side effects such as anaphylaxis, hypotension, or swelling of the throat or tongue have been reported. Because these potentially life-threatening reactions are possible, it is recommended that patients not be alone when they take their first dose of a 5-HT3 antagonist.

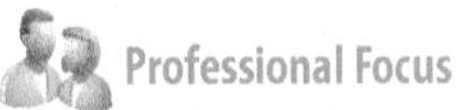

Cautions and Considerations Because 5-HT3 receptor antagonists may cause dizziness and drowsiness, patients should be reminded that activities such as driving may not be safe while taking these medications. You should place an auxiliary label on these prescriptions.

Ondansetron is available as a generic drug, but other 5-HT3 blockers currently are not. As a result, these medications are expensive. For a patient's insurance plan to cover these drugs, you may need to obtain a prior authorization from the physician.

Professional Focus

If you work in the inpatient setting, pay attention to the antiemetics you handle during unit dose preparation. How many are there? If you don't work in a hospital, see if you can arrange to shadow an inpatient pharmacy technician for a day. Make a note of each antiemetic dispensed. What were the doses and dosage forms being used? Why would a patient need to take an antiemetic medication via an alternative to the oral route?

Neurokinin 1 Inhibitor Aprepitant (Emend), the only **neurokinin 1 (NK1) inhibitor** on the market, is used to prevent nausea and vomiting induced by chemotherapy drugs or anesthesia. It works by blocking NK1 receptors, preventing substance P from stimulating nausea. Blocking NK1 receptors stops the nausea signal as it travels from the brain to the GI tract. Aprepitant is only available by prescription in oral capsules. Common side effects of aprepitant include fatigue, muscle weakness, and constipation. Hypotension, slow heart rate, diarrhea, GI pain, kidney and liver dysfunction, and blood abnormalities are rare but significant side effects. If the patient experiences severe side effects while taking aprepitant, he or she should call a physician immediately.

Aprepitant inhibits the metabolism of warfarin, corticosteroids, and chemotherapy medications. Patients may require lower doses of corticosteroids and chemotherapy medications, if they are taking aprepitant. Patients taking warfarin should be monitored closely after initiating aprepitant.

Hemorrhoids

The anus contains two sphincters that control defecation. The **hemorrhoidal cushion** protects the anal sphincters from becoming damaged over time. However, in response to straining during defecation and passing hard stools, blood vessels from the hemorrhoidal cushion can be forced into the anal cavity, where they are at risk of rupturing. **Hemorrhoids** can be thought of as varicose veins, except they occur in blood vessels near the anus rather than in the legs. Hemorrhoid disease is bleeding and irritation when a blood vessel of the hemorrhoidal cushion ruptures.

Drugs for Hemorrhoids

For mild hemorrhoids, increasing dietary **fiber** or taking a fiber product such as a bulk-forming laxative may make passing stool easier and resolve symptoms. Patients with hemorrhoids should increase water intake, avoid straining when defecating, take sitz baths, and treat constipation promptly. Serious hemorrhoids may require topical corticosteroids or surgery. **Topical hemorrhoid agents** are used to decrease symptoms of itching and pain caused by hemorrhoids. **Witch hazel** is an astringent that may also help stop bleeding. **Pramoxine** is a local anesthetic. It is available by itself (brand name Anusol) and in combination with a corticosteroid (brand name ProctoFoam). Topical foams need to be shaken well before use to ensure adequate mixing and proper dosing.

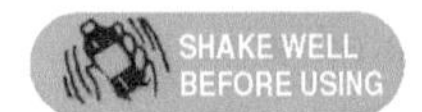

Most available hemorrhoidal products are over the counter. Medications for hemorrhoids decrease symptoms, but they do not reduce bleeding or cure the underlying problem.

Other GI Conditions

Irritable bowel syndrome (IBS) is a chronic disease that features frequent and painful constipation or diarrhea without any structural or dietary problems. There are three types of IBS: constipation-predominant, diarrhea-predominant, and mixed IBS. The exact cause of IBS is still unknown, but it is thought to be due to muscle dysfunction in the intestines, leading to altered GI motility. For reasons that are not well understood, IBS is more common in women than in men. Drug therapy options specifically for IBS are limited and have restricted distribution. Therefore, medications for IBS are not covered in this text.

Ulcerative colitis and **Crohn's disease** are two conditions that cause chronic diarrhea. Ulcerative colitis involves excessive inflammation of the GI tract, causing ulcers. This damage causes abdominal pain and weight loss as well as diarrhea. The damage tends to be limited to specific portions of the colon or large intestine, and some patients can be cured surgically by removing the affected portion. Crohn's disease is similar to ulcerative colitis in that it involves inflammation of the GI tract and causes chronic diarrhea. It also has manifestations outside the GI tract. However, it is different in that it is an autoimmune disease, where the immune system malfunctions and attacks tissue lining of the entire GI tract. Although surgery is sometimes performed, it cannot cure Crohn's disease like it can for ulcerative colitis. Despite these differences, ulcerative colitis and Crohn's disease share similar symptoms and many of the same treatments. Drug therapy includes immunosuppressants, salicylates, and anti-inflammatory drugs.

Herbal and Alternative Therapies

Ginger can be used to reduce nausea associated with surgery, vertigo, and motion sickness. It also has demonstrated benefit in pregnant women with morning sickness but has not undergone rigorous safety testing in this population. The mechanism of action of ginger is still poorly defined, but it may exert its effects by stimulating serotonin receptors (5-HT3) in a similar manner to other antiemetics. The standard dose for preventing nausea and vomiting is 500–1,000 mg. Ginger may cause heartburn, gas, bloating, mouth and throat irritation, and diarrhea. Because ginger has antiplatelet effects, its use should be avoided in patients taking aspirin, warfarin, or other anticoagulants (see Chapter 13).

Probiotics are products that contain live cultures of yeast or bacteria. They are commonly available in capsules, powders, beverages, or yogurts, some of which need to be refrigerated to keep the microorganisms alive. These products are used to colonize the GI tract with beneficial organisms for digestion and regular GI motility. Probiotics are used for diarrhea, constipation, *H. pylori* infection, and antibiotic-induced diarrhea. They may even be used for diarrhea associated with rotavirus, Crohn's disease, ulcerative colitis, and IBS. Probiotic organisms are not pathogenic. They compete with harmful bacteria, hopefully replacing or displacing them. They may enhance the immune response to pathogenic organisms and break down toxins. Patients with poor immune system function should not use probiotic products. Doses vary based on the product and indication.

Lactobacilli are gram-positive bacteria that are normal flora of the human GI tract. Common lactobacillus products contain *Lactobacillus acidophilus*, *Lactobacillus helveticus*, *Lactobacillus bulgaricus*, and *Lactobacillus rhamnosus*. Lactobacilli products are taken daily divided into three or four doses. They are usually well tolerated with few side effects, the most common of which are gas and bloating.

Saccharomyces boulardii (S. boulardii) (brand name Florastor) is a yeast organism that lives in the human GI tract. For prevention of antibiotic-associated diarrhea, 250–500 mg is taken two to four times a day. *S. boulardii* can cause gas, bloating, and constipation.

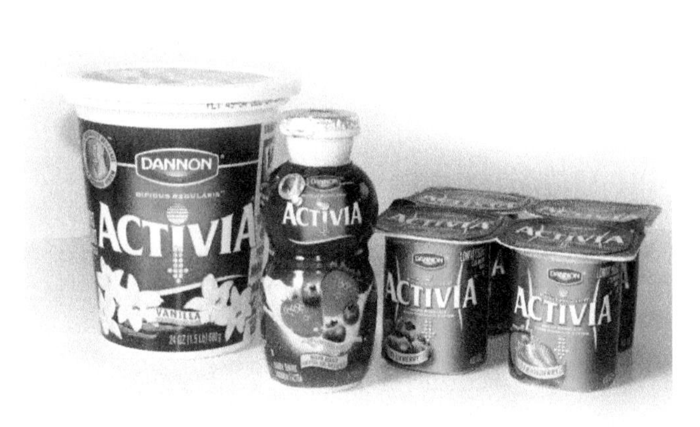

Activia, a line of functional food products that contain bifidobacteria, is an example of a probiotic culture.

Bifidobacteria agents are not as well studied as lactobacillus and *S. boulardii* products. However, they might be effective for diarrhea associated with a variety of causes. Doses vary based on specific products and indications. As with other probiotics, bifidobacteria are well tolerated in general but have the potential to cause gas and bloating.

Chapter Summary

Diarrhea, constipation, and hemorrhoids are common complaints from patients seeking self-treatment in the pharmacy. They can be caused by many conditions, including infection, food poisoning, medication, and chronic conditions. Diarrhea can be treated with OTC medicines such as loperamide, diphenoxylate plus atropine, and bismuth subsalicylate. Drugs that relieve constipation are known as laxatives and come in many varieties. Some take a few days to work, whereas others produce a bowel movement in less than an hour. Hemorrhoids are treated with topical agents.

GERD and PUD are caused by irritation and damage to the esophagus, stomach, or small intestine from stomach acid. GERD produces heartburn and is usually caused by eating large meals, fatty or spicy foods, or certain medications. PUD is usually caused by a bacterial organism called *H. pylori*, or drugs such as NSAIDs and aspirin. PPIs and H_2 blockers treat both GERD and PUD by increasing the pH of the stomach. If a patient has PUD secondary to *H. pylori* infection, he or she needs antibiotics in addition to a PPI or H_2 blocker. Antacids are commonly used for GERD to relieve heartburn associated with meals.

Nausea and vomiting are common problems associated with motion sickness, food poisoning, and anesthesia for surgery. They are also a common side effect of medications, most notably chemotherapy agents. Anticholinergic antiemetics are used for mild nausea and vomiting. General antiemetics such as promethazine are given to hospital patients who become nauseated. Patients taking chemotherapy are given powerful antiemetics known as 5-HT3 antagonists.

Chapter Review

For the following sets of exercises, write the exercise heading, exercise numbers, and your answers on a separate sheet of paper. Your instructor may direct you to turn in the sheet of paper or discuss your answers as a class.

REVIEW THE BASICS

Choose a, b, c, or d as the correct answer to each multiple-choice question.

1. In which part of the GI tract does the majority of nutrient (and medication) absorption occur?
   a. stomach
   b. small intestine
   c. large intestine
   d. liver
2. Which of the following best describes peristalsis?
   a. release of digestive enzymes from the pancreas into the small intestine
   b. secretion of acid from the stomach
   c. coordinated muscle contraction along the GI tract
   d. passing of stool
3. How does psyllium (and other bulk-forming laxatives) work to prevent constipation?
   a. contains fiber, which cannot be absorbed, drawing water into the GI tract
   b. stimulates the GI tract to speed up the passage of food
   c. softens stools, making their passage out of the GI tract easier
   d. clears the contents of the bowels by rapidly drawing water and electrolytes into the GI tract
4. Which of the following drugs is useful in treating nausea and vomiting due to motion sickness or vertigo?
   a. ranitidine
   b. loperamide
   c. hydroxyzine
   d. pantoprazole
5. Which of the following medications are available in both oral and IV dosage forms used in both outpatient and inpatient ulcer prevention?
   a. polyethylene glycol
   b. bismuth subsalicylate
   c. pantoprazole
   d. ondansetron
6. Which of the following best describes an enema?
   a. solution that is administered rectally to clear the bowels
   b. soft, torpedo-shaped dosage form that is inserted rectally and dissolves
   c. injectable solution for preventing stress ulcers
   d. functional food product containing probiotic bacteria
7. Which of the following should be kept in the refrigerator?
   a. bisacodyl
   b. lansoprazole
   c. ondansetron
   d. lactobacillus
8. Which of the following is a potent (and costly) medication for nausea and vomiting associated with cancer chemotherapy?
   a. lactulose (Enulose)
   b. dolasetron (Anzemet)
   c. promethazine (Phenergan)
   d. famotidine (Pepcid)
9. On which of the following medications should you place an auxiliary label for drowsiness?
   a. promethazine
   b. hydroxyzine
   c. granisetron
   d. all of the above
10. Which of the following is available in a transdermal patch?
    a. ondansetron
    b. prochlorperazine
    c. scopolamine
    d. meclizine

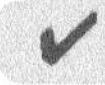

KNOW THE DRUGS

Match each brand name drug with its corresponding generic name and most common use. Your answers should follow this example format: Generic Name: 1. a; 2. b; 3. c; etc. Most Common Use: 1. h; 2. i; 3. j; etc.

Brand Name	Generic Name	Most Common Use
1. Colace	a. promethazine	h. diarrhea
2. Prilosec	b. ranitidine	i. GERD
3. Imodium	c. loperamide	j. constipation
4. Maalox	d. omeprazole	k. nausea and vomiting
5. Zantac	e. docusate	
6. Phenergan	f. calcium carbonate	
7. Compazine	g. prochlorperazine	

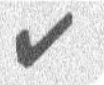

PUT IT TOGETHER

For each item, write down a short answer, a single term to complete the sentence, or true or false.

1. Distinguish the OTC and prescription strengths of omeprazole and lansoprazole.
2. _______________ is the only drug for GI problems that is a controlled substance.
3. Excluding the miscellaneous laxatives that have specialized uses, list the classes of laxative agents from quickest to slowest onset of action.
4. True or False: Oral laxative products work much faster than suppositories or enemas.
5. List the brand and generic names of the most expensive class of antiemetics. What class is this?
6. List the drug classes used for treating GERD.

THINK IT THROUGH

Read and think through each numbered scenario carefully and then write several sentences in reply to the question(s) presented. Question 4 requires you to undertake Internet research before completing your answer(s).

1. You are entering new medication orders into a patient's profile in the outpatient pharmacy of the day surgery pavilion. The patient and her family are waiting to go home with prescriptions for oxycodone, ibuprofen, and Phenergan. You see in her profile that she also takes iron supplements for anemia. Considering these medications and supplements, what are the most likely side effects that the patient will experience? Which OTC product is used for these side effects?
2. During a busy day in the pharmacy, a patient asks the pharmacist for a recommendation for treating "chest pain" that is experienced following meals. After asking some additional questions, the pharmacist concludes that the patient is experiencing GERD symptoms approximately once a week. The pharmacist asks for your help to assist this patient in locating an appropriate OTC remedy.
   a. Which OTC medicine would you recommend and why?
   b. Are there any nonmedication recommendations you can give to this patient?

3. When taking a new prescription order at the intake window, the patient complains that he has been prescribed three different prescription drugs for a suspected ulcer. He asks you why he needs three drugs, "Why can't I just take Pepcid or something? I see one of these is amoxicillin. My kid takes that for ear infections . . . . What are you, nuts?" His prescription is for omeprazole, clarithromycin, and amoxicillin. How should you respond?

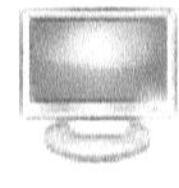

4. **On the Internet,** look up the cash price for each of the 5-HT3 receptor antagonists. Remember, only one of these products is available generically. One convenient way to obtain a price is to look online at some popular drugstore Web sites. What is the cash price for a typical ten-day supply of one of these medications? Why do you think that insurance companies require prior authorization for these medications?

Chapter 16 Nutrition and Drugs for Metabolism

LEARNING OBJECTIVES

- Describe the basic physiology of nutrition and weight management including intake of essential vitamins and minerals.
- Explain the therapeutic effects of vitamins and minerals.
- Identify recommended daily intake amounts and common doses of vitamin and mineral products.
- Explain the therapeutic effects of prescription medications, nonprescription medications, and alternative therapies commonly used to treat obesity.
- Describe the adverse effects of prescription medications, nonprescription medications, and alternative therapies commonly used to treat obesity.
- Identify the brand and generic names of prescription and nonprescription medications commonly used to treat obesity.
- State the doses, dosage forms, and routes of administration for prescription and nonprescription medications commonly used to treat obesity.

Interactive self-quizzes, games, audio files, and glossaries help you to learn drug names and facts.

Nutrition is important to overall health because it affects so many other disease states. Although few pharmacy professionals think of themselves as nutrition experts, numerous vitamins and nutritional supplements are sold in pharmacies throughout the United States. Patient interest in dietary supplements continues to grow. As scientists learn more about the connections between nutrition and disease, pharmacists and technicians will require access to useful and up-to-date nutritional information to help patients. Dietary supplements and nutrition services are becoming an area of special emphasis in some pharmacy practice sites. Considering the increasing number of stores that combine a grocery and drugstore under one roof, both patients and technicians will benefit from a basic understanding of nutrition. Nutrition-associated products and services related to weight loss and healthy living have become a billion-dollar industry. Consequently, pharmacy technicians encounter numerous over-the-counter (OTC) and some prescription drug and supplement products in these categories. A basic understanding of the place of nutrition-related products in therapy is valuable in helping patients obtain cost-effective care and achieve appropriate goals for body weight.

This chapter covers contributing factors and physiological processes that affect nutritional status and obesity. It also describes the roles of essential vitamins and minerals and other common pharmacologic therapies used to treat malnutrition and obesity.

Physiology of Nutrition

A variety of factors contribute to the maintenance of what is considered a normal body weight. Both external and internal physiological processes are involved in weight maintenance. Evaluating **nutrition status** requires comparing what is considered "normal" body weight for a patient's age and development with the patient's **actual body weight (ABW)**. Someone within the normal range shows no signs of vitamin or nutrient deficiency and maintains an appropriate body weight and makeup for his or her age and frame size. The best indicator of nutrition status in children is appropriate growth (including height and weight by age). Growth charts with population averages are used to determine whether a child is growing appropriately for his or her age, gender, and development. The 50th percentile for a particular age on a growth chart is considered ideal.

Ideal body weight (IBW) is the weight for a given height that is associated with maximum longevity and health. IBW is calculated in adults as follows:

$$\text{Males: IBW (kg)} = 50 + (2.3 \times \text{height in inches over 5 feet})$$

$$\text{Females: IBW (kg)} = 45.5 + (2.3 \times \text{height in inches over 5 feet})$$

Table 16.1 Evaluating ABW

	ABW ≤ 69% IBW	Severe malnutrition
Undernutrition	ABW 70–79% IBW	Moderate malnutrition
	ABW 80–90% IBW	Mild malnutrition
Normal	ABW 90–120% IBW	Normal
	ABW > 120% IBW	Overweight
Overnutrition	ABW ≥ 150% IBW	Obese
	ABW ≥ 200% IBW	Morbidly obese

Comparing a patient's ABW with the IBW enables a basic assessment of nutritional status (see Table 16.1). Some drugs are dosed based on weight. Sometimes, ABW can be used, but many times IBW is used to determine a proper weight-based dose.

Another way to assess appropriate weight for height is **body mass index (BMI)**. BMI is used to identify both undernutrition and overnutrition. Table 16.2 shows the general interpretations of BMI that have been accepted by most in the healthcare field. Due to increased muscle mass, some males and athletes may not be considered overweight until their BMI reaches 27. In children and teens, the BMI calculation is slightly different and takes into account age and gender differences. In these age-groups, BMI must be compared to averages in growth in order for age to be interpreted correctly.

$$\text{BMI} = \text{weight (kg)} / [\text{height (m)}]^2$$

Good nutritional status is maintained through appropriate energy intake and expenditure. Typically, energy intake is measured in **calories** (kcal/kg). Appropriate daily caloric needs depend on age. For adults, an intake of 25 kcal/kg of body weight a day is usually adequate to maintain the basal metabolic rate. Malnourished and critically ill patients need more calories.

In addition to calories, the body needs appropriate amounts of protein, carbohydrates, fluids, and micronutrients. Protein needs vary depending on age, disease state, and clinical condition. For instance, the elderly need relatively more protein to compensate for the lean muscle mass lost with advancing age. In patients with wounds or severe burns, healing and tissue growth is a high priority, and adequate protein is needed to form the building blocks for tissue regeneration. On the other hand, protein intake may be restricted in patients with kidney or liver failure, because nitrogen cannot exit the body normally. Proteins are made up of amino acids that contain nitrogen in their chemical structure. Albumin, prealbumin, and transferrin are proteins in the blood and can be measured via laboratory tests to assess protein and nutritional status. Low amounts of any of these substances in the blood usually indicate malnutrition.

Table 16.2 Evaluating Body Mass Index (BMI)

	BMI (kg/m²)	
Adults	< 16	Severe malnutrition
	16–17	Moderate malnutrition
	17–18	Mild malnutrition
	19–25	Normal
	25–30	Overweight
	> 30	Obese
Children and teens	BMI for age < 5th percentile	Underweight
	BMI for age 5–85th percentile	Healthy
	BMI for age > 85th percentile	At risk for overweight
	BMI for age > 95th percentile	Overweight

Micronutrients include **vitamins** and **minerals** (i.e., electrolytes and trace elements). They play a key role in many metabolic processes, such as supporting coenzyme and cofactor production. In 2005,

Table 16.3 Adult RDIs of Vitamins and Minerals

Vitamins	RDI
A (beta carotene)	3000 IU (800 mcg)
Thiamin (B_1)	1.2 mg
Riboflavin (B_2)	1.3 mg
Niacin (B_3)	16 mg
Pantothenic acid (B_5)	5 mg
Pyridoxine (B_6)	1.7 mg
Biotin (B_7)	30 mcg
Folate (folic acid or B_9)	400 mcg
Cyanocobalamin (B_{12})	2.4 mcg
C (ascorbic acid)	90 mg
D (cholecalciferol, ergocalciferol)	600 IU
E (alpha tocopherol)	15 mg
K (phytonadione)	120 mcg
Trace Elements	
Chromium	20–35 mcg
Copper	900 mcg
Iodine	150 mcg
Iron	8 mg males 18 mg females
Manganese	2.3 mg
Selenium	55 mcg
Zinc	11 mg

the U.S. Department of Agriculture and the Institute of Medicine published **recommended daily intakes (RDIs)** for vitamins and essential trace elements (see Table 16.3). These RDI values are different from the recommended daily allowances (RDAs) developed in the 1960s.

RDI values of micronutrients are sometimes measured in **international units (IU),** instead of milligrams (mg) or micrograms (mcg). IU are units of measurement developed for each substance based on its biological effect. Vitamins, hormones, and other medications, such as heparin, are measured in IU. Reading labels and dosing information is important for getting the appropriate RDI. When deficiency of a particular vitamin or trace element is present, intake may need to be much more than the RDI to replenish lost stores.

When someone receives too much or too little of the daily caloric, protein, or micronutrient needs for his or her age and size, either over- or undernutrition can result. **Obesity**, in basic terms, is overnutrition. More specifically, an obese body composition contains significantly more fat than is considered normal or healthy. **Malnutrition** is a lack of adequate nutrient intake to supply basic metabolic needs. It can be related to an overall lack of calorie or protein consumption or might be associated with a deficiency in a specific micronutrient (e.g., vitamins and minerals). Malnutrition is most prevalent in underdeveloped countries and in children. In the United States, malnutrition is most often encountered in the inpatient setting, where it is associated with disease states, acute illness, and even drug therapy.

Signs of malnutrition include weight loss, skin changes (to dry, shiny, or scaly), hair loss, fatigue, poor wound healing, pallor (pale skin), sunken eyes, dry mouth and eyes, visible loss of muscle mass, and fluid accumulation in the abdomen or around the ankles and tailbone. Some causes for malnutrition include:

- anorexia
- food allergies/intolerance
- chronic infection or inflammatory conditions
- cancer
- endocrine disorders
- pulmonary disease
- cirrhosis of the liver
- renal failure
- nausea/vomiting/diarrhea
- trauma, burns, or sepsis
- inflammatory bowel disease, Crohn's disease, or short bowel syndrome
- inadequate parenteral or enteral nutrition
- psychiatric/psychological conditions

Marasmus is a chronic condition caused by inadequate caloric and protein intake over a prolonged time. Muscle and fat tissue visibly waste away—this is called **cachexia**.

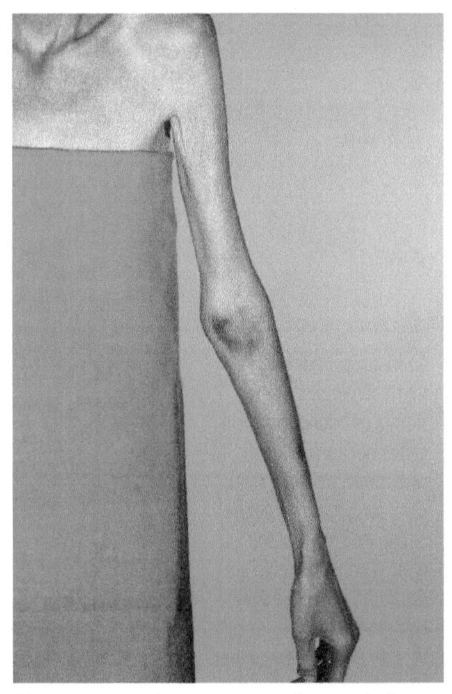

Often patients with malnutrition will appear to be wasting away, a condition called cachexia.

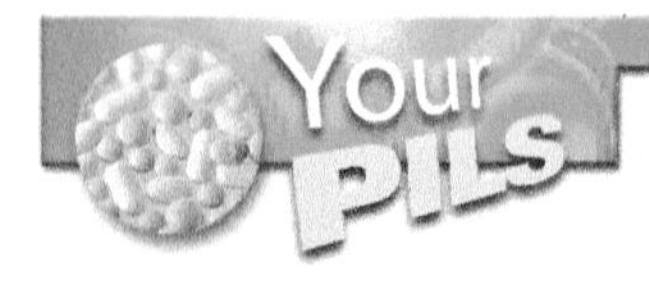

For those of you who like to learn things using hands-on, active methods—as do Enactors or Directors—take a look at the food labels you have around the home. Write down everything you have eaten for the past twenty-four hours. Then calculate how much calcium, vitamin D, and iron you have consumed. You may have to use additional resources (such as the Internet) to determine vitamin content of some foods. Did you achieve the RDI? If not, what changes could you make to ensure you get adequate amounts of these nutrients?

Starvation and wasting from cancer are causes of cachexia. **Kwashiorkor** is a condition in which caloric intake is adequate, but protein intake is deficient. These patients, paradoxically, usually appear well nourished, because heightened metabolic rates break down protein stores but leave adipose tissue intact. However, fluid can accumulate in the abdomen and feet in this kind of malnutrition. Physical trauma and critical illness can cause this kind of malnutrition.

Caloric and protein requirements increase during fever, sepsis, major surgery, trauma and burn recovery, and long-term chronic conditions. Even when patients are immobile and not perceived as expending much energy, their basal metabolic rate increases to handle stress and healing. Nutrient requirements in critically ill patients must be met appropriately. For instance, daily caloric needs increase to 30–40 kcal/kg a day in patients who are critically ill or have major burns. Special attention must be paid to protein and amino acid intake, because wound healing requires proteins, the building blocks of new tissue.

Micronutrient Abnormalities

Because vitamins, minerals, and essential fatty acids are integral to basic metabolic processes, deficiencies or excesses can cause significant morbidity. **Fat-soluble vitamins** (A, D, E, and K) accumulate in fatty tissue and can build up in the body over time. Although large doses are needed to ingest too much of a fat-soluble vitamin, it is possible. **Water-soluble vitamins** (eight B vitamins and vitamin C) are easily excreted from the body in the urine, and it is difficult to cause an overdose with these vitamins. They are not typically associated with toxicity other than occasional incidents of stomach upset or diarrhea. Table 16.4 describes the signs of deficiency and toxicity for common vitamins and trace elements.

Vitamin and mineral deficiencies can be measured with specially ordered laboratory tests. Diagnosis usually starts with clinical presentation of signs and symptoms.

Vitamins

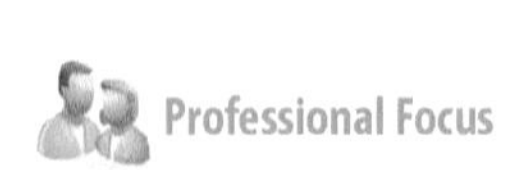

Some postulate that the myth of vampires stems from a deficiency of niacin, called pellagra. Though rare today, pellagra was common years ago before complete nutrition sources were readily available. Its symptoms, including sensitivity to sunlight, swollen mouth, and dementia, are thought to mimic those associated with vampires.

Vitamins and minerals are used either to treat or prevent malnutrition. Because these products are categorized as dietary supplements, labeling is not regulated for them like it is for prescription or OTC medicines. Pharmacy technicians can assist patients in reading labels for vitamin supplements. For instance, helping patients understand the difference between IU and milligrams is important for taking appropriate doses.

Vitamin A refers to a family of compounds called **retinoids**. Retinoids are needed for vision, growth, bone formation, reproduction, immune system function, and skin health. Vitamin A is found in eggs, whole milk, butter, meat, and fish. One compound in the retinol family, beta carotene, is found in vegetables (especially carrots), and fruits. Vitamin A is used primarily in cases of deficiency but has also been used for cataracts and reducing complications of HIV, measles, and malaria.

Thiamin (B_1) is an important coenzyme involved in carbohydrate metabolism. Thiamin is found in pork, cereal, grains, peas, beans, and yeast. Thiamin supplements are used for vitamin B_1 deficiency. Thiamin deficiency is most common during pregnancy and in Wernicke-Korsakoff syndrome, which occurs during alcohol withdrawal.

Table 16.4 Deficiencies and Toxicities of Common Vitamins and Minerals

	Signs of Deficiency	Signs of Toxicity
Water-Soluble Vitamins		
Thiamin (B_1)	**Beriberi** (numbness and tingling, edema, heart failure), impaired memory, lactic acidosis, visual disturbances, mental status changes	
Riboflavin (B_2)	Mucositis, skin rash, cracked lips, photophobia, tearing, poor vision, poor wound healing, anemia	
Niacin (B_3)	**Pellagra** (swelling of mouth and tongue, diarrhea, skin rash, sensitivity to sunlight, memory loss, headaches, dementia)	
Pantothenic acid (B_5)	Fatigue, malaise, headache, insomnia, vomiting, abdominal cramps	
Pyridoxine (B_6)	Skin rash, nerve pain, loss of reflexes, convulsions, anemia	
Biotin (B_7)	Skin rash, hair loss, change in hair color, depression, tiredness, hallucinations, numbness and tingling	
Folate (folic acid or B_9)	Anemia, diarrhea, swelling/painful tongue	
Cyanocobalamin (B_{12})	Anemia, swelling/painful tongue, nerve pain and degeneration	
Ascorbic acid (C)	**Scurvy** (anemia, hemorrhages, nosebleeds, spongy gums, enlargement of hair follicles), poor wound healing, fatigue, depression	
Fat-Soluble Vitamins		
A	**Keratomalacia** (skin rash, corneal degeneration, night blindness, dry eyes)	Nausea, vomiting, vertigo, blurry vision, hair loss, headache, irritability, skin peeling, bone and liver problems
D	**Rickets** (bone softening, muscle weakness)	High blood calcium, kidney stones, nausea, vomiting, thirst, increased urination, muscle weakness, bone pain
E	Hemolysis	Only in cases of very high doses: bleeding, stroke
K	Bleeding	Very rare: anemia, jaundice
Trace Minerals		
Chromium	Glucose intolerance, peripheral neuropathy, weight loss, elevated LDL cholesterol, sugar in the urine	Skin/nasal lesions, skin rash, lung cancer
Copper	Neutropenia, leukopenia, anemia, osteoporosis, hair/skin depigmentation, anorexia, diarrhea, mental status changes, high cholesterol	Diarrhea, vomiting, metallic taste, cirrhosis
Iodine	**Goiter**, hypothyroidism, neuromuscular problems, deafness, decreased mental function, bone softening/slowed growth	Metallic taste, sore teeth and gums, irritation of the mouth and throat, toxic thyroid, stomach upset, diarrhea, weight loss, tachycardia (rapid heartbeat), muscle weakness, fever, infertility
Iron	**Anemia**, fatigue, weakness, pallor, swelling/painful tongue, headache, difficulty swallowing, fingernail changes, numbness/tingling	Cirrhosis, heart problems, pancreatic damage, change in skin pigmentation
Manganese	Nausea, vomiting, skin rash, hair color changes, low cholesterol, growth retardation, problems with carbohydrate/protein metabolism	Parkinson's-like symptoms (changes in gait when walking), irritability, hallucinations, changes in libido
Selenium	Muscle weakness and pain, heart problems	Nausea, vomiting, hair and nail loss, tooth decay, skin lesions, irritability, fatigue, peripheral neuropathy
Zinc	Skin rash, loss of taste, hair loss, diarrhea, depression, growth retardation, poor wound healing, immunosuppression	Stomach upset, nausea, dizziness, decreased HDL cholesterol

Patients with known alcohol abuse may be given thiamin supplements while hospitalized to combat symptoms of alcohol withdrawal.

Riboflavin (B_2) is a coenzyme involved in tissue respiration and normal cell metabolism. Riboflavin is found in milk, cereal, green vegetables, and some meats. It is also made in the intestines by bacteria. Riboflavin is usually used for vitamin B_2 deficiency, but it can also be used in doses of 400 mg/day to decrease migraine headaches.

Niacin (B_3), also called nicotinic acid, is essential for reactions in the body that produce adenosine triphosphate, a critical molecule in cellular energy production. Niacin also helps regulate production and activity of cholesterol molecules in the blood. It is found in yeast, lean meats, peanuts, peas, beans, whole grains, and potatoes. Although niacin can be taken to treat vitamin B_3 deficiency, it is probably most often used for its beneficial effects on blood cholesterol. It lowers triglycerides and low-density lipoprotein (LDL) and raises high-density lipoprotein (HDL) (see Chapter 12). The dose required for these effects is at least 1,200–1,500 mg/day.

Pantothenic acid (B_5) is a precursor of coenzyme A, which is required for proper metabolism of carbohydrates, proteins, and lipids. Vitamin B_5 is found in vegetables, yeast, cereal, and organ meats (liver, kidney, heart). Pantothenic acid supplements are usually used for vitamin B_5 deficiency.

Pyridoxine (B_6) is converted in the body to the coenzymes responsible for amino acid metabolism. Pyridoxine is found in most foods of plant or animal origin. Pyridoxine is used for vitamin B_6 deficiency as well as for certain types of anemia and seizure disorders. It is also given to alcoholic patients with nerve damage and to patients who take isoniazid for tuberculosis. Isoniazid depletes vitamin B_6.

Biotin (B_7) is a coenzyme involved in metabolism. Deficiencies of it are associated with altered absorption, such as short gut syndrome. Biotin supplements are taken for vitamin B_7 deficiency.

Folate (B_9), or **folic acid**, plays a major role in intracellular metabolism and the breakdown of homocysteine, an amino acid associated with cardiovascular disease. It is also involved in the production of the neurotransmitter serotonin. Folic acid is frequently added to foods. Folate is naturally found in green leafy vegetables and red meat. Deficiencies in folic acid cause anemia and neural tube defects in a developing fetus and have deleterious effects on the cardiovascular system. Folic acid supplements are highly recommended for all women who are pregnant or planning to get pregnant. Taking folic acid can greatly reduce the incidence of birth defects. The RDI of 400 mcg is the amount that women of childbearing age should take. Folic acid is also used for patients with end-stage kidney disease to reduce homocysteine levels. Other uses include treatment for chronic fatigue syndrome, depression, and vitiligo.

Cyanocobalamin (B_{12}) is a coenzyme necessary for cell reproduction, normal growth, and red blood cell production. Vitamin B_{12} is essential to the proper use of folate within the body. Therefore, deficiency of it causes pernicious anemia. It is found in meats, fish, milk, and bread. Cyanocobalamin deficiency takes a long time to develop but is easily treated with supplements. It is most common in older adults and strict vegetarians. Cyanocobalamin is used for vitamin B_{12} deficiency, pernicious anemia, and conditions in which homocysteine levels are high (i.e., end-stage renal disease). Intestinal absorption of vitamin B_{12} requires **intrinsic factor**, which is made in the stomach.

Vitamin C (ascorbic acid) is best known for its role in immune system function and as an antioxidant. Antioxidants reduce DNA mutations that lead to cancer. Vitamin C is found in vegetables and fruits, especially citrus fruits. It is most effective for scurvy (vitamin C deficiency) and for improving iron absorption. It has also been used in premature infants (for protein metabolism), macular degeneration, seasonal allergies, and preventing illness such as the common cold. Some even use it for cancer, atherosclerosis, and sunburn. Small doses (100–250 mg/day) will correct a deficiency, whereas large doses (1–3 g/day) are used for preventing illness like a cold (see Chapter 3).

Vitamin D is important for maintaining calcium and phosphate levels in the blood. It also enhances intestinal absorption of calcium. Therefore, vitamin D has significant effects on bone health. Studies also show it may play a role in cardiovascular health, the development of cancer, and respiratory disease. Vitamin D has two active forms, **ergocalciferol** and **cholecalciferol**. Ergocalciferol is found in plants and yeasts, whereas cholecalciferol is made in the skin in response to sunlight. In fact, sunlight usually provides 80 to 90% of the body's vitamin D stores. In Northern regions, available

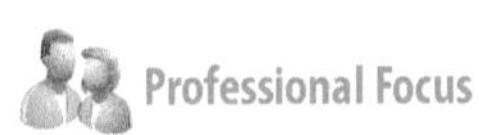

Professional Focus

The recommended dose for vitamin D deficiency has multiple approaches. Some recommend 1,100 mg/day on an ongoing basis, and some recommend mega-doses of 50,000 IU given weekly for a month to replenish bodily stores. After this loading dose, a daily dose of 1,100 mg/day is used to maintain vitamin D levels.

sunlight is not sufficient to allow for adequate vitamin D production in the skin. Therefore, supplements are often recommended. Foods that contain vitamin D are fortified milk, some eggs, and fatty fish, such as tuna and sardines. Although the RDI of vitamin D is 600 mg/day, many studies support doses of 1,100–1,200 mg/day as necessary to maintain good vitamin D stores. Vitamin D is commonly recommended to be taken along with calcium supplements to improve calcium absorption.

Vitamin E (alpha tocopherol) is fat-soluble and difficult to become deficient in, except in cases of very specific genetic or malabsorption disorders. Vitamin E is found in vegetable oils, cereals, grains, animal fat, meat, poultry, eggs, fruits, and vegetables. The physiologic role of vitamin E is controversial. Studies support the use of it for macular degeneration and Alzheimer's disease as well as to reduce the risk of developing some cancers and dementia. It is also used with varying success to improve immune system function. Some recommend vitamin E for diabetic retinopathy and cardiovascular disease (see Chapter 12). Therapeutic doses range between 400 and 2,000 IU a day. Although greater effects can be seen at high doses, long-term risks are associated with doses higher than 800 IU a day. Therefore, doses should not exceed 400 IU a day. Topical use of vitamin E can improve skin health, healing, and hydration (see Chapter 5).

Vitamin K (phytonadione) is a coenzyme for the hepatic production of blood clotting factors. It is found in green leafy vegetables, broccoli, brussels sprouts, plant oils, and margarine. Vitamin K deficiency can be caused by drug therapy (e.g., salicylates, sulfonamides, quinine, quinidine, and broad-spectrum antibiotics). Vitamin K is used in cases of deficiency or when enhanced blood clotting is desired. It is used most often to reverse the effects of warfarin, a common anticoagulant (see Chapter 13).

Side Effects Most side effects of vitamin supplements result from excess intake and mimic conditions of vitamin toxicity (see Table 16.4). Niacin products commonly cause flushing, hot flashes, and a sensation of prickly skin. Some prescription formulations slow the release and absorption of niacin, thereby reducing this effect. However, the effect is still quite common and can be the reason patients stop taking niacin. Taking niacin with food or swallowing an aspirin thirty minutes prior to taking niacin can reduce this effect. For this reason, doses are usually started at low levels and increased slowly. Instructions for use recommend taking niacin at bedtime so that if flushing occurs, the patient may not notice it while sleeping. Pharmacy technicians can help patients by ensuring that pharmacist counseling occurs for all new niacin prescriptions and by recommending an aspirin product along with any niacin purchases.

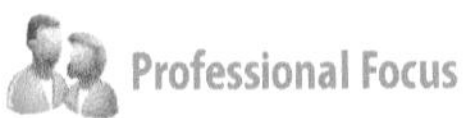

Professional Focus

Technicians in a food store retail setting may be able to detect potential interactions between vitamin K–rich foods and warfarin therapy. Patients taking warfarin should not widely vary their intake of green leafy vegetables, because dosing is based on typical dietary intake of vitamin K. If you see such patients purchasing more spinach, lettuce, broccoli, or other green vegetables than usual, point out this drug–food interaction. The pharmacist may need to get involved.

Cautions and Considerations Although vitamin A is necessary for appropriate fetal growth, doses in excess of 800 mcg a day have been associated with birth defects. Therefore, doses higher than the RDI are considered category X (contraindicated) in pregnant women.

Trace Elements

Trace elements are essential minerals needed for normal physiologic functions. Recommended daily intake of trace elements is relatively low and typically easy to obtain through normal food consumption (see Tables 16.3 and 16.4). Supplements are used primarily as additives to enteral and parenteral nutrition formulas. Because enteral and parenteral nutrition are artificial ways to feed a patient using methods other than swallowing, special care must be taken to include trace elements. It can be easy to underdose or overdose trace elements in nutrition formulas.

Chromium is part of a complex of molecules called glucose tolerance factor, which helps regulate glucose tolerance and insulin levels. It is found in canned foods, meat, fish, brown sugar, coffee, tea, whole wheat bread, and rye bread. Chromium levels are low in many patients with diabetes, but its role in diabetes is not fully understood. Chromium picolinate is taken in doses of 200–400 mcg a day to improve glucose tolerance and control in Type 1 and Type 2 diabetes. However, unless the patient is quite deficient (which is rare), the clinical effect may not be noticeable. True deficiency in chromium usually only happens in patients receiving parenteral nutrition. Glucose tolerance improves when taking chromium, but patients do not find that they can eliminate drug or insulin therapy for diabetes (see Chapter 17). Chromium has not been found to be useful in prediabetes to prevent the onset of this condition.

Copper is a catalyst and coenzyme in a wide variety of chemical reactions in the body. Without it, red blood cells (RBCs) and white blood cells decline, causing anemia, leukopenia, and neutropenia. Copper is found in organ meats, seafood, nuts, seeds, wheat bran cereals, grains, and cocoa. Copper deficiency is rare and usually only encountered in patients on parenteral nutrition. It is used almost exclusively for cases of deficiency.

Iodine is used in the body to make thyroid hormones, which regulate metabolic rates. Iodine is found in highest concentrations in seafood and seaweed and is added to salt in developed countries. Consequently, deficiencies there are usually rare. Iodine deficiency, which is more commonly seen in underdeveloped countries, may cause thyroid gland enlargement, or goiter. Iodine is used for some thyroid conditions and for radiation emergencies in which radioactive iodides have been used.

Iron is found in hemoglobin inside RBCs and myoglobin in muscles. It is a cofactor for neurotransmitter production and is a part of the functional groups of many important enzymes. Without iron, the production of RBCs is diminished, and the oxygen-carrying capacity of RBCs is reduced. Weakness and fatigue result from iron-deficiency anemia. Iron is found in red meat, poultry, and fish. It is found in some vegetables, but many cooking and storage methods reduce its availability. Vegetarians sometimes do not get enough iron. Iron is used to treat anemia of chronic disease and iron-deficiency anemia (see Chapter 13). Too much iron may cause a liver condition called hemochromatosis.

Manganese is a cofactor in many metabolic and enzymatic reactions in the body. Some believe it is involved in the development of osteoporosis. It is found in nuts, legumes, seeds, tea, whole grains, and green leafy vegetables. Manganese is used to treat deficiency.

Selenium is a metallic trace element that is incorporated into amino acids. It reduces oxidative stress in the body. It is found in broccoli, garlic, and onions. Selenium is used as an additive parenteral nutrition, and natural deficiencies of it are rare.

Zinc is a cofactor in many physiologic processes, including the synthesis of DNA and protein. It plays an important role in immune function, wound healing, blood clotting, reproduction, and appropriate growth. Zinc is found in meat, seafood, dairy products, nuts, legumes, and whole grains. It is used for zinc deficiency, boosting immune function, aiding in wound healing, and Wilson's disease. Zinc lozenges are used to reduce the symptom severity and length of the common cold (see Chapter 3). Zinc is also used topically to heal burn and skin wounds (see Chapter 5).

Side Effects Most side effects of trace element supplements result from excess intake. Thus, side effects mimic conditions of toxicity (see Table 16.4).

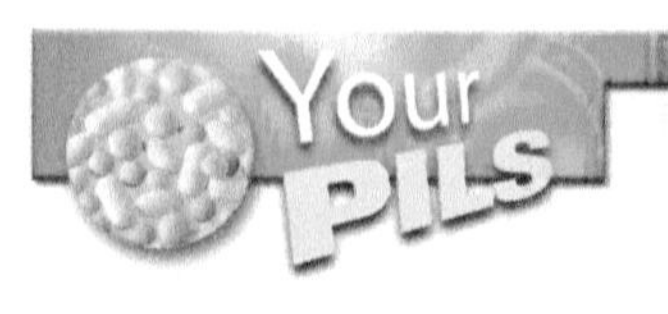

For those of you who enjoy outside-of-the-box learning activities and entertainment like Creators, develop a news story (either written or videotaped) on the claims made about the use of supplements to cure disease. Although scientific literature does not always support these claims, the media and the Internet heighten awareness with anecdotal stories about miraculous cures. You can see how easy it is for patients to become enamored with such products. Be sure to report both sides of the issue. Discuss with others their take on the information you find.

Enteral and Parenteral Nutrition

When a patient cannot be fed normally, alternative ways to supply nutrition must be employed. If a patient goes longer than a week to ten days without food or nutrition, malnutrition will ensue and negatively affect health outcomes.

Enteral Nutrition

Enteral nutrition is provided by feeding a patient through a tube into the gastrointestinal (GI) tract. The tube can be inserted manually (nasogastric [NG] tube) or surgically into the stomach (gastrostomy [G] tube) or jejunum (jejunostomy [J] tube) (see Figure 16.1). Liquid nutrient is put through the tube either in bolus doses to mimic eating a meal or continuously with an enteral pump. Indications for enteral feeding include bowel obstruction, short gut syndrome, and Crohn's disease. Patients in long-term care who are unable to swallow foods voluntarily (e.g., those with a severe stroke or in a prolonged coma) may have an enteral feeding tube placed to supply them with adequate nutrition. Intravenous (IV) fluids are usually given in addition to enteral feeding to maintain hydration status.

Professional Focus

Drugs can be administered through enteral feeding tubes. But restrictions apply because some drugs clog the tube, requiring surgical removal and replacement. For example, drugs that should not be crushed or chewed cannot be given via an enteral feeding tube.

Sometimes, pharmacy technicians prepare enteral feeding formulas; most often, they simply order them. In some locations, special nutrition services handle this responsibility. Specialized enteral feeding products are available for specific conditions, so patients must be matched with appropriate formulas. It is important to label enteral feeding preparations with a warning not to administer them through an IV. They are neither sterile nor formulated for that use. Enteral feeding is preferred to parenteral feeding because it keeps the GI tract functional and prevents abdominal infections.

Figure 16.1
Tube Feeding Sites
NG tubes are uncomfortable for patients, so such tubes are only for short-term use. If enteral feeding is necessary for more than a few days, a G tube or J tube will be placed surgically.

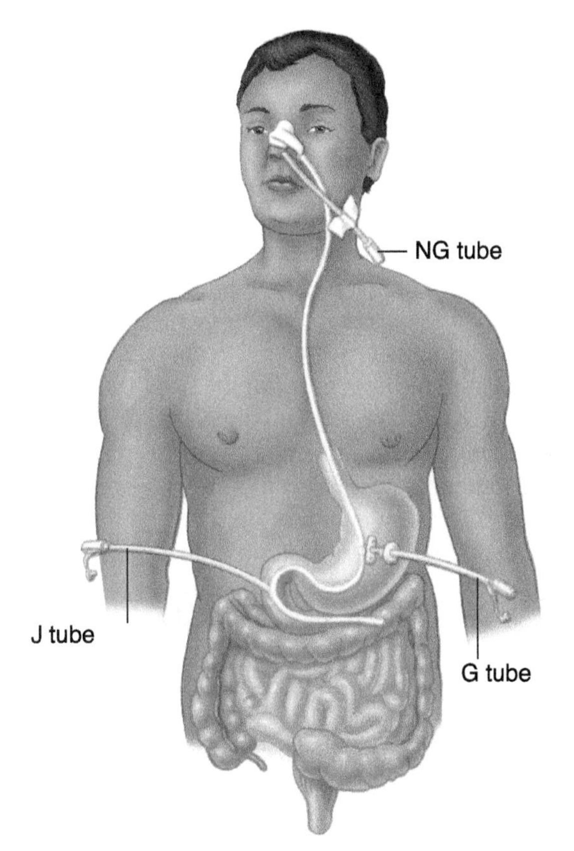

Parenteral Nutrition

Parenteral nutrition (often referred to as **total parenteral nutrition** or **TPN**) is provided by feeding a patient through an IV. It is used when the digestive tract cannot be used at all. Indications for TPN include severe burns, intolerance to enteral feeding, anorexia nervosa (refusal to eat), pancreatitis, severe gallbladder disease, inflammatory bowel disease, and severe diarrhea. TPN may also be necessary in pregnancy, AIDS, and cancer.

TPN carries risks for complications. TPN is complex in that it supplies all the fluids, electrolytes, nutrients (carbohydrates, proteins, and fats), vitamins, and minerals that a patient needs through a vein. If an essential nutrient or trace element is not included, a patient can easily become deficient or imbalanced. Regular laboratory monitoring is necessary to guide TPN therapy and protect against infection.

Pharmacy technicians, especially those working in specialty or home-infusion pharmacies, are involved in mixing TPN solutions. Careful calculations and mixing techniques must be used to ensure that the end product is both safe and appropriate for an individual patient. The order of mixing is important. All clear ingredients should be mixed before cloudy ingredients. Some electrolytes and trace minerals should be added separately to reduce the

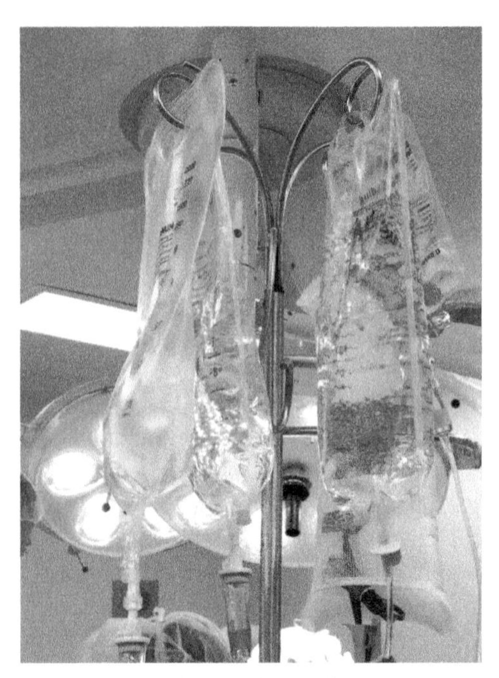

TPN may be infused from two bags at the same time to prevent precipitation problems.

chance of precipitating out of solution. When minerals precipitate out of solution, they bind together and form visible clumps or specks of material. These specks could block capillary blood flow and have dire consequences if introduced through an IV.

Vitamins are usually added to the solution last, just before administration. Proper agitation and mixing of each TPN bag is important to ensure even concentrations throughout. TPN bags are large, so this mixing takes special effort. TPN solutions can be infused temporarily through a peripherally inserted central catheter line but are most often administered through a surgically placed central line because they are hypertonic (higher concentration and osmolality than blood plasma).

TPN solutions can be mixed in two ways: two-in-one and three-in-one mixtures. Two-in-one mixtures contain only proteins (amino acids) and carbohydrate (dextrose); three-in-one mixtures also contain lipids (fats). Patients receiving TPN will need all three nutrient components (carbohydrates, proteins, and lipids), but adding the lipids into the same bag poses complications. In particular, lipids are cloudy and hide the appearance of precipitants, and TPN solutions with lipids are less stable and do not last as long as those with only amino acids and dextrose. TPN bags with lipids are good for seven days if refrigerated and for twenty-four hours if kept at room temperature. Two-in-one mixtures are good for twenty-one days if refrigerated and for seven days if kept at room temperature.

Obesity

The Centers for Disease Control and Prevention estimates that approximately 34% of adults in the United States are obese, an alarmingly high proportion of the population. This proportion has grown over the past few decades. In males, obesity is indicated when ABW is 25% or more above IBW. In females, the figure is 35% or more above IBW. **Morbid obesity** is when ABW is more than twice IBW. "Morbid" indicates that bearing this amount of added weight begins to cause disability. The weight itself causes other medical conditions to emerge.

The causes of obesity are multifactorial and not fully understood. Environmental, genetic, physiological, and psychological factors all contribute to development of obesity in different ways. Environmental factors contributing to obesity include leading a sedentary lifestyle, having a readily available food supply, consuming increased amounts of fat and refined sugar, and decreased amounts of fruits and vegetables. The United States' culture is said to promote weight gain and overnutrition because portion sizes are abnormally large, and the nature of many work settings involves less physical activity than was true just forty years ago. Genetic predisposition is a major factor in obesity and the distribution of body fat. For instance, obesity among first-degree relatives (parents and siblings) is a strong predictor of obesity in adulthood.

Physiologic factors affect appetite control. Peptides such as leptin and incretins as well as neurotransmitters such as serotonin, norepinephrine, and dopamine are involved in **satiety**, the sensation of feeling full and satisfied. As weight and adipose (fat) tissue accumulate, it is thought that normal release and sensitivity to these hormones and neurotransmitters are affected. Other physiologic contributors include medical conditions such as hypothyroidism and Cushing's syndrome. Drugs including corticosteroids cause fat redistribution and appetite changes that foster weight gain.

Obesity is associated with serious health risks and mortality (see Table 16.5). **Centrally distributed fat** is adipose tissue that accumulates in the abdominal area, rather than in the hips, thighs, or buttocks. This kind of fat distribution is linked to

Table 16.5 Comorbid Conditions of Obesity

Hypertension	Eating disorders
Congestive heart failure	Depression
Coronary artery disease	Gallbladder inflammation
Stroke	Gastroesophageal reflux disorder
High cholesterol	Hiatal hernia
Type 2 diabetes	Obstructive airway disease
Polycystic ovarian syndrome	Sleep apnea
Osteoarthritis	Pulmonary hypertension
Degenerative bone and joint disease	Skin tags and stretch marks
Breast and colon cancer	Other dermatologic problems

heart disease and diabetes. Obese people also suffer more from depression and psychological disturbances. Consequently, preventing and treating obesity is an important effort within healthcare.

Drugs for Obesity

The preferred treatment for obesity is lifestyle and dietary changes. Patients who restrict caloric intake and also perform physical activity will lose weight. However, such changes are easier to talk about than to make. Changes must be permanent to keep off lost weight. Consequently, providing products and services for weight loss and physical fitness is a billion-dollar industry.

Special diets tend to restrict specific components of nutrition to achieve weight loss. Popular weight loss programs include those that restrict the intake of carbohydrates or fats. These programs are not often sustainable because they do not represent a balanced way to eat that ensures adequate nutrition in the long term. The most successful and healthy diets are those that restrict caloric intake while maintaining a proper balance in nutrients.

Some patients are candidates for more aggressive therapy options. Medications and/or surgical intervention can achieve significant weight loss. Surgical options include (1) restrictive procedures (laparoscopic banding) that effectively make the stomach smaller and prevent eating excess food, and (2) malabsorptive techniques (gastric bypass) that bypass parts of the intestine, thus preventing food eaten from getting fully absorbed. Whether surgical or drug therapy is chosen for weight loss, patients must meet specific criteria first. Usually, surgical methods are limited to patients with a BMI over 40. Some patients with a BMI over 30 will be considered if they have comorbid health conditions.

Appetite Suppressants

One class of drugs to treat obesity, **anorexiants**, which is another name for **appetite suppressants,** stimulates the central nervous system (CNS) much like amphetamines do. They are used in conjunction with exercise, behavior modification, and reduced caloric intake to produce weight loss in patients with a BMI over 30 (or over 27 with the presence of other risk factors, such as high blood pressure, diabetes, or high cholesterol). These amphetamine derivatives stimulate dopamine and norepinephrine and prevent reuptake of serotonin. Increased neurotransmitter levels signal a sense of fullness and satisfaction. In effect, patients do not feel as hungry. Fast-acting dosage forms are taken thirty minutes to an hour prior to eating, and long-acting forms are taken once a day (see Table 16.6).

Side Effects Common side effects of CNS stimulants are headache, stomachache, insomnia, nervousness, and irritability. Taking these medications in the morning may help reduce insomnia, but other effects can be limiting if they are bothersome. CNS stimulants can also cause dry mouth, difficulty urinating, and constipation. Patients with

Table 16.6 Common Appetite Suppressants

Generic (Brand)	Dosage Form	Route of Administration	Common Dose
Benzphetamine (Didrex)	Tablet	Oral	25–50 mg 1–3 times a day
Diethylpropion (Ienuate)	Tablet	Oral	25 mg 3 times a day (1 hour prior to meals)
Phendimetrazine (Bontril)	Tablet, capsule	Oral	35 mg 2–3 times a day (1 hour prior to meals)
Phentermine (Ionamin, Pro-Fast, Adipex-P)	Tablet, capsule	Oral	15–30 mg once a day (2 hours prior to breakfast)
Sibutramine (Meridia)	Capsule	Oral	10–15 mg a day

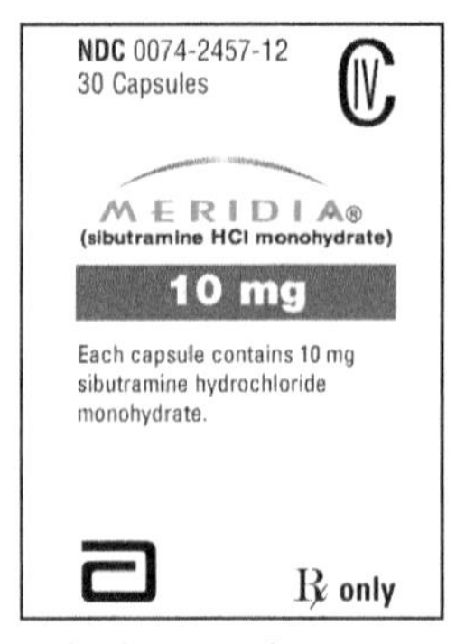

A plan between the physician, patient, and pharmacy should be established to appropriately handle controlled substance restrictions.

urinary problems should not take these medications, and drinking plenty of water can help with these effects. In males, CNS stimulants can cause impotence. Patients should discuss the risks versus benefits of CNS stimulants with their healthcare providers.

A possible serious side effect of CNS stimulants is serotonin syndrome, a condition causing a dangerous rise in blood pressure and heart rate. In fact, deaths have occurred from this syndrome when it is linked to the use of appetite suppressants. These medications should not be taken with other drugs that also increase serotonin (e.g., antidepressants). Cardiac function must be closely monitored. Some patients with cardiovascular problems may not be good candidates for this class of medications.

Cautions and Considerations All CNS stimulants are controlled substances (Schedules II–IV) and have addiction and abuse potential. For Schedule II stimulants, no refills are allowed, and limited supplies can be given at one time. Patients must be informed that a new written prescription is needed each time they need a refill.

Lipase Inhibitor Orlistat is a **lipase inhibitor** used to promote weight loss. Prescription dosing is used for patients with a BMI over 30 (or over 27 with the presence of other risk factors, such as high blood pressure, diabetes, or high cholesterol). OTC dosing is lower and can be used by patients who are overweight but not necessarily obese. Orlistat works by binding to gastric and pancreatic lipase enzymes in the intestines, preventing the enzymes from breaking down fats into a form that can be absorbed. Fat then passes on through the intestines and out of the rectum. Orlistat is taken up to three times a day with meals (see Table 16.7).

Side Effects Common side effects of orlistat include fatty or oily stools, fecal incontinence or urgency, gas, and diarrhea. Patients can reduce these effects by limiting fat intake to less than 30% of total calories. These effects may decrease over time. Patients will find that they must alter their diet by reducing fat intake if they wish to avoid or reduce these effects. If not, they may find the side effects become intolerable.

Cautions and Considerations Because orlistat interferes with the absorption of fat, it can also prevent absorption of fat-soluble vitamins. Patients should take multivitamin supplements to combat potential vitamin deficiency. Pharmacy technicians can help patients locate a suitable supplement containing fat-soluble vitamins.

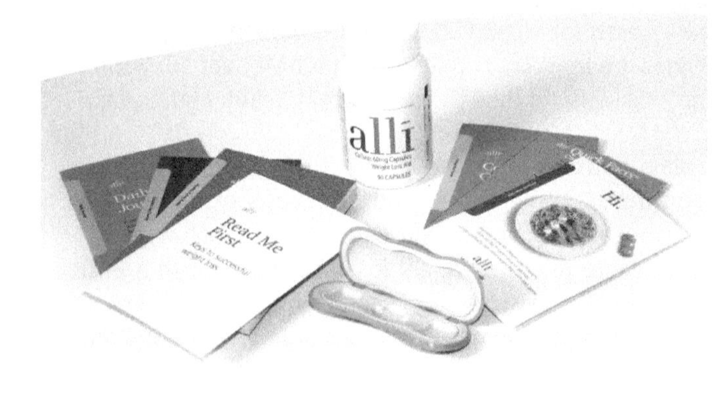

Alli is often advertised in lay literature. Knowing what this product packaging looks like, what it includes, and where it is located in the pharmacy will be useful in answering patient questions.

Table 16.7 Lipase Inhibitors

Generic (Brand)	Dosage Form	Route of Administration	Common Dose	Dispensing Status
Orlistat (Alli)	Capsule	Oral	60 mg with each meal	OTC
Orlistat (Xenical)	Capsule	Oral	120 mg with each meal	Rx

Herbal and Alternative Therapies

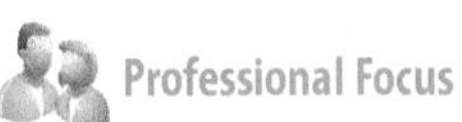

Ephedra use was connected with the death of a young baseball pitcher for the Baltimore Orioles in 2003. This news story prompted efforts to remove ephedra from the market. The Food and Drug Administration banned the sale of ephedra supplements in 2004.

Fiber is a natural substance in fruits and vegetables, which creates a sense of fullness and speeds GI motility, thus limiting fat and calorie absorption. Alone, it may not produce significant weight loss, but fiber can contribute to an overall diet program that results in weight loss. Patients can increase the fiber content of their diet by eating more fruits and vegetables (and reducing meat and carbohydrates). They can also take fiber supplements. Fiber has also been found to produce laxative effects (see Chapter 15), lower cholesterol, and promote colon health.

Ephedra (also known as ***ma huang***) is currently banned from sale in the United States. This natural supplement is a CNS stimulant with anorexiant effects. Serious effects, and even death, occurred from OTC use, so ephedra-containing supplements are no longer sold in the United States.

Chapter Summary

Appropriate nutrition includes the adequate intake of carbohydrates, proteins, fats, and other micronutrients such as vitamins and minerals. Malnutrition (or undernutrition) happens from a lack of appropriate intake or from disease states that affect absorption or digestion. Obesity is excess nutrition that results in a body composition that has too much fat tissue. The two most common methods for estimating body composition are comparing actual body weight (ABW) to a calculated ideal body weight (IBW) and the body mass index (BMI).

Recommended daily intake values are published for all vitamins and minerals. Lack of intake in these amounts can lead to deficiency and physiological consequences. Vitamins are either fat-soluble or water-soluble. A lack of vitamins can cause illness, whereas suffering from an excess of vitamins tends to occur only with fat-soluble vitamins, which accumulate in fatty tissue. Minerals are categorized into electrolytes and trace elements.

When malnutrition is a problem, enteral and parenteral nutrition may be needed. Enteral nutrition is feeding patients through a tube placed in the digestive tract. TPN is feeding patients through an IV. Special considerations and preparations are involved in both products; however, pharmacy technicians may find themselves more involved with TPN when they work in the inpatient or home infusion settings.

Treatment for obesity usually begins with diet and lifestyle changes but may progress to drug therapy if the obesity is severe enough. Medications for obesity include appetite suppressants and lipase inhibitors. Appetite suppressants are CNS stimulants and controlled substances because they can have addiction and abuse potential. They also can have significant cardiovascular side effects, so they are used only for patients with a BMI of 30 and higher. Lipase inhibitors are available as prescription and OTC products. They are easy to use but do come with undesirable side effects if the patient does not follow a diet low in fat. Last, fiber is a natural diet supplement that can promote weight loss. Pharmacy technicians can help patients read labels of vitamins and other dietary supplement products so that patients can make informed decisions about their healthcare.

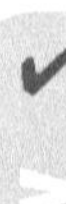

Chapter Review

For the following sets of exercises, write the exercise heading, exercise numbers, and your answers on a separate sheet of paper. Your instructor may direct you to turn in the sheet of paper or discuss your answers as a class.

REVIEW THE BASICS

Choose a, b, c, or d as the correct answer to each multiple-choice question.

1. Which of the following would be considered obesity?
   a. ABW > 110% IBW
   b. BMI = 25
   c. ABW > 150% IBW
   d. BMI = 27

2. Which of the following is a condition in which caloric intake is adequate but protein intake is deficient?
   a. marasmus
   b. kwashiorkor
   c. scurvy
   d. pellagra

3. Deficiency in which of the following vitamins can cause rickets (bone softening)?
   a. A
   b. B
   c. C
   d. D

4. Which of the following vitamins is needed to produce clotting factors and is used to reverse the effects of warfarin?
   a. A
   b. D
   c. E
   d. K

5. Excess of which of the following trace elements is associated with hypothyroidism?
   a. iodine
   b. iron
   c. manganese
   d. copper

6. Obesity can be treated by which of the following?
   a. caloric restriction
   b. increased exercise
   c. prescription anorexiants
   d. all of the above

7. Side effects of orlistat include which of the following?
   a. insomnia
   b. serotonin syndrome
   c. fecal incontinence
   d. all of the above

8. Which of the following is available only by prescription as a controlled substance?
   a. Alli
   b. Xenical
   c. Bontril
   d. ascorbic acid

9. Which of the following is given through an IV?
   a. enteral nutrition
   b. parenteral nutrition
   c. lipase inhibitors
   d. anorexiants

10. Which of the following works by blocking enzymes within the digestive tract from breaking down fat so that the fat can be absorbed?
    a. cyanocobalamin
    b. sibutramine
    c. phentermine
    d. orlistat

KNOW THE DRUGS

Match each brand name drug with its corresponding generic name and most common use. Your answers should follow this example format: Generic Name: 1. a; 2. b; 3. c; etc. Most Common Use: 1. e; 2. f; 3. e; etc.

Brand Name	Generic Name	Most Common Use
1. Xenical	a. benzphetamine	e. inhibiting lipase enzymes, which keeps fat from being absorbed in the intestines
2. Meridia	b. phentermine	f. stimulates dopamine, norepinephrine and enhances serotonin to stimulate the satiety center of the brain to create a sense of fullness
3. Ionamin	c. sibutramine	
4. Didrex	d. orlistat	
5. Alli		

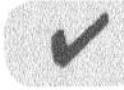

PUT IT TOGETHER

For each item, write down the matching answers, a short answer, a single term to complete the sentence, or true or false.

1. Match these vitamins to their chemical name.

Vitamin	Chemical Name
B_1	a. niacin
B_2	b. pyridoxine
B_3	c. cyanocobalamin
B_5	d. biotin
B_6	e. pantothenic acid
B_7	f. thiamin
B_9	g. riboflavin
B_{12}	h. folate

2. Describe the difference between enteral and parenteral nutrition. Which method is preferred? Why?
3. _______________ is a vitamin that is produced in the skin when exposed to sunlight.
4. Name the fat-soluble vitamins and a toxicity that could result from an excess of each.
5. True or False: Deficiency occurs more rapidly with the fat-soluble vitamins than with the water-soluble vitamins.
6. Describe the similarities and differences between Alli and Xenical.

THINK IT THROUGH

Read and think through each numbered scenario carefully and then write several sentences in reply to the question(s) presented. Question 4 requires you to do some Internet research before completing your answer(s).

1. Mrs. Dean comes to the pharmacy to pick up her prescription for Boniva and is about to purchase a bottle of calcium to go with it. She is eighty-two years old and says that she was just diagnosed with osteoporosis. She is hoping the new drug therapy will help with her back pain. What can you do to improve the effectiveness of her new regimen as you check her out at the register?
2. A forty-four-year-old patient comes to the pharmacy to purchase niacin for high cholesterol. He has an order from his physician for Niaspan (a prescription niacin product) but would like to save some money and get an OTC version. He seems to understand the dosage and instructions that his physician and the pharmacist gave him about taking niacin. What else can you do to help this patient get good results and remain adherent to therapy?
3. A patient who weighs 225 pounds and is 6 feet, 4 inches tall comes to the pharmacy and wants to know if he would be a candidate for Pro-Fast. He says his brother used this medication and lost more than sixty pounds. He wants to lose some weight and is considering a diet plan. He would like to take an appetite suppressant to help speed the weight loss. Calculate this patient's BMI and IBW. What can you do to assist this patient?

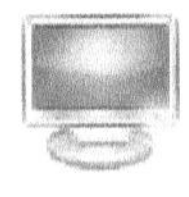

4. **On the Internet,** look up a few Web sites you would consider to be accurate and reputable resources that your pharmacy could recommend to patients to calculate their BMI. How might you use these Web sites with patients?

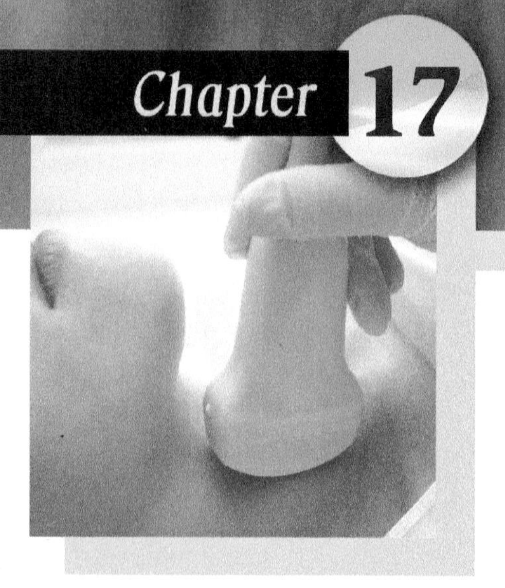

Chapter 17 The Endocrine System and Drug Therapy

LEARNING OBJECTIVES

- Describe the basic anatomy and physiology of the endocrine system.
- Explain the therapeutic effects of prescription medications, nonprescription medications, and alternative therapies commonly used to treat diseases of the endocrine system.
- Describe the adverse effects of prescription medications, nonprescription medications, and alternative therapies commonly used to treat diseases of the endocrine system.
- Identify the brand and generic names of prescription and nonprescription medications commonly used to treat diseases of the endocrine system.
- State the doses, dosage forms, and routes of administration of prescription and nonprescription medications commonly used to treat diseases of the endocrine system.

Interactive self-quizzes, games, audio files, and glossaries help you to learn drug names and facts.

Disorders of the endocrine system are on the rise. As obesity rates climb in the United States, the incidence of Type 2 diabetes is increasing dramatically. In fact, diabetes has been compared to an epidemic in scale and impact on the healthcare system. Myriad drug therapies treat diabetes, but none completely cure it. Therefore, the pharmacy field finds itself at the center of diabetes care efforts and is increasingly called on to aid in treatment and educational efforts for patients. As pharmacists move into direct patient care, pharmacy technicians must become familiar with an increasing number of pharmacologic options and devices sold in pharmacies. In some cases, technicians work directly with patients to teach them how to monitor blood glucose at home.

The endocrine system regulates many different bodily functions and includes several different organs. This chapter focuses on disorders with common drug therapies encountered most often in a pharmacy. These disorders include diabetes, thyroid disorders, and adrenal gland disorders. Pharmacologic options to treat diabetes are expanding, so these drug classes are covered in depth. Glucose monitoring systems are also mentioned, because technicians can help patients choose one system and learn to use it.

Anatomy and Physiology of the Endocrine System

The **endocrine system** is a collection of glands located in various parts of the body that produce hormones that regulate physiological functions (see Figure 17.1). Endocrine **hormones** are secreted substances that regulate metabolism, maintain fluid balance, control the life cycle, stimulate growth, and generate responses to stressful stimuli. Hormone release is regulated by a **negative feedback system**. As more hormones are released into the bloodstream, receptors detect the rise in concentration and signal the associated gland to slow further production. Often, this feedback loop includes a series of hormones, each one controlling release of the next. For instance, the **hypothalamus** produces hormones that regulate the pituitary gland, which in turn releases several different hormones.

The **pituitary gland** plays an important role in controlling several other endocrine glands and bodily functions. The hormones it produces vary widely in the target tissues they affect (see Figure 17.2). It is an integral part of the **hypothalamic-pituitary axis,** a core feedback mechanism that controls endocrine function.

The **thyroid gland** releases **tri-iodothyronine (T_3)** and **thyroxine (T_4)** in response to **thyroid-stimulating hormone (TSH)** released from the pituitary gland. Iodine is necessary for formation of thyroid hormones. Whereas T_3 is responsible for the majority

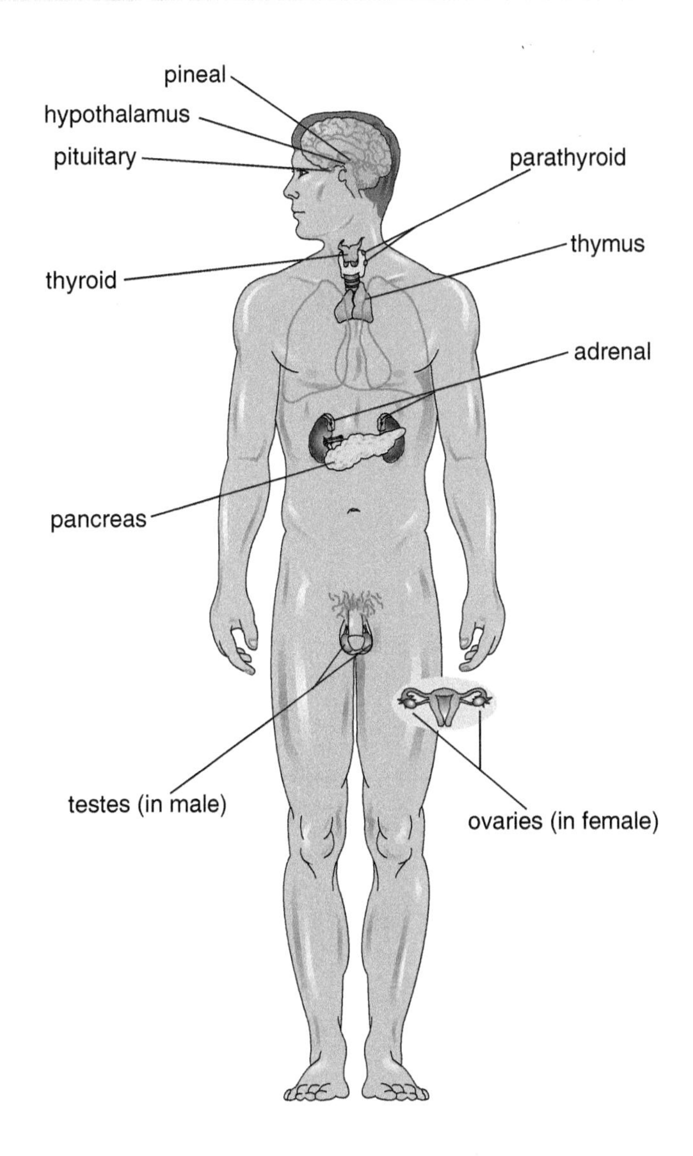

Figure 17.1
Endocrine System
Endocrine glands release hormones directly into the bloodstream, where they travel throughout the body to trigger responses in specific target tissues.

of the physiological action, both T_3 and T_4 regulate basal metabolic rate and affect metabolism of carbohydrates, fats, and proteins. Thyroid hormones increase conversion of food to energy and thereby raise body temperature. The thyroid gland is found in the neck surrounding the trachea (see Figure 17.3). The **parathyroid gland** is located on top of the thyroid. It releases **parathyroid hormone**, which regulates calcium and phosphorus balance within the body.

The **adrenal glands** are located on top of the kidneys. The inner layer, called the **adrenal medulla**, produces **adrenaline** (**epinephrine**). Heavy physical activity, stress, and low blood glucose trigger the medulla to produce adrenaline. Adrenaline, also called epinephrine, elevates blood pressure and diverts blood away from body organs to muscles (see Figure 17.4). It also prompts release of stored glucose and fats into the blood. These actions ready the body to "fight or flight" in a stressful situation.

The outer layer of the adrenal glands, called the **adrenal cortex**, releases **corticosteroids,** including mineralocorticoids and glucocorticoids. **Mineralocorticoids** regulate fluid and electrolyte balance; **glucocorticoids** affect day/night cycles and metabolism. The hypothalamus produces corticotropin-releasing factor, which stimulates the pituitary gland to make **adrenocorticotropic hormone (ACTH)**. ACTH travels through the blood to the adrenal glands, where it stimulates release of **cortisol**, the primary glucocorticoid, in a **circadian rhythm**. This rhythm cycles every twenty-four hours, peaking in the morning and decreasing at night (see Figure 17.5). Cortisol affects glucose metabolism, fat deposition, water retention, and anti-inflammatory action of the immune system. Although the ovaries and testes produce the vast majority of sex hormones,

Figure 17.2

Pituitary Gland

The pituitary gland plays a key role in growth, onset of puberty, and reproduction cycles.

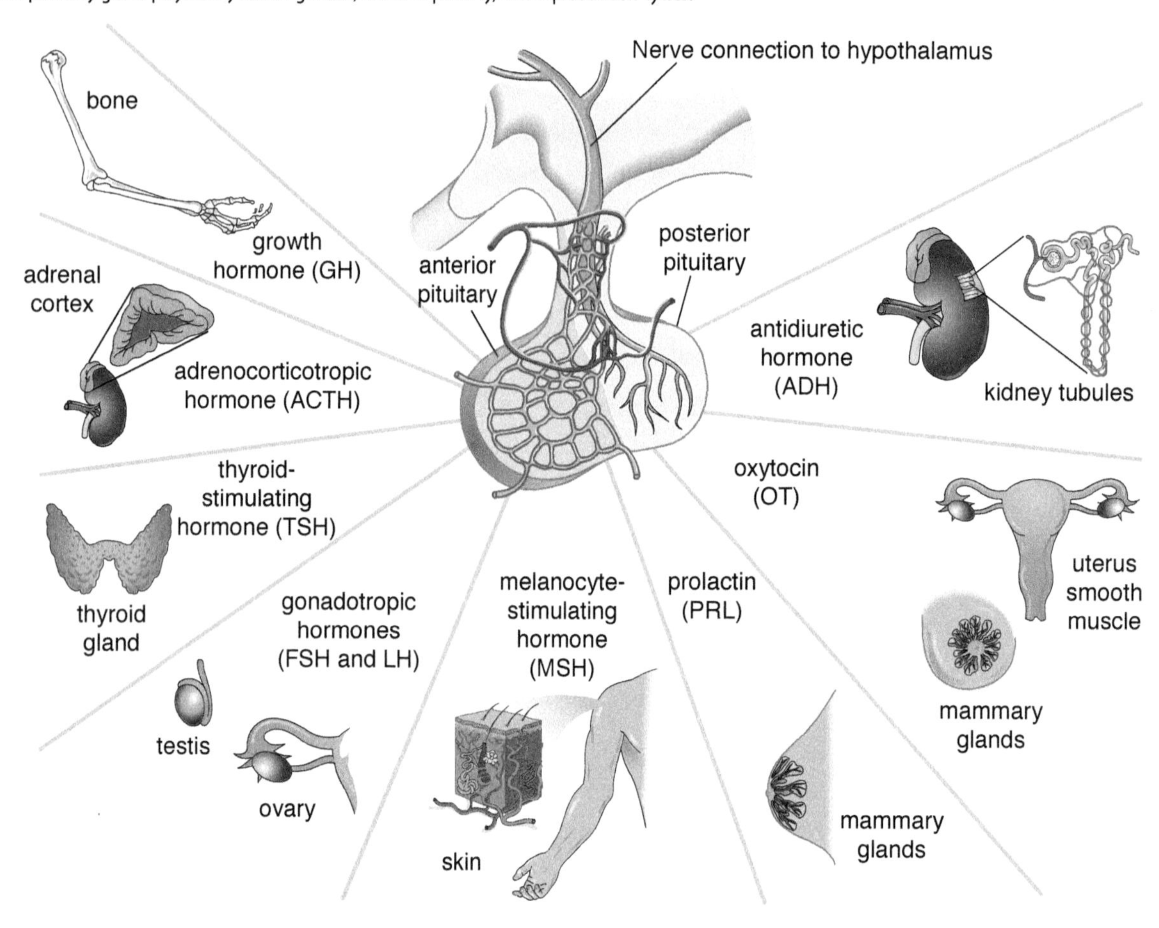

Figure 17.3

Thyroid Gland

Iodine deficiency causes the thyroid gland to enlarge and form a visible lump on the neck if not treated. Such a lump is called a goiter.

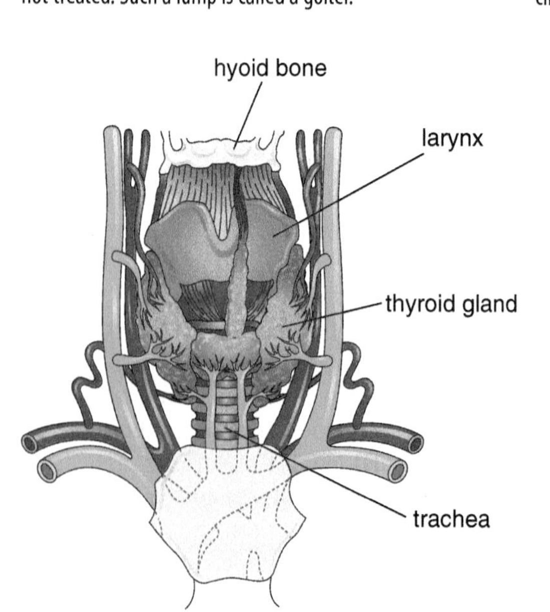

Figure 17.4

Adrenal Glands

Adrenaline can give someone tremendous strength or speed when encountering a fearful circumstance.

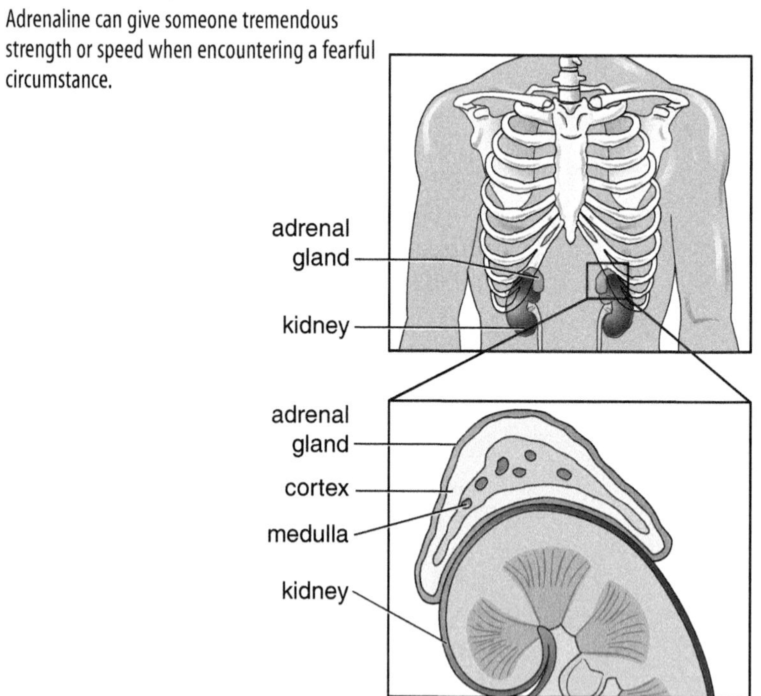

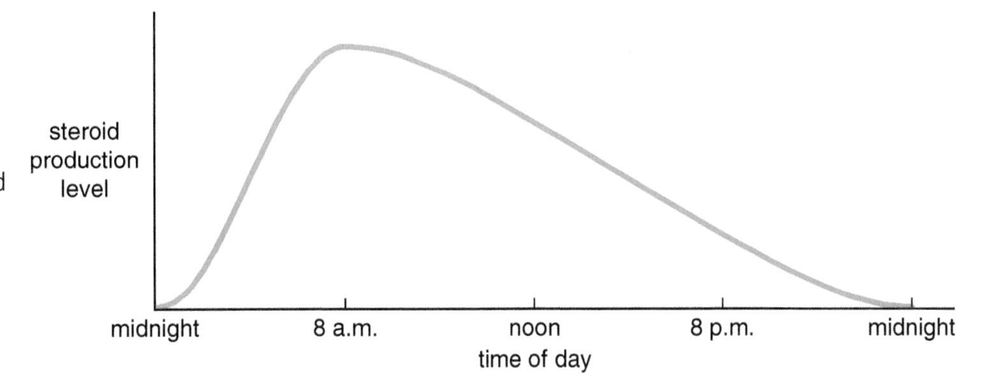

Figure 17.5
Circadian Rhythm of Cortisol
Cortisol ramps up metabolism in the morning in advance of daily activity and meals, and slows down for rest and sleep at night.

aromatase (an enzyme made by the adrenal glands) converts estrogen and testosterone to active forms in other parts of the body.

The **pancreas** is a large gland located in the abdomen, just under the stomach. In addition to producing digestive enzymes and releasing them into the intestine, the pancreas produces **insulin** and **glucagon**. **Alpha islet cells** produce glucagon, and **beta islet cells** produce insulin. Insulin is released in response to a rise in blood glucose, such as what happens after eating a meal, especially if that meal is high in **carbohydrates** (see Figure 17.6). Insulin connects with receptors on the surfaces of cells to activate channels in the membrane allowing glucose to enter. In effect, insulin is the key that opens the door allowing glucose to enter cells. Glucose provides the energy all cells need to live.

Glucagon, on the other hand, raises blood glucose levels. It activates liver cells to break down stored glycogen molecules into glucose and release it into the blood. Glucagon is released in response to low blood glucose, such as in between meals and overnight (see Figure 17.7). Glucagon also facilitates breakdown of fats and proteins as alternative sources of energy. Although this process is useful in the short term to maintain life, **ketones** (by-products of this alternative energy source) are produced. Ketones have toxic effects when they accumulate in the blood.

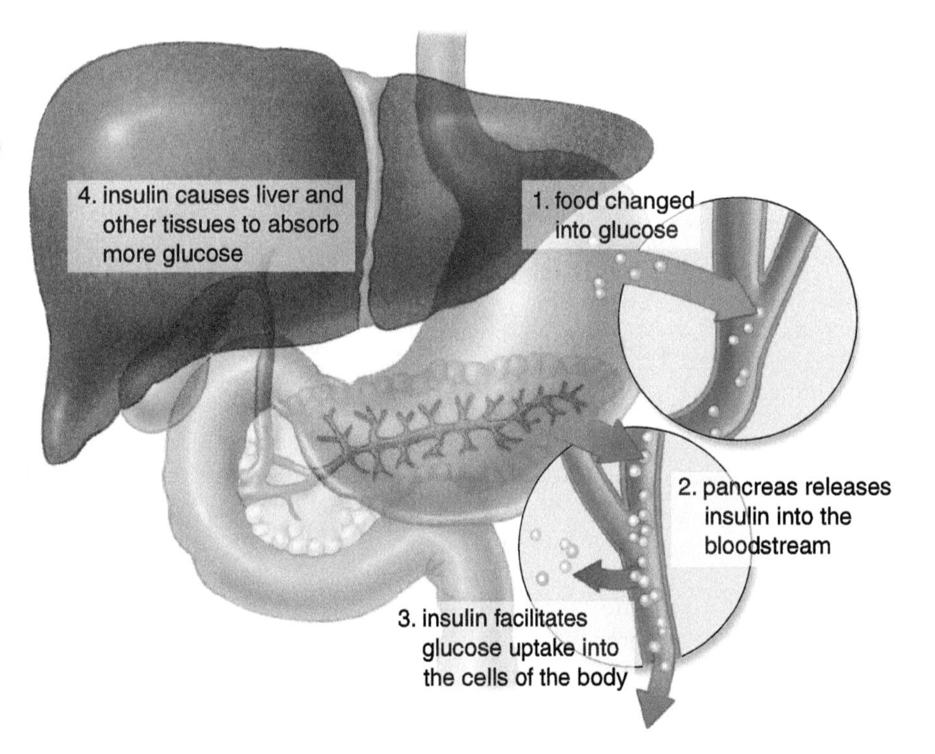

Figure 17.6
Pancreas and Normal Glucose Metabolism
The pancreas releases insulin after you eat to lower blood glucose and releases glucagon when you are fasting to maintain adequate blood glucose.

Figure 17.7
Maintaining Blood Glucose Levels
A variety of hormones produced by the pancreas, adrenal glands, and pituitary gland participates in maintaining appropriate blood glucose levels after eating and in between meals.

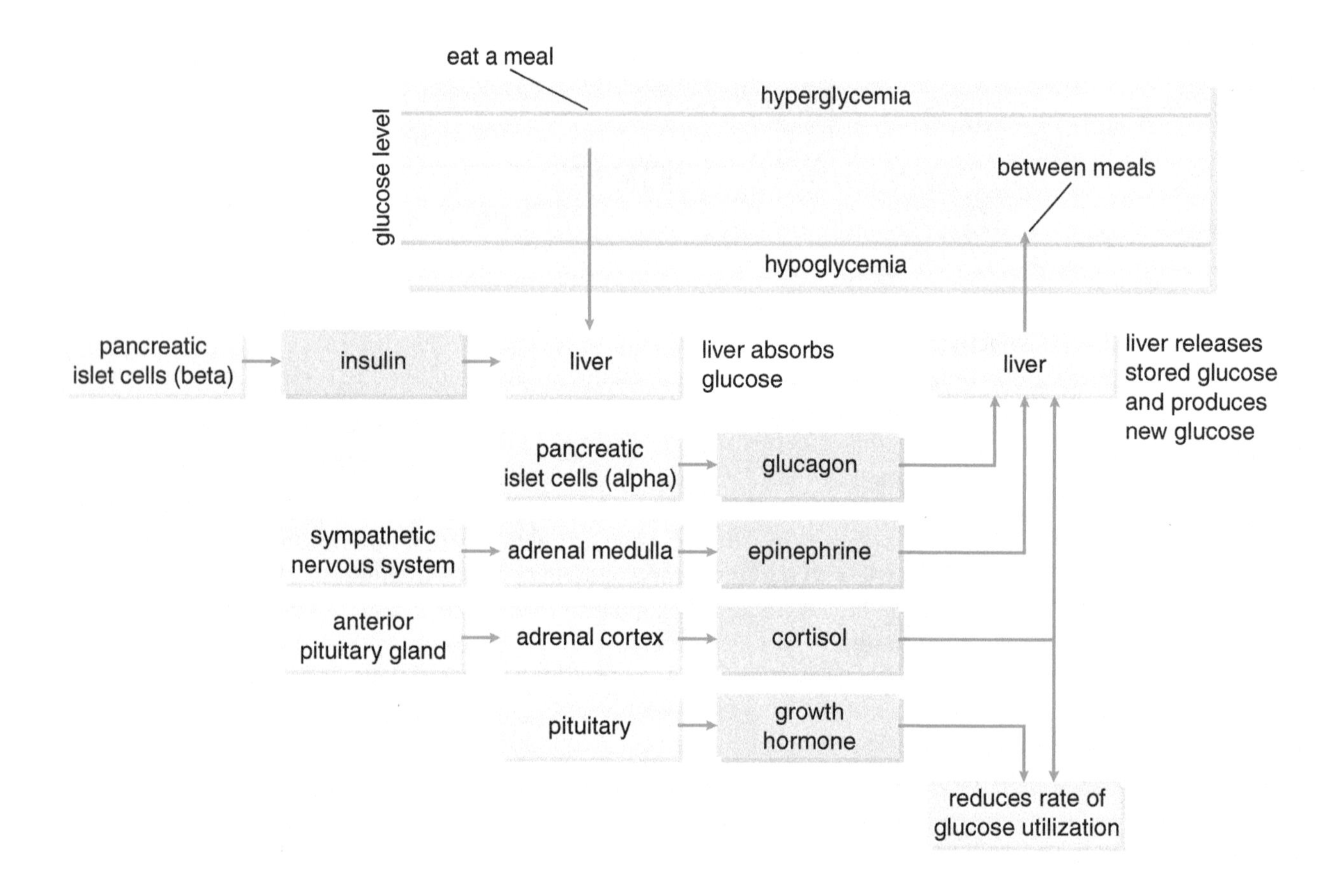

Diabetes

In simple terms, **diabetes mellitus** (commonly known as diabetes) refers to elevated blood glucose that results in damage to small blood vessels and nerve tissue that has significant and life-threatening effects. Diabetes has multiple causes and is categorized into Type 1, Type 2, and gestational diabetes. **Type 1 diabetes** (sometimes called juvenile diabetes) is the least common, affecting only about 10% of patients with diabetes. It is an autoimmune process that destroys the islet cells within the pancreas, impairing and eliminating the ability to make insulin (see Figure 17.8). Patients with Type 1 diabetes must be given insulin to stay alive. If insulin is not present, glucose remains in the blood and climbs to dangerous levels. The body also begins using alternative energy sources, producing ketones. **Ketoacidosis** is a life-threatening emergency in which ketones accumulate to toxic levels in the blood.

Type 2 diabetes is a multifactorial disorder causing high blood glucose (see Figure 17.9). It accounts for around 90% of patients with diabetes. Usually, Type 2 diabetes starts with accumulation of abdominal fat (**central obesity**), which is highly resistant to the effects of insulin. The pancreas still makes insulin, but the insulin does not work as well as it should. In fact, insulin receptors around the body become less sensitive to its effects. This **insulin resistance** triggers a cascade of other abnormal metabolic processes, one of which is overproduction of glucagon from the pancreas. Glucagon further increases blood glucose by promoting release of unneeded glucose from the liver into the blood. At first, the beta cells compensate for additional glucose by producing excess insulin, but eventually they cannot keep up and their ability to make insulin

Figure 17.8
Type 1 Diabetes
Insulin is given to patients with Type 1 diabetes because their pancreas no longer produces any insulin.

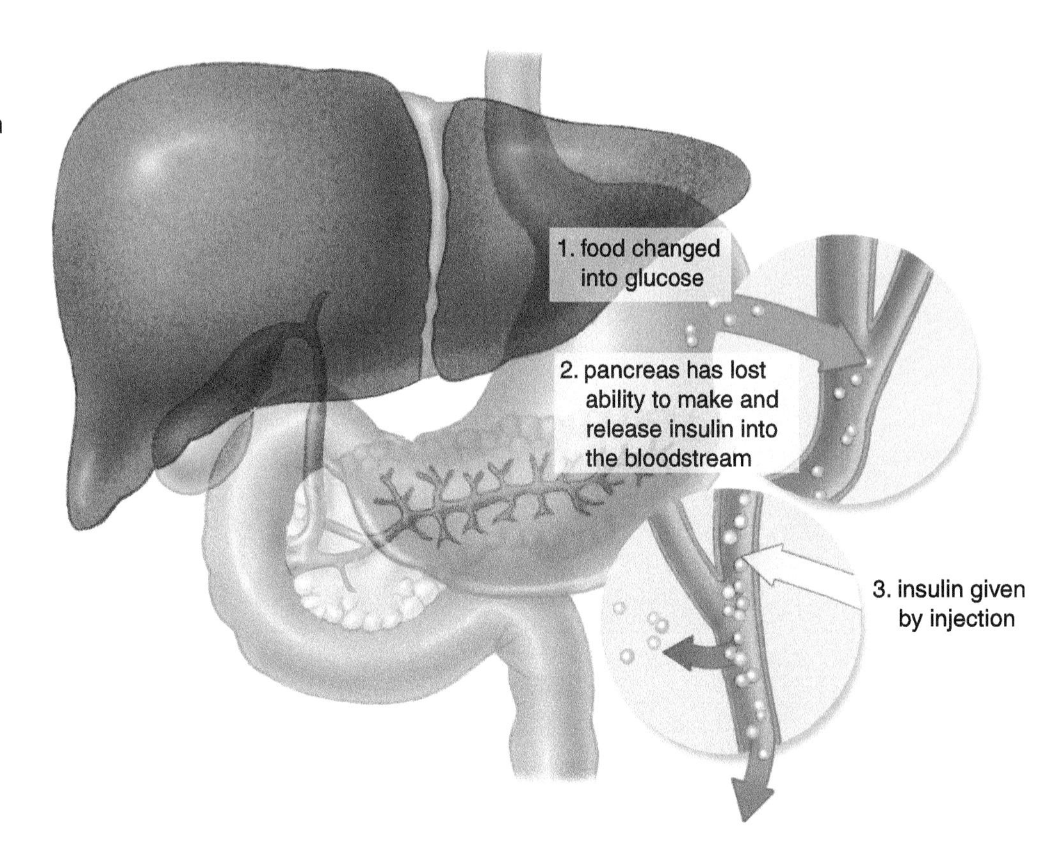

Figure 17.9
Type 2 Diabetes
Type 2 diabetes is a multifactorial disorder including insulin insensitivity, impaired insulin production, and altered glucagon release.

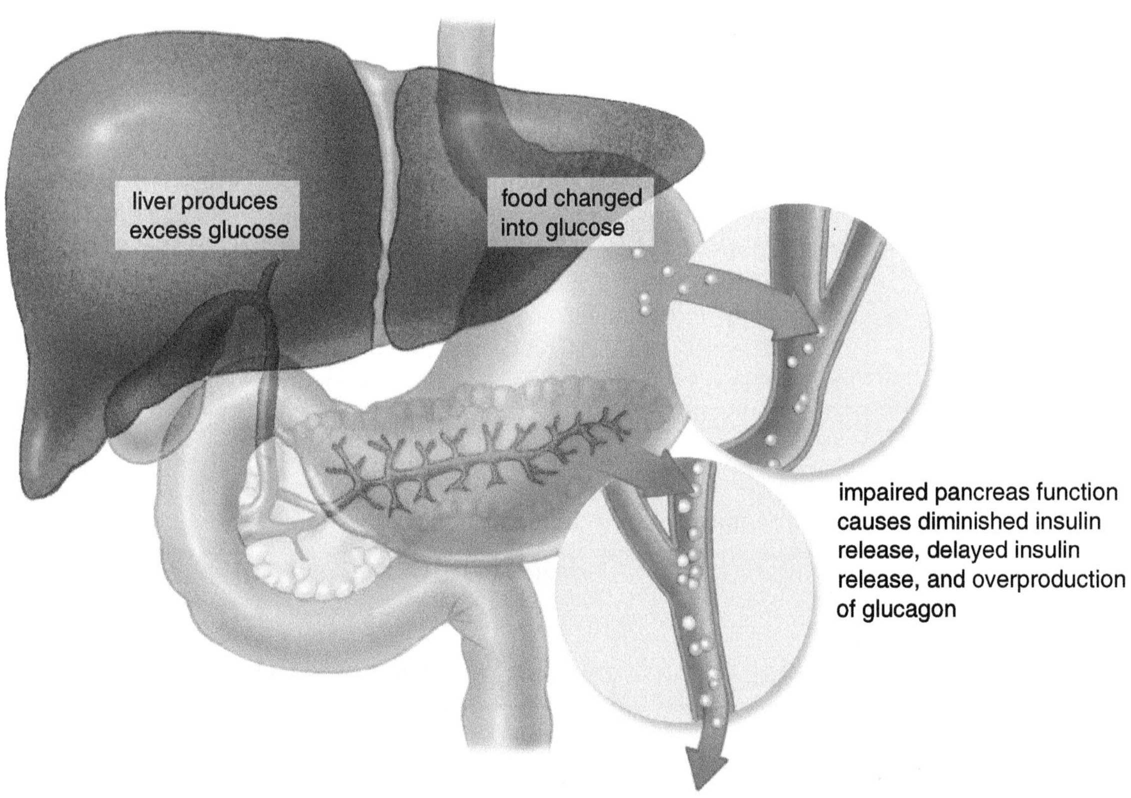

diminishes. Thus, Type 2 diabetes is characterized first by insulin insensitivity and then by **relative insulin insufficiency**. Type 2 diabetes is a progressive disease that worsens over time, necessitating changes in treatment every few years.

Many people with Type 2 diabetes have **metabolic syndrome**. This condition refers to a triad of problems: high blood pressure, high cholesterol and triglycerides, and high blood glucose. Patients do not have to be diagnosed with diabetes to have metabolic syndrome. Patients may not have high blood glucose all of the time. They may have impaired fasting glucose (elevated blood sugar on waking) or impaired glucose tolerance (elevated blood sugar after eating) along with hypertension and high triglycerides. Patients with metabolic syndrome are at high risk for cardiovascular disease.

Gestational diabetes results from insulin resistance caused by hormones produced in excess during pregnancy. Pregnancy hormones, especially progesterone, cause insulin resistance in the mother to preserve glucose availability for the developing fetus. Therefore, gestational diabetes mimics Type 2 diabetes and often precedes it.

Patients should be aware of risk factors for developing diabetes. Risk factors for Type 2 diabetes include:

- age over 45 years
- family history of diabetes (parents or siblings)
- overweight (body mass index over 25 kg/m^2)
- habitual physical inactivity
- race/ethnicity (African American, Asian, or Latino)
- impaired fasting glucose or impaired glucose tolerance
- hypertension (blood pressure over 140/90 mmHg)
- cholesterol abnormalities (low high-density lipoproteins and high triglycerides)
- history of gestational diabetes or birth of baby over nine pounds
- polycystic ovary syndrome

Prominent symptoms of diabetes, no matter the cause, include increased urination (**polyuria**), excessive urination at night (**nocturia**), glucose in the urine (**glycosuria**), thirst (**polydipsia**), hunger (**polyphagia**), blurred vision, and fatigue. Other symptoms and effects of diabetes include frequent infections, slow wound healing, weight gain or loss, and numbness and tingling in fingers and toes. Onset of these symptoms is sudden in Type 1 diabetes but is slow to appear in Type 2 diabetes. Unfortunately, many patients do not realize they have Type 2 diabetes until they have had it for years.

When glucose cannot enter cells, it remains in the bloodstream and causes damage to tiny blood vessels and capillaries in important organs such as the kidneys, eyes, and heart. These **microvascular complications** are leading causes of dialysis and kidney transplants, blindness, and lower leg amputations (see Table 17.1). **Macrovascular complications** of Type 2 diabetes include heart disease, heart attack, and strokes. Someone with diabetes is half as likely to survive a heart attack as someone without it. Consequently, the ultimate concern about diabetes is preventing long-term complications.

If a patient is taking insulin or other medication for diabetes, **hypoglycemia** (low blood glucose or low blood sugar reaction) is possible. Hypoglycemia commonly results from injecting too much insulin or skipping meals when taking medication for diabetes.

Table 17.1 Microvascular Complications of Untreated Diabetes

Nephropathy	Damage to kidneys, affecting their ability to filter the blood. If left untreated, it can lead to kidney failure. In fact, the leading cause of dialysis and kidney transplant is diabetic nephropathy.
Neuropathy	Damage to tiny nerves in the extremities. In the feet, loss of sensation can lead to ulcers, infection, and, ultimately, amputation. The leading cause of lower leg amputations is diabetic neuropathy.
Retinopathy	Damage to retina tissue in the eyes. If left untreated, it can progress to blindness. The leading cause of blindness (other than congenital causes) is diabetic retinopathy.

Symptoms of hypoglycemia include:

- shakiness
- dizziness
- sweating
- headache
- irritability
- confusion
- vision changes
- hunger

Patients experiencing these symptoms should test their blood glucose, if possible, and get something to eat or drink with sugar in it right away. To treat hypoglycemia, patients should ingest 15–30 g of carbohydrate in the form of simple sugar. Juice, nondiet soda, hard candy, and glucose tablets are good sources of such carbohydrates. Although foods such as pasta, bread, and rice are carbohydrates, they consist of complex carbohydrates (or starch) that take time for the body to break down. The glucose in foods or beverages with simple sugar will reach the bloodstream more quickly. Patients should understand that ingesting large amounts of food is not necessary and will raise blood glucose too much.

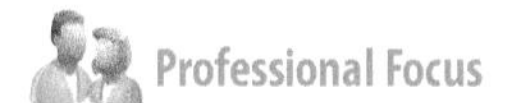

Patients are commonly sent from their prescriber to the pharmacy to buy a glucose meter, and you will frequently be asked which one they should purchase. Become familiar with the glucose meters available in your workplace so you can help patients select one. Take a few minutes to determine what the patient needs in a glucose meter and what they can afford to buy based on factors in the bulleted list to the right.

Measuring Blood Glucose

Diabetes is detected by measuring **blood glucose** (sugar) concentrations. Concentrations can be determined via laboratory blood tests or fingerstick technology at home. The normal range for blood glucose is 70–120 mg/dL. Any random blood glucose result of 200 mg/dL or greater or a fasting result (at least eight hours since eating) of 126 mg/dL or greater is diagnostic for diabetes. The purpose of measuring blood glucose is to determine trends in its concentration throughout the day. Many **glucose meters** are available for home use to allow patients to monitor their blood sugar levels. Immediate feedback about blood glucose level at any time of day can help patients determine trends for high and low concentrations. These results guide drug therapy as well as help the patient to make changes in diet and exercise. The goal is to maintain blood glucose concentrations within the normal range.

Pharmacy technicians can assist patients in choosing a glucose meter for purchase in the pharmacy and even teach patients hands-on how to use one. Factors that patients should consider when choosing a glucose meter are:

- cost (or third-party coverage for the meter and/or strips)
- ease of use
- patient comprehension of steps for operation and calibration
- size of drop of blood required (most meters require very little blood)
- patient preference for size and portability of meter and strips
- patient dexterity and eyesight (some strips are small, thus difficult to handle)
- patient preference for measuring sites other than fingertips (many meters perform alternate site testing on palms, arms, and legs)
- patient preference for meter memory, extra data functions, and ability to download results to a computer
- speed in producing results (time to results varies from five to forty-five seconds)

The test used to assess overall blood glucose control is the **hemoglobin A1C** test. Normal range for an A1C is 4–6%, but patients with untreated diabetes can have an A1C of 10% or greater. This test can be run via a blood draw in the laboratory or fingerstick technology in a clinic or pharmacy setting. The A1C measures the percentage of red blood cells (RBCs) with glucose stuck to the hemoglobin molecules contained inside. Glucose irreversibly binds to hemoglobin and remains there for the life span of the RBC. Because RBCs live for about three months in the body, this test provides an overall average of glucose concentration in the blood over the previous three months. Both blood glucose and A1C testing can be conducted in pharmacies with proper staff training and equipment.

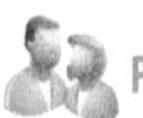

Professional Focus

Research the software packages and connection hardware your pharmacy would need to offer meter downloading services. Downloading and printing meter results provides a great service and teaching tool for patients and helps them take control of their diabetes.

Drugs for Diabetes

As the incidence of diabetes increases, drug therapy options available to treat it expand. Unfortunately, none cure the disorder. However, the variety of medication choices can be customized to achieve good outcomes for individual patients. Patients must often be reminded that although high blood sugar does not necessarily make them feel sick, it does cause long-term damage to vital organs. The leading cause of death in people with diabetes is heart disease and stroke. Fortunately, treating diabetes dramatically reduces risk of developing long-term complications.

Type 1 diabetes requires treatment with insulin, because these patients cannot make their own insulin. Treatment for Type 2 diabetes begins with **lifestyle modifications**: changes in diet to reduce carbohydrate, fat, and calorie intake; regular exercise for thirty minutes most days of the week; smoking cessation; and weight loss. Drug therapy begins with metformin, progresses to combination therapy, and eventually requires insulin to achieve goals for blood glucose and A1C.

Metformin Initial drug therapy for Type 2 diabetes is **metformin**. It can be used alone or in combination with other agents and works by inhibiting excess hepatic glucose production, a process that normally occurs at a slow rate overnight. Metformin also increases insulin sensitivity in muscle and other tissues of the body.

Metformin is typically taken two to three times a day with food or meals. When treatment begins, a low dose is prescribed so as to avoid stomach upset, abdominal cramps, and diarrhea. Slowly dosage is increased. Metformin can take as long as three weeks to reach full effect. It usually does not cause hypoglycemia unless it is taken in combination with other agents for diabetes. Metformin can also promote mild weight loss (five to six pounds) and improve cholesterol profiles. The best time to test blood glucose when taking metformin is in the morning, just after waking. See Table 17.2 for metformin products.

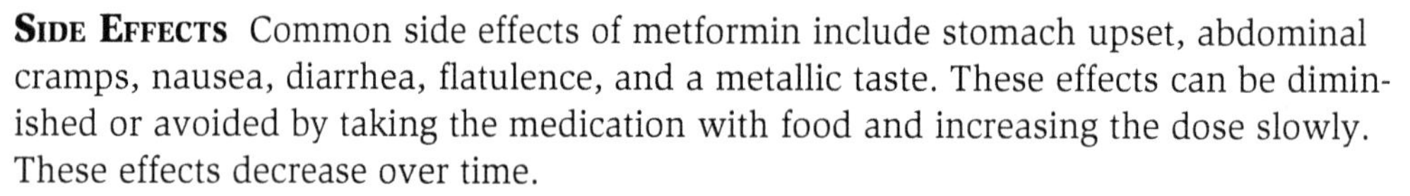

Side Effects Common side effects of metformin include stomach upset, abdominal cramps, nausea, diarrhea, flatulence, and a metallic taste. These effects can be diminished or avoided by taking the medication with food and increasing the dose slowly. These effects decrease over time.

Serious but rare side effects include **lactic acidosis**, a potentially fatal condition. Lactic acidosis only occurs if the patient becomes severely dehydrated or takes other medications that contribute to kidney impairment or altered fluid balance. It can usually be avoided altogether if patients stop taking metformin when they are severely ill or hospitalized.

Table 17.2 Metformin Products

Generic (Brand)	Dosage Form	Route of Administration	Common Dose
Metformin (Glucophage)	Tablet, oral solution	Oral	500–1,000 mg twice a day
Combination Products			
Glipizide/metformin (Metaglip)	Tablet	Oral	2.5 mg/250 mg to 5 mg/500 mg twice a day
Glyburide/metformin (Glucovance)	Tablet	Oral	1.25 mg/250 mg to 5 mg/500 mg twice a day
Pioglitazone/metformin (ACTOplus Met)	Tablet	Oral	15 mg/500 mg to 15 mg/850 mg once or twice a day
Repaglinide/metformin (Prandimet)	Tablet	Oral	1 mg/500 mg to 2 mg/500 mg 2 or 3 times a day
Rosiglitazone/metformin (AvandaMet)	Tablet	Oral	2 mg/500 mg to 4 mg/1,000 mg a day
Sitagliptin/metformin (Janumet)	Tablet	Oral	50 mg/500 mg to 50 mg/1,000 mg once or twice a day

Cautions and Considerations Patients should cease taking metformin treatment when undergoing procedures in which contrast dye or iodine substances are used. Such patients are usually instructed to stop taking metformin one or two days before their procedure. Drug interactions between these substances and metformin can precipitate kidney failure and lactic acidosis. Metformin is contraindicated in patients who have kidney dysfunction, liver problems, or heart failure, because these conditions raise the risk for lactic acidosis.

Insulin Secretagogues Agents that stimulate insulin production from the pancreas to directly lower blood sugar are known as **insulin secretagogues**. Two common classes of insulin secretagogues are **sulfonylureas** and **glinides**. The difference between sulfonylureas and glinides is the onset and duration of action. Sulfonylureas can take thirty minutes or more to start working and last for eight hours or longer. Glinides act within ten minutes and last for around two hours.

Sulfonylureas are used alone or in combination with other agents to treat Type 2 diabetes. They are taken prior to breakfast each day and sometimes again before dinner. Glinides are used in combination with other agents for Type 2 diabetes. They are taken just prior to eating and give an extra boost of insulin for a specific meal. Table 17.3 provides information on common insulin secretagogues.

Side Effects Low blood sugar reactions (hypoglycemia) are the most common side effect of these medications. Hypoglycemia tends to occur when a patient takes the medication but then skips a meal or does more physical activity than usual. Patients can avoid this by not skipping meals or omitting a dose when they anticipate eating significantly less than usual on a particular day. Other side effects include nausea, diarrhea, and constipation.

Cautions and Considerations Because sulfonylureas and glinides increase the risk of hypoglycemia, patients should be informed of the symptoms of low blood sugar and know how to treat it. Special glucose tablets can be purchased in the pharmacy to have on hand in case such a reaction occurs. Patients should monitor their blood glucose at home regularly and whenever they feel they may be low. The best time to check blood sugar when taking sulfonylureas is when waking in the morning before eating (fasting) and occasionally before other meals during the day. The best time to check blood sugar when taking glinides is 1–2 hours after meals.

Patients with liver or kidney disease may not be able to take sulfonylureas depending on the agent chosen. Patients with these conditions should talk with their prescribers before taking one of these agents.

Table 17.3 Common Insulin Secretagogues

Generic (Brand)	Dosage Form	Route of Administration	Common Dose
Sulfonylureas			
Glimepiride (Amaryl)	Tablet	Oral	2–4 mg a day
Glipizide (Glucotrol)	Tablet	Oral	5–10 mg a day
Glyburide (DiaBeta, Micronase, Glynase)	Tablet	Oral	5–10 mg a day
Glinides			
Nateglinide (Starlix)	Tablet	Oral	60–120 mg prior to meals
Repaglinide (Prandin)	Tablet	Oral	0.5–2 mg prior to meals

Thiazolidinediones (Glitazones or TZDs) Agents known as **glitazones (thiazolidinediones, or TZDs)** are used in combination with metformin or sulfonylureas for Type 2 diabetes (see Table 17.4). They work by directly increasing insulin sensitivity in cells of the body. TZDs connect with intracellular receptors to stimulate production of more insulin receptors. This process can take weeks to months to occur, thus onset of effect is not immediate. The best time to check blood sugar when using TZDs is in the morning, before eating (fasting), and occasionally after meals during the day.

Table 17.4 TZDs

Generic (Brand)	Dosage Form	Route of Administration	Common Dose
Pioglitazone (Actos)	Tablet	Oral	15–30 mg a day
Rosiglitazone (Avandia)	Tablet	Oral	4–8 mg once or twice a day

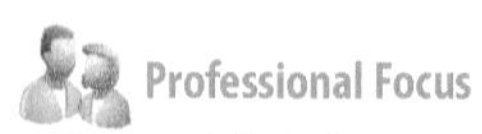

Professional Focus

You can help diabetes patients take good care of themselves by reminding them to get an eye exam, cholesterol test, flu shot, and foot exam annually.

Side Effects Common side effects of TZDs include fluid accumulation (edema) and weight gain. If patients notice rapid weight gain or swelling, especially with shortness of breath, they should talk with their prescribers right away.

Rare but serious effects include liver toxicity and macular edema (swelling of the eye, resulting in distorted vision). If patients experience unexplained nausea, vomiting, abdominal pain, fatigue, or dark urine, they should report these symptoms to a healthcare provider. Regular blood tests will be conducted to monitor liver function. Patients with diabetes should see an eye doctor annually to receive an exam in which their pupils are dilated and retinas are examined.

Cautions and Considerations Because TZDs can cause fluid retention and edema, they can worsen heart failure. Patients with heart failure should not take TZDs. Patients with edema or other heart problems may not be good candidates for TZD therapy.

In some women with fertility problems, TZDs have increased ovulation and increased pregnancy rates. Patients who are sexually active but do not want to become pregnant should use birth control to avoid the chance of pregnancy.

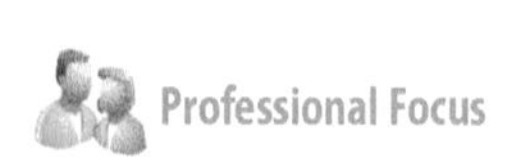

Professional Focus

Incretin therapies tend to be expensive, so many insurance plans require prior authorization. Insurance coverage may not pay for one of these products until other, less expensive ones have been tried first. You can reduce frustration by helping patients understand this process.

Incretin Therapies Incretin drugs either mimic endogenous incretin hormones or change the metabolism of them to increase their activity. **Glucagon-like peptide-1 (GLP-1)** and **glucose-dependent insulinotropic polypeptide** are **endogenous incretin hormones**, which are produced in response to glucose arriving from the gut. They have multiple physiological effects. First, incretins facilitate proper timing and function of phase I and II insulin response. **Phase I insulin** response refers to the immediate burst of insulin that occurs just as, or even slightly before, the first bite of food. **Phase II insulin** response refers to the continued but somewhat slower release of insulin in the hours after eating. In Type 2 diabetes, both phase I and II insulin responses are blunted. Second, incretins inhibit glucagon production from the pancreas that otherwise promotes an undesirable increase in blood glucose. Third, incretins have some effect on appetite and produce **satiety**, a sensation of fullness and satisfaction. For this reason, these agents promote weight loss. Other medications such as sulfonylureas, TZDs, and insulin are associated with weight gain. Many patients experience significant and sustained weight loss on incretin mimetics. Incretin drug therapies are used most often in combination with other medications for Type 2 diabetes. Common incretin drugs are listed in Table 17.5.

Exenatide and liraglutide are injectable products that mimic the action of GLP-1. Because this substance is released only when glucose is introduced to the bloodstream, it does not cause hypoglycemia between meals. Exenatide is injected twice a day, thirty minutes before breakfast and dinner. Liraglutide is injected once a day.

Table 17.5 Incretin Therapies

Generic (Brand)	Dosage Form	Route of Administration	Common Dose
Exenatide (Byetta)	Injection	SC	5–10 mcg twice a day
Liraglutide (Victoza)	Injection	SC	0.6–1.2 mg a day
Pramlintide (Symlin)	Injection	SC	15–120 mcg per dose
DPP-4 Inhibitors			
Saxagliptin (Onglyza)	Tablet	Oral	2.5–5 mg a day
Sitagliptin (Januvia)	Tablet	Oral	100 mg a day

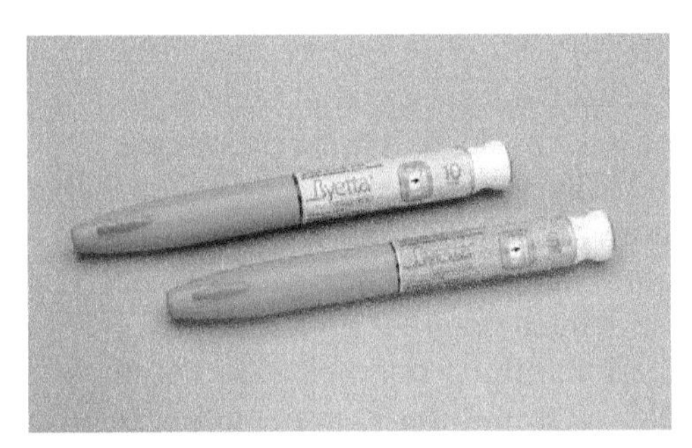

Exenatide is available in a self-injector pen device that patients can easily learn to use.

Pramlintide mimics amylin, a hormone co-produced with insulin that reduces glucagon production, slows gastric emptying, and produces satiety. This incretin mimetic can be used by patients with Type 1 diabetes to supplement insulin. Addition of pramlintide to the insulin regimen can dramatically reduce the amount of insulin a patient has to take. Pramlintide is injected thirty minutes prior to each meal or snack containing at least 30 g of carbohydrate. Pramlintide is available in vials and uses typical insulin syringes for injection. This drug is dosed in micrograms, not insulin units. Therefore, measuring the correct amount can be tricky.

Saxagliptin and sitagliptin are oral **dipeptidyl-peptidase (DPP-4) inhibitors** that slow inactivation of incretin hormones, allowing them to persist longer and produce beneficial effects. Satiety does not seem to be as pronounced with these agents, and thus weight loss is not usually an added benefit. They are taken daily without regard to food.

Side Effects Common side effects of GLP-1 drugs include nausea, vomiting, diarrhea, dizziness, fatigue, and headache. Nausea is quite common at the beginning of therapy but diminishes over time. Side effects can be minimized by beginning treatment at a low dose and increasing slowly. Timing injections immediately before eating can reduce nausea, vomiting, and upset stomach. Over a period of several weeks, the patient can move the time of injection further ahead of eating until reaching thirty to sixty minutes prior to a meal.

Common side effects of DPP-4 inhibitors include headache, nasopharyngitis (runny nose and sore throat), and upper respiratory tract infections. The reason for these somewhat odd side effects is not fully understood.

Cautions and Considerations Doses of DPP-4 inhibitors are renally cleared, so they must be adjusted for patients with kidney disease. Patients with kidney problems should alert their prescribers, so that proper dosing is ordered.

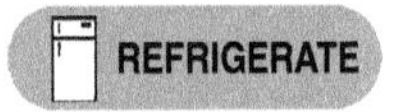

Injectable incretin products must be stored in the refrigerator until dispensed. Once they come to room temperature, they begin to degrade. Injectable incretin products are good at room temperature for only thirty days. Therefore, patients should keep these products in the refrigerator until they begin using them. Once opened, they can be kept at room temperature. Patients should protect these products from heat or freezing.

Insulin Insulin is generally produced in a combination of basal and bolus rates to maintain steady glucose concentrations in the blood (see Figure 17.10). **Basal insulin** is slowly released throughout the day and night to allow energy for basic cellular function. In contrast, **bolus insulin** is released at mealtimes to react with glucose entering the body from food intake. When giving insulin by injection, the goal is to mimic this natural physiological insulin production. For patients with Type 1 diabetes, multiple injections each day of combination basal and bolus insulins are necessary to achieve physiological insulin

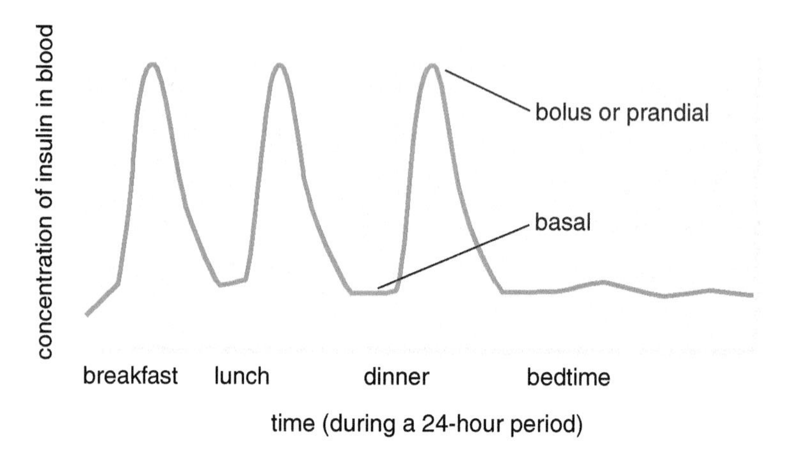

Figure 17.10
Normal Glucose Production
The timing of bolus insulin released with meals is called prandial, which means with meals.

dosing. Patients with Type 2 diabetes may be given insulin in a similar physiological dosing schedule or one injection at bedtime of long-acting insulin added to oral medications.

Insulin is essential for survival in someone with Type 1 diabetes. In Type 2 diabetes, insulin is used later in the course of disease treatment as an adjunct to other therapies. **Rapid-acting insulin** begins to work in ten minutes and, for practical purposes, lasts as long as two hours. It is given just before meals to reduce prandial rises in blood glucose. **Short-acting insulin** begins to work in around thirty minutes and lasts up to four hours in most cases. It is taken prior to meals as well. **Intermediate-acting insulin** begins to be effective in thirty to sixty minutes and lasts six to eight hours in most cases. It is used either once or twice a day. **Long-acting insulin** works for approximately twenty-four hours and is injected once a day (see Table 17.6 and Figure 17.11).

Insulin is available by injection only because it is a protein. If taken orally, the protein structure is denatured and deactivated by stomach acid before it reaches the bloodstream. Therefore, patients who need insulin must learn to self-inject into the subcutaneous (SC) tissue. Figure 17.12 shows places where SC injections of insulin are given. The abdomen is the preferred **insulin injection site** because rate of absorption into the blood is most consistent there. Physical activity increases blood flow to large leg muscles, dramatically increasing insulin absorption. Patients using this site should inject immediately before bedtime, when they will be inactive for a few hours.

Insulin is available in **vials** for use with **syringes** as well as in **self-injector pen devices**. Patients must be instructed how to use a pen injector or draw up insulin into a

Table 17.6 Commonly Used Insulins

Generic (Brand)	Onset of Action	Maxiumum Peak and Duration	Appearance and Dispensing Status
Rapid-Acting			
Insulin aspart (NovoLog)	10–15 minutes	1–2 hours; 4 hours	Clear; Rx only
Insulin glulisine (Apidra)	Few minutes	1 hour; 2 hours	Clear; Rx only
Insulin lispro (Humalog)	10–15 minutes	1–2 hours; 4 hours	Clear; Rx only
Short-Acting			
Regular insulin (Humulin R, Novolin R)	30 minutes	4 hours; 8 hours	Clear; OTC
Intermediate-Acting			
NPH insulin (Humulin N, Novolin N)	1 hour	6–8 hours; 24 hours	Cloudy; OTC
Long-Acting			
Insulin detemir (Levemir)	1 hour	Peak is possible with Levemir but absent with Lantus; 24–36 hours	Clear; Rx only
Insulin glargine (Lantus)	1 hour	None; 24–36 hours	Clear; Rx only

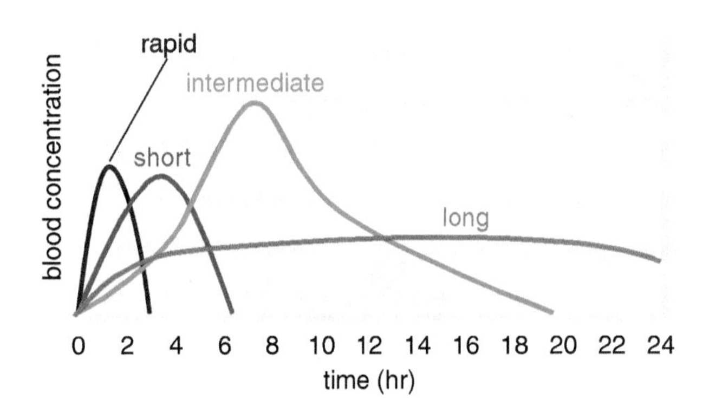

Figure 17.11
Onset and Duration of Action for Insulin
Rapid (bolus) insulins are used most often with long-acting (basal) insulins to mimic normal pancreatic function.

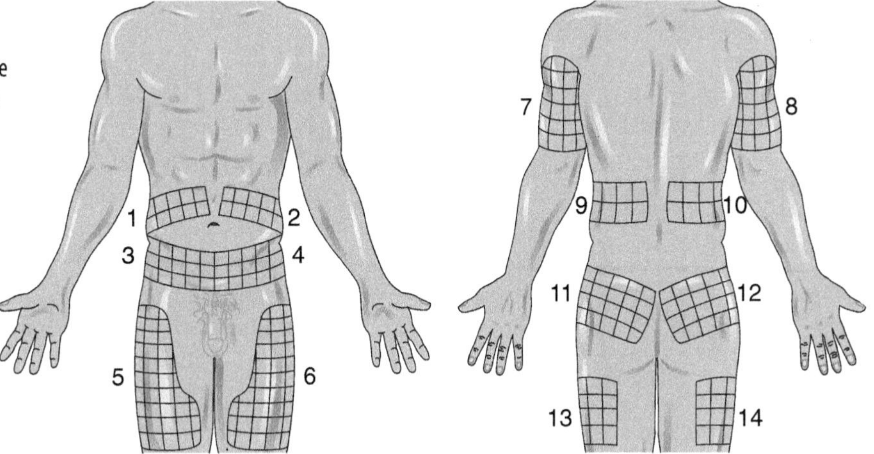

Figure 17.12
Insulin Injection Sites
Patients should rotate injection sites on areas of the body, keeping injections at least one to two inches away from previous injections on the skin.

syringe, measure the correct amount, prepare the injection site appropriately, and inject into an appropriate site on the body. **Insulin pumps** are also available; these deliver insulin through a tiny tube inserted just under the skin. These pumps can be programmed to deliver just the right amount of insulin each hour of the day for an individual patient. The tube must be reinserted every three days. Pumps eliminate the need for multiple injections a day, but must be well understood and properly maintained to work effectively. Inhaled insulin was available for a short while but was taken off the market due to limited market performance. Other inhaled insulins are currently in clinical trials and are expected to reach the market soon.

Side Effects The most common "side effect" of insulin is hypoglycemia. Though often listed as a side effect, hypoglycemia is, in fact, the intended effect of insulin. However, someone using insulin is at increased risk of developing serious hypoglycemia when doses are too high or meals are skipped. If blood glucose concentrations are lower than 40 mg/dL, loss of consciousness and brain damage can occur. Diabetic coma is life-threatening if not treated immediately. Patients must be educated about signs and symptoms of hypoglycemia and know how to treat it if symptoms occur.

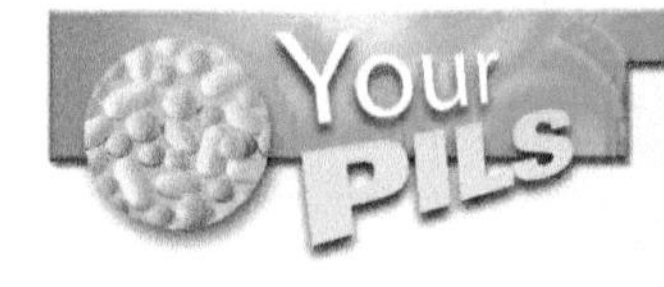

If you like working with abstract concepts, as Creators do, copy Figure 17.11 onto a piece of paper and label each line representing insulin with its corresponding generic and brand name insulin products. For each type of insulin, identify the time of day and frequency patients should check their blood glucose to see if the medication is working.

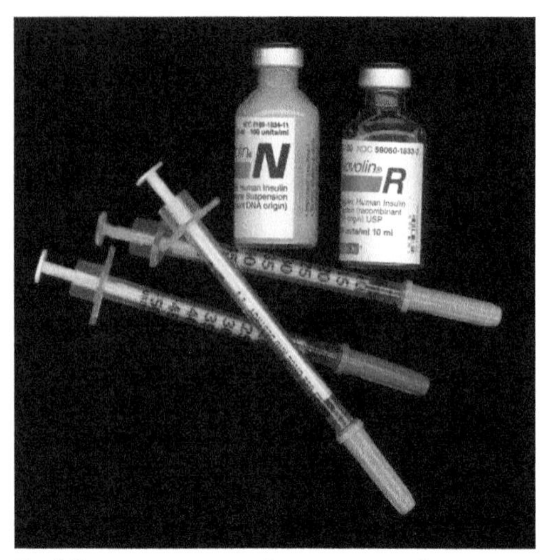

The difference in appearance between intermediate-acting and short-acting insulins is easy to see. Intermediate-acting insulins are cloudy (see the N-insulin vial) and short-acting insulins are clear (see the R-insulin vial). Because long-acting insulins (not shown) are also clear, they are distinctively packaged in a vial that is taller and thinner than those containing the other insulins.

Other side effects are rare but can include lipodystrophy (fat accumulation or depletion at injection site). This effect can be largely avoided by rotating injection sites.

Cautions and Considerations Because most hospitalizations and emergency room visits for patients with Type 1 diabetes result from hypoglycemic events, the risk of hypoglycemia cannot be overemphasized. Patients must be instructed how to recognize and treat low blood sugar when it happens. Family members of someone who uses insulin should be taught how to administer glucagon. It is given when the patient is unconscious from hypoglycemia and cannot self-treat by eating or drinking something with sugar in it.

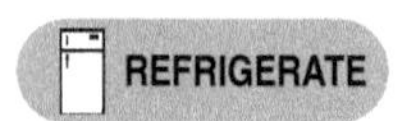

All insulin products must be stored in the refrigerator until dispensed. Once insulin warms to room temperature, the protein begins to degrade. Therefore, patients should keep insulin vials or pens in the refrigerator until they use them. Once opened, insulin vials will expire in twenty-eight to thirty days. Most insulin pens are also good for one month after opening, but a few expire in fourteen days. If exposed to extreme heat or cold, insulin can become damaged. Patients should protect insulin from heat (e.g., do not keep it in a car during the summer) or freezing temperatures. Keeping insulin with them in a carry-on bag when flying is recommended, as air cargo areas on planes are not climate controlled. Patients should discard any insulin package that contains clumps or appears frosty.

It is easy to confuse insulins that have different onsets of action, even for pharmacy staff. Such mistakes pose potentially life-threatening effects for patients. Boxes of insulin look the same and are all the same size, so be sure to double-check the label when dispensing insulin.

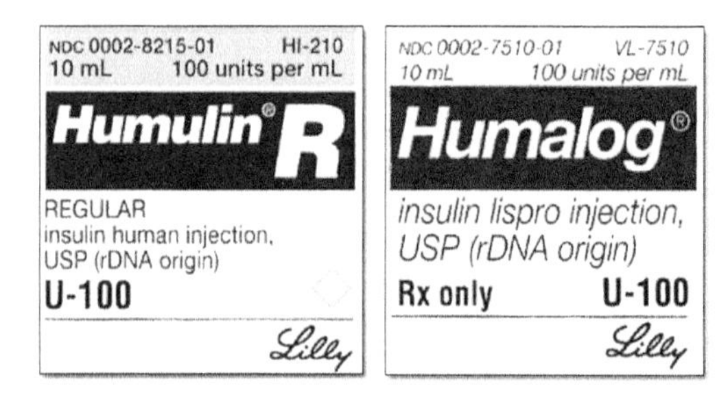

Humulin and Humalog have look-alike, sound-alike names. Be sure to select the correct insulin package every time you dispense.

Alpha-Glucosidase Inhibitors

Acarbose and miglitol are **alpha-glucosidase inhibitors**, adjunctive treatment choices for Type 2 diabetes. They work by inhibiting digestion of carbohydrates within the gastrointestinal system, which reduces glucose absorption. Alpha-glucosidase inhibitors are taken with the first bite of each meal to keep carbohydrates within the food from entering the bloodstream in high amounts. Use of these agents is often limited by side effects, which include abdominal pain, gas, bloating, and diarrhea. These effects can be minimized by starting with low doses and increasing gradually; even so, many patients find them too bothersome.

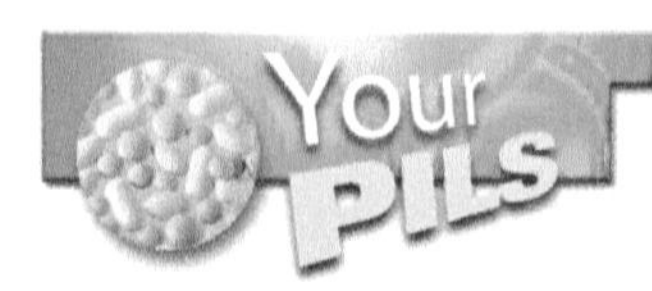

If you are a visual learner or like to learn in small groups, as do Directors and Enactors, try using pictures to learn the drugs for Type 2 diabetes. Draw a diagram of the organs and abnormal functions involved in diabetes, then write the drug names that address each abnormal process next to the organ involved. Explain your diagram to a classmate and ask him or her to do the same for you. Teaching someone else is one of the best ways to solidify concepts in your own mind.

Thyroid Disorders

Thyroid disorders include hyperthyroidism, whereby too much thyroid hormone is produced, and hypothyroidism, in which too little thyroid hormone is produced. Hypothyroid conditions are more common than hyperthyroid. Causes of **hypothyroidism** other than general dysfunction include autoimmune destruction of thyroid tissue (known as **Hashimoto's disease**), radioactive iodine therapy, surgical removal of the thyroid, or pituitary and hypothalamus dysfunction. Symptoms of hypothyroidism include constipation; bradycardia; depression; fatigue; dry skin, nails, and scalp; tremors; reduced mental acuity; memory loss; intolerance to cold; lower voice pitch; and weight gain.

Causes of **hyperthyroidism** include **Graves' disease**, thyroid nodules or tumors, or pituitary nodules or tumors. Symptoms of hyperthyroidism include diarrhea, skin flushing, nervousness, hyperactivity, insomnia, heat intolerance, perspiration, tachycardia, decreased menses, and weight loss. One visible sign of hyperthyroidism is **exophthalmos**, a condition in which fat collects behind the eyeball, causing protrusion and inability for eyelids to fully close. In addition to natural causes of hyperthyroidism, too much thyroid hormone can cause someone to experience these symptoms.

Figure 17.13
The Hypothalamic-Pituitary Axis and Thyroid Hormones
A high TSH test results means that T3 and T4 are low (hypothyroid).

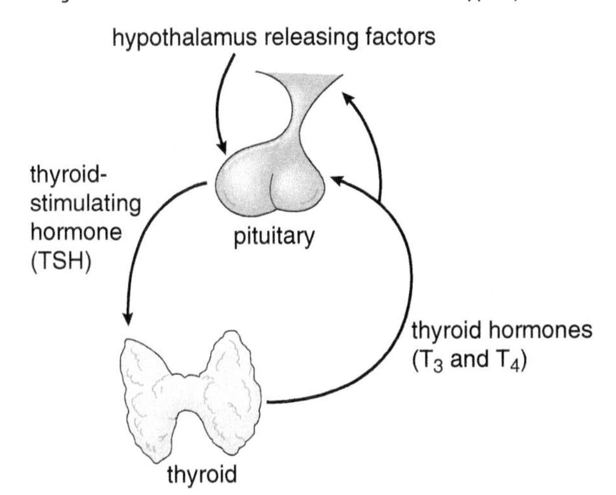

Thyroid disorders are diagnosed through combining symptom history with interpretation of laboratory tests. The primary lab test used to detect and monitor thyroid disorders is TSH. TSH is released from the pituitary gland to stimulate the thyroid to make T_3 and T_4 (see Figure 17.13). If TSH is high, the pituitary gland is sensing low T_3 and T_4 levels in the blood (via the feedback loop) and producing extra TSH to stimulate the thyroid.

Drugs for Thyroid Disorders

Treatment for hyperthyroid disease usually involves surgery, which removes or reduces the malfunctioning gland, or **ablation**, which destroys the thyroid gland via radioactive iodine. Afterward, **oral thyroid supplementation** is given to artificially provide adequate hormone levels. In hypothyroidism, thyroid hormone supplementation is needed and accomplished with the same oral medications as used after thyroid ablation in hyperthyroid disease.

Even though the Food and Drug Administration has approved generic substitution for thyroid hormone products, variability between products is still possible, Therefore, patients are instructed to chose one brand or generic version of thyroid hormone and continue with it consistently. Switching between brands and generic forms of thyroid hormone can result in variability in drug delivery and corresponding hormone levels measured in the laboratory. Because doses are adjusted and maintained on results obtained from one product, the patient should not switch products if at all possible.

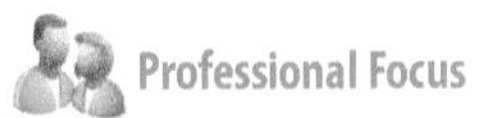

Make a reference card to keep in your pocket with the tablet colors and corresponding strengths for thyroid products. Such a tool comes in handy when talking to patients and answering questions about thyroid supplements. Patients generally remember the color of their tablet more easily than the strength.

Thyroid Hormone Drug treatment for hyperthyroidism and hypothyroidism is generally the same: oral thyroid medication. The difference is that in hyperthyroidism the thyroid gland is removed or ablated (destroyed) using radiation first. Then, supplementation with oral thyroid hormone (see Table 17.7) is used to maintain appropriate levels of T_3 and T_4 in the blood. Hypothyroidism is treated simply with oral thyroid hormone supplementation. Doses are individualized to each patient using blood tests to measure hormone levels. Once an appropriate dose is found for a patient, it is taken daily.

Table 17.7 Common Thyroid Hormone Products

Generic (Brand)	Dosage Form	Route of Administration
Levothyroxine (Synthroid)	Tablet	Oral
Liothyronine (Cytomel)	Tablet	Oral
Liothyronine (Triostat)	Tablet, solution for injection	Oral, injection
Liotrix (Thyrolar)	Tablet	Oral
Thyroid extract (Armour Thyroid)	Tablet	Oral

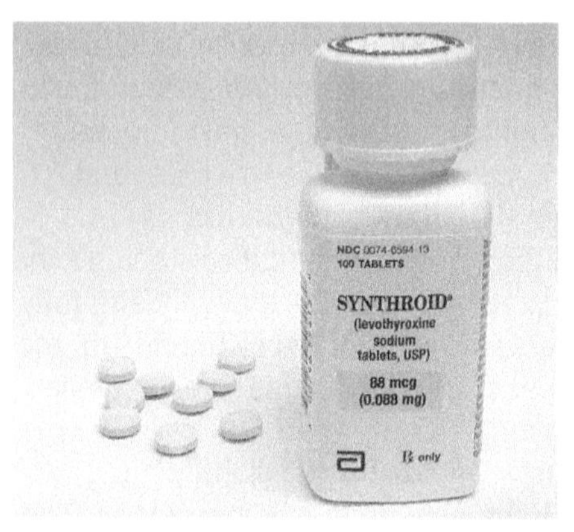

Each tablet strength of thyroid hormone is color-coded to help patients identify their dose by tablet color. The pale green tablets in this photo correspond with the strength of 88 mcg.

Side Effects Common side effects of thyroid hormone are usually related to therapeutic overdose, when someone exhibits hyperthyroid symptoms due to excess thyroid hormone. Such symptoms include heart palpitations, fast heartbeat, elevated blood pressure, fever, tremors, headache, nervousness, insomnia, anxiety, hyperactivity, irritability, diarrhea, vomiting, abdominal cramps, flushing, sweating, heat intolerance, and weight loss. Patients should notify their prescribers if any of these effects begin to happen. Long-term overdosage can also cause loss of bone density and impair fertility. If gross overdosing continues, cardiac arrest can happen.

Cautions and Considerations Patients should be reminded to get regular, periodic blood tests to check thyroid hormone levels. When filling thyroid products, pharmacy technicians should use the same product for the same patient for each refill. Various brands of thyroid hormone may contain slightly different amounts, enough for changes in therapy to be felt by individual patients. Once one brand of thyroid hormone is chosen, the patient should continue receiving that brand at each refill.

Adrenal Gland Disorders

As with thyroid disorders, **adrenal gland disorders** can be categorized by either the overproduction or the underproduction of hormones.

Addison's disease is a deficiency, or underproduction, of glucocorticoids and mineralocorticoids. Symptoms include weakness, hyperkalemia (high potassium levels), hyperpigmentation of skin, low blood sodium, low blood glucose, low blood pressure, and weight loss. This condition can be serious and must be treated with oral corticosteroids. See Chapter 4 for more details on oral corticosteroid therapy.

Cushing's disease, on the other hand, is an overproduction of steroid hormones. Symptoms include round, puffy face (called moon face); abdominal weight gain; osteoporosis; mood changes and psychosis; hypertension; cataracts; peptic ulcer disease; and fat accumulation over the shoulder blades (called buffalo hump). Normal sleep and wake cycles may also be affected as the circadian rhythm is disrupted. Cushing's disease is often caused by tumors of some kind in the adrenal glands, but elevated steroid hormones can also be caused by overmedication with corticosteroids. Surgery is used most often to remove tumors causing Cushing's disease, and sometimes cytotoxic drug therapy is used. See Chapter 21 for more details on cytotoxic drug therapies.

Herbal and Alternative Therapies

Chromium is an essential trace element that has been used for diabetes prevention and treatment. Its effectiveness is somewhat controversial in that patients should not expect dramatic reductions in blood glucose from taking it. Patients with diabetes have been found to be deficient in chromium, but little definitive evidence is available to verify that correcting chromium deficiency is beneficial for improving blood glucose levels. Typical doses range from 200 mg to 1,000 mg a day. Side effects are rare but may include headache, insomnia, diarrhea, and hemorrhage/blood loss. Patients with kidney or liver disease should not take chromium.

Cinnamon is often taken for Type 2 diabetes, but research shows that it has minimal effects on blood glucose. One initial study showed potential benefits, but all subsequent trials have shown that cinnamon has little effect on blood sugar. Even though sellers of cinnamon products claim benefits, patients should know that taking cinnamon may not produce any noticeable effect on their blood glucose or A1C results. Patients with liver disease probably should not take cinnamon because it has the potential to exacerbate hepatic conditions.

Chapter Summary

The endocrine system regulates various bodily functions via hormone production. This system of glands regulates metabolism, growth, and fluid balance in a variety of ways. The thyroid gland controls the metabolic rate, which has effects on weight, heart rate, and digestion. Hypothyroidism is treated with oral thyroid hormone supplementation. The adrenal glands produce steroid hormones that affect metabolism, appetite, daily wake/sleep cycles, and fat deposition in the body. Addison's disease is a deficiency of steroid hormones, whereas Cushing's disease is overproduction of these hormones.

The pancreas produces insulin and glucagon, which regulate blood glucose levels. Without glucose, cells in the body die from lack of energy. Type 1 diabetes is an autoimmune disorder that destroys beta cells in the pancreas, eliminating their ability to produce insulin. Type 2 diabetes begins with central obesity that causes insulin insensitivity. Eventually, insulin and glucagon production are altered, and blood glucose rises. Insulin is used exclusively to treat Type 1 diabetes. Type 2 diabetes is treated with oral agents first, but most patients end up needing insulin at some point. Oral agents for Type 2 diabetes include metformin, sulfonylureas, TZDs, and incretins. Because Type 2 diabetes is so prevalent in our population, medications for it are among the top 100 drugs dispensed in pharmacies. Pharmacy technicians can help patients learn to use glucose meters and test their blood glucose at home.

Chapter Review

For the following sets of exercises, write the exercise heading, exercise numbers, and your answers on a separate sheet of paper. Your instructor may direct you to turn in the sheet of paper or discuss your answers as a class.

REVIEW THE BASICS

Choose a, b, c, or d as the correct answer to each multiple-choice question.

1. Which of the following is a deficiency of steroid hormones?
   a. Addison's disease
   b. hypothyroidism
   c. Cushing's disease
   d. Type 1 diabetes
2. Which of the following glands makes glucagon?
   a. adrenal cortex
   b. adrenal medulla
   c. pancreas
   d. thyroid gland
3. Which of the following drugs is used to treat Type 1 diabetes?
   a. exenatide
   b. insulin
   c. levothyroxine
   d. metformin
4. Which trace element is necessary for production of thyroid hormone?
   a. zinc
   b. chromium
   c. iron
   d. iodine
5. Which of the following drugs has the predominant side effect of stomach upset and diarrhea that can be relieved by taking it with food?
   a. Glucophage
   b. Actos
   c. Humalog
   d. Synthroid
6. Which of the following is the route of administration for insulin?
   a. IV
   b. SC
   c. IM
   d. PO
7. Which type of insulin is injected ten minutes prior to meals and lasts up to two hours?
   a. rapid-acting (i.e., Humalog)
   b. short-acting (i.e., Humulin R)
   c. intermediate-acting (i.e., Novolin N)
   d. long-acting (i.e., Lantus)
8. Which of the following pairs of drugs contains two agents, both of which can cause hypoglycemia?
   a. levothyroxine, metformin
   b. metformin, glyburide
   c. glimepiride, insulin lispro
   d. insulin glargine, sitagliptin
9. Which of the following agents works by stimulating beta cells in the pancreas to produce insulin?
   a. Actos
   b. Amaryl
   c. Avandia
   d. Januvia
10. Which of the following medications is an SC injection given once a day for diabetes?
   a. saxagliptin
   b. liraglutide
   c. NPH insulin
   d. thyroid extract

KNOW THE DRUGS

Match each brand name drug with its corresponding generic name and most common use. Your answers should follow this example format: Generic Name: 1. a; 2. b; 3. c; etc. Most Common Use: 1. i; 2. j; 3. k; etc.

Brand Name	Generic Name	Most Common Use
1. Synthroid	a. insulin aspart	i. Type 1 diabetes
2. Amaryl	b. exenatide	j. Type 2 diabetes
3. Glucophage	c. insulin glulisine	k. Hypothyroidism
4. Apidra	d. levothyroxine	
5. Januvia	e. metformin	
6. Byetta	f. insulin glargine	
7. NovoLog	g. sitagliptin	
8. Lantus	h. glimepiride	

PUT IT TOGETHER

For each item, write down either a short answer or a single term to complete the sentence.

1. Describe the difference between Type 1 and Type 2 diabetes. Why can't patients with Type 1 diabetes use oral medication to treat their condition?
2. Vials of insulin expire after _________ days at room temperature. How should they be stored in the pharmacy?
3. When will insulin kept in the refrigerator expire?

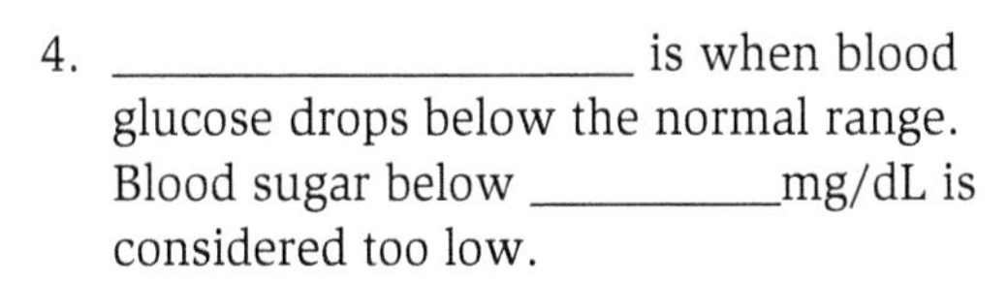

4. ____________________ is when blood glucose drops below the normal range. Blood sugar below __________mg/dL is considered too low.
5. List five potential symptoms of low blood glucose a patient may exhibit.

THINK IT THROUGH

Read and think through each numbered scenario carefully and then write several sentences in reply to the question(s) presented. Question 4 requires you to do some Internet research before completing your answer(s).

1. A new customer visits the pharmacy to inquire about insulin. She says she is here from out of state, visiting her daughter and grandchildren, and her luggage did not arrive with her flight. She has diabetes and uses a Lantus insulin pen. Her pen injector is almost out of insulin, and she only has another day or two left. Her backup supply was in her lost luggage. She says she heard that insulin is available over the counter and would like to purchase a week's supply. What should you tell this patient to do?
2. You notice a patient in the clinic is acting oddly. He is staggering as he walks, seems confused, and is argumentative. You recall dispensing glyburide, metformin, and NPH insulin to him recently and recognize that he has diabetes. You overhear him tell another technician that he cannot wait to get out of here because his doctor appointment went overtime and he is hungry because he has not had lunch yet. What concerns should you have, and what should you do?
3. A patient drops off a new prescription for a glucose meter. The patient says her doctor told her to go to the pharmacy to buy a meter, but she has no idea what to get. What should you ask, and how can you help this patient?

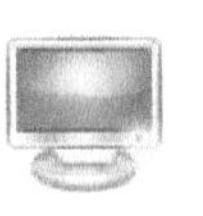

4. **On the Internet,** look up the Web site for the American Diabetes Association (ADA) and look through the information. What information is there for patients versus healthcare providers? Locate the practice standards for diagnosing and treating diabetes. Take some time to read these standards and find a classmate to discuss your findings. These standards are lengthy, so memorizing them is not necessary. Discussing them with others can help you understand the complexity of treating and caring for patients with diabetes.

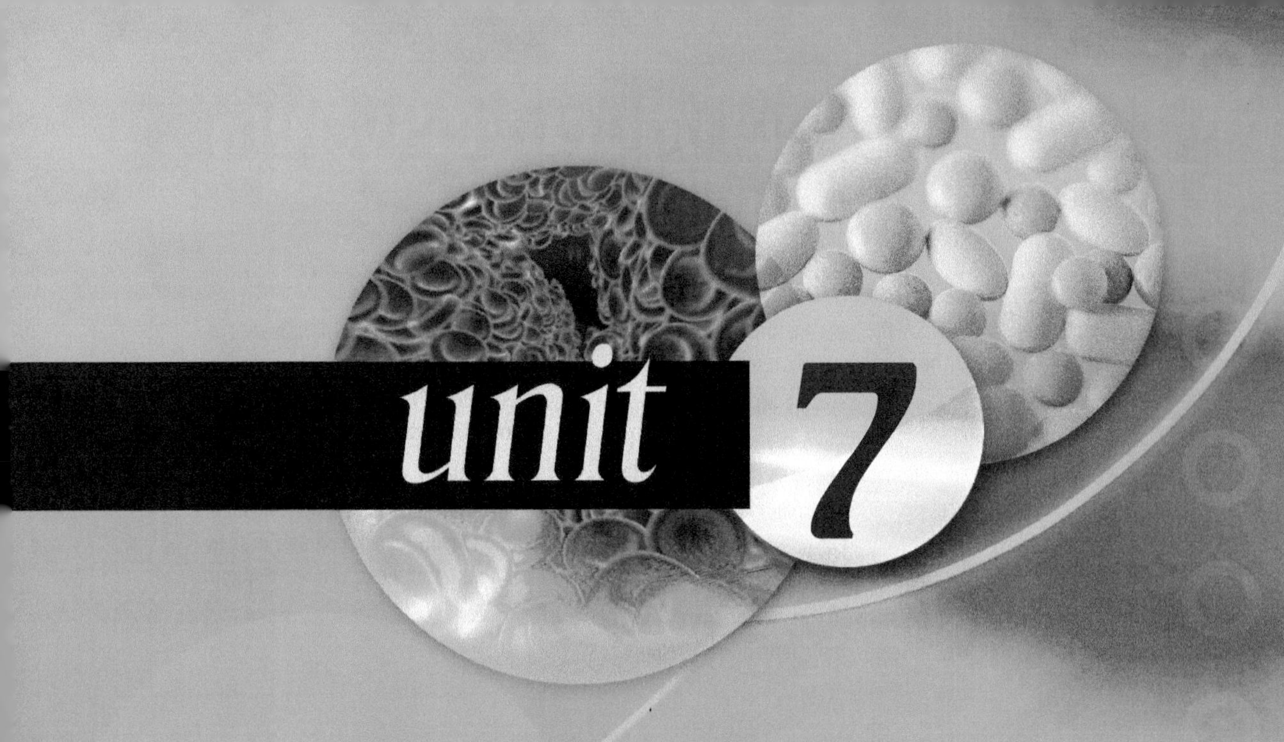

Drugs for the Genitourinary System

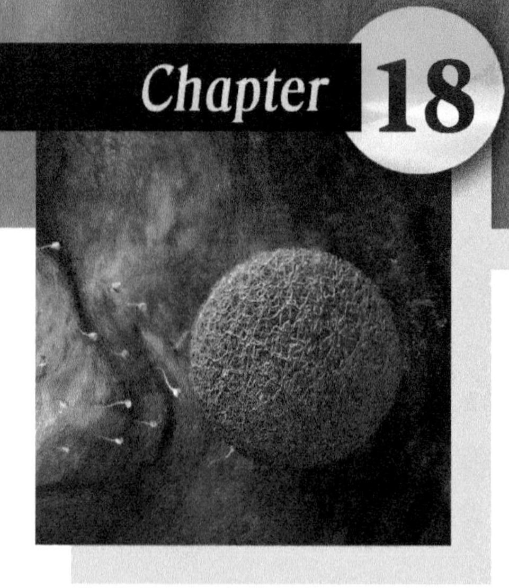

Chapter 18 The Reproductive System and Drug Therapy

LEARNING OBJECTIVES

- Describe the basic anatomy and physiology of the reproductive system.
- Explain the therapeutic effects of prescription medications, nonprescription medications, and alternative therapies commonly used to treat diseases of the reproductive system.
- Describe the adverse effects of prescription medications, nonprescription medications, and alternative therapies commonly used to treat diseases of the reproductive system.
- Identify the brand and generic names of prescription and nonprescription medications commonly used to treat diseases of the reproductive system.
- State the doses, dosage forms, and routes of administration for prescription and nonprescription medications commonly used to treat diseases of the reproductive system.

Interactive self-quizzes, games, audio files, and glossaries help you to learn drug names and facts.

Oral contraceptives, drugs for erectile dysfunction, and antibiotics for sexually transmitted diseases are dispensed every day in pharmacies across the United States. Due to the sensitive nature of the conditions that they treat, these products generate many questions from patients. Pharmacy technicians should be prepared for the issues relating to confidentiality that are associated with these medications. Armed with information, you should feel confident in helping pharmacists dispel myths and help patients with their reproductive healthcare needs.

This chapter begins with an overview of the anatomy and function of the reproductive systems of males and females, followed by descriptions of common disorders affecting these systems. Because the reproductive system is regulated by hormones, many of the drugs used to treat issues in this system contain these chemical messengers. This chapter distinguishes the uses, similarities, and differences in hormone therapies. Infertility, erectile dysfunction, and sexually transmitted diseases are all abnormal conditions for which prescription medication is used. In contrast, menopause is considered a natural part of a woman's life cycle and reproductive health. Finally, contraception is commonly a central concern for women's reproductive health. Drug therapy is used frequently to prevent pregnancy and to relieve menopausal symptoms. Oral contraceptives and estrogen replacement therapies are among the top 200 most commonly dispensed medications in the United States.

Anatomy and Physiology of the Reproductive System

The **reproductive system** is responsible for procreation and fetal development. Males and females have **gonads** (specialized reproductive organs) that make **gametes**, a kind of cell containing single strands of DNA (the code for life and cell function). These cells are generated specifically so that when they combine—one from the male and one from the female—they produce a **zygote** (a normal cell containing double-stranded DNA). Females produce **ova** (the plural of "**ovum**") from the **ovaries** and males produce **sperm** from the **testes**. The ovum and sperm combine during **fertilization** to form an **embryo**. If properly supported inside the female uterus, an embryo grows into a fetus and is born.

Both male and female reproductive systems are regulated by the **hypothalamic-pituitary-adrenal (HPA) axis** (see Figure 18.1). In response to a negative feedback

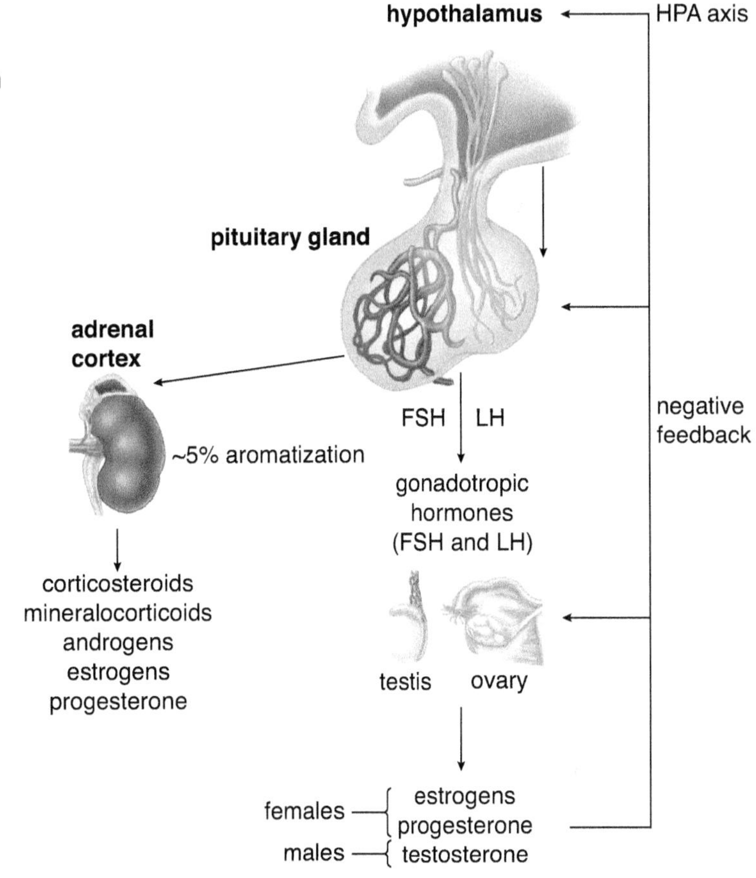

Figure 18.1
Sex Hormone Production and Control
Because breast and prostate cancer grow in response to estrogen and testosterone, drug therapy is used to interrupt the HPA axis to shut off androgen production from the ovaries and testes.

loop, the pituitary gland releases **follicle-stimulating hormone (FSH)** and **luteinizing hormone (LH)**, which stimulate sex hormone production from the ovaries and testes. The sex hormones include **estrogen, progesterone,** and **testosterone**. **Androgens** (which include estrogen and testosterone) are made by both males and females. However, testosterone is more prominent in men, and estrogen is more prominent in women. Although sex hormones are produced primarily from the ovaries and testes, approximately 5% of them come from a process called **aromatization**. This process occurs peripherally, in tissues other than the ovaries and testes.

Female Reproductive System

The female reproductive system includes the **ovaries, fallopian tubes, uterus, cervix,** and **vagina** (see Figure 18.2). These organs develop and present mature ova for fertilization and then support the growth of the embryo and fetus when fertilization occurs.

The ovaries produce ova in response to FSH from the pituitary gland. After release from the ovary, the ovum travels through the fallopian tube to the uterus. If sperm is present, fertilization typically happens within the fallopian tube. If fertilized, a zygote is formed and travels to the uterus. It implants into the endometrial lining (see Figure 18.3) and begins dividing into a clump of cells that gradually develops into an embryo. If not fertilized, the egg passes through the uterus and out through the cervix to the vagina. The uterine lining then sloughs off, and the whole process starts over. This sloughing of the endometrial tissue is called **menstruation** (commonly referred to as a woman's period or monthly cycle).

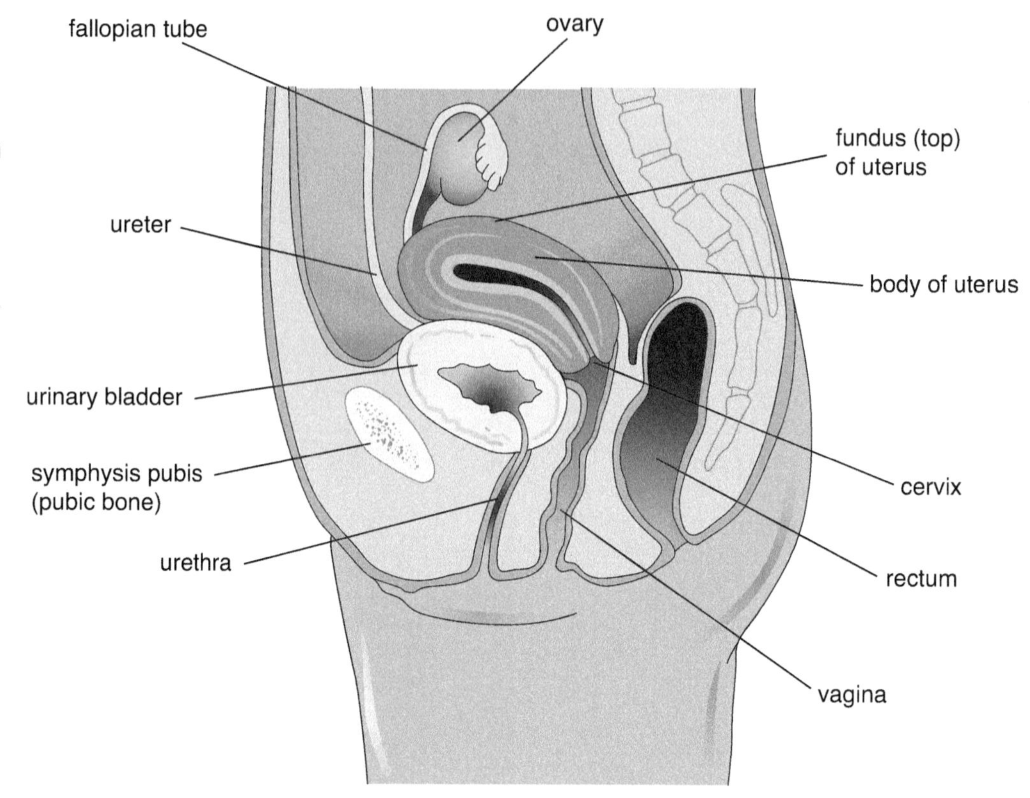

Figure 18.2
Female Reproductive Anatomy
Vaginal yeast infection creams are applied into the vagina with an applicator. Diaphragms for contraception are inserted into the vagina and positioned to cover the cervix, preventing sperm from entering the uterus.

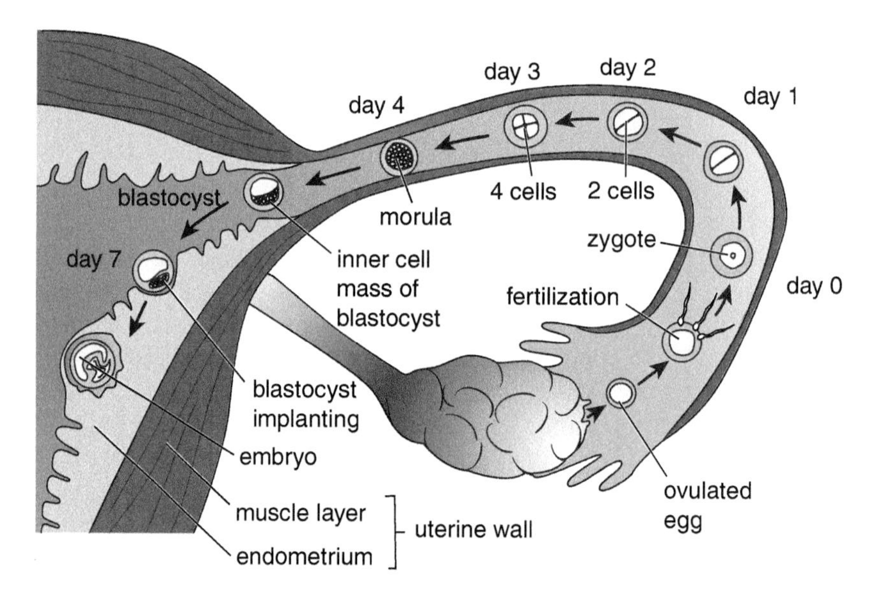

Figure 18.3
Fertilization and Implantation
Fertilization typically occurs in the fallopian tube within a day or two of ovulation if sperm are present. When fertilization does not occur, the ovum travels through the fallopian tube and uterus and leaves the body.

The **menstrual cycle** is regulated by FSH, LH, estrogen, and progesterone. It restarts about every twenty-eight days, unless pregnancy occurs (see Figure 18.4). The cycle begins with FSH production from the pituitary gland. FSH stimulates **follicles** in the ovaries to grow and produce estrogen. Even though a handful of follicles begin to grow with each cycle, generally only one will release an ovum. As ova inside the follicles reach maturity, the pituitary gland senses a rise in estrogen in the bloodstream and releases LH. The surge in LH causes the most mature follicle to burst and release an ovum. Ovulation occurs approximately every 28 days from puberty to menopause adding as many as 450–650 released ova over a lifetime. However, decreased ovum reserve and poor quality of aging oocytes begin to affect a woman's fertility in her late thirties and forties. LH also stimulates the leftover follicle tissue (**corpus luteum**) to begin releasing progesterone, which facilitates endometrial lining growth and supports

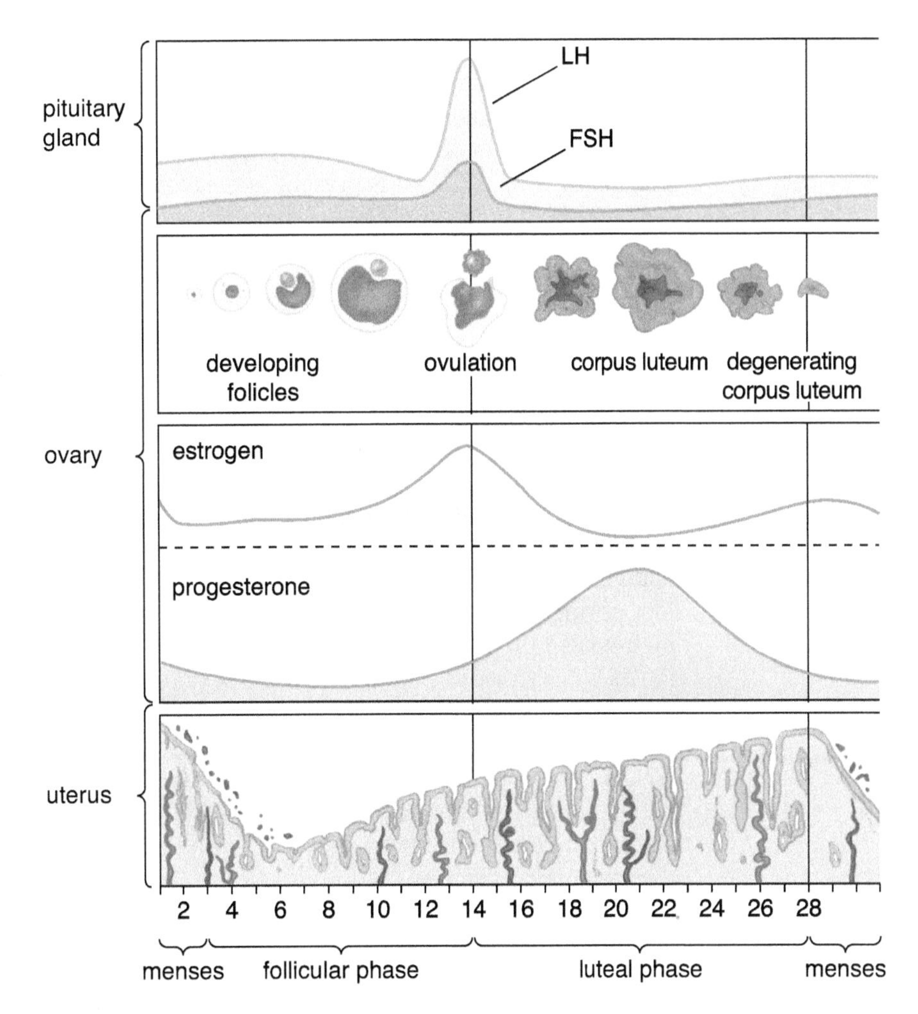

Figure 18.4

Female Menstrual Cycle

In pregnancy, the estrogen and progesterone levels continue to rise (instead of fall at the end of the luteal phase) to support embryo implantation and uterine/placental growth.

embryo implantation. If sperm reaches the egg in the fallopian tube and fertilizes it, the embryo will begin to release **human chorionic gonadotropin (HCG)**, the pregnancy hormone. In the presence of HCG, progesterone and estrogen levels continue to rise. Without fertilization and the presence of HCG, progesterone levels drop and menstruation ensues.

Sex hormone production varies throughout a woman's life cycle. Production begins significantly at puberty and generally tapers off during the fifth decade (ages 40–49) of a woman's life; that is, during menopause. Estrogen is considered the primary female sex hormone because it is responsible for female sex characteristics, such as breast enlargement. It is also responsible for endometrial growth, production of cervical mucus, vaginal mucosa maintenance, bone health, and cessation of growth in height for girls. Estrogen has effects on sodium retention, skin blood vessel function, cholesterol levels, blood coagulation, calcium utilization, and carbohydrate metabolism. A rise in estrogen levels coincides with bloating, weight gain, cravings, headaches, and mood swings during the days leading up to menstruation. When estrogen levels decline with age, menopausal symptoms (described later in this chapter) begin. Estrogen is prescribed for women for contraception and relief of menopausal symptoms. In men, estrogen can be used to treat prostate cancer.

Progesterone, also referred to as progestin when produced in the body, is the hormone necessary for embryo implantation and maintaining pregnancy. Progesterone suppresses LH production, thickens cervical mucus, and alters the endometrial lining to support implantation. It has effects on insulin levels, glucose tolerance, fat deposition, and body temperature, all changes that prepare a woman's body for pregnancy. Progesterone levels rise in pregnancy and decline in menopause. Progesterone is prescribed for women for contraception, infertility, and menopausal symptoms.

HCG is considered the pregnancy hormone because its presence indicates that an embryo has implanted in the uterus and a placenta has started to form. The steep rise in this hormone signals pregnancy to the body, which starts the physiological changes that prepare for and maintain pregnancy. Thus, HCG is the hormone measured by home pregnancy tests. When it is present in measurable concentrations in the blood or urine, a diagnosis of pregnancy can be made.

Male Reproductive System

The male reproductive system includes the **testes, epididymis, ductus deferens** (also called **vas deferens**), **seminal vesicles, prostate gland, urethra**, and **penis** (see Figure 18.5). The function of these organs overlaps with those of the urinary system; their purpose facilitates sexual reproduction as well as eliminating urine from the body. Trillions of sperm cells are made in the testes (testicles) over a man's lifetime. After maturing in the epididymis, sperm move through the ductus deferens. During sexual stimulation, sperm combine with semen, the fluid produced by the seminal vesicles, and are ejaculated through the urethra. The purpose of ejaculation is to deliver sperm into a woman's vagina near the cervix, thus enabling these cells to travel to the fallopian tubes to fertilize an ovum.

As with female sex hormones, male sex hormones are produced in response to FSH and LH from the pituitary gland. However, in men this process is continual and does not cycle every twenty-eight days. FSH and LH stimulate androgen production from **Leydig cells** in the testes. Testosterone, the primary androgen in males, is responsible for sperm production and maturation of male genitalia. Testosterone is also associated with secondary sexual characteristics that develop during puberty in males, including pubic hair growth, increased libido (sex drive), fat distribution away from hips and thighs to the abdomen, and development of greater bone and muscle mass than women. Testosterone is also responsible for male pattern hair growth (such as on the chest) and baldness. Testosterone levels decline with age but do not typically cause the dramatic symptoms in men that menopause causes in women. Changes men may experience with reduced testosterone associated with age include decreased testicular size, muscle weakness, reduced bone density, and decreased energy, mood, and libido.

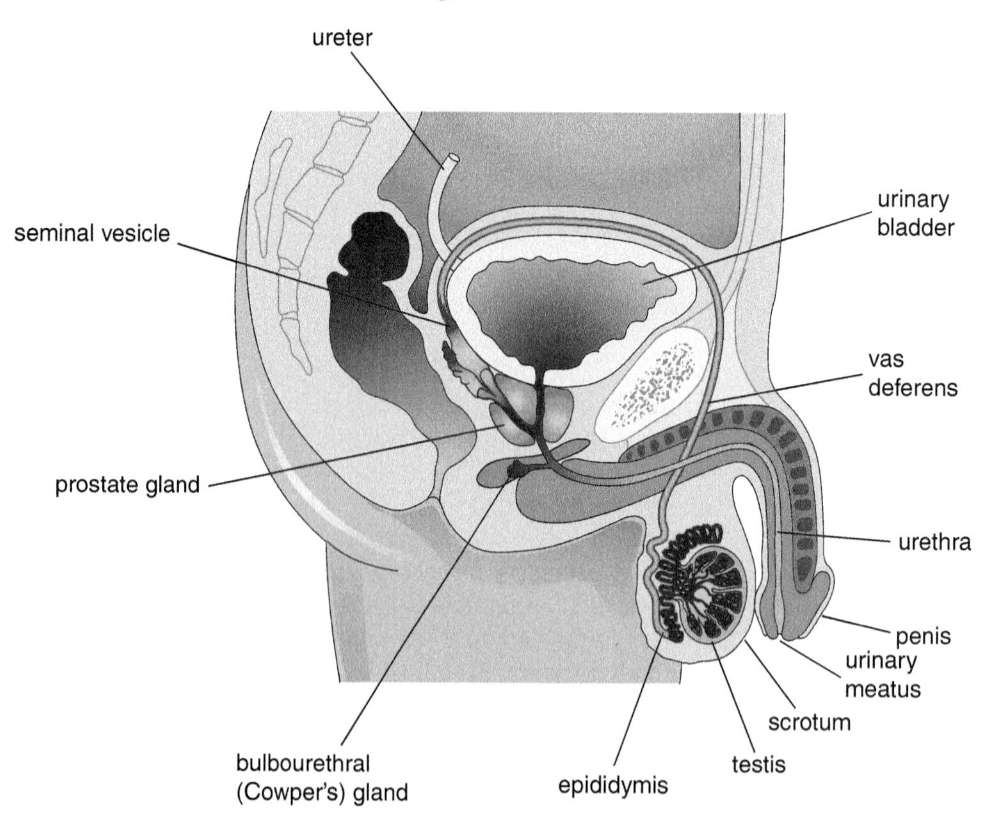

Figure 18.5
Anatomy of the Male Reproductive System
In a vasectomy, the vas deferens is cut, thereby interrupting the flow of sperm from the epididymis to the urethra.

Menopause

The life change of **menopause**, or cessation of sex hormone production in females, is not an abnormal physiological process. Rather, it is part of the normal life cycle of a woman and typically occurs during her fifth decade. This process begins with perimenopause, a period of three to five years during which menstrual cycles become erratic, hormone levels fluctuate, and fertility declines. Menopause is permanent cessation of menstruation, defined by the absence of menses for at least twelve months. During menopause, ovarian follicle activity stops, estrogen levels drop 40 to 60%, and progesterone levels fall dramatically. The release of FSH and LH, in fact, increases due to the negative feedback loop, but the ovaries lose sensitivity to these chemicals.

Menopause has significant impact on quality of life. Lack of estrogen causes vasomotor spasms (hot flashes), irregular menstrual bleeding, vaginal dryness and atrophy (tissue shrinkage), weight gain, insomnia, fatigue, loss of libido, depression, mood swings, and memory impairment. To mitigate the impact of these effects, many women take estrogen supplements (i.e., **hormone replacement therapy** or **HRT**).

Menopause is associated with several adverse outcomes, such as osteoporosis (bone thinning) and increased risk for heart disease and stroke. Because estrogen has beneficial effects on bone resorption, cholesterol metabolism, and blood coagulation, lack of estrogen after menopause causes bone thinning; elevations in blood cholesterol that contribute to atherosclerosis and heart disease; and increased potential for blood clot formation, resulting in stroke. Prior to menopause, estrogen provides protection against these conditions. Incidences of osteoporosis, heart disease, and stroke increase dramatically after menopause.

Hormone Replacement Therapy (HRT)

For many years, HRT was prescribed as a method that offered protection against life-threatening conditions, such as heart disease, stroke, and osteoporosis, in addition to providing relief from some menopausal symptoms. However, research has shown that HRT is not without risks. For instance, increased rates of breast cancer are observed in women who take estrogen after menopause. Recent well-designed studies now report that the potential benefits and protections against heart disease and stroke originally thought to be associated with HRT are not accurate. Therefore, risks and benefits of HRT must be weighed for each patient individually. The general consensus is that HRT is acceptable for women without any contraindications when necessary for symptomatic relief. However, doses should be kept as low as possible, and length of therapy should be as short as possible to minimize adverse effects.

Estrogen and Progesterone Even though most people think of estrogen when referring to HRT, both progesterone and estrogen are taken for relief of menopausal symptoms. The current standard of practice is to use the lowest dose necessary for the shortest time possible. Women who have had a hysterectomy (removal of the uterus) can take estrogen alone. For the majority of women (those retaining the uterus), both estrogen and progesterone are taken in combination to reduce risk of endometrial cancer, which can occur when taking estrogen alone. Dosing is individualized to each patient (see Table 18.1).

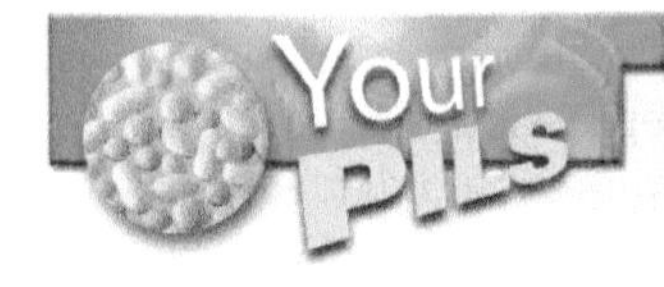

If you like to learn by discussing topics in a small group as do Creators or Enactors, get together with at least two others and discuss the pros and cons of HRT. What are some reasons why women choose or refuse to take HRT?

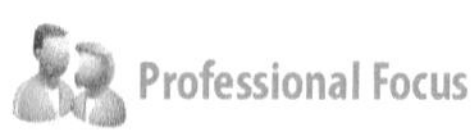
Professional Focus

Some pharmacies specialize in compounding and may make a number of natural estrogen and progesterone creams. Special training in compounding is available for technicians who work in such pharmacies.

Estrogen products usually include **ethinyl estradiol,** either from natural or equine (horse) sources. Conjugated estrogens are sodium salt forms of estrogen collected from pregnant mare urine. Progesterone preparations include synthetic agents such as medroxyprogesterone acetate or natural progesterone. Synthetic hormone products are available commercially and are taken orally or applied transdermally. Natural-source estrogen and progesterone products are specially compounded in the pharmacy and are often used topically (on the skin). Some controversy exists about whether HRT compounded in the pharmacy has the same risks that synthetic products carry. Most likely, they pose the same long-term risks. Natural HRT is an attractive choice for some women because it may produce fewer short-term side effects.

Side Effects Common side effects of HRT agents include dizziness, abdominal pain or bloating, diarrhea, nausea, headache, breast tenderness, vaginal discharge, fluid retention, hair loss, and depression. Reducing alcohol intake can decrease dizziness. The other effects may subside with continued therapy. Sometimes, HRT can cause dark skin patches, called melasma, on the face. Patients should inform their prescribers about these effects so that necessary dose changes can be made. Some women find that compounded forms of estrogen and progesterone produce fewer such effects.

Cautions and Considerations Due to the increased risks for breast, endometrial, and ovarian cancer associated with HRT, patients with a history of these conditions should not begin this kind of therapy. Patients with no personal history but with a significant family history of cancer should discuss risks and benefits of HRT with their prescribers.

Patients with cardiovascular disorders, such as heart attack, deep-vein thrombosis, or pulmonary embolism, probably should not begin HRT. Patients with a family history of these conditions should discuss the risks versus benefits with their prescribers.

Table 18.1 Commercially Available Female Hormone Replacement Products

Generic (Brand)	Dosage Form	Route of Administration
Conjugated estrogen (Premarin)	Tablet	Oral
Estradiol (Estrace, Femtrace)	Tablet	Oral
Estropipate (Ogen)	Tablet	Oral
Progesterone (Prometrium)	Capsule	Oral
Combination Products		
Conjugated estrogen/medroxyprogesterone (Prempro, Premphase)	Tablet	Oral
Estradiol/levonorgestrel (Climara Pro)	Patch	Transdermal
Ethinyl estradiol/norethindrone (Femhrt, Activella)	Tablet	Oral
Ethinyl estradiol/norethindrone (CombiPatch)	Patch	Transdermal

Hypogonadism

Hypogonadism is underproduction of testosterone in males. **Andropause** is the decline in androgen (testosterone) production that occurs with age. Symptoms include fatigue, low sexual desire, weakness, erectile dysfunction, poor sleep, depression, irritability, and memory loss. Many men attribute these symptoms simply to getting older. Recent research shows that hypogonadism is associated with obesity and Type 2 diabetes. Treatment of this condition can significantly improve quality of life.

Testosterone

Testosterone is taken most commonly for testosterone deficiency (hypogonadism) in males. In females, testosterone is used either for metastatic breast cancer or occasionally as an adjunct to HRT. Because these uses are specialized, this text does not go into great detail on testosterone treatment other than to make technicians aware of the special handling and storage these products require.

Testosterone is a controlled substance (Schedule III), because it can be used as a physical performance enhancement drug. Athletes, as reported in the media, use such agents to produce larger muscle mass and improve strength and speed. In general, testosterone and related compounds are referred to as **anabolic steroids**. Unfortunately, many serious risks are associated with testosterone when it is not medically needed and is improperly used. The pharmacist should consult with patients individually regarding these products.

Pharmacy technicians should be aware of federal and state laws regarding dispensing testosterone products. Besides special storage, labeling, and handling issues related to controlled-substance laws, some states also require that prescriptions written for testosterone state the patient's medical diagnosis on the face of the document. Without this wording, a prescription is not considered legal and cannot be filled.

Erectile Dysfunction (ED)

Erectile dysfunction (ED) is the failure to initiate or maintain an erection until ejaculation. Another phrase for it is male impotence. Causes include testosterone deficiency, high blood pressure, heart disease, alcoholism, cigarette smoking, diabetes with microvascular (blood vessel) problems, psychological factors, and medication. Cardiovascular disease is probably the condition most closely associated with erectile dysfunction. Some studies show that 40 to 50% of patients with heart disease suffer from some form of erectile dysfunction.

Medications are commonly associated with ED (see Table 18.2). Many blood pressure medications have been studied for effects on sexual function. Not all these drugs cause problems with sexual function, but some researchers believe that drugs, such as beta blockers, can contribute to the problem.

Drugs for ED

Table 18.3 lists common ED medications. By far the most frequently used drugs for ED are the **phosphodiesterase-5 (PDE-5) inhibitors**. In fact, they are usually listed in the top fifty drugs dispensed in pharmacies today. Much media attention is paid to them. PDE-5 inhibitors work by relaxing smooth muscle in the corpus cavernosum of the penis, which eases blood flow into the area, facilitating erection. This effect, however, only occurs on excitatory or sexual stimulation. Contrary to the exaggerated depictions in movies and media, these drugs do not cause erection directly or immediately. Instead, they create conditions whereby erection is allowed to occur more easily if sexual stimulation is applied. These medications are taken at least one hour or more prior to sexual activity, depending on the agent. The duration of action varies among products, so planning for sexual activity must occur.

Alprostadil is considered a second-line choice of therapy. It is a prostaglandin that works by relaxing

Table 18.2 Drugs that Can Cause ED

Drugs that Can Cause ED
Alcohol
Antidepressants, especially selective serotonin reuptake inhibitors (SSRIs)
Cimetidine
Clonidine
Ketoconazole
Methyldopa
Nicotine
Spironolactone
Thiazide diuretics

smooth muscle in the vasculature of the penis. After drug injection, blood flow increases to the corpus cavernosum, causing erection. Alprostadil is injected into the base of the penis or inserted as a pellet into the urethra, and erection occurs in five to twenty minutes. The route of administration for these products is not as convenient as that for the oral PDE-5 inhibitors. However, alprostadil is an alternative when PDE-5 inhibitors are contraindicated. Patients must be appropriately instructed in preparation and administration of alprostadil.

Yohimbine, a third choice, works by blocking alpha-2 receptors and enhancing parasympathetic nervous system effects. It is taken three times a day continuously to promote conditions conducive to erection on sexual stimulation. It does not cause erection directly or immediately.

Side Effects Common side effects of PDE-5 inhibitors include headache, heartburn, nausea, and flushing. If an erection lasts longer than four hours or is painful (a condition called priapism), the patient should seek medical attention so that permanent tissue damage does not occur.

Common side effects of alprostadil include pain or burning in the penis, urethra, or testes. These effects are brief and go away once activity of the drug wears off but can be a reason patients stop therapy. To avoid the potential of priapism, patients should use alprostadil a maximum of three times per week.

Common side effects of yohimbine include changes in blood pressure, nervousness, irritability, tremor, dizziness, nausea, headache, and skin flushing. Patients with hypertension probably should not take yohimbine.

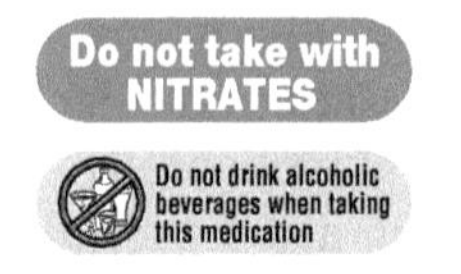

Cautions and Considerations PDE-5 inhibitors are contraindicated in patients who take nitrates or alpha blockers. Combination of PDE-5 inhibitors and these other medications can cause a dangerous drop in blood pressure. Patients taking other medications for blood pressure should first discuss use of PDE-5 inhibitors with their prescribers. Drinking alcohol while taking a PDE-5 inhibitor can worsen these blood pressure effects. Patients may experience increased heart rate, dizziness, and headache.

PDE-5 inhibitors interact with several other medications. The patient should be sure that his or her pharmacist and prescriber know all medications and over-the-counter (OTC) dietary supplements he or she takes to avoid any dangerous interactions. You can help by obtaining thorough medication histories for patients who bring in prescriptions for PDE-5 inhibitors.

Yohimbine can interact with several antidepressant medications. Patients taking antidepressants should not take yohimbine.

Table 18.3 Common ED Medications

Generic (Brand)	Dosage Form	Route of Administration	Duration of Action	Common Dose
Alprostadil (Caverject, Edex)	Injection	Intracavernosal injection	1 hour	0.2–140 mcg, individualized to patient at physician's office
Alprostadil (Muse)	Pellet	Urethral insertion	1 hour	125–1,000 mcg
Yohimbine (Aphrodyne, Yocon)	Tablet	Oral	—	1 tablet (5.4 mg) 3 times a day
PDE-5 Inhibitors				
Sildenafil (Viagra)	Tablet	Oral	4 hours	50–100 mg taken 1–4 hours prior to sexual activity
Tadalafil (Cialis)	Tablet	Oral	36 hours	40 mg taken 1–36 hours prior to sexual activity
Vardenafil (Levitra)	Tablet	Oral	4 hours	10 mg taken 1 hour prior to sexual activity

Contraception

The prevention of pregnancy through artificial means is called **contraception. Birth control** products on the market today generally apply one or more of the following three contraception approaches:

1. Physical or pharmacologic barriers that prevent sperm and egg from coming into contact.
2. Drug therapy that prevents ovulation from occurring.
3. Drug therapy that prevents implantation of a fertilized egg in the uterus.

Choosing a contraception method is a personal decision and must include consideration for effectiveness and ease of use. Patients should understand that rates of effectiveness for preventing pregnancy reported in product labeling refer to "perfect use." These rates are only achieved when the patient follows instructions exactly and uses the product every time she or he engages in sexual intercourse. If a product is difficult to use or undesirable for a particular patient, compliance will not be ideal. Perfect use is not representative of actual use in many cases, and all products have some failures, even if such failures are rare. Despite perfect compliance with the oral contraceptive pill, sometimes certain drugs and conditions will adversely affect its efficacy.

A couple can use temporary abstinence from intercourse as a birth control method. This is often referred to as the rhythm method, and it calls for avoiding sexual intercourse during days in the menstrual cycle when conception is likely to occur. Fertility is highest during the days surrounding ovulation, when a mature ovum is present. Basal body temperature and changes in cervical mucus can be indicators of this fertile period, but they are not exact predictors. An ovum lives for twenty-four hours, and sperm can live for up to five days inside the female reproductive system. Consequently, predicting exactly when ovulation occurs and knowing with certainty when a live ovum and active sperm are present is nearly impossible. Consequently, this method of birth control has a relatively high pregnancy rate compared with other methods.

Condoms, Diaphragms, and Other Barrier Methods

Barrier methods of birth control are used when intercourse is anticipated. They form a physical barrier that prevents sperm from entering the uterus through the cervix. These methods are put in place prior to intercourse, left there for a specific amount of time, and then removed. They do not alter normal ovulation, cervical mucus, or endometrial lining formation.

The male **condom** is placed over the erect penis before penetration into the vagina. Condoms collect the ejaculate (semen and sperm) and prevent it from coming into contact with the vagina or cervix. The female condom is worn by a woman and also forms a physical barrier between the penis and the vagina. When either type of condom is used properly, ejaculate material is removed along with the condom. Condoms are the only birth control method that also prevent or lower the risk of **sexually transmitted disease (STD)** transmission. Latex and polyurethane (for patients allergic to latex) condoms provide the best protection because they are impermeable. **Diaphragms** and **cervical caps** are made of rubber, latex, or silicone and are bordered by a rounded ring that fits over the cervix inside the vagina. They form a barrier that covers the cervical opening and prevents sperm from entering the uterus and traveling to the fallopian tubes. A diaphragm is larger than a cervical cap and covers a larger area over the cervix. These products work best when used with a **spermicide** that kills sperm cells on contact. Diaphragms and cervical caps are prescription items that must be fitted or sized to a woman's internal anatomy by her prescriber. They are self-inserted prior to sexual intercourse and left in place for at least six hours.

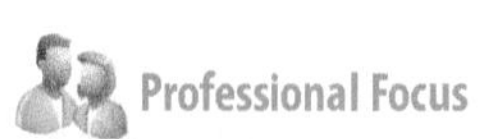

Although diaphragms are fitted (sized) by a gynecologist, they are dispensed in the pharmacy. Be sure to pay particular attention to sizes on the packaging for these items.

Oral Contraceptives

Pharmacologic contraception involves manipulating hormones to prevent ovulation and change cervical mucus texture. They contain ethinyl estradiol, a synthetic estrogen, and one of several synthetic progesterones. **Oral contraceptives** that contain synthetic estrogens work by suppressing production of LH, the hormone that triggers ovulation. Oral contraceptives that contain progesterones suppress LH production and thicken cervical mucus, making travel difficult for sperm.

Oral contraceptives are taken on a daily basis to maintain a steady and elevated hormone level. Depending on the product chosen, patients begin therapy on the first day of their menstrual flow, the first Sunday after their menstrual flow, or whenever desired. In any case, backup birth control, such as a barrier method, must be used to prevent pregnancy for at least the first seven days of therapy, if not for the entire first cycle.

Oral contraceptives contain either a combination of estrogen and progestin or progestins only (see Table 18.4). The advantage of products containing only progestin is that the lower hormone dose reduces side effects, such as headaches and elevated blood pressure. These products are commonly used in patients for whom oral contraceptives are typically not appropriate (i.e., women who have high blood pressure or heart disease, women older than thirty-five years old, women with blood clotting disorders, and especially those who smoke). The disadvantage with this kind of pill is that missed doses more quickly affect failure rate. If a dose of a progestin-only pill is missed by more than three hours, the patient should take it as soon as she remembers and use a backup birth control method, such as condoms, for at least forty-eight hours.

Combination oral contraceptives come in monophasic, biphasic, and triphasic dosing regimens. Monophasic regimens contain the same dose throughout the cycle, whereas biphasic and triphasic regimens increase the dosage once or twice during a menstrual cycle. The color of the tablet usually changes as the dose changes.

New approaches to oral contraception have brought about extended oral regimens. Such products (Seasonale and Seasonique) involve taking a steady dose for eighty-four days before allowing a hormone-free week during which menstruation occurs. In effect, patients experience bleeding only once every three or four months. Although concern about endometrial thickening exists, such a regimen works well for patients who have menstrual cycle–related migraines, severe premenstrual symptoms (PMS), endometriosis, or polycystic ovarian syndrome (PCOS). Prescribers occasionally order a similar extended regimen of monophasic oral contraceptives. The patient skips using the placebo pills in the dose pack until the end of the extended regimen.

Emergency contraception (Plan B and Preven) is taken within seventy-two hours of unprotected intercourse or the failure of another form of birth control, followed by a second dose twelve hours later. Emergency contraceptives work by preventing ovulation (if it has not occurred), altering tubal transport of sperm and ovum, or inhibiting implantation. It is not effective if implantation of a fertilized egg has already begun and will not affect a pregnancy if it has already started. This OTC product is available over the counter to patients at least eighteen years old. It is kept behind the counter at the pharmacy. Technicians should refer patients inquiring about emergency contraception to the pharmacist, because only a pharmacist or a prescriber can order it. It is not intended to be used as a primary method of birth control. Preven is packaged with a pregnancy kit. The pregnancy kit is intended to confirm whether pregnancy has already occurred from an earlier sexual encounter, as Preven is ineffective if the patient is already pregnant.

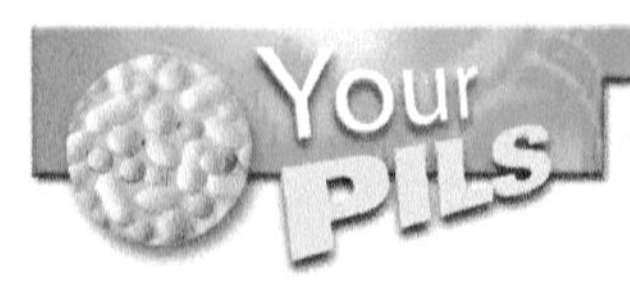

If you are particularly musical or kinesthetic (as are Creators), you may find that putting the brand and generic drug names for oral contraceptives to a rhyme, tune, or dance will help you recall them better.

Table 18.4 Common Oral Contraceptive Agents

Generic Name(s)	Brand Name(s)	Dispensing Status
Ethinyl estradiol/desogestrel	Apri, Azurette, Caziant, Cesia, Cyclessa, Desogen, Kariva, Lovelle, Marvelon , Mircette, Ortho-Cept, Oviol, Solia, Velivet	Rx
Ethinyl estradiol/drospirenone	Ocella, Yasmin, Yaz	Rx
Ethinyl estradiol/ethynodiol diacetate	Demulen, Kelnor, Zovia	Rx
Ethinyl estradiol/levonorgestrel	Alesse, Aviane, Enpresse, Levlen, Levlite, Levora, Lutera, Min-Ovral, Ovral, Preven, Seasonale, Seasonique, Tri-Levlen, Triphasil, Triquilar	Rx
Ethinyl estradiol/norethindrone	Brevicon, Estrostep, Femcon Fe, Femhrt, Genora, Loestrin, Microgestin, Necon, Nelova, Norethin, Norinyl, Nortrel, Ortho, Ortho-Novum, Ovcon, Tri-Norinyl	Rx
Ethinyl estradiol/norgestimate	Cyclin, MonoNessa, Ortho-Cyclen, Ortho-TriCyclen, Ortho-TriCyclen Lo, Previfem, Sprintec, TriNessa	Rx
Ethinyl estradiol/norgestrel	Cryselle, Lo/Ovral, Norgestrel, Ogestrel, Ovral	Rx
Levonorgestrel	Plan B, Preven EC	OTC, Rx
Norethindrone	Camila, Errin, Jolivette, Nor-QD, Ortho Micronor	Rx

Side Effects Common side effects of oral contraceptives include weight gain, nausea, vomiting, bloating, increased appetite, tiredness, fatigue, breast tenderness or enlargement, headaches, and edema (fluid retention). These effects tend to subside with continued use but can be a reason to stop or change therapy if bothersome. Patients should discuss these effects with their prescribers.

Breakthrough bleeding (blood flow in the middle of a menstrual cycle) can occur, especially at the start of therapy. If it continues, the patient should talk with her prescriber.

Increase in blood pressure can occur in the first few months of oral contraceptive therapy. Patients with high blood pressure should be encouraged to use other methods of contraception if possible.

Cautions and Considerations Patients with clotting disorders should not take oral contraceptives because these agents can increase the formation of blood clots. Patients with heart or cerebral vascular disease should not take oral contraceptives. A clot in either of these locations could be fatal.

Patients taking oral contraceptives should not smoke, especially if they are more than thirty-five years old. Smoking in conjunction with hormone therapy increases the risk of heart attack, blood clots, and stroke.

Patients with a history of breast, endometrial, ovarian, or cervical cancer should discuss the risks and benefits of oral contraceptives with their healthcare providers. Some controversy exists about whether oral contraceptives increase a woman's risk of cancer in these organs, so patients should make informed decisions about their own care.

This drug interferes with the effectiveness of oral contraceptives

Other medications can interact with oral contraceptives and reduce their effectiveness. These drugs include antibiotics (especially penicillins and tetracyclines), barbiturates, carbamazepine, lamotrigine, phenytoin, protease inhibitors, fluconazole, and St. John's wort. Many pharmacies prefer that auxiliary warning labels about antibiotic interactions be used when dispensing antibiotics to patients on oral contraceptives. Pharmacy technicians should be familiar with all medications that reduce the effectiveness of oral contraceptives and the policy their pharmacy has on use of auxiliary warning labels. Patients should use other methods of birth control while taking these interacting medications to prevent pregnancy. When patients have questions regarding this warning, the pharmacist should counsel them appropriately.

Oral contraceptives have special packaging and dispensing regulations, which state that all patients must receive a patient information leaflet that has been approved by the Food and Drug Administration (see the following photo).

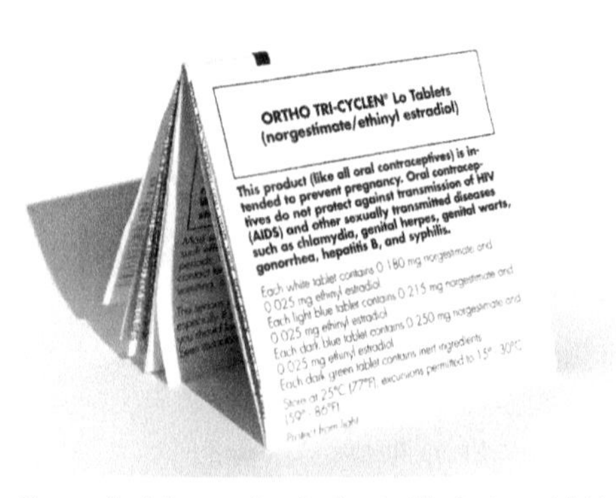

You can find these patient leaflets inside the box with birth control products. Do not throw these small packets away.

One of these leaflets should be given to each patient receiving oral contraceptives.

Patients who have disorders that affect potassium levels, such as kidney disease, liver dysfunction, or adrenal insufficiency, should not take Yasmin. Yasmin contains drospirenone, which acts similar to a diuretic that adversely affects potassium levels.

Oral contraceptives do not protect against STDs. Take care to notice whether patients confuse prevention of STDs with pregnancy prevention.

Transdermal and Vaginal Contraceptives

Transdermal contraceptives use a stick-on patch to deliver a combination of estrogen and progesterone in a steady supply through the skin (see Table 18.5). As is true for oral contraceptives, the hormones that are delivered alter the menstrual cycle and prevent follicle maturation and ovulation. They also thicken cervical mucus, making it difficult for sperm to pass through the cervix. One patch is applied each week for three weeks and then left off for one week while menstruation occurs. The patch should be removed and replaced the same day of the week. It is placed on a clean, dry, intact area of the skin on the buttock, abdomen, upper outer arm, or upper torso (not the breasts).

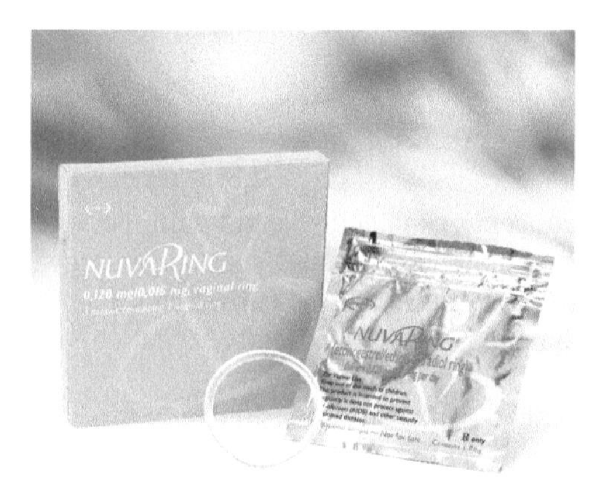

Placement of the ring in the vagina does not have to be precise. The mechanism of action comes from hormone absorption, not from the physical location of the ring.

The **vaginal ring** is a combination birth control that contains synthetic estrogen and progesterone. It is inserted into the vagina every three weeks. The hormones are absorbed through the vaginal mucosa. One ring is inserted and left in place for three weeks and then removed for a week while menstruation occurs.

The **sponge** is made of a latex porous material that is infused with a spermicide that kills sperm on contact. Although the sponge forms a partial barrier over the cervix, the true mechanism of action comes from the spermicidal foam that is released on insertion of the sponge into the vagina. It should be inserted prior to sexual intercourse (twelve to twenty-four hours in advance) and left in place for six hours after intercourse. The sponge is available OTC.

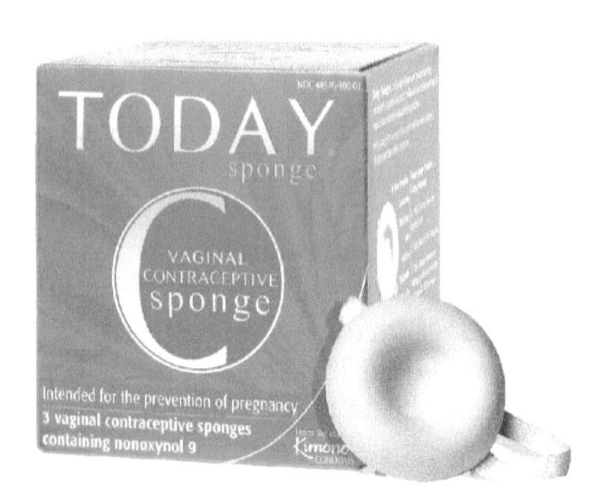

The sponge is wetted with water to start the foaming process, then rolled (dimple side in) and inserted into the vagina.

Side Effects Common side effects of transdermal contraceptives are similar to those of oral contraceptives and include breast tenderness, headache, irritation at application site, nausea, menstrual cramps, and abdominal pain. These effects tend to subside with continued use. If these effects remain bothersome, an alternative contraceptive agent should be tried.

Common side effects of the vaginal ring include headache, nausea, vaginal secretion, vaginitis, bloating, cramps, and weight gain. These effects seem to be less than those experienced with oral contraceptives, presumably because the ring delivers a lower dose of hormone to a local area. These effects may subside with continued use. If these effects continue to be bothersome, the patient should discontinue therapy and talk with her prescriber.

Table 18.5 Transdermal and Vaginal Hormonal Contraceptives

Brand Name	Active Ingredient	Dosage Form	Route of Administration
NuvaRing	Etonogestrel and ethinyl estradiol	Ring	Intravaginal
Ortho Evra	Norelgestromin and ethinyl estradiol	Patch	Transdermal
Today	Nonoxynol 9	Sponge	Intravaginal

Common side effects of the sponge include vaginal irritation. If this effect is bothersome, an alternative choice of contraception is recommended.

Cautions and Considerations As with all estrogen and progesterone hormone products, benefits and risks of therapy must be weighed. Hormone therapy can increase risk of cardiovascular events, stroke, and blood clots. Risk of blood clots is especially high for patients thirty-five years and older who smoke. These hormones can exacerbate depression and migraine headaches. Patients with these conditions should discuss use of hormone contraception with their healthcare providers.

If the patch detaches (fully or partially) from the skin, it should be reapplied if possible. If detachment lasts for less than a day, no backup birth control is needed. If detached for longer than a day, then backup (barrier) method birth control should be used for seven days. If the patch cannot be reapplied, a new patch should be used and backup birth control used for seven days. A new cycle then begins and the patch change day changes.

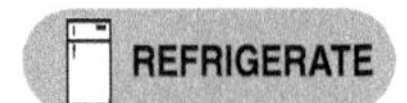

When stored in the pharmacy, the vaginal ring must be kept in the refrigerator to maintain its potency. You should put these products into the refrigerator when checking in new inventory. The NuvaRing should also be kept in the refrigerator until patients pick up their orders. If the patient will not be using the ring immediately, she should keep it in the refrigerator at home until she plans to use it. This warning is especially important to tell patients when they are picking up a ninety-day or three-month supply.

If the vaginal ring is removed or expelled, it can be replaced within three hours with no problems. If removal is longer than three hours during the first two weeks of a cycle, the ring should be replaced and a backup (barrier) method of birth control used for at least seven days. If removed during the third week, a new ring should be inserted or left out entirely and menstruation allowed to begin. Backup (barrier) birth control methods must be used for seven days.

If the sponge is left in the vagina longer than twenty-four hours, risk of infection and toxic shock syndrome increases. The sponge should be left in place for six hours after sex, to avoid pregnancy, but it should be removed as soon as possible after that to avoid bacterial growth and infection.

Injections, Implants, and Intrauterine Devices (IUDs)

Injections, implants, and **intrauterine devices (IUDs)** are contraception methods used to prevent pregnancy for long periods of time (i.e., months to years). All of these methods use hormonal therapy in some way. The advantage is that the patient does not have to remember to take or use the product regularly to prevent pregnancy. Once administered, these methods continue working for a period of time during which the patient is protected without having to think about it.

Medroxyprogesterone (Depo-Provera) is an injection given every three months, and **etonogestrel** (Implanon) is an implant placed just under the skin on the inner upper arm every three years to prevent pregnancy. Both of these agents are administered by a healthcare provider and work by inhibiting ovulation, thickening the cervical mucus, and changing the endometrium to inhibit implantation.

Multiple kinds of IUDs are available. An IUD is a small device placed into the uterus by a healthcare provider every five years. Most IUDs contain progesterone, the hormone that alters the endometrium to disallow implantation.

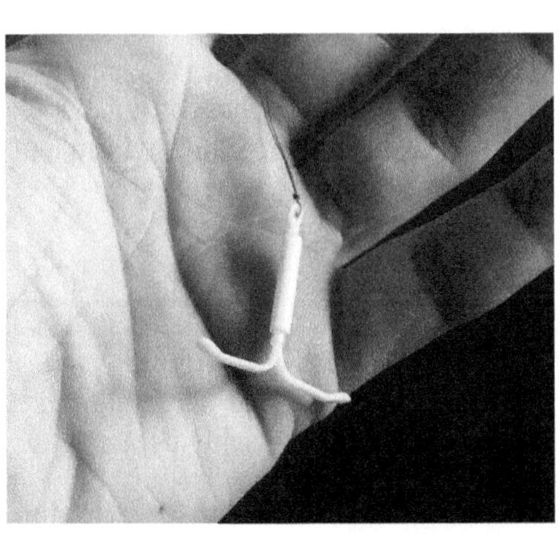

The presence of the IUD within the uterus changes the endometrium itself, and the drug that leaches out of the device affects ovulation.

Side Effects Common side effects of medroxyprogesterone injection include menstrual irregularity, abdominal pain, weight changes, dizziness, headache, weakness, fatigue, and nervousness. Also possible are decreased libido, inability to achieve orgasm, pelvic pain, backache, breast pain, leg cramps, hair loss, depression, bloating, nausea, rash, insomnia, edema, hot flashes, acne, sore joints, and vaginitis. Patients should understand the risks of these potential side effects along with the benefits when choosing this contraception option. Because the drug is long-acting, these effects are unavoidable once they occur and will probably continue for three months.

Common side effects of etonogestrel include changes in menstrual bleeding, weight gain, and mood swings. Other potential side effects include upper respiratory tract infection, vaginitis, breast pain, acne, and abdominal pain. These effects, if particularly bothersome, can be sufficient reason to have the implant removed.

Common side effects of IUDs can include spontaneous abortion, septicemia, pelvic infection, perforation of the uterus, vaginitis, abnormal menstrual bleeding, anemia, pain, cramping, backaches, tubal damage, and more. These effects can be serious and should be fully discussed and understood before patients choose this contraception method.

Professional Focus

Traditionally, Depo-Provera shots are given in the physician's office, but now some pharmacies are administering them under certain protocols. Technicians should be prepared to order appropriate inventory for such services.

Cautions and Considerations None of these contraception methods should be used during pregnancy. For this reason, the patient may be required to take a pregnancy test before administration. Because all of these agents are long-term options for contraception, patients should understand the risks and potential complications of these therapies before choosing one.

Mifepristone and Misoprostol

Mifepristone (Mifeprex) and **misoprostol** (Cytotec) are taken to terminate a uterine pregnancy during the first forty-nine days of pregnancy. Treatment with one of these agents requires three visits to a prescribing physician in a clinic, medical office, or hospital where gestational age of the embryo can be determined. Mifepristone is only supplied to physician offices that agree to abide by strict monitoring and therapy guidelines. Pharmacies do not dispense mifepristone. Pharmacists and technicians can help patients understand that emergency contraception (i.e., Plan B) is not mifepristone or misoprostol. Emergency contraception attempts to prevent ovulation or implantation, thereby preventing pregnancy. Mifepristone and misoprostol terminate a pregnancy once it has already begun.

Home Pregnancy Tests

Professional Focus

You can help patients get accurate results from their pregnancy test by regularly checking expiration dates on products stocked on the shelf and removing expired stock.

Home pregnancy tests measure the presence of HCG in the urine. HCG is produced by the embryo and placenta once implantation has occurred. It can be detected as soon as six to eight days after conception, so home pregnancy tests can be used on day one of a missed period. A variety of home pregnancy tests is available on the market. Although each is slightly different in the technique and time to result, most patients get reliable results with these products. Testing for pregnancy at home allows a woman to make informed decisions about lifestyle and healthcare early in a pregnancy. Because vital organs begin to develop in the fetus in the first weeks of gestation, a woman's diet, alcohol consumption, caffeine intake, and medication use can affect this critical development. Early confirmation of pregnancy allows a woman to make choices that will improve her prenatal care.

Infertility

Infertility is the inability to achieve pregnancy after one year of regular, unprotected sexual intercourse. For women over thirty-five years old, infertility may be diagnosed sooner, after only six months, because egg production and quality quickly decline after that age. Infertility can be associated with problems in the female's, male's, or both reproductive systems. It is estimated that up to 10% of the U.S. population faces fertility issues at some point.

Common causes for infertility in women include pelvic inflammatory disease, hormonal imbalance, anatomic abnormalities, and PCOS. **Endometriosis** is another common cause of infertility in women and has a negative effect on general health and well-being. This condition is the presence of endometrial tissue outside of the uterus. It can be in the fallopian tubes, ovaries, or pelvic abdominal cavity. Why this tissue grows outside of the uterus in some women is not fully understood, but such growth can cause pelvic or abdominal pain, heavy menstrual flow, severe cramping, and painful intercourse. Women with endometriosis tend to have more problems with irritable bowel symptoms and infections of the urinary tract and vagina than women without it. Endometriosis can also be silent—a woman may not realize she has it until she encounters problems when trying to become pregnant.

Common causes of infertility for men include infectious diseases, anatomic abnormalities, immunologic factors, and anything that hinders sperm production or prevents semen (and sperm) from exiting through the urethra. Lifestyle factors—such as excessive alcohol or caffeine consumption, tight-fitting clothes or hot tubs (which increase temperature of the testes), and use of street drugs, such as cocaine or marijuana—can affect growth and maturation of sperm.

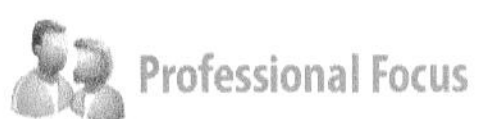

Just one cycle of drug therapy for ovulation induction can cost the patient $5,000 out of pocket.

Drugs for Infertility

Assistive reproductive technology (ART) is a complicated and specialized practice that matches drug therapy and other modes of treatment to the specific cause for infertility. **Ovulation induction** is the process of using hormones (such as FSH and LH) to stimulate the ovaries to produce and release multiple ova. **Artificial insemination** is the process of collecting semen containing sperm from a man and introducing it into a woman's uterus during peak ovulation. These two methods are often used together to bring more ova and eggs into potential contact and improve chances for fertilization. **In vitro fertilization** is a procedure whereby multiple eggs are retrieved from a woman (after ovulation induction) and artificially fertilized with sperm (from a designated man) in a laboratory. The fertilized embryos are then placed into the woman's uterus for implantation. Additional drug therapy (such as progesterone), given after fertilization, may be needed to improve chances of implantation and to help maintain a pregnancy once initiated.

Although a few medications in ART are taken orally, many agents in this specialty are costly injectables that require precise dosing and close monitoring. Insurance generally does not cover ART or the medications involved, so patients pay their own costs. Due to their high cost and specialized use, these agents are usually dispensed by specialty pharmacies. Pharmacy technicians who have the opportunity to work with these products should be mindful of the emotional and financial toll ART has on patients.

Home Ovulation Tests

Ovulation tests are used to identify the twenty-four- to forty-eight-hour period when ovulation occurs. If intercourse is timed to take place during the ideal period of ovulation, the likelihood of sperm and egg meeting in the fallopian tube is increased and the chances of pregnancy improved. **Home ovulation predictor kits** typically measure either body temperature or hormonal fluctuation to predict when ovulation is about to occur. Immediately before ovulation, a slight decrease in body temperature occurs, followed by a slight rise after the egg is released. By measuring basal body temperature daily and charting the results over time, patients can detect trends and predict when ovulation is most likely to occur.

Urine test kits detect the LH surge that occurs just prior to ovulation. These tests tend to be more sensitive and are used more often than temperature charting. Urine tests are easy to use, but the instructions should be followed closely. Most kits include five to seven tests, so it is important to test appropriately—on those days when ovulation is expected. A meter with test strips is available but is not usually covered by insurance. Patients should determine how often they plan to use ovulation tests to be sure that purchasing a meter is cost-effective.

Sexually Transmitted Diseases (STDs)

Sexually transmitted diseases (STDs) are infections that affect the reproductive system in males and females; they are transmitted through sexual contact. Although abstinence from sexual activity is the only sure way to prevent transmission, some barrier methods (such as the male or female condom) have shown some effectiveness in preventing transmission of some STDs. Causes of STDs include bacteria and viruses. Bacterial infections can be cured, but viral STDs can only be treated symptomatically. Once someone contracts a viral STD, goals of treatment change from curing to reducing the severity of symptoms and chance of transmission.

Chlamydia

Chlamydia trachomatis, an organism with characteristics of both bacteria and viruses, causes the STD **chlamydia.** This is the most common STD in the United States. It can also infect the eyes and pharyngeal (throat) tissue. Babies born to women with chlamydia or gonorrhea can become infected in the eyes during a vaginal delivery. Cesarean birth can reduce transmission, but most newborns receive either erythromycin or silver nitrate treatment on their eyes to prevent infection and blindness. In males, common symptoms of chlamydia include painful urination, urinary frequency, and urethral discharge. These symptoms occur seven to twenty-one days after exposure. Women are often asymptomatic and do not realize they have the disease. The infection can progress to involve the entire pelvic region (i.e., pelvic inflammatory disease, [PID]). Women with PID have abdominal pain and can suffer from infertility as inflammation scars and blocks fallopian tubes. Chlamydia frequently accompanies gonorrhea, so testing for both diseases when either one is suspected is standard procedure.

Gonorrhea

Gonorrhea is a gram-negative bacterial infection caused by *Neisseria gonorrhoeae* that attaches to mucosal tissue in the reproductive tract of males and females, rectum, eyes, and oropharyngeal (throat) area. Symptoms are most pronounced in males who have painful urination and pus-like discharge from the urethra (i.e., urethritis). These symptoms usually develop within two to eight days of exposure, prompting most men to seek treatment and avoid further complications. Women are usually asymptomatic but can have vaginal discharge and abdominal pain that develop within 7 to 14 days from exposure. If left untreated, the bacterial infection can progress to PID in women and can affect the heart, brain, eyes, pharynx, and joints.

Syphilis

Syphilis is a bacterial infection cause by *Treponema pallidum*. It is contracted through contact with reproductive mucous membranes and/or genital skin lesions. If left untreated, syphilis can slowly progress to affect the central nervous and cardiovascular systems. Primary syphilis develops first, within ten to ninety days after exposure. At this stage, a painless lesion or chancre appears as a round or oval red lump or blister in the genital area, ulcerates, and then heals on its own within one to eight weeks.

If not treated during the primary phase, syphilis continues to the secondary phase, two to eight weeks after the first phase is over. In this phase, multiple lesions appear on the skin, often on the palms of the hands or soles of the feet. Swelling, fever, headache, sore throat, loss of appetite, and joint pain usually accompany these skin lesions. Most patients seek treatment before or at this secondary phase of the disease.

However, when treatment is not sought, the patient enters the latent phase, during which no symptoms are present; the disease can remain latent for years. Patients are contagious to others through the early part of this latent phase. Tertiary syphilis is the final stage of disease, in which a generalized inflammatory response occurs throughout the body. In this stage, patients can develop blindness, deafness, dementia, aortic aneurysm, and destructive skin lesions. Because antibiotic treatment is easy, inexpensive, and highly successful, few patients reach the tertiary stage of syphilis.

Vaginosis

Inflammation and infection of the vaginal mucosa is known as **vaginosis**. It can be caused by bacteria, such as *Gardnerella vaginitis* and *Trichomonas vaginalis*, or by yeast-like fungus, such as *Candida albicans*. Symptoms of bacterial vaginosis include frothy or discolored vaginal discharge, fishy odor, and vaginal itching and pain. Symptoms of vaginal yeast infection include white discharge (often described as looking like cottage cheese) in addition to vaginal odor, itching, and irritation. All vaginosis infections can be transmitted sexually, and yeast infections can develop even without sexual activity. Poor exposure to air, such as from wearing tight underwear and/or wet clothing, can create a damp atmosphere conducive to yeast growth. Taking antibiotics can also kill normal vaginal flora, allowing yeast and other bacteria to grow and cause infection. Vaginal yeast infections can be treated with OTC or prescription antifungal products; bacterial infections usually need prescription antibiotic treatment.

Genital Herpes

Genital herpes is a viral infection caused by the herpes simplex virus. Herpes simplex virus type 1 (HSV-1) is associated with canker sores in and around the mouth, whereas HSV type 2 (HSV-2) is associated with genital herpes. HSV-2 appears as painful blister-like lesions on the skin, typically in the pubic region, within two to fourteen days after exposure. Vesicles (or blisters) containing infectious material form and then heal in about two weeks. Fever, headache, and body aches can also occur in this phase. Once healed, the lesions become latent but can reappear at any time. Recurrent outbreaks are less severe but tend to happen in response to stress, menstruation, or times of illness. Up to half of patients are asymptomatic, however. Genital herpes is not curable and usually recurs. Although patients are most contagious during an outbreak, they can pass the virus to someone else through sexual contact at any time. Antiviral drug therapy can reduce frequency and severity of outbreaks but does not completely eliminate the possibility of transmission.

Human Papillomavirus

The most common viral STD infection in the United States is **human papillomavirus (HPV)**. Although not all patients with HPV have them, wart-like lesions can be caused by the virus and appear in the genital region. The warts are not usually painful but are unsightly and difficult to remove. The virus is closely linked to development of cervical cancer in women, and no cure is available. A vaccine for preventing HPV is now available for females and males ages 9–26. The vaccine helps reduce transmission of HPV and thus significantly reduces cervical cancer risk.

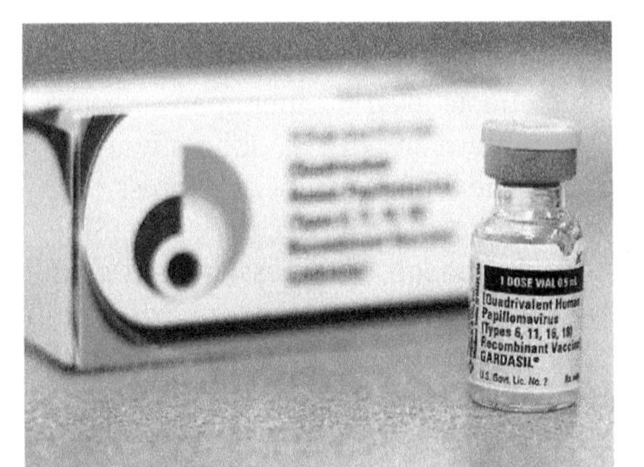

Some pharmacies offer HPV immunizations, so you should be prepared to order and store this vaccine appropriately.

AIDS

Acquired immunodeficiency syndrome (AIDS) is a viral infection that is transmitted through exchange of bodily fluids, such as during sexual activity. It can also be passed via blood transfusion and from an infected mother to her developing fetus, if not treated. AIDS is a retrovirus that attacks the DNA of T cells, destroying their ability to attack foreign cells and fight infection. Thus, AIDS not only destroys the body's ability to rid itself of the virus but also damages the immune response to all infections. Although drug therapy is possible to subdue the virus to almost unmeasurable levels, there is no cure for this condition. AIDS is deadly for infected individuals because the immune system cannot fight infection, and patients eventually die from opportunistic infections. See Chapter 3 for more details.

Drugs for STDs

Bacterial STDs are treated with antibiotics. Viral STDs are treated with antiviral therapy, which does not cure the disease but decreases symptom severity and reduces recurrent outbreaks. Table 18.6 provides an overview of the most commonly used drugs for the STDs discussed in this chapter. Refer to Chapter 3 for additional discussion of the antibiotics, antivirals, and vaginal candidiasis agents listed in Table 18.6. Drugs for human immunodeficiency virus (HIV) are also discussed in Chapter 3.

Table 18.6 Common Drug Therapy for STDs

Disease Treated	Drugs of Choice
AIDS	NRTIs, NNRTIs, PIs, and enfuvirtide
Chlamydia	Doxycycline, azithromycin, or erythromycin
Genital herpes	Acyclovir, valacyclovir, or famciclovir
Gonorrhea	Ceftriaxone or a fluoroquinolone
HPV	Imiquimod, podofilox, or other therapies applied by healthcare provider
Syphilis	Penicillin, doxycycline, or tetracycline
Vaginosis (bacterial)	Metronidazole, clindamycin
Vaginosis (yeast)	OTC or prescription vaginal candidiasis products

Herbal and Alternative Therapies

Soy, also known as isoflavone or **phytoestrogen**, is a plant source of protein used for several conditions. In the United States, it is used most frequently for hot flashes associated with menopause. Soy is a source of fiber and protein found most commonly in milk and dairy substitutes. It can be obtained from dietary sources alone or from a combination of food and oral supplements. It has estrogenic effects that can be beneficial for menopausal symptoms, diabetes, high cholesterol, osteoporosis, kidney disease, and possibly breast cancer prevention. Soy is usually well tolerated but can cause stomach upset, diarrhea, constipation, bloating, nausea, and even insomnia in some cases. It can also worsen migraine headaches, especially for women whose headaches are related to hormonal fluctuations of the menstrual cycle.

Black cohosh is a plant product with estrogenic effects used for menopausal symptoms such as hot flashes. It is sometimes used in combination with St. John's wort for psychological symptoms that may be associated with menopause such as depression and mood swings. Studies have not produced standard dosing, so success varies. Side effects of black cohosh include stomach upset, rash, headache, dizziness, weight gain, cramping, breast tenderness, and vaginal spotting (bleeding). Some concern exists about black cohosh and liver disease because some women have experienced hepatitis-type symptoms after taking black cohosh. Women with liver disease or who are pregnant or breast-feeding should probably avoid black cohosh.

Evening primrose oil is sometimes used to reduce symptoms of menopause or PMS. However, studies have found mixed results and do not currently support its effectiveness for these conditions. Evening primrose oil has, however, been found to be beneficial for osteoporosis when taken with fish oils and calcium. It is considered safe to take and has few side effects reported.

Wild yam, also called Mexican yam, is a phytoestrogen similar to soy with mild estrogenic effects. It is applied topically or ingested orally as a tincture. Some use it for menopausal symptoms such as hot flashes. Published research does not recommend a formulation or dose that is consistently effective. Ingestion of large amounts can cause vomiting. More research is needed to determine clinical usefulness of wild yam.

Chapter Summary

The male and female reproductive systems are complex sets of organs regulated by hormones, such as estrogen, testosterone, progesterone, FSH, and LH. Female ovaries produce ova, and male testes produce sperm. Conditions affecting the female reproductive system are pregnancy, menopause, infertility, and STDs. Conditions affecting the male reproductive system are erectile dysfunction, infertility, and STDs. Drug therapies used for the reproductive system include a variety of contraceptive products, hormones (primarily estrogen, progesterone, and testosterone), and PDE-5 inhibitors. Oral contraceptives and their transdermal, vaginal, and subcutaneous counterparts are among the most commonly dispensed medications in pharmacy today. Understanding the hormones used in contraception is not an easy task. Familiarity with the normal female reproductive cycle provides a good start to understanding how estrogen or progesterone can prevent ovulation. Familiarity with these agents is useful because they are a source of many patient questions. In addition, drug therapies for these conditions have significant risks associated with them. You can help pharmacists identify potential problems and help dispel myths patients commonly have about reproductive drugs.

Chapter Review

For the following sets of exercises, write the exercise heading, exercise numbers, and your answers on a separate sheet of paper. Your instructor may direct you to turn in the sheet of paper or discuss your answers as a class.

REVIEW THE BASICS

Choose a, b, c, or d as the correct answer to each multiple-choice question.

1. Which of the following hormones is responsible for stimulating release of mature ova from the ovary in females?
   a. estrogen
   b. FSH
   c. LH
   d. progesterone
2. Which of the following hormones is produced by the pituitary gland and stimulates maturation of ova and sperm?
   a. estrogen
   b. FSH
   c. progesterone
   d. testosterone
3. Which of the following medications is an oral contraceptive agent?
   a. Depo-Provera
   b. Ortho-Cyclen
   c. Ortho Evra
   d. Premarin
4. Which of the following medications contains progesterone?
   a. Climara Pro
   b. Cialis
   c. Premarin
   d. all of the above
5. Which of the following is the active ingredient in the contraceptive sponge (Today)?
   a. ethinyl estradiol
   b. nonoxynol
   c. norethindrone
   d. b and c only
6. Which of the following medications should be kept in the refrigerator in the pharmacy?
   a. Prempro
   b. Ortho Evra
   c. NuvaRing
   d. Yasmin
7. Which of the following ED medications can be taken the day before sexual intercourse and be effective?
   a. alprostadil
   b. vardenafil
   c. tadalafil
   d. yohimbine
8. Which of the following medications should receive an auxiliary warning label notifying patients of a potentially life-threatening drug interaction with nitrates?
   a. sildenafil
   b. tadalafil
   c. vardenafil
   d. all of the above
9. Which of the following STDs is treated with valacyclovir to reduce symptoms and outbreaks but not cure the disease?
   a. chlamydia
   b. genital herpes
   c. gonorrhea
   d. HPV
10. Which of the following contains phytoestrogens that can be used for relief of menopausal symptoms, such as hot flashes?
    a. soy
    b. black cohosh
    c. evening primrose oil
    d. all of the above

KNOW THE DRUGS

Match each brand name drug with its corresponding generic name and most common use. Your answers should follow this example format: Generic Name: 1. a; 2. b; 3. c; etc. Most Common Use: 1. h; 2. i; 3. j; etc.

Brand Name	Generic Name	Most Common Use
1. Viagra	a. ethinyl estradiol/desogestrel	h. Contraception
2. Depo-Provera	b. ethinyl estradiol/levonorgestrel	i. Hormone replacement therapy
3. Premarin	c. ethinyl estradiol/norgestimate	j. Erectile dysfunction
4. Mircette	d. medroxyprogesterone	
5. Cialis	e. conjugated estrogen	
6. Seasonique	f. sildenafil	
7. Ortho-TriCyclen Lo	g. tadalafil	

PUT IT TOGETHER

For each item, write either a single term to complete the sentence or a short answer.

1. ________________ is an important hormone that prepares the body for pregnancy and prepares the endometrial lining to support implantation of a fertilized egg.
2. ____________________ is the hormone detected in home pregnancy tests that indicates pregnancy has begun.
3. Which controlled substance schedule includes testosterone products? Why? What is the proper medical use of testosterone?
4. How many days should alternative methods of birth control be used if a transdermal contraceptive patch is removed or falls off and is left off for twenty-four hours?
5. Name the two natural/herbal products used for menopausal symptoms that seem to be supported by studies as most likely to be effective for hot flashes.

THINK IT THROUGH

Read and think through each numbered scenario carefully and then write several sentences in reply to the question(s) presented. Question 4 requires you to do some Internet research before completing your answer(s).

1. A young, timid female patient approaches you at the counter in the pharmacy. She is hesitant to ask you but inquires, "I've heard about something . . . a pill, like for abortion. I think it's called something like Plan B. How does someone get it?" What should you do?
2. You are entering a prescription for vardenafil into the computer. A warning comes up on the screen alerting you to a potential interaction with nitrates. You see that the patient's cardiologist has prescribed nitroglycerin, and his primary care provider has written a prescription for Levitra. Is this an important interaction? What should you do?
3. A female patient approaches you to ask where the yeast infection creams are. What should you do?

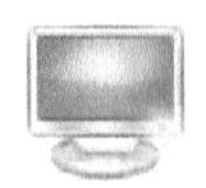

4. **On the Internet,** use the government Web site for PubMed to review publications about the Women's Health Initiative study. This large study is ongoing and looks at several outcomes, including cancer prevention and nutrition. However, in 2002 significant results were announced that long-term HRT increases risk of cardiovascular disease. This information contradicted conventional wisdom and medical practice at the time about use of HRT for menopausal symptoms and its perceived benefits on cardiovascular risk. The study changed practice recommendations to limit HRT for short-term relief of menopausal symptoms. From the information you find, can you determine reasons for the controversy and why women might be concerned about long-term use of HRT? Be sure you use publications dated 2002 or later.

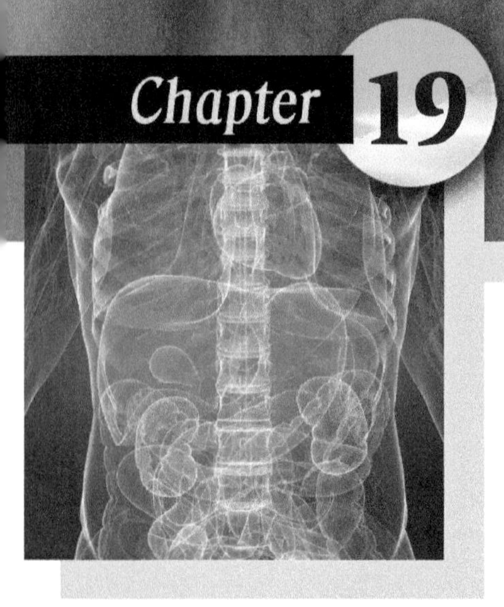

Chapter 19 The Renal System and Drug Therapy

LEARNING OBJECTIVES

- Describe the basic anatomy and physiology of the renal system.
- Explain the therapeutic effects of prescription medications, nonprescription medications, and alternative therapies commonly used to treat diseases of the renal system.
- Describe the adverse effects of prescription medications, nonprescription medications, and alternative therapies commonly used to treat diseases of the renal system.
- Identify the brand and generic names of prescription and nonprescription medications commonly used to treat diseases of the renal system.
- State the doses, dosage forms, and routes of administration for prescription and nonprescription medications commonly used to treat diseases of the renal system.

Interactive self-quizzes, games, audio files, and glossaries help you to learn drug names and facts.

Understanding the renal system is important in the field of pharmacy, because this system plays an essential role in eliminating drugs from the body. Most drugs or their metabolites eventually exit the body through the kidneys into the urine. Elimination, how fast and how much of a drug leaves the body, greatly affects how well a drug works and how often the patient must take it. Therapy choices are also affected by how much a desired medication relies on the renal system for excretion. In fact, kidney dysfunction is a frequent reason for dose adjustments. If the medication cannot exit the body, side effects and toxicities accumulate. As a pharmacy technician, you will see pharmacists alter doses to account for kidney function. Some drugs are directly damaging to the kidneys, and close monitoring is necessary. Pharmacists may ask you to assist in gathering laboratory results to assess kidney function.

Renal and urinary tract problems account for several frequently dispensed medications. Conditions such as urinary tract infections, spastic bladder, and prostate enlargement all have common drug treatments. Diuretics are used to treat high blood pressure and heart failure, but their site of action is in the kidneys and upon the regulatory systems that affect renal function. This chapter begins by describing the anatomy of the renal system and then explains how the nephron (the functional unit of the kidney) works. Common disorders and diseases of the urinary system and kidney function are covered along with the drug treatments for them. Drug classes such as antispasmodics and diuretics are described, along with treatments for benign prostatic hyperplasia (BPH).

Anatomy and Physiology of the Renal System

The **renal system**, also called the urinary system, is responsible for clearing waste products from the blood while maintaining proper fluid and electrolyte balance. The **kidneys** are the primary filter for this process. Blood flows through the kidneys, which clear it of metabolic by-products and waste substances. These compounds build up and become toxic if not eliminated from the body. The kidneys are responsible for balancing fluids and electrolytes, such as sodium, potassium, and calcium, in the body. The kidneys can affect acidity, or blood pH, as well as blood pressure. They also produce erythropoietin, which stimulates red blood cell production (as discussed in Chapter 13).

The kidneys perform the filtering function, and then the **ureters** transport the waste products and excess fluid to the **urinary bladder**, where these substances are held until voiding (urination) (see Figure 19.1). Urine exits the body through the **urethra**. In

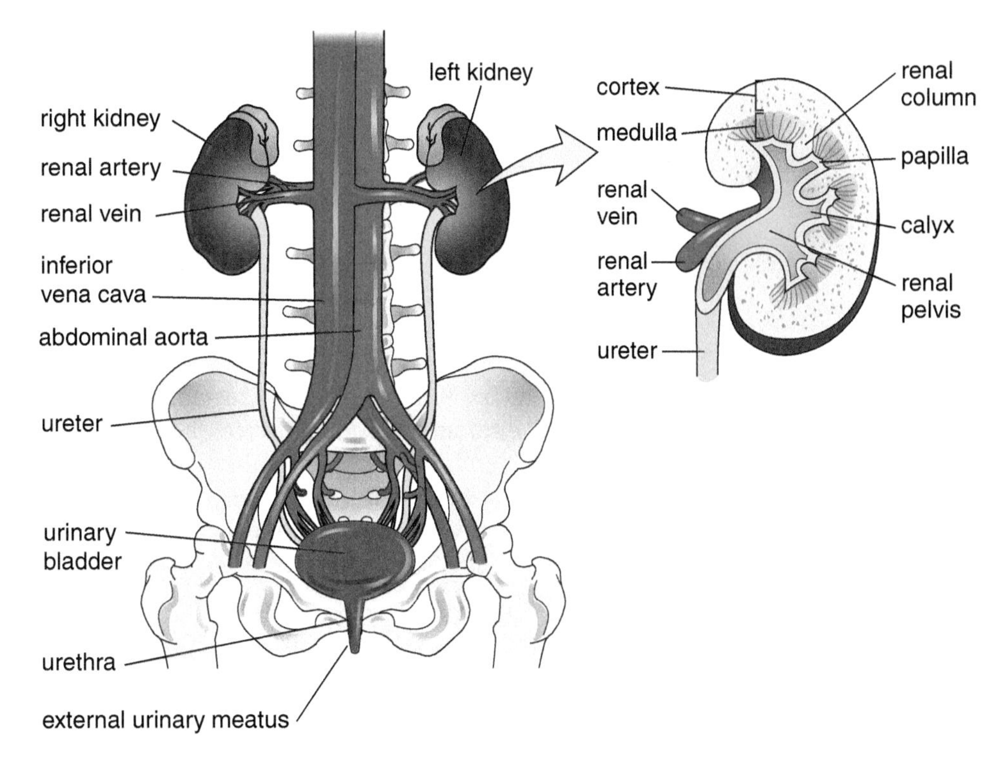

Figure 19.1
Anatomy of the Renal System
The proximity of the kidneys to the abdominal aorta, the largest artery in the body, makes these delicate organs highly susceptible to changes in blood pressure. High blood pressure damages the kidneys' filtering ability, and low blood pressure can cause acute renal failure.

females, the urethra is short, and in males, the urethra is long and passes through the center of the prostate gland before exiting the body.

The kidneys are bean-shaped organs located in the rear upper torso just below the ribs. Although they are in the abdominal region, they are not inside the peritoneal cavity, where the stomach, pancreas, and intestines are located. The adrenal glands (as discussed in Chapter 17) are located on top of the kidneys, almost like two little caps. The renal artery branches off from the abdominal aorta and brings blood into the kidneys. Blood that has been filtered in the kidneys returns to the bloodstream via the renal vein (see Figure 19.2).

The **renal cortex** is the outer layer of the kidneys and is responsible for hormone production. The **renal medulla**, in the body of each kidney, is made up of many

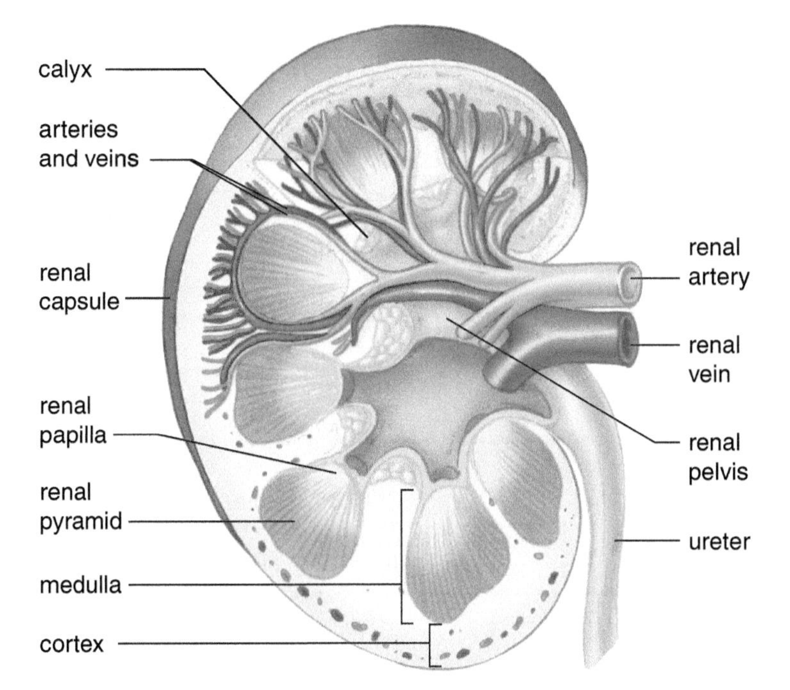

Figure 19.2
Kidney Anatomy
Erythropoietin, the hormone that stimulates red blood cell production, is released from the renal cortex.

triangle-shaped sections that perform filtration. Each triangular section is made up of thousands of microscopic-sized **nephrons**, the functional filtering units of the kidney. Urine formation begins in the nephron (see Figure 19.3). Urine production is a multistep process including (1) glomerular filtration, (2) tubular reabsorption, and (3) tubular secretion.

Blood containing fluid and waste products enters the nephron through the **afferent arteriole** into the **Bowman's capsule**. Here, the capillary is tightly folded, forming the **glomerulus**. The tight folding in the glomerulus and the small amount of space inside the capsule create the high pressure that forces fluid and other substances out of the blood. **Glomerular filtration** is the first step in urine production and the maintenance of fluid balance. Large molecules, such as proteins, are not filtered out in the glomerulus, but most fluids and other smaller substances are. Blood leaves the Bowman's capsule via the **efferent arteriole**. **Filtrate**, the fluids and by-products filtered out of the blood in the glomerulus, continues on through the nephron.

As filtrate passes through the tubules and **loop of Henle**, molecules selectively reenter the bloodstream via several mechanisms. Some substances are reabsorbed

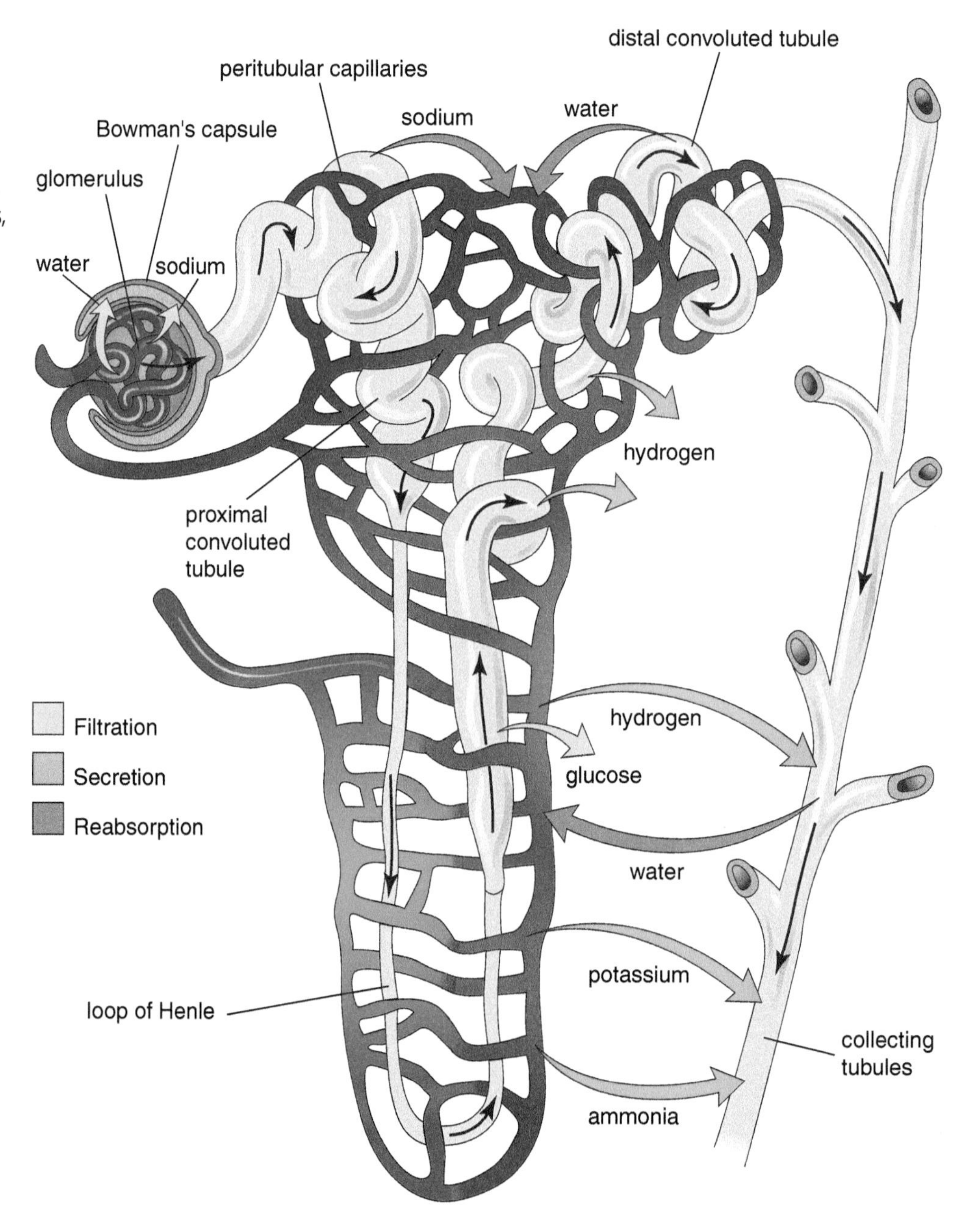

Figure 19.3
The Nephron and Urine Formation
Each part of the microscopic-sized nephron performs specific functions: filtration, reabsorption, and secretion of select electrolytes, fluids, and other substances.

through simple diffusion. Others are exchanged between blood and urine via secretion, an active transport process. Others move across the membranes due to force of pressure, which is another way to describe **filtration**. Those substances that are filtered out or secreted into the urine (but that do not reenter the blood) are then eliminated from the body.

Proper urine production and maintenance of fluid balance rely on the tubular **reabsorption** and **secretion** processes. In fact, reabsorption of water and sodium is essential for maintaining good hydration. If kidney failure occurs, the proper balance of excretion and reabsorption is not maintained. Inability to produce urine is called **anuria**. It signals kidney failure, which results in toxins building up in the blood and poisoning the body.

Hormones such as **aldosterone** and **antidiuretic hormone (ADH)** regulate the rate and volume of urine production. These hormones are released in response to changes in fluid status, blood pressure, and the concentrations of various substances in the blood. They can stimulate or inhibit urine production in the nephron and maintain overall body fluid status.

The urinary bladder is located in the pelvic region. It collects and holds urine until the fluid exits the body during urination. The bladder is made of stretchy epithelial and smooth muscle cells, which allow it to expand and contain up to a liter of fluid. The **internal urinary sphincter** muscle is an involuntary muscle that keeps urine from flowing back into the ureters once it enters the bladder. In contrast, the **external urinary sphincter** is a voluntary muscle that holds urine in the bladder before it exits the body.

When the bladder is full and distended, stretch receptors sense the pressure and cause the **detrusor muscles** in the bladder to contract and the external sphincter to relax. Urine is pushed out, and the bladder empties (see Figure 19.4). This urination process is called **micturition**. **Urinary retention** occurs when the kidneys make urine but the micturition process does not function properly and, consequently, urine accumulates in the bladder. This problem is a malfunction in the bladder. The inability to control the external urinary sphincter, thus allowing urine to leak out of the bladder, is called **incontinence**.

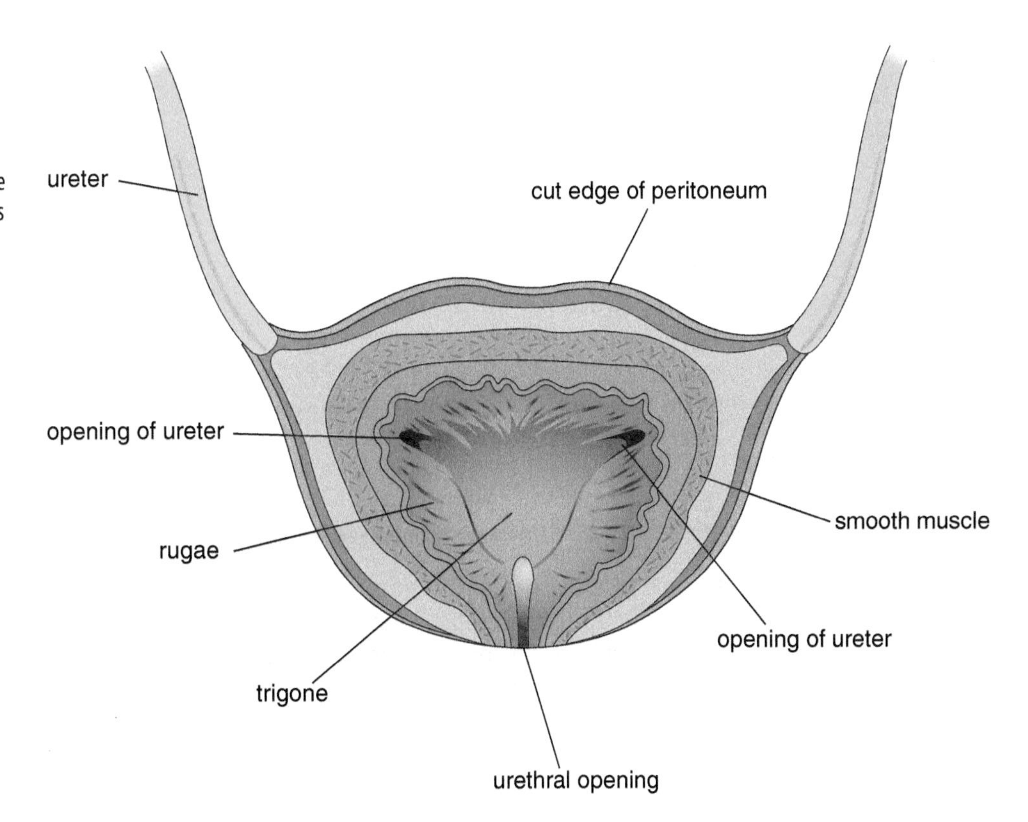

Figure 19.4
The Bladder
While the bladder can hold up to a liter of urine, stretch receptors typically trigger the urge to urinate when only 20% of that volume has accumulated.

Nephrotoxicity and Renal Dosing

Drug accumulation in the blood leads to side effects and toxicities. Drugs can cause direct damage, called **nephrotoxicity**, to kidney tissue. Examples of drugs commonly considered to be nephrotoxic or potentially nephrotoxic under certain conditions (including dehydration) include:

- nonsteroidal anti-inflammatory drugs
- amphotericin B
- contrast media (dye for imaging procedures)
- aminoglycosides
- vancomycin

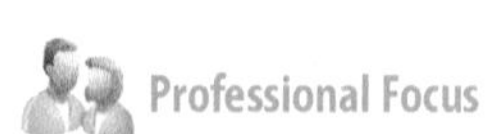

Learning which drugs require kidney function tests can help you anticipate the pharmacists' needs. If you work in the inpatient setting where you have access to lab test results, keep a list of these drug names on a card in your pocket and check it frequently. Take an extra moment to pull relevant lab results together and present them to the pharmacist first thing each morning.

Nephrotoxicity is usually reversible, but if it is not addressed quickly, it can cause kidney failure. Typically, renal function is monitored closely, and doses of these drugs are kept low to avoid negative effects.

Because so many drugs are eliminated from the body through the kidneys, dosing calculations must take into account the reduced renal function in patients with kidney problems. Even with drugs that are not directly harmful to the kidneys, doses for such patients must be adjusted because the drugs still require good renal function for elimination. Dose adjustment often depends on the degree of renal dysfunction present. Some drugs need dose adjustment only in the case of severe renal failure, whereas others cannot be used (are contradicted) even in mild kidney impairment. In some settings, pharmacy technicians may assist pharmacists in gathering kidney function laboratory tests for patients taking drugs that require renal dose adjustment.

Urinary Tract Infections

Urinary tract infections (UTIs) usually occur in the bladder but can affect any part of the urinary system. **Cystitis** is a lower UTI involving the bladder, and **pyelonephritis** is an upper UTI affecting the kidneys. **Prostatitis** is a prostate infection in men. Symptoms of UTIs include pain or burning during urination, a frequent urge to urinate, abdominal pain, fever, chills, and cloudy urine. Symptoms of pyelonephritis may also include flank pain (pain in the back, just under the ribs), nausea, and vomiting.

UTIs happen most often in sexually active women because the opening of the urethra is in close proximity to the vagina and anus, where bacteria are commonly found. The urethra is short in women, so bacterial access to the bladder is relatively easy. Most UTIs in women are considered uncomplicated in that they do not involve structural or neurologic problems in the urinary system. Bladder infections in men, however, are rare and considered complicated infections to treat. Complicated UTIs involve structural, obstructive, or other problems that contribute to their development. Treatment modalities other than drug therapy, such as surgery or prostate resection, may be required in these cases. Treatment of UTIs usually involves prescription antibiotics, such as penicillins, nitrofurantoin, sulfamethoxazole-trimethoprim, and ciprofloxacin. See Chapter 3 for more information on these antibiotics.

Spastic or Overactive Bladder

Spastic bladder is a malfunction of the detrusor muscles in the bladder, causing contraction and frequent urination. Patients feel the urge to urinate often and may also feel pain in the bladder. The condition can be embarrassing because it can cause frequent trips to the restroom and incontinence.

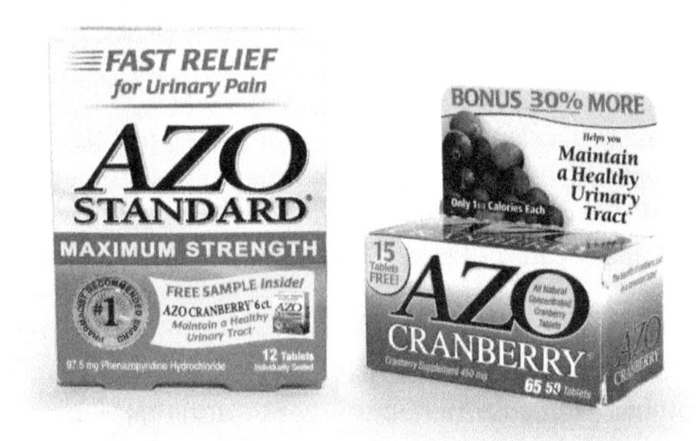

Technicians can help patients suffering from the discomfort of UTIs by showing them where to find a phenazopyridine product on the shelf.

Drugs for Spastic or Overactive Bladder

Urinary **antispasmodics** are used to treat spastic bladder and urinary frequency. Most of them work by inhibiting acetylcholine in the autonomic nerves that control involuntary bladder contraction and emptying. In effect, they relax the smooth detrusor muscles and enhance muscle waves in the ureters. Some drugs also have local anesthetic and analgesic effects to relieve pain. Most of these drugs work best on an empty stomach, so they should be taken a half hour prior to eating or two hours after eating.

Phenazopyridine is an over-the-counter agent with anesthetic effects specifically used for the pain, burning, itching, and urinary urgency associated with UTIs. Methenamine is a prescription product with similar indications (see Table 19.1).

Side Effects Common side effects of antispasmodics include dry mouth, constipation, blurred vision, and urine retention. These effects can subside over time but may not completely disappear. Drinking plenty of water or sucking on hard candy can help alleviate dry mouth. Staying hydrated and taking a stool softener may help with constipation. Other side effects can include drowsiness and stomach upset. If abdominal pain, eye pain, or difficulty urinating occurs, the patient should consult his or her prescriber. Allergic reactions are rare but can happen. Patients should inform their doctors if they experience skin rash while taking one of these medications.

May Discolor Urine

Cautions and Considerations Phenazopyridine can turn the urine orange and stain clothing. It also should be limited in length of use to two to three days only. Methenamine can turn urine blue. Patients, especially those using one of these agents for the first time, should be warned of this harmless but sometimes alarming effect. You should use appropriate auxiliary warning labels when dispensing these medications.

Table 19.1 Commonly Used Antispasmodics

Generic (Brand)	Dosage Form	Route of Administration	Common Dose
Darifenacin (Enablex)	Tablet	Oral	7.5 mg a day
Fesoterodine (Toviaz)	Tablet	Oral	4–8 mg a day
Flavoxate (Urispas)	Tablet	Oral	100 mg 3–4 times a day
Methenamine (Hiprex, Urex)	Tablet	Oral	1 g twice a day
Oxybutynin (Ditropan)	Tablet, syrup, patch	Oral, transdermal	Oral: 5 mg 2–3 times a day Transdermal: 3.9 mg patch applied every 3–4 days
Phenazopyridine (Azo, Pyridium)	Tablet	Oral	200 mg 3 times a day
Solifenacin (Vesicare)	Tablet	Oral	5 mg a day
Tolterodine (Detrol)	Tablet, capsule	Oral	2–4 mg a day
Trospium (Sanctura)	Tablet, capsule	Oral	20 mg twice a day or 60 mg extended-release form once a day

Benign Prostatic Hyperplasia (BPH)

Benign prostatic hyperplasia (BPH) is a chronic condition that happens in men as the prostate gland enlarges with age. Enlargement happens in all males, but it may not result in the same incidence of symptoms for all men (see Figure 19.5). Especially for men aged approximately sixty to eighty-five years, BPH is quite common. Although prostate enlargement is not harmful in itself, the enlarged gland can impinge on the urethra and obstruct urine flow.

Symptoms of BPH include a weak or slow urine stream, a delayed start of urination, and straining to urinate. Because urine flow is obstructed, the bladder cannot be fully emptied. This incomplete or partial emptying can cause frequent urges to urinate. Men with this condition find themselves feeling as if they need to urinate often, but they void only small amounts each time. The condition is diagnosed by a review of symptoms and a digital rectal exam, in which a gloved finger is inserted into the rectum to feel the prostate directly. **Prostate-specific antigen (PSA)** is a laboratory test that can screen for BPH and more serious prostate problems. When properly interpreted, elevations in PSA can indicate whether the enlargement is benign or potentially malignant (prostate cancer).

Some drug therapies cause urinary retention (see Table 19.2). These agents can exacerbate urination problems and should not be used by patients with BPH.

Though usually benign, prostate tissue growth can become a malignant process. Prostate cancer is the second most common type of cancer in men, just behind skin cancer. It is estimated that one in six men will be diagnosed with prostate cancer in their lifetime. Fortunately, prostate cancer is highly treatable, especially when caught early. Symptoms of prostate cancer are similar to those of BPH and include difficulty starting or stopping urination, frequent urination, painful urination, and blood in the urine.

Table 19.2 Agents to Avoid for Patients with BPH

Avoid	Instead Try . . .
Anticholinergics	H_2 blockers, sucralfate, antacids
Oral bronchodilators	Inhaled bronchodilators
Tricyclic antidepressants (TCAs)	Selective serotonin reuptake inhibitors (SSRIs)
Calcium-channel blockers	Alpha blockers
Disopyramide	Quinidine

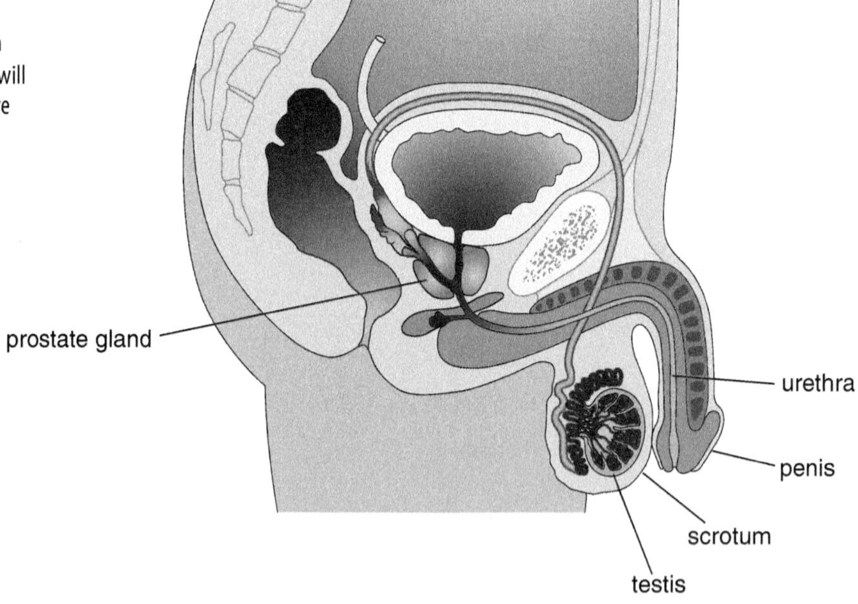

Figure 19.5
Anatomy of the Male Urinary System
Unvoided urine can promote infection. Most males will not have UTIs, but men with BPH may find they have bladder infections frequently.

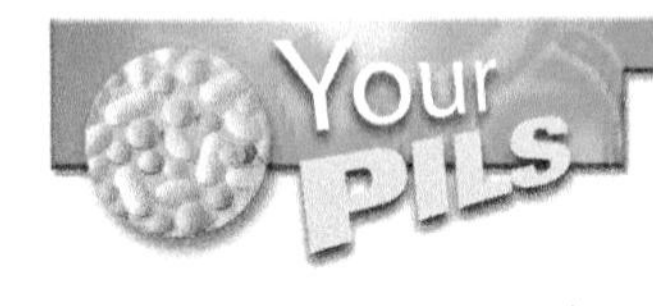

Enactors and Creators may enjoy this particular learning activity to help them remember the drugs used for urinary bladder problems. Antispasmodic agents and 5 alpha-reductase inhibitors (drugs for BPH) are frequently advertised on television and in magazines. Take some time to locate a few such ads and make note of the brand names mentioned. Think of the generic name for each drug and then describe how each drug works.

Drugs for BPH

Treating BPH first involves watchful waiting. When symptoms become bothersome, drug therapy is initiated. If symptoms become severe or cause complications, more invasive action may be needed. Procedures to remove part of the prostate and open an obstructed urethral lumen include transurethral resection of the prostate and transurethral needle ablation, among others.

Alpha Blockers This class of drugs is used for patients with BPH, especially those who also have high blood pressure. **Alpha blockers** work by inhibiting the alpha-1 receptors that relax smooth muscle in the prostate and bladder (as well as relax blood vessels in the rest of the body). Because hypertension plus BPH is a common combination in older men, these agents are used when treatment for both conditions is needed. Commonly used alpha blockers appear in Table 19.3. Other alpha blockers used primarily for hypertension include doxazosin, prazosin, and terazosin (see Chapter 7). In the urinary system, alpha blockers reduce urinary resistance and improve urine flow. They are sometimes used to help pass kidney stones that have become lodged in the ureters.

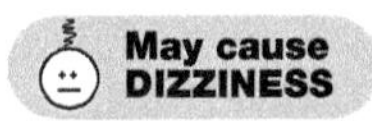

Side Effects Common side effects of alpha blockers include dizziness, drowsiness, fatigue, headache, fainting, and orthostatic hypotension, which is a drop in blood pressure that causes dizziness on sitting or standing up. Getting up slowly from a seated or lying position can alleviate this effect. Patients should be careful about driving or operating machinery until they know how the medication affects them. Patients should take these medications at night, before sleeping.

Alpha blockers also have sexual side effects that are very rare but serious. One such effect is priapism, a prolonged and painful erection. If this happens, patients should seek medical attention immediately or permanent damage and impotence could occur.

Cautions and Considerations Alpha blockers can have a first-dose effect whereby blood pressure drops dramatically, causing dizziness or fainting. Patients are often closely observed during the first dose to monitor for this effect. Repeated blood pressure measurement may be required for four to six hours after taking the first dose.

Alpha blockers interact with several other prescription medications. The patient should inform his or her prescriber and pharmacist of all medications he or she takes so that interactions can be detected and evaluated appropriately. Pharmacy technicians should not disregard any computer alerts or warnings regarding drug interactions. If you receive such an alert, stop and notify the pharmacist before filling the order.

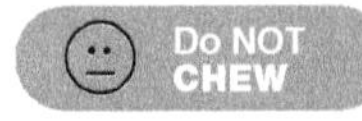

Tamsulosin and alfuzosin should be swallowed whole, not crushed or chewed. Affixing an auxiliary warning label to this effect is useful.

These agents must be used with caution in patients with gastrointestinal (GI) disorders, liver disease, or kidney impairment. Alpha blockers can exacerbate GI motility disorders. Patients should inform their prescribers if they have any of these conditions before taking an alpha blocker.

Table 19.3 Commonly Used Alpha Blockers

Generic (Brand)	Dosage Form	Route of Administration	Common Dose
Alfuzosin (Uroxatral)	Tablet	Oral	10 mg a day
Tamsulosin (Flomax)	Capsule	Oral	0.4–0.8 mg a day

5-Alpha Reductase Inhibitors This class of drugs is used for BPH, but it can also be used for male-pattern hair loss. The **5-alpha reductase inhibitors** (see Table 19.4) work by inhibiting the conversion of testosterone into dihydrotestosterone (DHT). Reducing this active form of testosterone reduces the size of the prostate, because prostate tissue growth is testosterone-dependent. Although blocking testosterone altogether would reduce prostate size, the side effects of reduced androgen production in the body are undesirable for most patients. With this class of drugs, only DHT is blocked, thereby reducing prostate size while allowing adequate levels of testosterone to remain in the bloodstream.

Side Effects Common side effects of 5-alpha reductase inhibitors include decreased libido, erectile dysfunction, and ejaculation disorders. They can also cause breast enlargement. If these effects are bothersome, the medication should be stopped.

Table 19.4 Common 5-Alpha Reductase Inhibitors

Generic (Brand)	Dosage Form	Route of Administration	Common Dose
Dutasteride (Avodart)	Capsule	Oral	0.5 mg a day
Finasteride (Propecia, Proscar)	Tablet	Oral	5 mg a day

Women DO NOT TOUCH with bare hands

Cautions and Considerations Because these agents block an active form of testosterone production, they could be harmful to a developing fetus in utero. Women of childbearing age must not handle these agents with bare skin. They should wear gloves to prevent measurable absorption of 5-alpha reductase, especially if handling broken tablets or opened capsules.

Kidney Failure

Kidney failure can be acute or chronic in nature. **Acute renal failure** generally occurs as a result of some type of damage, either physical or chemical, or lack of blood supply to the kidneys. Often, the insult is temporary or short-lived. If supportive care is provided and the cause for failure resolved, renal function typically returns to normal. If the insult is severe enough, acute renal failure can be life threatening and might leave some level of permanent damage. **Chronic kidney disease (CKD)**, on the other hand, involves progressive damage or results in the death of kidney tissue over time. CKD is irreversible.

Renal Function Tests

Laboratory blood tests are used to diagnose and monitor renal function. The most common tests are **blood urea nitrogen** and **serum creatinine (SCr)**. When renal function is impaired, the elimination of urea, nitrogen, and creatinine (a by-product of muscle metabolism) is also impaired, and their concentrations rise in the blood. Although results of these tests vary based on age, weight, and gender, as well as other factors such as exercise, these tests are good markers for renal function. Typically, the normal range for SCr is 0.5–1.5 mg/dL. SCr can be used to calculate **creatinine clearance (CrCl)** which estimates **glomerular filtration rate (GFR)**. CrCl and GFR estimate the level of kidney function while taking into account such factors as age and gender. The most common formula used to calculate CrCl is the **Cockcroft and Gault equation**:

$$\text{CrCl (mL/min)} = \underbrace{\frac{[(140 - \text{age}) \times \text{IBW}]}{\text{SCr} \times 72}}_{\text{multiply the result of this side of the equation by 0.85 for females}}$$

Where IBW is ideal body weight in kg and SCr is in mg/dL.

Although other formulas for estimating glomerular function exist, the Cockcroft and Gault equation is used most often when adjusting drug dosing for impaired renal function. For instance, the dose is decreased or the interval between doses is increased for many drugs when CrCl drops below 30 or 60 mL/min.

Pharmacists in the inpatient setting find themselves calculating GFR many times a day when monitoring drug therapy. As a technician, you can help pharmacists by retrieving these lab results and performing these calculations for those drugs requiring dose adjustment in renal impairment. Supplying the pharmacist with this information can help with efficiently monitoring those patients needing close follow-up.

Stages of CKD

CKD is more common than acute kidney failure. Common cases for CKD include diabetes and untreated hypertension. As stated earlier, chronic renal failure is irreversible, and it is progressive. As it worsens, it can be categorized into stages that guide the approach and degree of urgency for treatment (see Table 19.5). Drug therapies, such as diuretics and other renal-protective medications, can help slow the progression of the disease in early stages, but in later stages these agents are of no use. Eventually, dialysis and kidney transplant are the only means of treatment.

Table 19.5 Stages of Renal Disease

Stage	Disease State	Symptoms
Stage I	Loss of renal reserve	Patient is asymptomatic.
Stage II	Renal insufficiency	Patient is generally asymptomatic, but may experience nocturia (rising in the night to urinate) from inability to concentrate urine and hypertension. BUN and SCr are slightly elevated, and mild anemia is present.
Stage III	Chronic renal insufficiency	Patient has symptoms: easily fatigued, intolerance to cold, abnormal taste sensation, anorexia, anemia worsens, uremia (high levels of urea in the urine) begins, and dialysis may be indicated. BUN and SCr are clearly elevated.
Stage IV	End-stage renal disease	Patient requires chronic dialysis for survival. Patient may be candidate for renal transplant.

Dialysis

Dialysis is an artificial method of filtering blood and correcting the electrolyte imbalances caused by renal failure. When indicated, dialysis is accomplished by one of two common methods: hemodialysis or peritoneal dialysis. **Hemodialysis** is accomplished by diverting blood flow through a machine that mechanically filters the blood and returns the blood to the body (see Figure 19.6). **Peritoneal dialysis** is accomplished by putting dialysate (a special fluid that draws toxins from the body into itself) into the abdominal cavity and leaving it there for a period of time (usually a few days) (see Figure 19.7). During this time, toxins and electrolytes diffuse into the dialysate fluid from the many capillaries in the abdominal cavity. The dialysate fluid can be drained and changed at home with proper instruction. Risk of infection and other complications is greater with peritoneal dialysis.

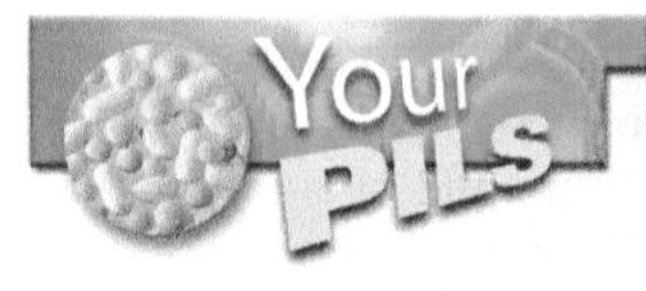

For those who like to observe others (such as Producers) or apply real-life experiences to what you learn from textbooks (as do Enactors or Directors), contact a local dialysis center and arrange a tour. Meet with a pharmacist who works with dialysis patients to talk about the drug therapy he or she sees most often in patients with kidney failure. Connecting real-world people and places to what you are learning makes it easier to grasp concepts and remember facts.

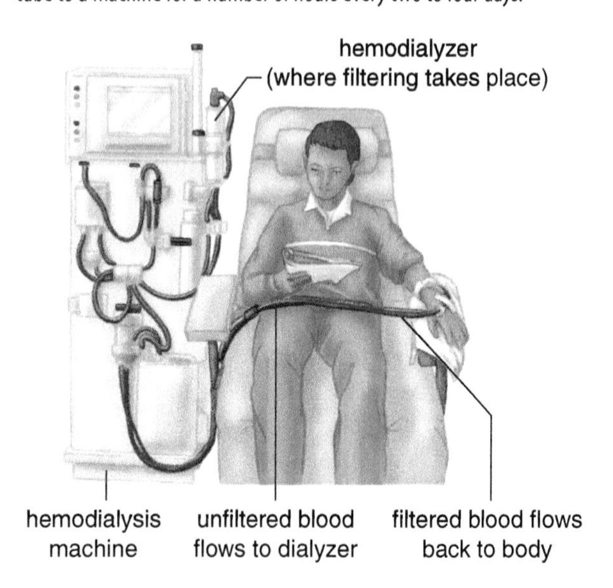

Figure 19.6
Hemodialysis
In hemodialysis, patients must be connected through an intravenous tube to a machine for a number of hours every two to four days.

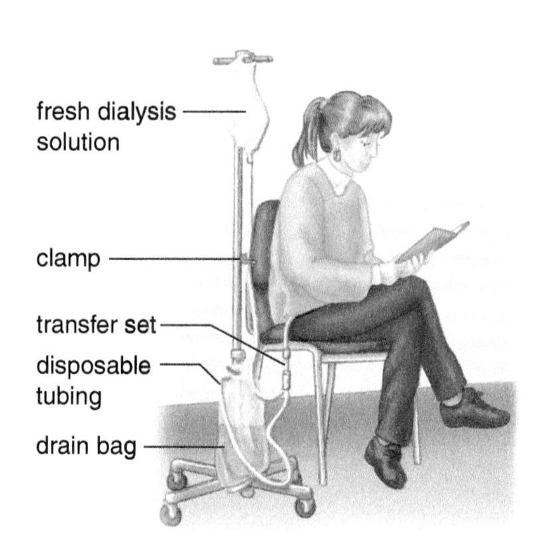

Figure 19.7
Peritoneal Dialysis
Peritoneal dialysis allows more freedom for patients because they do not have to return regularly to the dialysis center and remain hooked to a machine there for hours at a time.

Drugs for Renal Failure

Acute renal failure typically improves or reverses as its cause is resolved. Therefore, drug treatment for acute renal failure is limited and short term. CKD is more frequently treated with medication. Diuretics are used to improve urine output, but eventually CKD in advanced stages may require dialysis. In end-stage kidney failure, imbalances of sodium, potassium, calcium, phosphorus, aluminum, and vitamin D become problematic. Various drugs are needed in addition to dialysis. Anemia is also a problem as erythropoietin production from the renal cortex declines. Patients eventually need hemopoietic therapy and iron supplementation (see Chapter 13).

Diuretics These medications are used either to improve urine output in renal failure or to reduce blood volume in high blood pressure. Thiazides and potassium-sparing **diuretics** tend to be used more for hypertension, whereas loop diuretics are used more for renal failure or reducing edema. Combinations of these diuretic classes may be used in certain renal failure situations to maximize urine output. Figure 19.8 shows the site of action for the commonly used diuretics.

Thiazide diuretics work by inhibiting reabsorption of sodium and chloride ions in the distal tubule of the nephron. Because water follows sodium, water is excreted along with the sodium. In effect, water is pulled into the urine and eliminated from the body, thereby reducing blood volume. The loss of both water and sodium contributes to the decline in blood pressure. Because of a sodium-potassium exchange mechanism in the distal tubule, most diuretics cause potassium, in addition to sodium, to be lost. Especially at low doses, thiazide diuretics are cost-effective antihypertensives that are the drug of choice for newly diagnosed patients with high blood pressure.

Loop diuretics work by inhibiting reabsorption of sodium, chloride, and water in the ascending loop of Henle. This unique site of action produces fast and profound diuresis (urine production). Sodium, chloride, magnesium, calcium, and potassium are all excreted quickly and efficiently with use of a loop diuretic. For this reason, loop diuretics are used to pull fluid out of the body rapidly. Typically, these agents are used to treat swelling and fluid accumulation due to heart or kidney failure.

Potassium-sparing diuretics work by blocking the exchange of potassium for sodium that takes place in the distal tubule. Therefore, more sodium is excreted while potassium is preserved in the body. Water follows sodium, so water is excreted along

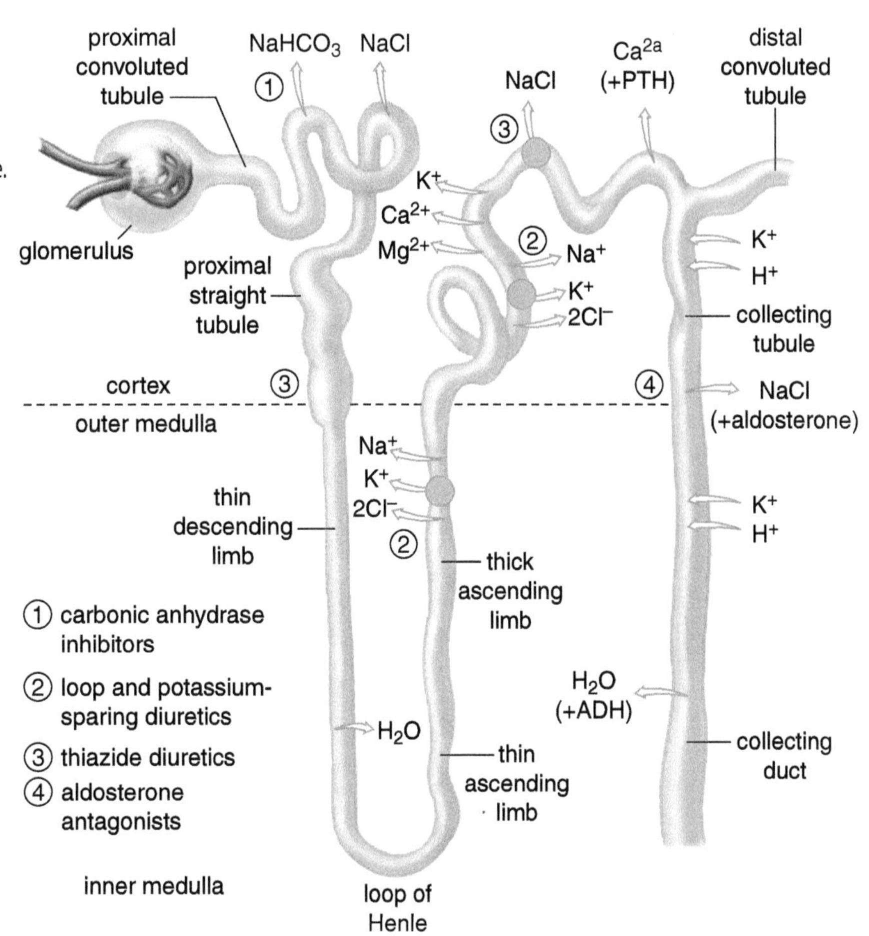

Figure 19.8
Diuretic Sites of Action
Thiazide diuretics work in the distal convoluted tubule, and loop diuretics work in the loop of Henle.

with sodium ions without depleting the body of potassium, as may happen with thiazide and loop diuretics. These drugs are primarily used to treat hypertension.

Aldosterone antagonists can be considered to be potassium-sparing, but they work by inhibiting a hormone that promotes fluid retention. Spironolactone, an older medication with this activity, has regained favor in recent years. It works by inhibiting aldosterone, which promotes sodium and water reabsorption in the distal tubule and collecting duct of the nephron. Spironolactone is primarily used for hypertension and heart failure and sometimes may be used in hyperaldosteronism (a condition in which the body produces too much aldosterone).

Carbonic anhydrase inhibitors work in the nephron by increasing excretion of bicarbonate ions, which carry sodium, potassium, and water into the urine. They are similar to sulfonamides in their chemical structure. Carbonic anhydrase inhibitors are used more commonly for open-angle glaucoma (see Chapter 11) but are occasionally used for diuresis in congestive heart failure.

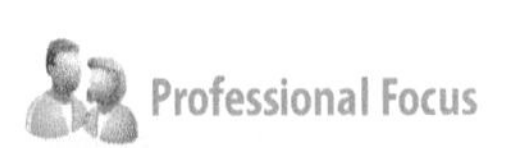
Professional Focus
Hydrochlorothiazide is a generic diuretic that is usually abbreviated HCTZ. Listen and look for it on prescriptions and medication orders.

Table 19.6 lists the commonly used diuretics by class. Combination products that contain diuretics from multiple drug classes are also available. Examples include Aldactazide, which contains spironolactone and hydrochlorothiazide (HCTZ), as well as Maxzide and Dyazide, which both contain triamterene and HCTZ.

Side Effects Common side effects of thiazide and loop diuretics are similar; they are also rare at low doses. Possible side effects include hypotension, dizziness, headache, rash, hair loss (alopecia), stomach upset, diarrhea, and constipation. Getting up slowly from sitting or lying down can help with dizziness and drops in blood pressure.

Common side effects of potassium-sparing diuretics include gynecomastia (breast enlargement). If bothersome, this effect may limit therapy because there is no treatment for it, other than to stop taking the drug. Other, less common side effects include stomach upset, headache, confusion, and drowsiness.

Common side effects of carbonic anhydrase inhibitors include tinnitus (ringing in the ears), tingling, nausea, vomiting, diarrhea, drowsiness, and changes in taste.

Table 19.6 Commonly Used Diuretics

Generic (Brand)	Dosage Form	Route of Administration	Common Dose
Thiazides			
Chlorothiazide (Diuril)	Tablet, suspension, injection	Oral, IV	Varies by age
Chlorthalidone (Thalitone, Hygroton)	Tablet	Oral	30–120 mg a day
Hydrochlorothiazide	Tablet, capsule	Oral	12.5–50 mg a day
Indapamide	Tablet	Oral	1.25–2.5 mg a day
Methyclothiazide (Enduron)	Tablet	Oral	2.5–10 mg a day
Metolazone (Zaroxolyn)	Tablet	Oral	2.5–20 mg a day
Loop Diuretics			
Bumetanide (Bumex)	Tablet, injection	Oral, IM, IV	Individualized to patient
Ethacrynate (Edecrin)	Tablet, injection	Oral, IV	Individualized to patient
Furosemide (Lasix)	Tablet, oral solution, injection	Oral, IV	Individualized to patient
Torsemide (Demadex)	Tablet	Oral	Individualized to patient
Potassium-Sparing Diuretics			
Amiloride (Midamor)	Tablet	Oral	5–20 mg a day
Spironolactone (Aldactone)	Tablet	Oral	25–200 mg a day
Triamterene (Dyrenium)	Capsule	Oral	200–300 mg a day
Carbonic Anhydrase Inhibitors			
Acetazolamide (Diamox)	Tablet, capsule, injection	Oral, IV	250–375 mg a day or every other day

Cautions and Considerations Thiazide and loop diuretics deplete potassium levels in the body. Taking **potassium supplements** is often necessary with these diuretics to maintain proper electrolyte balance. Patients should understand that taking these supplements is important because potassium is essential for good cardiac function.

On the other hand, some potassium-sparing diuretics, such as spironolactone, can cause hyperkalemia (high potassium levels) because they promote potassium retention. Periodic lab tests are needed to monitor for this effect.

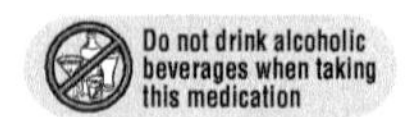

Thiazide diuretics can interact with alcohol to contribute to drops in blood pressure. Patients should use caution when drinking alcohol while taking these medications. Thiazides also interact with drugs for diabetes, because they can raise blood sugar levels. However, this is not a concern at low doses. In addition, thiazides interact with corticosteroids and lithium, so they are not usually used in conjunction with them.

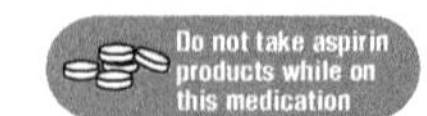

Carbonic anhydrase inhibitors can cause sulfa allergy and Stevens-Johnson syndrome. If patients experience rash while taking one of these agents, they should notify their prescribers right away.

Carbonic anhydrase inhibitors interact with aspirin to cause difficulty breathing, lethargy, coma, and even death. These agents should not be used in combination with each other.

Potassium Supplements Prescription potassium supplements are used to replenish a deficiency in this electrolyte as caused by diuretics (thiazides and loops). They are taken in tablet form on a daily basis. Most potassium tablets are quite large and can be difficult to swallow. Brand names include K-Lor-con, K-Tab, K-Dur, K-Lyte, Micro-K, Kaon-Cl, and K-lor. Common side effects of potassium supplements include nausea, vomiting, diarrhea, gas, and stomach upset. These effects are usually mild and can be reduced by taking the supplement with food or a full glass of water. Most potassium supplements are extended-release formulations, so they should be swallowed whole, not chewed or crushed. Effervescent tablets should be dissolved in three to eight ounces of water and then drunk slowly.

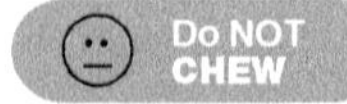

Because most salt substitute products contain potassium rather than sodium, patients who take potassium supplements should not use salt substitutes. If they do, they can ingest too much potassium, which is harmful to cardiac function. Patients with digestive problems that affect the motility of stomach or intestinal contents should not take potassium supplements. If the potassium tablet gets stuck, the lining of the digestive tract can become irritated and damaged.

Osmotic Diuretics This class of drugs has specialized use in severe trauma, cardiac operations, and elevated intracranial pressure (such as from a head injury). **Osmotic diuretics** work by increasing the concentration of the filtrate which hinders reabsorption of water into the bloodstream from the renal tubules. Mannitol is the osmotic diuretic used most frequently, but you may also see urea, glycerin, and isosorbide used in the inpatient setting.

Herbal and Alternative Therapies

Saw palmetto is used for BPH symptoms, such as frequent or painful urination, as well as urination hesitancy and urgency. Clinical studies have shown that this herbal treatment may have efficacy similar to that of finasteride in reducing these symptoms. Saw palmetto does not shrink overall prostate size; it works by reducing the thickness of the inner layer. It inhibits 5-alpha reductase, which prevents conversion of testosterone to DHT. It has some anti-inflammatory effects but does not reduce PSA levels. Side effects are mild and include dizziness, headache, nausea/vomiting, constipation, and diarrhea. Drug interactions with anticoagulants and some hormone therapies are possible. Patients should inform their physicians and pharmacists if they take saw palmetto. Typical doses are 160 mg twice a day or 320 mg once day. Saw palmetto teas do not generally provide a high enough dose to be effective.

Cranberry juice is used for prevention of recurrent UTIs. When consumed on a daily basis, it has been shown in clinical trials to be effective in preventing UTIs in elderly females, pregnant women, and inpatients. Oral capsules are not as effective. Although initially thought to acidify urine, cranberry juice is now thought to work by adhering to bacterial cells and preventing them from attaching to the inner walls of the bladder. Cranberry juice does not release bacteria that has already adhered to the bladder wall, so it does not treat an active UTI. In studies, patients drank sixteen ounces of cranberry juice daily. Although side effects are few, cranberry juice, when consumed in large quantities, can cause stomach upset and diarrhea. Cranberry juice can interact with warfarin, so patients drinking it on a regular basis or in large amounts should let their prescribers know.

Chapter Summary

Concepts regarding renal function are particularly important to know in pharmacy, because so many drugs rely on kidney function for their elimination from the body. Kidneys are the primary organs filtering the blood and removing toxins, metabolic by-products, and drugs. The nephron is the part of the kidney responsible for filtration. The blood concentration of SCr is used as a laboratory marker for kidney function. It is used to calculate GFR, a guide to estimating renal function and dosing drug therapy. Kidney damage can be acute or chronic in nature. Acute kidney failure is often reversible, whereas chronic kidney failure is irreversible and progressive. Stages of chronic renal disease have been established to guide treatment. Stage IV CKD is an indication for renal transplant. Other problems with the urinary system include UTIs, bladder spasticity, and prostate enlargement. Antispasmodics are used to treat spastic or neurogenic bladder. Alpha blockers, 5-alpha reductase inhibitors, and saw palmetto (a natural plant product) are used to treat BPH. Diuretics are used to improve kidney function and urine production. At low doses, they are used most often for hypertension, but at high doses can treat early stages of renal failure. Thiazide, loop, and potassium-sparing diuretics work in different parts of the nephron and are used in different situations. Thiazides and potassium-sparing diuretics are used most for high blood pressure, and loop diuretics are used when large amounts of fluid need to be pulled from the body in patients with heart or kidney failure.

Chapter Review

For the following sets of exercises, write the exercise heading, exercise numbers, and your answers on a separate sheet of paper. Your instructor may direct you to turn in the sheet of paper or discuss your answers as a class.

REVIEW THE BASICS

Choose a, b, c, or d as the correct answer to each multiple-choice question.

1. Which part of the kidney is responsible for filtering blood and producing filtrate?
   a. renal cortex
   b. glomerulus
   c. loop of Henle
   d. urinary bladder
2. Which part of the renal system carries urine from the kidney to the bladder?
   a. Bowman's capsule
   b. ureter
   c. urethra
   d. nephron
3. Which of the following is a potassium-sparing diuretic?
   a. tolterodine
   b. tamsulosin
   c. furosemide
   d. triamterene
4. Which of the following diuretics produces the most profound diuresis?
   a. HCTZ
   b. furosemide
   c. spironolactone
   d. amiloride
5. Saw palmetto is most similar in mechanism of action to which of the following?
   a. terazosin
   b. oxybutynin
   c. finasteride
   d. phenazopyridine
6. Which of the following drugs cannot be handled by women of childbearing age?
   a. Detrol
   b. Flomax
   c. Propecia
   d. Bumex
7. Which of the following drugs works by promoting sodium reabsorption in the distal tubule?
   a. acetazolamide
   b. spironolactone
   c. doxazosin
   d. solifenacin
8. Patients taking which of the following drugs may likely need to take a potassium supplement?
   a. flavoxate
   b. HCTZ
   c. spironolactone
   d. triamterene
9. Which of the following drugs can cause gynecomastia?
   a. spironolactone
   b. prazosin
   c. methenamine
   d. HCTZ
10. A patient in which stage of chronic kidney disease would most likely be on dialysis?
    a. Stage I
    b. Stage II
    c. Stage III
    d. Stage IV

KNOW THE DRUGS

Match each brand name drug with its corresponding generic name and most common use. Your answers should follow this example format: Generic Name: 1. a; 2. b; 3. c; etc. Most Common Use: 1. g; 2. h; 3. i; etc.

Brand Name	Generic Name	Most Common Use
1. Lasix	a. finasteride	g. urinary spasticity
2. Avodart	b. oxybutynin	h. BPH
3. Propecia	c. acetazolamide	i. diuresis
4. Detrol	d. tolterodine	
5. Ditropan	e. furosemide	
6. Diamox	f. dutasteride	

PUT IT TOGETHER

For each item, write down either a short answer or a single term to complete the sentence.

1. Name two drugs that can cause nephrotoxicity. List drug names, not drug classes.
2. Name the classes of diuretics used most often for the treatment of hypertension. Which class is used to pull fluid from the body quickly when someone has edema due to heart or kidney failure?
3. During which stage of CKD are patients generally asymptomatic, except maybe for some nocturia?
4. Thiazide diuretics work primarily in the __________ of the nephron, whereas loop diuretics work primarily in the __________ of the nephron.
5. List at least four side effects for urinary antispasmodics. What can patients do to alleviate these effects?
6. In what dosage form(s) are potassium supplements available?

THINK IT THROUGH

Read and think through each numbered scenario carefully and then write several sentences in reply to the question(s) presented. Question 4 requires you to do some Internet research before completing your answer(s).

1. While picking up a refill for Lasix, Mr. Monroe tells you that he is glad he was finally placed on the waiting list for a kidney transplant. He says he is tired of going to dialysis three times a week and can't wait to feel better after the surgery. What stage of CKD is Mr. Monroe likely to be in? What type of dialysis is he most likely receiving?
2. Severe infections, fluid imbalances, and chronic disease are common in patients admitted to hospitals. In the inpatient setting, kidney function is altered in many patients, so pharmacists must adjust drug dosing for these patients regularly. Describe two ways that drug dosing may be changed to accommodate reduced drug elimination through the kidneys.
3. A female customer approaches you at the counter to inquire about an oral cranberry product she found on the shelf in the aisle. She says she has heard that cranberry helps treat urinary tract infections. She complains that she has a lot of UTIs and would like to take something more natural for them. What should you do?

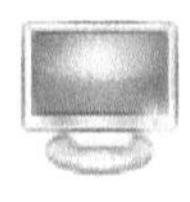

4. **On the Internet,** look up the FDA-approved labeling (often called full prescribing information) for the top ten drugs dispensed in your workplace. If you aren't working in a pharmacy, see Chapter 1 for how to locate a published list of commonly dispensed medications on the Internet and then pick ten such drugs. You can find prescribing information by going to the manufacturer's Web site for each drug product. See if recommendations are made for adjusting the dose in patients with renal impairment. (You can find this information in the section labeled Use in Specific Populations.) What could you do as the technician to facilitate this dose-adjustment process? Are there any drugs in this chapter that need to be dose-adjusted for renal impairment?

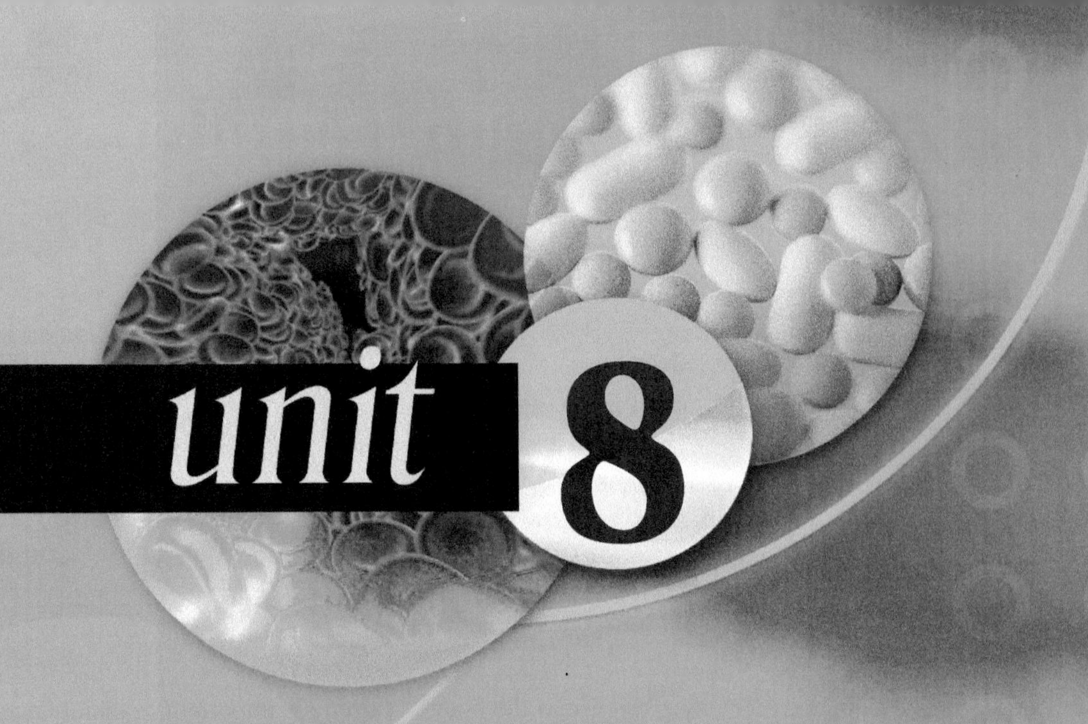

Drugs for Specialized Therapies

Chapter 20 Fluids and Electrolytes

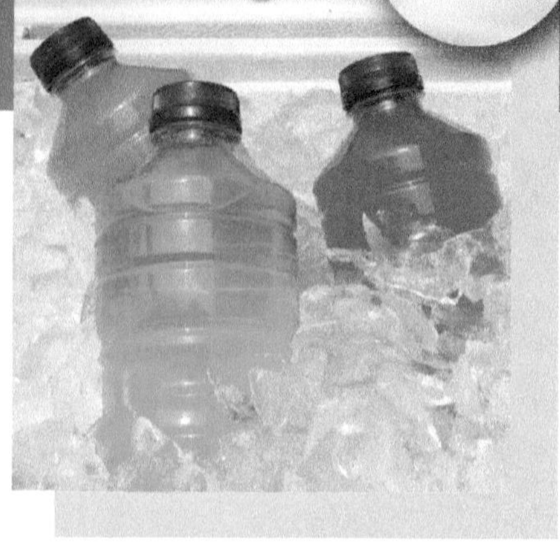

LEARNING OBJECTIVES

- Describe the basic physiological effects of fluids and electrolytes.
- Explain the therapeutic effects of fluids and electrolytes.
- Describe the adverse effects associated with treatment for fluid and electrolyte imbalance.
- State the dosage forms and routes of administration of fluid and electrolyte products.

Interactive self-quizzes, games, audio files, and glossaries help you to learn drug names and facts.

Fluid and electrolyte balance in the body is extremely important to maintaining life. Severe dehydration, for instance, can lead to organ failure and death. Water, the most abundant fluid in the body, is a major component of living cells. Typically, daily needs for water and minerals are met through normal nutrition and fluid intake. When fluid intake is altered or other disease processes affect normal balance, supplementation is needed. Consequently, several types of intravenous (IV) fluids and electrolyte products are used to prevent and treat fluid imbalances. Some of these fluids, such as normal saline and dextrose in water, are also used as delivery vehicles for IV drug therapy. Therefore, inpatient pharmacies use IV fluids and electrolytes every day when mixing and compounding sterile products. Because misuse of IV fluids and electrolytes can have dire consequences, pharmacists and technicians must emphasize special mixing parameters when working with such products. Appreciation for the benefits and limitations of these products is essential to providing high-quality patient care.

Physiology of Fluid and Electrolyte Balance

Fluids and electrolytes are highly related and dependent on each other. A change in one component usually causes subsequent changes to the other. Electrolytes are **solutes** dissolved in a **solvent**, usually water. **Water** moves from areas of low solute concentration to areas of high solute concentration in an attempt to maintain equilibrium. Fluids and electrolytes move around the body in relation to each other. A loss of fluids in one area of the body prompts a shift in fluids from another area to replace what was lost. During this shift, electrolytes are exchanged in an effort to balance the concentration of solutes between fluid compartments of the body.

Fluids

Fluid in the body is compartmentalized into intracellular and extracellular spaces. Two-thirds of body fluid is **intracellular fluid**, or contained inside the cellular membrane, and-one third is **extracellular fluid**, or located outside of the cells (see Figure 20.1). The volume of intracellular fluid remains relatively constant. In contrast, extracellular fluid volume varies and contains the majority of substances that are active in maintaining proper solute concentrations. Of the extracellular fluid, three-quarters of it resides in the **interstitial spaces** between the cells in tissues. The balance is part of the **plasma** inside the vasculature. Extracellular fluid plays a major role in maintaining overall fluid balance and hydration status.

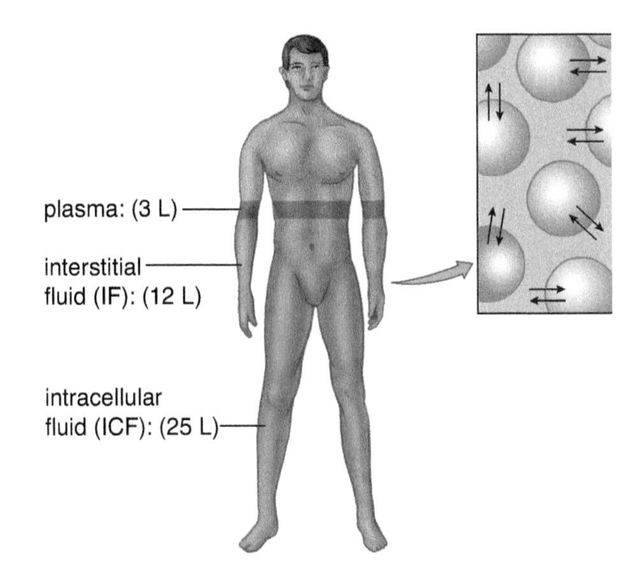

Figure 20.1
Body Fluid Compartments
Extracellular fluid, the active fluid that maintains hydration status, consists of plasma and interstitial fluid. Average quantities of water are given in liters (L) for each compartment in the body.

Most fluid in the body is water. In fact, one-half or more of body weight is water. As Figure 20.2 shows, 60% of body weight in men is water, whereas in women, this figure is 50%. Water is a crucial medium for dissolving substances essential for life and transporting these important molecules throughout the body. Water content changes with age and body makeup.

Homeostasis, which involves proper fluid balance, is maintained by multiple systems that regulate water intake and output as well as distribute water into the various body compartments. Typically, water intake roughly matches output (see Figure 20.3). Most adults take in approximately two liters of water a day by drinking fluids and eating food. A small amount of water is also produced during normal metabolism and breakdown of substances in the body. This water intake and production is necessary to replenish fluid lost through urination, feces production, and insensible loss (i.e., respiration and sweating).

Electrolytes

Electrolytes are molecular compounds that form ions when dissolved in water. Because water forms the majority of body fluid, electrolytes exist throughout the body as positively or negatively charged ions. For example, sodium chloride (table salt) dissociates into sodium (Na^+) and chloride (Cl^-) when dissolved in water. Positively charged ions

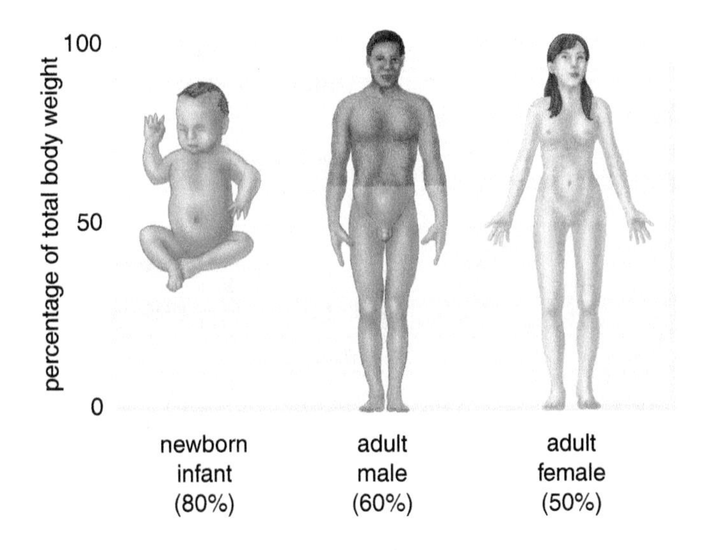

Figure 20.2
Body Water Content
In infants, water constitutes as much as 70–80% of the body by weight; in the elderly, water content is much lower.

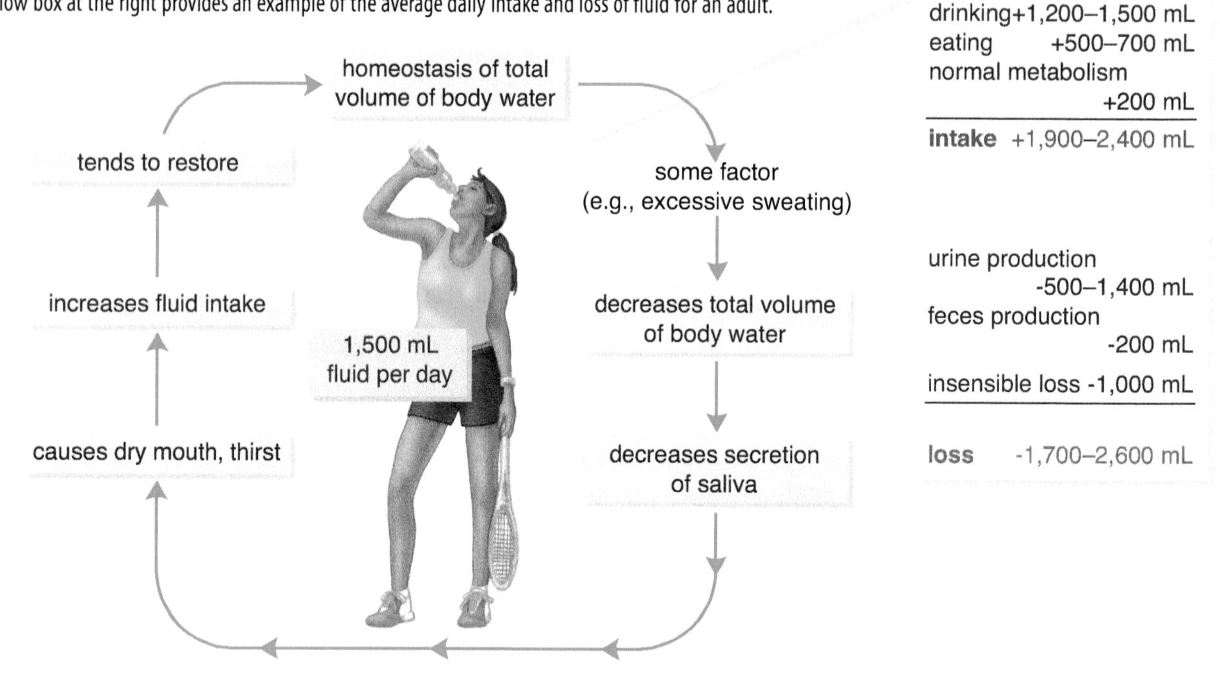

Figure 20.3
Daily Fluid Balance
Regulation mechanisms such as thirst and urine output help the body maintain proper fluid balance. The yellow box at the right provides an example of the average daily intake and loss of fluid for an adult.

are called **cations**, and negatively charged ions are **anions**. Important cations in the body are sodium (Na^+), potassium (K^+), calcium (Ca^{2+}), and magnesium (Mg^{2+}). Important anions include chloride (Cl^-), bicarbonate (HCO_3^-), and, at times, phosphate (PO_4^-). Concentration of electrolytes is measured in **milliequivalents (mEq)** per liter (L). Electrolytes are present in both intracellular and extracellular fluid, though in differing concentrations, depending on the ion (see Table 20.1). Specific ion pumps (e.g., sodium/potassium ion pumps) and channels (e.g., chloride channels) in cellular membranes maintain these concentrations.

Water passively moves across cellular membranes by **osmosis** to maintain the overall equilibrium in concentration of total molecules on both sides. If a solute (for example, an ion) is added to one side of the membrane, water moves to that side to keep concentration constant on both sides. More often than not, concentration of intracellular and extracellular fluid remains constant.

Sodium is the most abundant cation in the extracellular fluid. Sodium retains fluid in the body, helps generate and transmit nerve impulses, assists with acid-base balance, regulates enzyme activity, and serves as the primary active ion in maintaining fluid **isotonicity.** Isotonicity is a state of balanced concentration across cell membranes.

Table 20.1 Normal Electrolyte Concentrations

	Extracellular Fluid		Intracellular Fluid (mEq/L)
	Plasma (mEq/L)	Interstitial Fluid (mEq/L)	
Sodium (Na^+)	136–145	146	15
Potassium (K^+)	3.5–5.5	5	150
Calcium (Ca^{2+})	4.3–5.3	3	2
Magnesium (Mg^{2+})	1.5–2.5	1	27
Chloride (Cl^-)	100–106	144	1
Bicarbonate (HCO_3^-)	27	30	10

Potassium is the primary cation in intracellular fluid. Potassium is important in generating and transmitting nerve impulses and muscle contraction, such as in cardiac function and rhythm. Potassium also assists with acid–base balance, regulates enzyme activity, and is involved in carbohydrate metabolism.

Calcium is most often associated with bone formation, and it is also essential for muscle contraction and conducting impulses. Proper blood coagulation depends on sufficient intake of this electrolyte. Calcium is a positively charged ion that is highly bound to albumin, a protein in the plasma. Low albumin levels can therefore result in hypocalcemia.

Magnesium is an abundant intracellular cation. Most magnesium in the body is inside cells. It activates enzymes and facilitates normal nerve impulse production and muscle contraction. It is important in cardiac function.

Chloride is an anion that transports carbon dioxide, forms hydrochloric acid in the stomach, and retains potassium. It is important in controlling acid–base balance.

Bicarbonate is an anion that helps to maintain pH balance in the blood. Its most common salt form, sodium bicarbonate, is used in IV preparations in the inpatient pharmacy setting for patients with acidosis (low blood pH).

Phosphate is an anion that plays an important role in energy production within cells. Without sufficient phosphate, normal cell function is not possible. Phosphate commonly exists in counterbalance with calcium in the bloodstream. Excessive intake of phosphate can deplete calcium levels and affect bone health.

Acid-Base Balance

In addition to impacting fluid status, electrolytes affect the balance of **hydrogen ions (H^+)** in the bloodstream. The concentration of hydrogen ions is reported on the **pH scale** (see Chapter 2) and determines **acidity** or **alkalinity** of body fluids. Low pH represents acidic, and high pH represents basic properties. The pH of blood is maintained between 7.35 and 7.45. The body uses an **acid–base pair buffer** system to keep pH in this narrow range. **Carbonic acid** (acid) and **sodium bicarbonate** (base) are constantly produced through normal metabolism and respiration. This acid–base pair works together to mitigate, or buffer, large changes in pH. If acid is added to the blood, sodium bicarbonate reacts and neutralizes it. Likewise, carbonic acid neutralizes bases.

Acid–base balance is also maintained by kidney and lung function. Kidneys regulate retention and excretion of electrolytes in the urine. For instance, retaining acidic electrolytes, such as phosphate and ammonium, lowers blood pH. Respiration can correct pH imbalance more quickly than can kidney action. Carbon dioxide combines with water in the blood to make carbonic anhydrase, an acid. Breathing faster or slower changes the rate at which carbon dioxide is exhaled and eliminated from the blood. The body then makes more or less carbonic acid, which changes blood pH.

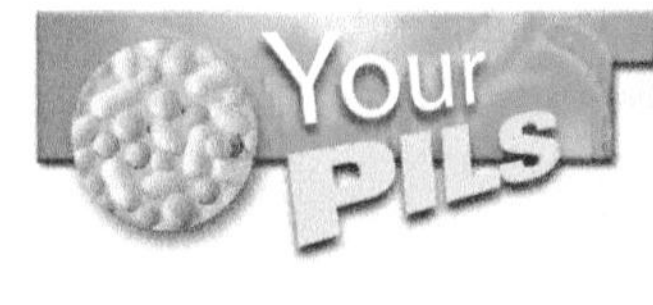

If you like learning with other people, as Creators and Enactors do, find a classmate with whom to discuss acid–base balance. Explain to each other what happens if an acid or a base is added to the bloodstream. Talking through this mechanism out loud is a way to solidify this concept. Teaching it to someone else helps you better understand the concept yourself.

Dehydration and Edema

Dehydration is the excessive loss of bodily fluids, primarily water. It can occur from vomiting, diarrhea, sweating from heat or fever, or excessive urine output. Symptoms of dehydration include thirst, dry mucous membranes, weakness, dizziness, dry skin, reduced skin elasticity (turgor), hypotension, rapid heartbeat, and reduced or absent urine production. Treatment of mild dehydration can be accomplished by drinking fluids. Moderate to severe dehydration requires IV fluids and electrolytes. Simply drinking or administering water alone will not correct the imbalance. In fact, water alone can be harmful. Fluids supplied for rehydration should be balanced with electrolytes so as not to cause further electrolyte imbalance while fluid status is being corrected.

Edema is an accumulation of excessive fluid in the interstitial tissue space. In edema, fluid most commonly accumulates in the lower extremities, the lungs, and sometimes the brain. Edema generally manifests as swelling in the ankles and legs or as difficulty breathing when it affects the lungs. One of the most common causes for edema is sodium (and fluid) retention in the extracellular compartment. Another cause of edema is renal failure. As the kidney function weakens, fluid cannot exit the body and begins to collect in interstitial spaces. Yet another cause for edema is reduced tissue perfusion, such as that which occurs in congestive heart failure. When the heart cannot efficiently pump blood through the vasculature, it pools in the capillaries. The resulting blood pressure buildup causes fluid to squeeze or leak into surrounding tissue. Treating edema requires both removal of excessive fluid as well as correction of electrolyte imbalances. Diuretics are the most common drug treatment for edema (see Chapter 19). They eliminate fluid from the body via the kidneys and urination.

Fluids and Solutions

IV fluid products are used to replace lost fluids and electrolytes due to dehydration as well as in parenteral nutrition solutions to supply essential trace minerals. They are also used as a liquid vehicle for administering IV drug therapy. IV fluids can be categorized by tonicity or content (i.e., colloids versus crystalloids).

Tonicity refers to the concentration of a solute (dissolved substance) in a solvent (liquid vehicle such as water) and how that concentration affects movement of water across membranes. The concept of tonicity refers only to molecules, such as ions and electrolytes, that do not move easily across membranes. Fluid and electrolyte products in the pharmacy have labeled concentrations in grams of solute per 100 mL of solvent, which is displayed as percent concentration.

Another related concept that affects tonicity is osmolarity. **Osmolarity** refers to the concentration of all molecules, both those that move across membranes and those that do not, in a set volume of fluid. Osmolarity is measured in milliosmoles (mOsm) per liter (L). The osmolarity of plasma is approximately 280–300 mOsm/L.

Isotonic solutions have a concentration similar to blood plasma. Isotonic fluid products replace daily fluid and electrolyte loss and prevent dehydration. When administered IV, normal balance between the vascular volume and interstitial spaces is maintained. Isotonic solutions are sometimes referred to as maintenance solutions. The most common isotonic IV solution used is normal saline (0.9% NaCl). Figure 20.4 shows what can happen when cells in the blood or body are exposed to solutions that are not isotonic.

Hypertonic solutions contain a higher concentration of solute than bodily fluids. Osmolarity of these products is usually over 350 mOsm/L. These products are used when urgent sodium replenishment is needed as part of hydration. They are indicated for severe sodium depletion from excess sweating, vomiting, or diarrhea. They are also used for excessive water intake, overuse of enemas or irrigating solutions (during surgery), and when sodium-free fluids and electrolyte products have been used for fluid replacement. Cells placed in a hypertonic solution shrivel and shrink as water passes out of the cell membrane (see Figure 20.4).

Hypotonic solutions contain a lower concentration of solute than bodily fluids. Osmolarity of these products is usually less than 280 mOsm/L. These solutions treat dehydration by diluting the concentration within the bloodstream, which decreases osmolarity. Water leaves the blood and enters interstitial and intracellular spaces. Cells placed in a hypotonic solution swell and burst as water rushes into the cell. Hypotonic solutions are commonly referred to as hydrating solutions, because they are used to correct dehydration.

Figure 20.4
Tonicity Effects on Cells in Solution
Body cells can be bathed with isotonic solution without a net change between intracellular and extracellular concentrations.

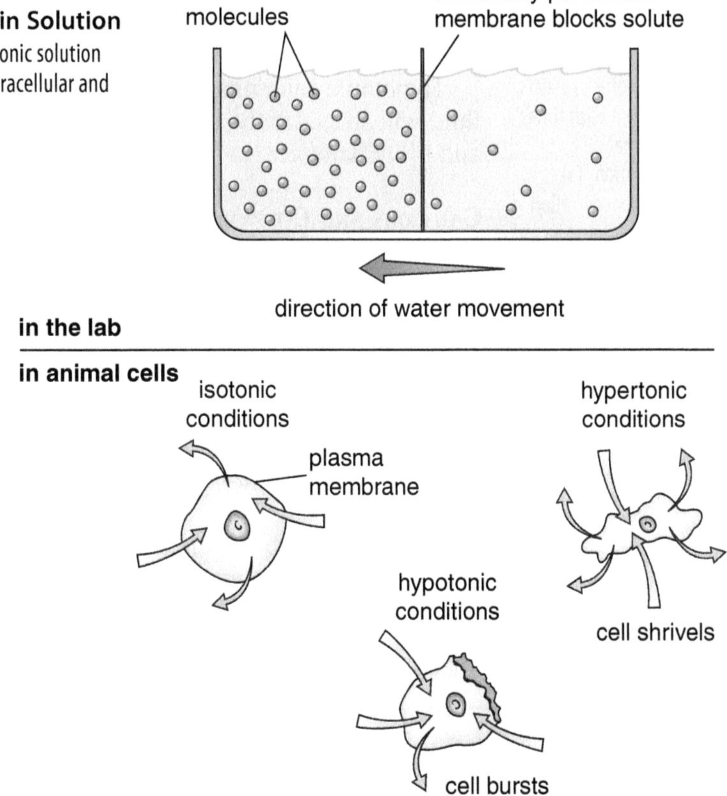

Crystalloid IV solutions contain electrolytes and **colloids**, which contain proteins and other large molecules (such as fats). Molecules in colloid products are so large that they do not quickly or easily move from the bloodstream to surrounding tissues. In that way, colloids act similarly to hypertonic solutions. They increase osmolarity of blood plasma, which pulls fluid from interstitial spaces. They are commonly referred to as blood volume expanders. Examples of colloids include albumin, dextran, and blood itself.

Crystalloid solutions contain small ions and molecules. They are used to replace lost fluid and treat dehydration. They are used on a daily basis as a liquid vehicle for administering IV drugs. Both normal saline and dextrose in water are crystalloid solutions. Dextrose is desirable when a patient has need for caloric energy (such as in malnutrition) or glucose levels are low. Table 20.2 contains examples of common crystalloid solutions along with their associated osmolarity.

Table 20.2 Common Crystalloid Solutions

Tonicity	Solution	Osmolarity
Hypotonic (hydrating) solutions	0.45% NaCl (½ NS)	155 mOsm/L
	Dextrose 2.5% in sterile water ($D_{2.5}W$)	140 mOsm/L
Isotonic solutions	Dextrose 2.5% in 0.45% NaCl ($D_{2.5}W$ in ½ NS)	280 mOsm/L
	Dextrose 5% in sterile water (D_5W)	300 mOsm/L
	0.9% NaCl (normal saline [NS])	310 mOsm/L
	Lactated Ringer's solution (LR)	275 mOsm/L
Hypertonic solutions	Dextrose 5% in 0.45% NaCl (D_5W in ½ NS)	405 mOsm/L
	Dextrose 5% in 0.9% NaCl (D_5W in NS)	560 mOsm/L
	Dextrose 10% in sterile water ($D_{10}W$)	600 mOsm/L
	3, 5, 14.6, and 23.4% NaCl concentrates	varies

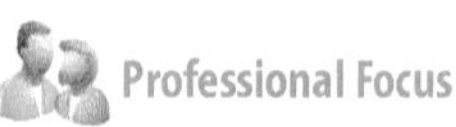
Professional Focus

If you work in the inpatient setting where you compound sterile products, take a moment each time you use normal saline or dextrose solution. Take note of the concentration and recall whether it would be considered isotonic, hypertonic, or hypotonic.

Side Effects Hypertonic solutions must be administered slowly and monitored closely. If given too quickly, the mass exodus of fluid from vital tissues can cause damage. Resulting fluid overload inside the blood vessels can cause heart failure.

Hypotonic solutions must also be used with caution. If administered too quickly, fluid will shift into the cerebral compartment and cause increased intracranial pressure and brain damage.

Cautions and Considerations Hypertonic solutions can be quite irritating and corrosive to tissues and blood vessels. They must be administered via a central IV line (i.e., surgically inserted into a port in a central vein), not a peripheral IV line placed in the arm or hand.

Sterile water for injection is a product available in the pharmacy. It is used for diluting other IV drugs or fluids and should never be administered by itself. Injecting or administering pure water through an IV line causes mass hemolysis as water rushes from the plasma into red blood cells, quickly bursting them. Hemolysis destroys the blood and releases intracellular material in mass amounts, causing death. Any order written for hydration therapy containing pure water must be questioned immediately. Careful attention to calculations and mixing procedures is vital to ensure that final products have the intended tonicity and to ensure patient safety.

Electrolyte Imbalances

Electrolyte imbalances can be caused by loss or excessive production of the electrolyte itself, or from a relative reduction or excess of fluid. Normal ranges for common electrolyte laboratory values in plasma are shown in Table 20.1. Measuring electrolyte concentration in plasma is a close estimate of extracellular levels. Intracellular levels cannot be directly measured, so lab values must be combined with clinical signs and symptoms to determine when deficits exist. Pharmacy technicians can retrieve laboratory values and flag results that are outside of the normal range. Knowing the conditions for which fluid and electrolyte status is monitored can be valuable. Retrieving relevant lab results and presenting them to the pharmacist can speed up effective patient care.

Hyponatremia is low sodium concentration, and **hypernatremia** is elevated sodium concentration relative to normal range. Hyponatremia is related to sodium loss or a relative excess of water in the extracellular space. It can be caused by excessive water intake, overuse of salt-wasting diuretics, adrenal gland insufficiency, and kidney or liver failure. Low sodium concentrations can also occur with fluid loss caused by excessive sweating or vomiting. Hypernatremia can be caused by dehydration from lack of fluid intake, diarrhea, and deficiency of antidiuretic hormone. Heart disease and kidney failure can also cause this condition.

Hypokalemia is a condition of lower than the normal potassium concentration. Potassium can be lost through overuse of potassium-wasting diuretics, vomiting or gastric suctioning, or excessive urine output. Signs of hypokalemia include reduced muscle tone (decreased reflexes), weakness, confusion, drowsiness, depression, low blood pressure, and cardiac arrhythmias. **Hyperkalemia** results from an increase in potassium levels. High potassium is a dangerous condition because cardiac function and contractility are greatly affected. Cardiac arrest can occur when potassium levels are too high. Hyperkalemia can be caused by kidney failure, diarrhea, excessive use of potassium-sparing diuretics, Cushing's syndrome, severe burns, and septic shock (severe systemic infection). Signs and symptoms include depressed breathing, diarrhea, nausea, vomiting, irritability, confusion, anxiety, intestinal upset, and cardiac arrhythmias.

Hypocalcemia is a depletion in calcium levels in the body. Low calcium can be caused by insufficient calcium intake or parathyroid disease. Signs and symptoms of hypocalcemia include hyperexcitability of nerves and muscle contraction (tetany). Muscle spasms and seizures and even death can occur. **Hypercalcemia** is an excess of calcium in the blood. It can be caused by excessive intake of calcium supplements and by some cancerous tumors. When calcium levels are high, crystals form in the urine and cause kidney stones.

Hypomagnesemia is a depletion of magnesium in the body. Magnesium can be lost through alcohol abuse, pregnancy-induced hypertension, or drug therapy that causes increased magnesium excretion. Digoxin, estrogen, and diuretics can deplete magnesium. Signs and symptoms of hypomagnesemia include muscle cramps, confusion, hypertension, tachycardia, arrhythmias, tremors, hyperactive reflexes, hallucinations, and seizures. **Hypermagnesemia** is too much magnesium in the body. It can be caused by renal failure, an overdose of IV magnesium infusion, or the use of enemas containing magnesium. Symptoms of hypermagnesemia may not immediately be apparent to patients. Signs include reduced deep tendon reflexes and changes in cardiac function.

Hypochloremia is a depletion of chloride in the body, and **hyperchloremia** is an excess of chloride. Hypochloremia can be caused by loss of fluid from excessive production of urine or sweat and from gastric suctioning. Some diuretics also deplete chloride. Hyperchloremia can be caused by diarrhea, kidney disease, or diabetes.

Hypophosphatemia is a drop in phosphate in the bloodstream. It can be caused by anorexia or severe malnutrition. It may also be altered in patients with kidney failure. Signs and symptoms include weakness, respiratory failure, heart failure, hemolysis, and rhabdomyolysis (mass muscle tissue breakdown). **Hyperphosphatemia** can be caused by tumor lysis syndrome (a condition that can occur when receiving chemotherapy drugs for large cancer tumors), rhabdomyolysis (massive muscle breakdown), lactic acidosis, or diabetic ketoacidosis. Taking bisphosphonates or too much vitamin D, or overusing bowel prep products containing phosphate can also cause hyperphosphatemia. Symptoms of hyperphosphatemia are not always apparent to patients but often include kidney damage or failure.

Electrolytes

Electrolytes are most commonly prescribed for patients with an electrolyte deficiency, or if a deficiency is anticipated. They are not administered in high doses to prevent disease, as is commonly the case with vitamins. Large quantities of electrolytes can be harmful.

Electrolytes in body fluids can be replaced in a variety of ways. In parenteral nutrition, electrolyte solutions are combined with carbohydrates, proteins, and fats in large-volume bags and infused through an IV line. In some cases, correcting the underlying cause for an imbalance is enough to correct an abundance or a deficiency of a particular electrolyte. In other cases, replacement or supplementation is needed. When depletion is mild, replacement can happen by changing the diet to include the absent mineral or taking an oral supplement. For instance, athletes use sports drinks to replenish fluids and electrolytes lost from sweating. Oral liquid electrolyte mixtures are available over the counter to treat mild dehydration from vomiting or diarrhea (see Table 20.3). These products are safe to use because they contain only small amounts of electrolytes. You can help patients locate these items in the pharmacy and alert the pharmacist when intervention is needed. The pharmacist should assess patients for signs and symptoms to determine severity of dehydration. If moderate to severe dehydration is suspected, the patient should be referred for medical attention.

When immediate correction is needed or severe deficiencies exist, IV electrolyte products are used. Electrolytes are added to IV fluids, such as normal saline or dextrose in

Table 20.3 Common Oral Liquid Electrolyte Mixtures

Product	Electrolyte Content	Other content
Infalyte	Na, K, Cl	Rice syrup
Naturalyte	Na, K, Cl	Dextrose
Pedialyte	Na, K, Cl	Dextrose
Pedialyte Freezer Pops	Na, K, Cl	Dextrose
Rehydrate	Na, K, Cl	Dextrose
Resol	Na, K, Cl, Ca, Mg, phosphate	Glucose

water, and administered. Laboratory results are used to guide therapy. Dosing must be individualized depending on the reason for the electrolyte imbalance and fluid status of the patient. Ensuring the appropriate labs are ordered and alerting the pharmacist to abnormal results are jobs that some technicians perform in the inpatient setting.

Oral potassium supplements are typically used to replace potassium lost from diuresis. Some diuretics deplete potassium, so patients must take a potassium supplement while on those drug therapies. Doses are individualized to patients.

Oral calcium products are used to prevent and treat bone loss from osteoporosis, rickets (calcium deficiency), and osteomalacia. They are also used for tetany. Calcium products are listed in Table 20.4, and more information about their use in osteoporosis is provided in Chapter 6. They are absorbed more efficiently when taken with vitamin D.

Other than treating a deficiency, oral magnesium products have been used with some controversy in people with heart disease and diabetes. Phosphorus products are used primarily in cases of malnourishment. Some patients do not acquire sufficient phosphorus due to gastrointestinal (GI) absorption abnormalities.

Side Effects Common side effects of sodium include water retention and high blood pressure. Patients should talk with their prescribers if edema, swelling, or rapid weight gain occur, because the dose may need to be reduced or stopped altogether.

Table 20.4 Common Electrolyte Replacement Products

Generic (Brand)	Dosage Form and Strength	Route of Administration
Sodium		
Sodium chloride (Slo-Salt, Sustain)	Tablet 600 mg, 650 mg, 1 g, 2.25 g (+ other combinations with potassium)	Oral
Sodium chloride	IV solution 0.9% (NS), 0.45% (1/2 NS), 3%, 5% Injectable concentrate 14.6%, 23.4% Solution for injection 2.5 mEq/mL, 4 mEq/mL	IV infusion
Potassium		
Potassium acetate	IV additive 10.2 mEq/g (diluted to 40–80 mEq/L)	IV infusion
Potassium chloride (K-Dur, K-Lor, K-Lyte, Klor-Con, Micro-K)	Tablet, capsule, liquid, effervescent powder (varying strengths 8–25 mEq a dose)	Oral
Potassium chloride	IV additive 13.4 mEq/g (diluted to 40–80 mEq/L)	IV infusion
Calcium		
Calcium carbonate (Caltrate, Os Cal, Tums)	Tablet 500 mg, 600 mg, 750 mg, 1,250 mg Suspension 500 mg/5 mL, 1,250 mg/mL	Oral
Calcium chloride	Injection 1 g/10 ml	IV infusion
Calcium citrate (Cal-Citrate)	Tablet 250 mg	Oral
Calcium gluconate	Tablet 500 mg, 650 mg, 972 mg	Oral
Calcium lactate (Ridactate)	Tablet 650 mg	Oral
Magnesium		
Magnesium chloride (Chloromag)	Injection solution 200 mg/mL	IV infusion
Magnesium gluconate (Maox, Mag-G, Magtrate, Magonate)	Tablet 500 mg Liquid 3.52 mg/mL, 1,000 mg/5 mL	Oral
Magnesium lactate (Mag-Tab)	Tablet 84 mg	Oral
Magnesium oxide (Mag-Cap, Uro-Mag, Mag-Ox)	Capsule 140 mg	Oral
Magnesium sulfate (Mag-200)	Tablet Injection solution 40 mg/mL, 80 mg/mL	Oral, IV infusion
Phosphate		
Phosphorus (Uro-KP, K-Phos, PHOS-NaK)	Capsule and powder packets 250 mg plus potassium and sodium	Oral

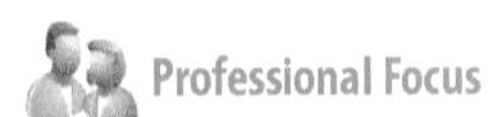

Professional Focus

Injectable electrolyte products are used in IV fluids and parenteral nutrition. If you do not work in a setting that handles sterile products, interview a pharmacist or technician who does. Ask which electrolytes they most commonly work with and about their procedures for mixing potassium and calcium salts in IV bags.

Common side effects of potassium include nausea, vomiting, diarrhea, and abdominal pain. In some cases, potassium supplements have been associated with GI ulceration. At a minimum, they can be irritating to the GI tract. Patients should take oral potassium products with a full glass of water to reduce these effects. Effervescent powder products should be mixed with plenty of water to avoid stomach and intestinal irritation. Taking potassium supplements with food may also decrease stomach upset.

Common side effects of calcium include constipation. Taking calcium supplements with food and drinking plenty of water may diminish occurrences of constipation. If hypercalcemia occurs, kidney stones can form. Patients should seek medical attention if they have back or flank pain and/or difficult or painful urination, especially if associated with nausea and vomiting. These can be signs of kidney stone formation.

Common side effects of magnesium include diarrhea. Taking magnesium supplements with food can decrease this effect. Over time, this effect usually improves.

Common side effects of phosphorus include stomach upset or diarrhea. Over time, this effect usually improves. Phosphorus supplements have also been associated with kidney stones. Patients should seek medical attention if they have back or flank pain and/or difficult or painful urination, especially if associated with nausea and vomiting. These can be signs of kidney stone formation.

Cautions and Considerations Most electrolyte products cannot be used in patients with kidney failure or impairment. If they are used in these cases, they must be monitored closely. Patients with kidney problems should notify their pharmacists and healthcare providers before taking an electrolyte supplement.

Injectable potassium products must be diluted before administration. Potassium is diluted, added to large-volume IV solution, and mixed well before administration. Such infusions must also be administered slowly because they can be irritating to the veins and painful for the patient. Usually, 40 mEq of potassium is added to 1 L IV fluid. Maximum safe concentration is 80 mEq/L. Administering too much potassium can be fatal because it will interfere with heart function and cause cardiac arrest. For this reason, vials of potassium concentrate have black tops. Pharmacy technicians should be aware of these parameters and take caution whenever handling injectable potassium products. In some pharmacies, potassium vials are physically separated in storage from other vials to emphasize safety and prevent errors and mistakes.

Injectable potassium products must be mixed well, so that the entire IV bag has a consistent concentration. Fully agitating the IV bag once potassium is added will help ensure consistent mixing. Do not add potassium to an IV bag or bottle in the hanging position. Potassium should usually be mixed in normal saline, not dextrose solutions.

Calcium and phosphate salts cannot always be mixed in the same IV bags. They can **chelate** (bond chemically to form an insoluble precipitate). The **precipitate** appears as small white specks or lumps of material within the bag. If infused through an IV, the precipitate clogs capillaries and has severe adverse effects for the patient. Technicians should follow accepted procedures at their institution for mixing any products containing these electrolytes. If calcium and phosphate are mixed together, the correct order of mixing must be followed strictly. For example, these substances may be mixed into some parenteral nutrition solutions. They are added to the bag before the opaque lipid material is added so that if a precipitate forms, you will be able to see it. If a precipitate forms, the IV bag must be discarded.

Acidosis and Alkalosis

Acidosis occurs when extracellular fluid (i.e., blood) contains excess hydrogen ions (commonly from an abundance of carbon dioxide), which causes the pH to drop below the normal range. **Metabolic acidosis** occurs when excess acid is produced; bicarbonate is lost (such as with diarrhea); or the kidneys do not excrete enough acid. **Respiratory acidosis** results from slow breathing and retention of carbon dioxide in the blood.

Alkalosis is typically caused by a loss in hydrogen ions, producing a relative increase in bicarbonate, which increases blood pH. Hydrogen ions can be lost from the GI tract (e.g., by vomiting) or in urine. **Metabolic alkalosis** takes place when excess acid is excreted via the kidneys (such as in overdiuresis) or acid is lost from the stomach (either from vomiting or gastric suction). **Respiratory alkalosis** occurs when breathing becomes more rapid, and more carbon dioxide is exhaled and eliminated from the blood.

When either a metabolic or respiratory process is contributing to an acid/base imbalance, the other pathway makes adjustments for it. Correction in pH can occur quickly with respiratory changes, but metabolic correction takes time. In either case, drug therapy may be needed to address the imbalance if severe or urgent.

Acidifying and Alkalinizing Agents

Some electrolyte products are used primarily for their acidic or basic properties in acidosis or alkalosis rather than for electrolyte deficiencies. Acidic electrolyte products are used to treat alkalosis, and basic products are used to treat acidosis (see Table 20.5).

Ammonium chloride is an acidic substance used for hypochloremia and metabolic alkalosis. It is typically administered in doses of 100–200 mEq mixed with 500–1,000 mL normal saline and then infused slowly during approximately three hours. This infusion prompts the kidneys to use ammonium in place of sodium in excretion processes. Less sodium is then available to combine to make sodium bicarbonate.

Sodium bicarbonate is a basic substance used as an antacid for heartburn and acid indigestion, a systemic alkalinizer for treating metabolic acidosis, and a urinary alkalinizer when treating hemolytic emergencies and drug overdoses (i.e., salicylates and lithium). When using it as an antacid, adult patients take one to two tablets every four hours, up to twenty-four tablets in twenty-four hours. Patients sixty years and older should not take more than twelve tablets in twenty-four hours. The oral powder is used by mixing ½ teaspoonful in half a glass (120 mL) of water and drinking as often as every two hours. When using it as an oral systemic alkalinizer, twelve to twenty-four 650 mg tablets are dissolved in one to two liters of water and consumed during an hour. When using the IV form for systemic alkalinization, 2–5 mEq/kg are given during four to eight hours, which allows pH to be adjusted upward gently. Using it as a urinary alkalinizer, the dose is six 650 mg tablets initially, and then two to four tablets every four hours under supervision of a physician.

Side Effects Close supervision and monitoring must accompany use of any acidifying or alkalinizing agent to prevent overcorrections in pH. Most side effects are related to overshooting pH goals. Ammonium chloride can result in ammonium toxicity. Patients must be watched for pallor, sweating, retching, irregular breathing, changes in heart rate, twitching, and convulsions. If left untreated, coma and death could occur. Sodium bicarbonate can result in sodium toxicity, which causes fluid overload. Renal function and cardiac function are impaired when sodium and water retention occurs.

Sodium bicarbonate is a hypertonic solution that can cause extravasation (ulceration of local tissue at the injection site). As is true of chemical burns, this process causes tissue necrosis (death) and skin sloughing. To prevent extravasation, any pain experienced during infusion should be given prompt attention and treatment.

Table 20.5 Common Acidifying and Alkalinizing Products

Generic (Brand)	Dosage Form and Strength	Route of Administration
Acidifying Agent		
Ammonium chloride	Injection 5 mEq/mL (diluted and then infused)	IV infusion
Alkalinizing Agent		
Sodium bicarbonate	Injection 4.2%, 5%, 7.5%, 8.4%	IV infusion

Cautions and Considerations Pharmacy technicians should be diligent when mixing and labeling acidifying and alkalinizing agents. The concentrations and rates of infusion must be precise to avoid adverse effects. For instance, the maximum concentration of ammonium chloride when mixed should be 1–2%. The maximum infusion rate of ammonium chloride is 5 mL/min to avoid venous irritation and ammonium toxicity. For this same reason, sodium bicarbonate is typically given slowly. In these cases, healthcare providers must be very attentive to signs of extravasation. Controlled infusion rates and frequent laboratory tests are necessary to prevent dramatic swings in pH and allow for gradual, safe correction of acidosis or alkalosis situations.

Herbal and Alternative Therapies

Because electrolytes are essential trace minerals that everyone should acquire from a nutritious diet, they are often categorized as dietary supplements rather than traditional OTC or prescription drug products. Oral dosage forms are indicated for situations when immediate correction of an electrolyte imbalance is not necessary. Many electrolyte drinks are available on the market for rehydration after physical exercise or diarrhea and vomiting associated with intestinal illness. Some of these products are listed in Table 20.3, and others are also available. You should become familiar with the rehydration products and electrolyte supplements available where you work.

Chapter Summary

Fluids and electrolytes depend on each other. Water is the primary body fluid and is compartmentalized into intracellular and extracellular space in the body. Extracellular fluid occurs either in interstitial spaces or in blood vessels. Electrolytes are salts and minerals dissolved in water. They contain molecules that easily dissociate into charged ions in water. Concentrations of electrolytes in the various fluid compartments are specific and help maintain equilibrium. When either fluid or molecules (such as electrolytes) are added or lost in one compartment, water shifts to compensate. Common electrolytes in the body include sodium, potassium, calcium, magnesium, phosphate, and chloride. Excess or loss of any of these ions can produce significant illness if not addressed. Other ions such as hydrogen ions (H^+) and bicarbonate help maintain acid–base balance.

Dehydration is the loss of water primarily from extracellular compartments. Edema is the accumulation of fluid in the interstitial space. Imbalances in electrolytes themselves may be related to fluid imbalances or other conditions. Each imbalance must be addressed individually for the patient and the electrolyte in question. Imbalances in electrolytes can cause changes in blood pH. A decrease in pH produces acidosis, which is an excess of acidic molecules, such as carbon dioxide or a relative absence of basic molecules, such as bicarbonate. An increase in pH results in alkalosis, which implies depletion of acidic molecules or an increase in bicarbonate molecules. IV electrolyte solutions containing ammonium chloride and sodium bicarbonate are used to treat acid–base disorders.

IV electrolyte products are used and prepared based on their tonicity (concentration compared with that of blood). Hypertonic solutions have a higher concentration than blood, and hypotonic solutions have a lower concentration. These solutions are used to hydrate patients. Isotonic solutions have the same concentration as blood and are used to maintain fluid status in the normal range.

IV fluids and electrolytes are products that pharmacy technicians work with on a daily basis in the inpatient setting. Whether they are used in drug therapy treatment or in mixtures as delivery vehicles for other medications, all of these products have significant effects on patients. Appreciation for the use, limitations, and special handling required of these products will help technicians provide safe and effective care.

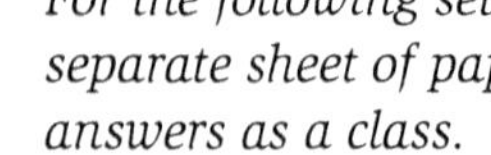

Chapter Review

For the following sets of exercises, write the exercise heading, exercise numbers, and your answers on a separate sheet of paper. Your instructor may direct you to turn in the sheet of paper or discuss your answers as a class.

REVIEW THE BASICS

Choose a, b, c, or d as the correct answer to each multiple-choice question.

1. Which of the following fluid compartments contains the most fluid but is the least active in affecting overall fluid status?
   a. extracellular
   b. intracellular
   c. interstitial
   d. plasma
2. Which of the following electrolytes exists in body fluid as a negatively charged ion?
   a. sodium
   b. potassium
   c. calcium
   d. chloride
3. Which of the following is a condition caused by vomiting or gastric suctioning that results in a drop in potassium levels in the body?
   a. hyponatremia
   b. hypokalemia
   c. acidosis
   d. edema
4. What strength of sodium chloride is isotonic with blood?
   a. 0.45%
   b. 0.9%
   c. 5%
   d. 9%
5. Which of the following is caused by retention of sodium and water in the extracellular space?
   a. dehydration
   b. edema
   c. hypernatremia
   d. alkalosis
6. Which of the following best describes D_5W?
   a. hypotonic
   b. hydrating
   c. isotonic
   d. hypertonic
7. Which of the following electrolytes can cause constipation as a common side effect?
   a. calcium
   b. magnesium
   c. potassium
   d. phosphate
8. Which of the following must be diluted, added to an IV fluid bag, and agitated well before administering to a patient?
   a. sodium chloride
   b. potassium chloride
   c. magnesium chloride
   d. ammonium chloride
9. Which of the following is an acidifying agent used to treat alkalosis?
   a. sodium chloride
   b. potassium chloride
   c. magnesium chloride
   d. ammonium chloride
10. Which of the following is only available in an oral dosage form?
    a. potassium acetate
    b. calcium chloride
    c. magnesium sulfate
    d. phosphorus

KNOW THE DRUGS

Match each brand name drug with its corresponding generic name and most common use. Your answers should follow this example format: Generic Name: 1. a; 2. b; 3. c; etc. Most Common Use: 1. d; 2. e; 3. f; etc.

Brand Name	Generic Name	Most Common Use
1. Caltrate	a. Na, K, Cl + dextrose	d. Rehydration after mild fluid loss
2. K-Dur	b. Potassium chloride	e. Replacing K^+ lost via diuresis
3. Pedialyte	c. Calcium carbonate	f. Osteoporosis prevention

PUT IT TOGETHER

For each item, write down either a short answer or a single term to complete the sentence.

1. List the available strengths of normal saline and dextrose in water IV solutions. Then indicate which ones are hypotonic, isotonic, and hypertonic.
2. ______________________ can be caused by alcohol abuse or pregnancy-induced hypertension.
3. ______________________ can cause kidney stones.
4. ______________________ can happen when the kidneys excrete too many acids. Name a drug class that, if overused, could cause this condition.
5. Name the maximum safe concentration of potassium mixtures.
6. For the following laboratory result values, indicate whether each is high, low, or normal.

Na	151 mEq/L
K	3.2 mEq/L
Ca	4.8 mEq/L
Cl	101 mEq/L
Bicarb	31 mEq/L

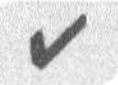

THINK IT THROUGH

Read and think through each numbered scenario carefully and then write several sentences in reply to the question(s) presented. Question 4 requires you to do some Internet research before completing your answer(s).

1. You receive an order from a medical resident asking for hydration therapy for a patient admitted to the emergency room. The order asks for sterile water 1 L to be infused over two hours as well as monitoring for fluid and electrolyte status. What should you do?
2. In the OTC aisle, you encounter a worried mother with her crying toddler and a tube of diaper rash cream in her hand. She asks you whether she should get some Gatorade or Pedialyte for her daughter, who has had diarrhea for two days. What should you do?
3. You mix a total parenteral nutrition IV bag for delivery to the floor. After adding the ordered electrolytes, you notice a white particulate matter inside the bag. What might this be? Explain how it got there and what you should do with the bag now that you have discovered this situation.

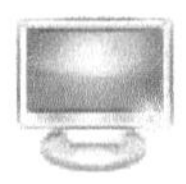

4. **On the Internet,** find the Web site for the American Society for Parenteral and Enteral Nutrition (ASPEN) and locate the Safe Practices for Parenteral Nutrition that have to do with Stability and Compatibility of Parenteral Nutrition Formulations. This document describes the incompatibility problems with calcium salts forming precipitates in parenteral nutrition formulations. Briefly summarize the recommendations for avoiding this incompatibility problem with calcium salts.

Chapter 21 Cancer and Chemotherapy

LEARNING OBJECTIVES

- Explain the basic physiology of malignancy and tumor cell growth.
- Explain the therapeutic effects of medications commonly used to treat cancer.
- Describe the adverse effects of medications commonly used to treat cancer.
- Identify the brand and generic names of medications commonly used to treat cancer.
- State common dosage forms and routes of administration of medications commonly used to treat cancer.
- Describe the required safety equipment for safely handling hazardous drugs.
- Explain strategies that pharmacy technicians can employ to help prevent chemotherapy-related errors.

Interactive self-quizzes, games, audio files, and glossaries help you to learn drug names and facts.

In the United States, cancer is the second leading cause of death, behind heart disease. Each year, approximately 1.5 million people are diagnosed with cancer. It is estimated that one of every two people in the United States will develop cancer in his or her lifetime. It is easy to see how cancer can have an impact on everyone professionally, personally, or both.

Chemotherapy drugs represent a complicated group of medications with a narrow window between safe therapeutic use and the potential for great toxicity. Many healthcare practitioners are uncomfortable working with these drugs due to a lack of understanding about how they work and the potential hazards associated with them. This chapter provides an overview of cancer and the pharmacology of drugs used in cancer treatment. It also summarizes safety measures that should be employed to optimize patient and personnel safety in the preparation, handling, and administration of these drugs. Because of the high number of patients who are affected by cancer, the continuous development of new drugs for cancer treatment, and the inherent risks associated with these agents, it is important for all pharmacy technicians to have a basic understanding of chemotherapy drugs and the unique issues associated with them.

Chemotherapy drugs are traditionally administered in a hospital or outpatient chemotherapy infusion center by the intravenous (IV) route. Most IV chemotherapy drugs are prepared by pharmacy technicians in these settings. Over the past ten years, however, the number of orally administered chemotherapy agents has increased. Many of these oral drugs have the same toxicity and side effect profiles as the IV agents. Consequently, the care of patients with cancer is expanding into community practice.

Pathophysiology of Cancer and Malignancy

Cancer is a term that describes a group of diseases characterized by the uncontrolled growth of dysfunctional cells. Normally, cells multiply only until there are enough of them to meet the needs of the body (for example, epidermal cells multiply to replace lost skin cells due to damage or aging). Cancer is thought to originate from a single cell (defined as **monoclonal**) that has lost its normal ability to control growth and proliferation.

In the past fifteen to twenty years, research has revealed the role of genes in the cancer process. The two major classes of these genes are **oncogenes** and **tumor-suppressor genes**. Oncogenes promote cancer formation, and tumor-suppressor genes turn off or downregulate the proliferation of cancer cells. Oncogenes develop from **proto-oncogenes**.

All cells possess proto-oncogenes for normal function. These are genes that code for growth factors or their receptors. Alterations of proto-oncogenes via exposure to chemicals, viruses, radiation, or hereditary factors can activate the oncogene that promotes abnormal cell growth. One example of an oncogene is the *erb-B2* (also called HER-2*neu*), which codes for a growth factor receptor found in some forms of breast cancer.

Tumor-suppressor genes are the brakes that inhibit inappropriate cell growth. Mutations or deletions of tumor-suppressor genes can also result in uncontrolled cell growth. One of the most common tumor-suppressor genes is *p53*. The normal gene product of *p53* halts cell division and induces **apoptosis** (cell death) in abnormal or aging cells. Mutations of *p53* are linked to resistance to many chemotherapy drugs.

It would make sense that cancerous cells must have at least two gene mutations in a single cell. In reality, many cancers express multiple oncogenes and mutations of tumor-suppressor genes. As the ability to identify these genes grows, the potential for using them in early cancer screening or as targets for drug therapy development continues to improve the treatment of the cancer patient.

Cell Proliferation and Gompertzian Kinetics

Gompertz was a German insurance statistician who came up with a mathematical model to show a relationship between age and expected death. This model is now widely accepted as an approximation of **tumor cell proliferation** (see Figure 21.1). Early cancer growth is considered to be exponential. One cell divides to two, two cells divide to four, and so on. It normally takes about thirty divisions to make 1 gram (about 1 cm^3) of tumor mass, which is the smallest clinically detectable tumor (10^9 = 1 billion cells). During the exponential phase, the tumor is most sensitive to those chemotherapy agents that attack and destroy rapidly dividing cells. After the tumor has reached a certain size, growth slows, possibly due to restrictions in space, decreased blood supply, and decreased nutritional supply. However, take note that only ten more divisions will make a 1 kg mass (about 10^{12} cells), which is considered a lethal **tumor burden.**

Tumor burden (or size) relates to response to chemotherapy. A predominant hypothesis applied in cancer treatment is the **cell-kill hypothesis**. This hypothesis presumes that each cycle of chemotherapy kills a certain percentage of cancer cells. If a tumor has 10 billion cells and a chemotherapy cycle kills 95% of them, then 0.5 billion cells remain. The second cycle kills 95% more, leaving 25 million cells, and the third would leave 1.25 million cells. Using this theory, tumor cell count will never reach zero from treatment alone, but once the number of cancer cells is low enough, normal host defense mechanisms take over to eradicate the remaining cells.

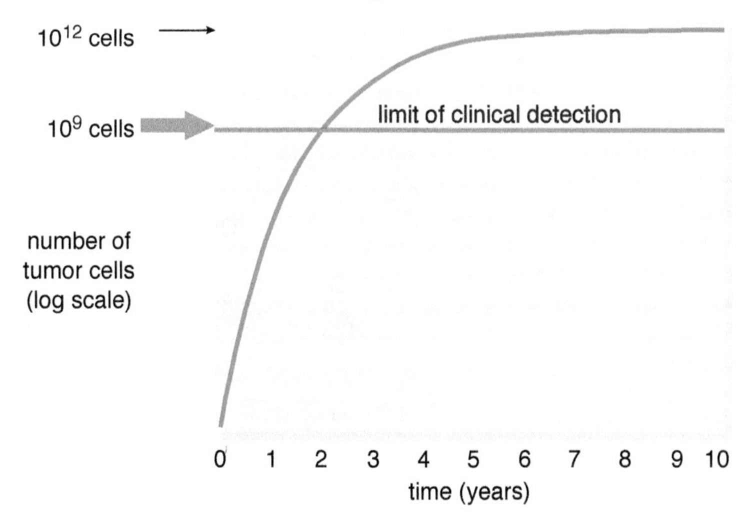

Figure 21.1
Tumor Cell Growth
A tumor must reach a certain size before it can be detected. Unfortunately, chemotherapy drugs can kill only a percentage of cancer cells in the tumor after this point, instead of completely eradicating it.

(Adapted from Schorge et al., *Williams Gynecology*, http://www.accessmedicine.com).

Drugs for Cancer

Chemotherapy is the use of drugs to treat disease. The term most often refers to drugs used to treat cancer. These drugs may be **cytotoxic drugs** (toxic to cells), hormonal therapies, or one of the newer targeted therapies for cancer. Many consider cytotoxic drugs to be synonymous with the term chemotherapy. Multiple factors affect tumor response to chemotherapy. Examples include the size of the tumor (tumor burden), cell resistance to the chemotherapy agent, the amount of chemotherapy given, and the condition of the patient prior to chemotherapy. To reduce the chances of the cancer becoming resistant to treatment, chemotherapy is usually given in combination regimens. These regimens are designed to include drugs that have shown efficacy against the tumor being treated, those that do not have overlapping toxicities, and medications that have different mechanisms of action.

The **cell cycle** describes the process by which both normal and cancer cells divide. Because most cancer cells have lost their checks and balances on the rate of cellular replication, they are usually most sensitive to drugs that interfere with the cell cycle (see Figure 21.2). These chemotherapy agents are known as **cell cycle–specific drugs**. Because cancer cells are constantly dividing, chemotherapy regimens take advantage of cell cycle–specific drug activity by administering them as continuous infusions (e.g., continuous infusion fluorouracil or cytarabine) or in repeated bolus doses (e.g., weekly bleomycin). Adjusting the administration and scheduling of cell cycle–specific drugs helps them target effects on rapidly dividing cells as those cells move into the susceptible phase of the cell cycle while minimizing exposure to normal cells that may be in a resting phase of the cell cycle. These drugs are considered schedule-dependent.

Other chemotherapy agents can work at any point in the cell cycle and are called **cell cycle–nonspecific drugs**. Cyclophosphamide, an alkylating agent, is an example of a nonspecific agent. The activity of these agents tends to be more dose-dependent (higher dose provides higher cell kill) than schedule-dependent.

In general, the smaller the tumor burden, the more effective chemotherapy will be. Rapidly dividing cells are generally the most sensitive to chemotherapy. **Combination chemotherapy** can maximize the effectiveness of the chemotherapy regimen while minimizing toxicity and resistance.

Chemotherapy may be described as primary, adjuvant, or palliative, depending on the goals of therapy.

1. **Primary chemotherapy** refers to the initial treatment of cancer with chemotherapy and **curative** intent. Examples of some of the cancers that can be cured with primary chemotherapy are Hodgkin's disease, lymphoma, leukemias, and testicular cancer.

2. **Adjuvant chemotherapy** refers to the treatment of residual cancer cells after removal or reduction of the tumor by surgery. Sometimes, if the tumor is too large to remove, a patient may be given **neoadjuvant chemotherapy** in an attempt to shrink the tumor so that it can be safely and completely removed with surgery. Both adjuvant and neoadjuvant chemotherapy can be curative if the tumor is effectively removed. One example of adjuvant therapy is administering chemotherapy and/or hormone therapy following lumpectomy or mastectomy (types of surgical removal) in breast cancer. The patient is given adjuvant chemotherapy and radiation after surgery to ensure that any remaining cancer cells are eradicated.

3. **Palliative chemotherapy** is given for cancer that is not curable. The usual purpose of palliative chemotherapy is to prolong life and improve quality of life by decreasing tumor size and reducing the symptoms caused by the tumor.

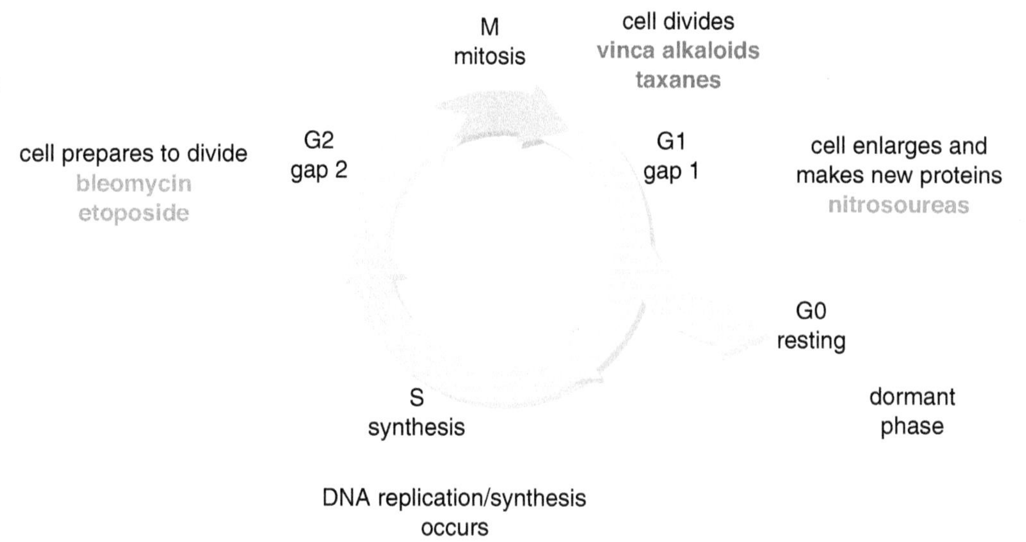

Figure 21.2
Cell Cycle
Often, multiple agents (shown in colored type) acting on different phases of cell growth and proliferation are used together to increase effectiveness and kill more cancer cells.

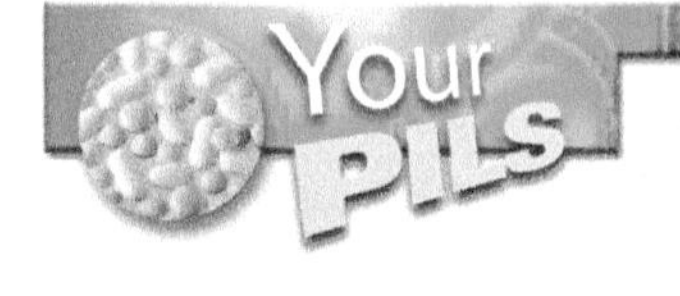

If you like working with others, as Enactors and Directors do, get together with someone and describe the difference between cell cycle–specific and cell cycle–nonspecific chemotherapy drugs. How are they different in their mechanisms of action? How can you change the administration schedule of cell cycle–specific drugs to enhance their cytotoxic effects on tumor cells? Try explaining this concept in two different ways to each other. Which way makes more sense? Think about how you would explain this concept to a patient with a question about how these medications work.

Traditional Chemotherapy and Cytotoxic Drugs

Cytotoxic drugs work by interfering with some normal process of cell function or proliferation (see Figure 21.2). Table 21.1 outlines the various categories of cytotoxic drugs and lists examples and common side effects of drugs within each category. Although cytotoxic drugs exert the majority of their effects on cancer cells, these agents don't target tumor cells specifically. As a result, chemotherapy drugs cause a lot of side effects related to normal cell function. Side effects from traditional chemotherapy drugs might include **bone marrow suppression** (decreased production of blood cells, increased risks of infections and bleeding), hair loss (**alopecia**), nausea and vomiting, and mucosal damage to the lining of the mouth and intestinal tract (**mucositis**). Table 21.2 describes some of the unique side effects of specific chemotherapy drugs as well as measures that are commonly employed to prevent these toxicities. Although there are many risks associated with traditional chemotherapy agents, the use of these powerful drugs continues to either cure many patients of cancer or provide relief from their disease, which prolongs their lives. Cytotoxic drugs remain a critical component of cancer treatment.

Alkylating Agents The oldest category of traditional cytotoxic drugs contains the **alkylating agents**. The first drug identified in this category as having anticancer activity was **mechlorethamine**, or nitrogen mustard, a derivative of mustard gas. The accidental release of mustard gas during World War II was only later discovered as playing a role in decreasing the activity of lymphocytes in soldiers who were exposed to the gas. The discovery of this reaction led to the development of this agent as a treatment for lymphoma, a cancer of the lymphatic system.

Alkylating agents work by binding to and damaging DNA during the cell division process, ultimately preventing cell replication. Examples of alkylating agents are listed in Table 21.1. Alkylating agents have a very broad spectrum of anticancer activity and

Table 21.1 Traditional Chemotherapy and Cytotoxic Drug Categories

Category	Drugs	Major Side Effects
Alkylating agents	Busulfan Carboplatin Carmustine (BCNU) Chlorambucil Cisplatin Cyclophosphamide Dacarbazine Ifosfamide Lomustine Mechlorethamine Melphalan Oxaliplatin Procarbazine Temozolomide	Bone marrow suppression Hair loss Nausea/vomiting Infertility Secondary cancers
Antimetabolites	Capecitabine Cladribine Clofarabine Cytarabine Fludarabine Fluorouracil Gemcitabine Hydroxyurea Mercaptopurine Methotrexate Pemetrexed	Bone marrow suppression Immune system suppression Mucositis
Topoisomerase inhibitors	Daunorubicin Doxorubicin Epirubicin Etoposide Idarubicin Irinotecan Mitoxantrone Teniposide Topotecan	Bone marrow suppression Nausea/vomiting Mucositis Hair loss
Antimicrotubule agents	Docetaxel Paclitaxel Vinblastine Vincristine Vinorelbine	Bone marrow suppression Mucositis Hair loss Nerve toxicity

are used to treat a wide variety of cancer types. **Cisplatin** is an alkylating agent used to treat many diseases, including lung, ovarian, and bone cancers. Cisplatin is a critical component of the chemotherapy regimens for testicular cancer. **Cyclophosphamide** is an alkylating agent that plays an important role in treating lymphomas, leukemias, and breast cancer. See Tables 21.3 and 21.4 for examples of other types of cancer treated with alkylating agents.

Side Effects The most common side effect of alkylating agents is bone marrow suppression. Alkylating agents also cause nausea, vomiting, and alopecia. Because alkylating agents cause damage to DNA, they are also **mutagenic**, meaning that they have the ability to cause changes in genetic material. As mutagens, these drugs have the potential to cause certain types of secondary cancers in patients who have received the drugs. This is a rare but very serious potential side effect. Alkylating agents are also known to cause damage to reproductive tissue, and patients who receive them may become infertile. Some alkylating agents are absorbed through the skin, so extreme caution must be used in handling them.

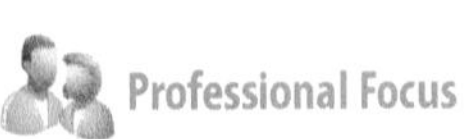

Professional Focus

Ifosfamide causes severe hemorrhagic cystitis and must *always* be given with the protective agent mesna. When preparing doses of ifosfamide, look for an accompanying order for mesna. You should question orders for ifosfamide without mesna in the preparation process.

Cautions and Considerations Many alkylating agents cause unique toxicities. Cisplatin is notorious for causing kidney damage and depleting potassium and magnesium levels. This side effect is minimized by providing patients with potassium and magnesium supplements as well as adequate amounts of fluid before and after administration. Cisplatin can also cause very painful damage to the nerves that affect the hands and feet (**peripheral neuropathy**) and the nerves that affect hearing (**ototoxicity**). Patients must be carefully assessed for these side effects between cycles of treatment, and doses should be decreased or stopped when symptoms develop. Maximum limits are placed on dosing cisplatin to avoid overdose and severe toxicities. Ifosfamide is known to cause **hemorrhagic cystitis** (damage and bleeding of the urinary bladder). This side effect can be prevented by co-administering the protective medication, mesna. Other unique toxicities of alkylating agents are outlined in Table 21.2.

Antimetabolites This class of cytotoxic drugs works in the synthesis phase of the cell cycle. They are called **antimetabolites**, and they work by a variety of different mechanisms. Some antimetabolites inhibit enzyme production or activity that is needed for DNA/RNA synthesis. **Methotrexate, cytarabine,** and **fluorouracil** are antimetabolite drugs that interfere with the enzymes that are essential for tumor cell proliferation. Antimetabolites may also act as false nucleotides and get falsely incorporated into DNA during synthesis because they look like DNA nucleotides. **Mercaptopurine** is an antimetabolite drug that interferes with cell synthesis by replacing normal nucleotides in DNA/RNA production.

Professional Focus

Even in very low doses, methotrexate can be one of the most toxic chemotherapy drugs administered if given inappropriately. Methotrexate is *never* administered daily. Daily orders for even very low doses of methotrexate (e.g., 2.5 mg PO once a day) should ALWAYS be questioned.

Antimetabolite drugs are used to treat a wide variety of tumors (see Tables 21.3 and 21.4). Methotrexate is commonly used to treat leukemias, bone cancer, breast cancer, and lymphomas. Methotrexate suppresses immune system function and is used to treat a variety of nonmalignant immunologic conditions, such as rheumatoid arthritis, lupus, and psoriasis (see Chapters 5 and 6). Fluorouracil and its oral counterpart, capecitabine, are commonly used to treat colon cancer. A topical form of fluorouracil also exists to treat some low-grade skin cancers and precancerous skin lesions. Gemcitabine is an antimetabolite used to treat lung and pancreatic cancers. Hydroxyurea is an orally administered antimetabolite drug that is commonly used to rapidly lower white blood cell counts in patients who have leukemia. Hydroxyurea is also used to help decrease painful crisis episodes for people with sickle cell anemia.

Methotrexate is one of the most complicated antimetabolites to administer. It is given in a very wide range of doses, from 5 mg once a week for rheumatoid arthritis to 20 g per treatment once or twice a month when used for bone cancer. If administered incorrectly, methotrexate can result in very serious and sometimes fatal toxicities. One of the most serious toxicities of this drug is kidney damage. When methotrexate is given in doses above 1 g, it can accumulate in the kidneys and form damaging crystals. To prevent such accumulation, patients are given IV fluids containing sodium bicarbonate or sodium acetate to alkalinize (increase the pH of) the urine. Increasing urine pH makes the methotrexate more soluble and prevents the crystals from forming.

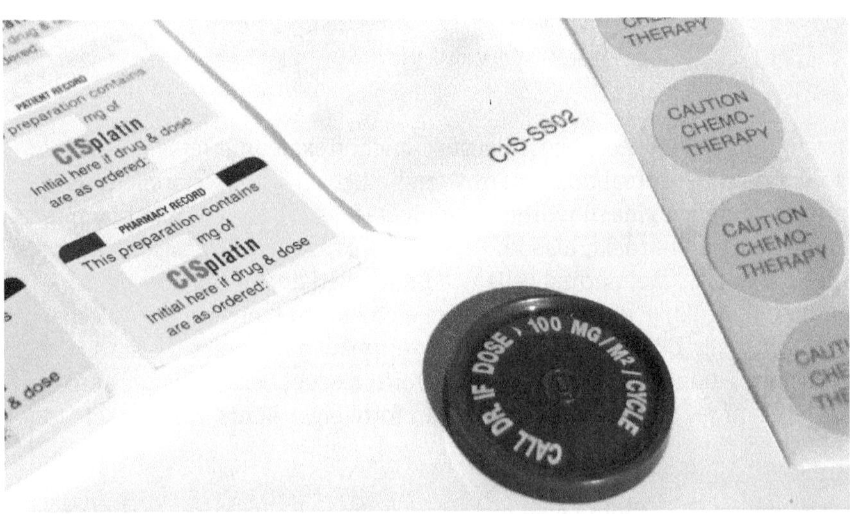

The vial lid on cisplatin prompts you to check the dose to be sure it does not exceed the maximum per cycle. Affix special warning stickers to cisplatin preparations to prompt the user to check the strength and dose against the prescriber's orders.

In high doses, methotrexate can also cause severe bone marrow suppression and mucosal injury in

Table 21.2 Unique Toxicities of Chemotherapy Agents

Agent	Toxicity	Preventive Measures
Bleomycin	Lung damage	Track and limit cumulative doses to < 400 units Limit individual doses to ≤ 30 units Avoid giving to patients with kidney dysfunction
Capecitabine	Hand-foot syndrome Diarrhea	Advise patients to use emollients on hands and feet Limit doses or stop therapy if symptoms develop
Cisplatin	Kidney damage Potassium and magnesium loss Nerve pain/damage	Aggressive IV fluids before and after each dose Potassium and magnesium supplements Assess level of nerve damage with each treatment. Stop treatment at onset of symptoms Limit doses to ≤ 100 mg/m^2 a cycle of treatment
Cytarabine	Conjunctivitis	Administer steroid eyedrops during treatment whenever patients receive doses > 1,000 mg/m^2
Daunorubicin Doxorubicin Epirubicin Idarubicin	Heart failure	Track and limit cumulative doses Monitor heart function Stop treatment if symptoms develop
Ifosfamide	Hemorrhagic cystitis	Give IV fluids during and after treatment Give mesna (bladder protectant) during and after treatment
Irinotecan	Severe diarrhea	Give atropine for diarrhea that occurs during drug administration Educate patients about how and when to take antidiarrheal agents (e.g., Imodium, Lomotil) after treatment
Methotrexate	Kidney damage Severe bone marrow and mucosal toxicity	Aggressive IV fluids Urinary alkalinization with sodium bicarbonate Leucovorin rescue
Oxaliplatin	Nerve pain/damage (hands, feet, throat)	Avoid cold temperatures Avoid cold beverages Limit doses or stop treatment if symptoms do not reverse
Paclitaxel	Allergic reaction Nerve pain/damage	Premedication with: Diphenhydramine Cimetidine Dexamethasone Decrease dose or stop treatment if symptoms occur
Pemetrexed	Severe bone marrow suppression Skin rash	Give folic acid and vitamin B_{12} supplements starting 5–7 days before treatment Give dexamethasone, starting 1 day before treatment
Vincristine	Nerve damage	Cap individual doses at 2 mg Stop treatment if symptoms develop

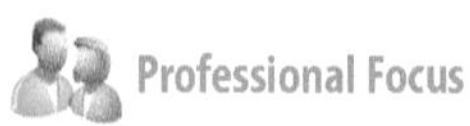

Folinic acid, or leucovorin, is sometimes confused with folic acid. Folic acid will *not* provide the same benefit as leucovorin. Orders substituting folic acid for leucovorin (folinic acid) should be immediately questioned.

the intestinal tract. These side effects occur because methotrexate interferes with an enzyme that is important in normal bone marrow and mucosal cell development. **Folinic acid** is a by-product of the enzyme dihydrofolate reductase, which is inhibited by methotrexate. By administering folinic acid, also known as **leucovorin**, to patients who have received high-dose methotrexate, normal cells will be rescued and allowed to resume their normal proliferation. To give the methotrexate a chance to work on cancer cells, leucovorin rescue is usually initiated twenty-four to thirty-six hours after the start of the methotrexate infusion. Timing is essential for leucovorin rescue, because if cells are exposed to high levels of methotrexate for more than forty-eight hours, it is too late to rescue them.

Side Effects The major overlapping side effects of antimetabolite drugs include bone marrow suppression, immune system suppression, and mucositis. Antimetabolite drugs also exhibit some unique toxicities. Capecitabine, the oral antimetabolite, can cause a debilitating reaction called palmer-plantar erythema, better known as **hand-foot**

Table 21.3 Commonly Used Oral Chemotherapy Drugs

Generic (Brand)	Common Use
Busulfan (Myleran)	Leukemia
Capecitabine (Xeloda)	Breast cancer, colon cancer
Chlorambucil (Leukeran)	Chronic lymphocytic leukemia
Cyclophosphamide (Cytoxan)	Breast cancer, immune system diseases (e.g., arthritis, lupus)
Dasatinib (Sprycel)	Chronic myelogenous leukemia
Erlotinib (Tarceva)	Lung cancer
Hydroxyurea (Hydrea, Droxia)	Leukemia, sickle cell anemia
Imatinib (Gleevec)	Chronic myelogenous leukemia
Lomustine (CeeNU)	Brain tumors
Melphalan (Alkeran)	Multiple myeloma
Mercaptopurine (Purinethol)	Leukemia
Methotrexate (Various)	Immune system diseases (e.g., arthritis, psoriasis, lupus)
Procarbazine (Matulane)	Brain tumors, Hodgkin's disease
Sunitinib (Sutent)	Kidney cancer
Temozolomide (Temodar)	Brain tumors, melanoma
Thalidomide (Thalomid)	Multiple myeloma
Tretinoin (Vesanoid)	Acute promyelocytic leukemia

syndrome. In hand-foot syndrome, patients experience painful sloughing and peeling of skin on the palms of the hands and soles of the feet. The appearance of this condition in patients taking capecitabine necessitates a pause in treatment as well as a reduction in subsequent doses. Cytarabine is an antimetabolite used in a wide range of doses. When it is given at doses above 1,000 mg/m^2 of body surface area, cytarabine is excreted in tears and causes a chemical irritation of the eye, or conjunctivitis. To prevent this side effect, patients receiving high-dose cytarabine must also receive steroid eyedrops (e.g., dexamethasone, prednisolone) during and for twenty-four to forty-eight hours after completion of therapy. See Table 21.2 for additional information on the unique toxicities of antimetabolites.

Topoisomerase Inhibitors Some enzymes important in the process of DNA synthesis and cell replication are **topoisomerases**. DNA structure is tightly coiled and must be unwound during the replication process. Topoisomerases produce temporary breaks and repairs in DNA strands, which help unwind the DNA and allow the transcription process to occur. There are two types of topoisomerase enzymes. Topoisomerase I enzymes produce single-strand breaks in DNA, and topoisomerase II enzymes produce double-stand DNA breaks. Topoisomerase inhibitors interfere with the DNA repair function of topoisomerases and disrupt the cell replication process. These agents are very important components of cancer treatment and are used to treat many different types of cancer (see Tables 21.3 and 21.4). Common side effects of topoisomerase inhibitors are bone marrow suppression, mucositis, nausea and vomiting, and alopecia.

Topoisomerase I inhibitors include **topotecan** and **irinotecan**, both of which are derived from the *Camptotheca* tree. Topotecan is commonly used to treat ovarian cancer and lung cancer. Irinotecan is most frequently used to treat lung and colon cancers. Irinotecan causes the unique side effect of severe diarrhea (see Table 21.2). If not managed quickly, diarrhea from irinotecan can lead to serious complications. Patients who experience this type of diarrhea are managed with atropine, which is an injectable

Table 21.4 Commonly Used Injectable Chemotherapy Drugs

Generic (Brand)	Common Use
Arsenic trioxide (Trisenox)	Acute promyelocytic leukemia
Asparaginase (Elspar)	Leukemia
Azacitidine (Vidaza)	Myelodysplastic syndrome
Bevacizumab (Avastin)	Lung cancer, breast cancer, colon cancer
Bleomycin (Blenoxane)	Testicular cancer, lymphoma
Bortezomib (Velcade)	Multiple myeloma
Busulfan (Busulfex)	Stem cell/bone marrow transplant
Carboplatin (Paraplatin)	Lung cancer, ovarian cancer, breast cancer
Carmustine (BiCNU)	Brain tumor, lymphoma
Cetuximab (Erbitux)	Colon cancer, head and neck cancer
Cisplatin (Platinol)	Testicular cancer, ovarian cancer, cervical cancer, bladder cancer, sarcoma
Cyclophosphamide (Cytoxan)	Breast cancer, lymphoma, leukemia, immune system diseases
Cytarabine (Cytosar U)	Leukemia, lymphoma
Daunorubicin (Daunomycin, Cerubidine)	Leukemia
Docetaxel (Taxotere)	Breast cancer, lung cancer, prostate cancer
Doxorubicin (Adriamycin)	Breast cancer, lymphoma, leukemia, sarcoma, bone cancer, multiple myeloma
Epirubicin (Ellence)	Breast cancer, stomach/esophageal cancer
Etoposide (VePesid)	Leukemia, lymphoma, testicular cancer, lung cancer
Fludarabine (Fludara)	Leukemia, lymphoma
Fluorouracil (Adrucil)	Colon cancer, breast cancer, some skin cancers and pre-malignant skin conditions
Gemcitabine (Gemzar)	Pancreatic cancer, lung cancer, breast cancer, ovarian cancer, bladder cancer
Ifosfamide (Ifex)	Lymphoma, testicular cancer, sarcoma
Irinotecan (Camptosar)	Colon cancer, lung cancer, brain tumor
Mechlorethamine (Mustargen)	Hodgkin's disease, lymphoma
Melphalan (Alkeran)	Multiple myeloma
Methotrexate (Various)	Bone cancer, leukemia, lymphoma, immune system diseases
Mitoxantrone (Novantrone)	Leukemia, lymphoma, breast cancer
Oxaliplatin (Eloxatin)	Colon cancer
Paclitaxel (Taxol)	Breast cancer, ovarian cancer, lung cancer
Pemetrexed (Alimta)	Lung cancer
Rituximab (Rituxan)	Lymphoma, leukemia, immune system diseases
Topotecan (Hycamtin)	Ovarian cancer, lung cancer
Trastuzumab (Herceptin)	Breast cancer
Vinblastine (Velban)	Testicular cancer, lymphoma
Vincristine (Oncovin)	Leukemia, lymphoma
Vinorelbine (Navelbine)	Breast cancer, lung cancer

anticholinergic drug. The most serious form of diarrhea occurs in the days following administration of irinotecan. Patients must be adequately warned about the potential for this side effect and educated on how to appropriately administer antidiarrheal agents, such as loperamide, at the first onset of symptoms.

Anthracyclines represent a large category of **topoisomerase II inhibitors** that are commonly used. They inhibit topoisomerase activity by inserting themselves (or intercalating) into strands of DNA. Anthracyclines are also referred to as DNA **intercalating agents**. These agents include **daunorubicin, doxorubicin, epirubicin,** and **idarubicin**. They are derived from a microorganism species, *Streptomyces*, which is found in soil and produces a red pigment. The –rubicin portion of their name comes from the French word *rubis*, which describes the red color of anthracycline agents. Doxorubicin is part of curative chemotherapy regimens for breast cancer and lymphoma. It is also used in treating bone cancer, leukemia, multiple myeloma, and sarcomas. Daunorubicin and idarubicin are primarily used to treat leukemia. Epirubicin is most frequently used to treat breast and stomach/esophageal cancers.

Side Effects The most serious toxicity that can occur in patients who receive anthracyclines is heart or **cardiac toxicity**. Cardiac toxicity from the anthracyclines typically occurs many years after patients have received the drug. The risk of cardiac toxicity with anthracyclines is cumulative, increasing with each dose the patient receives. The best way to limit the risk of cardiac toxicity with these drugs is to track the patient's cumulative exposure and stop treatment after he or she has reached a threshold dose. The threshold dose is different for each anthracycline drug. For example, the lifetime cumulative dose limit for doxorubicin is approximately 450 mg/m^2, whereas the cumulative dose limit for idarubicin is approximately 225 mg/m^2.

Professional Focus

Make sure that liposomal daunorubicin and doxorubicin are not stored next to regular anthracycline formulations. Very serious errors have occurred when these products have been mixed up with the regular daunorubicin and doxorubicin products.

Cautions and Considerations Anthracyclines can also cause severe tissue damage if the infusion leaks under the skin during administration. This leaking and the damage it causes are called **extravasation**. Drugs that cause extravasation injury are referred to as **vesicants** (see Table 21.5). As such, anthracyclines require special precautions to prevent extravasation during administration. Veins must be chosen carefully for administration of vesicant drugs. Patients must be carefully observed during administration so the infusion can be stopped immediately at the first sign of pain or other symptoms of drug leakage under the skin. If vesicant drugs are to be administered in a prolonged infusion, patients must have central venous catheters or surgically placed implanted ports to decrease the risk of extravasation. Some anthracycline drugs have been prepared in lipid formulations, known as **liposomal** products, to help decrease toxicity. Both daunorubicin and doxorubicin have liposomal formulations. Liposomal daunorubicin is known as DaunoXome, and liposomal doxorubicin is known as Doxil.

Mitoxantrone and etoposide are two other topoisomerase II inhibitors. Etoposide is derived from the American mayapple plant. Mitoxantrone is similar in activity to the anthracyclines but has a dark, ink-like blue color. Table 21.4 lists some of the cancers that these agents are commonly used to treat.

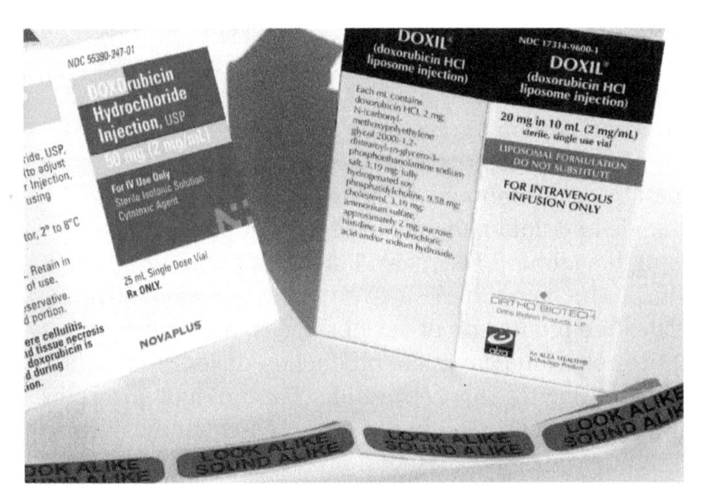

Notice that the strengths for doxorubicin and liposomal doxorubicin are different.

Table 21.5 Chemotherapy Vesicant Drugs

Daunorubicin	Mitomycin
Doxorubicin	Vinblastine
Epirubicin	Vincristine
Idarubicin	Vinorelbine
Mechlorethamine	

Antimicrotubule Agents **Microtubules** are important to cell function. They play a role in maintaining cell shape and structure and are critical elements in the process of cell division or mitosis. **Antimicrotubule agents** interfere with the formation and function of microtubules, ultimately preventing cell growth and division.

Most antimicrotubule drugs are derived from plant sources. **Paclitaxel** and **docetaxel**—the **taxanes**—are derived from the bark and needles of yew trees. **Vincristine**, **vinblastine**, and **vinorelbine**—the **vinca alkaloids**—are derived from periwinkle plants. Antimicrotubule agents are important components in the treatment of lung, breast, ovarian, prostate, and testicular cancers, as well as for some types of leukemia and lymphoma.

Side Effects As plant derivatives, paclitaxel and docetaxel are commonly associated with allergic reactions during drug administration. Patients typically require premedication with antihistamines and corticosteroids to prevent severe allergic reactions to these drugs. Because microtubules also play an important role in nerve function, many antimicrotubule agents cause peripheral neuropathy. Patients must be carefully assessed for this side effect while receiving paclitaxel or vincristine.

Miscellaneous Cytotoxic Drugs Two commonly used chemotherapy drugs that don't fit into the other cytotoxic drug categories are **bleomycin** and **asparaginase**. Bleomycin works by causing cuts or breaks in DNA strands, preventing the process of cell proliferation. It is part of the curative chemotherapy regimens used to treat testicular cancer and Hodgkin's disease (a type of lymphoma). One advantage to bleomycin is that it does not cause bone marrow suppression like other chemotherapy agents do. However, bleomycin can cause a deadly type of lung toxicity, known as pulmonary fibrosis. It is important to track and limit cumulative doses of bleomycin to decrease the risk of pulmonary fibrosis.

Asparaginase is a drug with a very narrow spectrum of activity. Asparaginase is used to treat a common and often curable type of leukemia in children, acute lymphocytic leukemia. Leukemia cells require a large amount of the amino acid asparagine to proliferate. Unlike normal cells, leukemia cells are not able to make asparagine. Asparaginase is an enzyme that breaks down asparagine, depriving leukemia cells of this essential amino acid. Asparaginase products are made from two different bacterial sources. Patients who develop an allergic reaction to one type of asparaginase can often safely switch to the other product.

Hormonal Drug Therapies

Some types of cancer depend on naturally occurring hormones for growth (see Chapter 18 for human sex hormones). Estrogen and progesterone are hormones that frequently stimulate breast tumors. Prostate cancer is often dependent on androgens, such as testosterone, for growth. In tumors that are known to be dependent on specific hormones for proliferation, one treatment strategy is to block the activity of those hormones. When breast cancer is diagnosed on biopsy, tests are run on the tissue to determine whether the tumor has estrogen receptors. **Antiestrogens**, such as tamoxifen, anastrazole, letrozole, and exemestane, are commonly used to treat breast cancer. **Antiandrogens**, such as bicalutamide and flutamide, are used to treat prostate cancer.

Luteinizing hormone releasing hormone (LHRH; also known as gonadotropic-releasing hormone) stimulates the production of both male and female reproductive hormones. LHRH initially stimulates the production of sex hormones, but over time, continuous exposure to LHRH ultimately shuts down the production of sex hormones through a negative feedback loop (see Chapter 18). **Leuprolide** (Lupron) and **goserelin** (Zoladex) are analogs of naturally occurring LHRH. These drugs are frequently given to patients with hormone-sensitive tumors, such as breast and prostate cancers, to eliminate the source of endogenous estrogen, progesterone, and testosterone production.

Targeted Drug Therapies

As scientists have learned more about the biology of cancer, they have identified specific features of certain types of cancer that are critical for tumor cell growth. These critical components have become targets for more sophisticated cancer treatment. **Targeted therapies** are directed at specific molecular entities that are required for tumor cell development, proliferation, and growth. By targeting specific features of tumor cells, these therapies exert fewer effects on normal cells and are usually much better tolerated than are traditional cytotoxic drugs. Table 21.6 outlines some basic categories of targeted therapies.

Some targeted therapies were developed to affect the molecular abnormalities associated with specific tumor types. Many of the **signal transduction inhibitors** fit into this category. **Imatinib** and **dasatinib** were developed to target a specific chromosomal mutation associated with chronic myelogenous leukemia (CML). These drugs have revolutionized the way CML is treated and have been extremely successful in controlling this disease. However, because they work against the specific abnormality associated with CML, imatinib and dasatinib have not been very useful in the treatment of other types of cancer.

A **monoclonal antibody** is an antibody that has been developed from a single type of immune cell that was cloned from a parent cell. These antibodies are directed against a specific marker or antigen on target cells. Monoclonal antibodies are developed from a variety of sources, including mouse, bacterial, and human cell lines. Some of those designed to target specific markers on tumor cells have a limited range of activity.

Trastuzumab is a monoclonal antibody developed to target the HER2/neu receptor commonly found on breast cancer cells, but it does not have as much activity in treating other types of tumors. **Rituximab** targets a specific marker (CD20) on B lymphocytes. Rituximab was developed to treat non-Hodgkin's lymphoma. Because lymphocytes are active in various immunologic diseases, such as rheumatoid arthritis, rituximab has become important in treating many nonmalignant conditions by the same mechanism.

Although some targeted therapies have narrow therapeutic application, many agents have been developed to target a wider variety of cancers. Bevacizumab, an **angiogenesis inhibitor**, has significant anticancer activity in an array of diseases, including breast, lung, colon, and brain cancers. Additionally, bevacizumab seems to enhance the effects of cytotoxic drugs when administered in combination. Cetuximab is a monoclonal antibody that targets a growth factor receptor present on many types of cancer cells. Cetuximab has shown activity in treating head and neck, colon, lung, and pancreatic cancers.

Side Effects Targeted therapies are usually much better tolerated than are traditional cytotoxic drugs, but they are not entirely free of side effects. Many targeted therapies

Table 21.6 Targeted Anticancer Therapy

Category	Anticancer Effect	Examples
Signal transduction inhibitors	Prevent transmission of intracellular signals that stimulate cell proliferation	Dasatinib (Sprycel) Erlotinib (Tarceva) Imatinib (Gleevec) Sunitinib (Sutent)
Angiogenesis inhibitors	Prevent formation of blood vessels that allow for tumor growth and invasion of surrounding tissue	Bevacizumab (Avastin) Thalidomide (Thalomid)
Monoclonal antibodies	Are directed at a specific marker or receptor on the surface of tumor cells, leading to destruction of those cells	Cetuximab (Erbitux) Panitumumab (Vectibix) Rituximab (Rituxan) Trastuzumab (Herceptin)

cause acne-like skin reactions. Sometimes, the rash from targeted therapies is a sign that the treatment is working. For example, patients who develop a rash while receiving cetuximab generally have a better response to treatment than those who do not develop a rash. These rashes can usually be managed with topical creams and antibiotic gels. On some occasions, the rash may be so severe that treatment must be stopped.

Monoclonal antibodies are frequently derived from animal sources and for that reason can cause allergic reactions. Reactions, such as fever, chills, and flushing, occur most commonly during administration. Infusion reactions with rituximab and cetuximab can be prevented by premedicating patients with acetaminophen, diphenhydramine, and sometimes corticosteroids. More serious allergic reactions, such as anaphylactic shock, necessitate a change in therapy.

Although most side effects associated with targeted therapies are less severe and more manageable than those seen with cytotoxic drugs, some of these drugs can cause very serious reactions. Bevacizumab has the potential to interfere with blood vessel formation. It can prevent wound healing and must not be given to patients within four weeks of a surgical procedure. Bevacizumab may also *cause* bleeding, such as gastrointestinal bleeding, nose bleeding, and central nervous system bleeding. Patients must be carefully monitored for bleeding and treatment stopped if symptoms develop. Bevacizumab can also cause high blood pressure and kidney damage, so blood pressure and urine samples must be evaluated prior to treatment.

Because targeted therapies are relatively new agents in the armamentarium of cancer-fighting drugs, oncologists are still learning about them. Despite the fact that they have some serious and unusual side effects, targeted therapies typically offer patients a much more direct treatment for their cancer, with fewer side effects than accompany traditional cytotoxic drugs. Targeted therapies are the wave of the future in anticancer treatment.

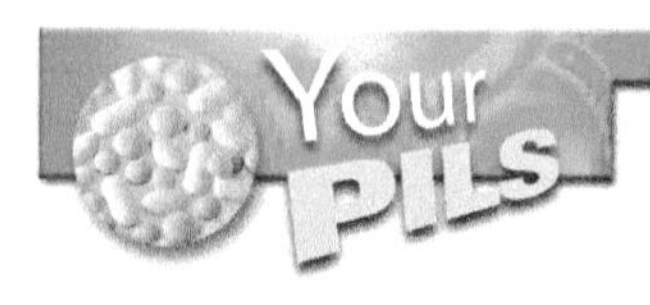

No matter your preferred learning style, you may find it useful to approach learning chemotherapy drugs from the patient's point of view. Start with a list of the common types of cancer (such as breast, prostate, colon, and lung). For each type, list the chemotherapy, hormonal, and targeted drug therapies mentioned in this chapter. Last, for each drug, add a chart entry on the potential side effects that a patient with that type of cancer may face. Completing such a chart not only helps you remember the drugs, their uses, and their adverse effects, it also puts into perspective the choices patients with cancer have before them. Imagine that you are the patient and think about the choices you would make and the adverse effects you would face if given each therapy.

Preparing and Handling Cytotoxic Drugs

The potential consequences of long-term exposure to cytotoxic drugs require special precautions in the handling, preparation, and administration of these agents. The compounding of oral or injectable hazardous drugs must be done in either a **Class II Biological Safety Cabinet (BSC)** or a **Compounding Aseptic Containment Isolator (CACI** or **glove box)** for product, personal, and environmental protection. Because this protection is very technique-dependent, it is crucial to adhere to strict aseptic and negative pressure techniques as well as regulations for wearing personal protective equipment (PPE). An additional form of protection is the **Closed System Transfer Device (CSTD)**. This is a vial-transfer system that allows no venting or exposure of hazardous substances to the environment. It is used inside a BSC or a CACI as added protection.

All unused hazardous drugs—such as expired tablets, capsules, and suspensions; vials with pourable amounts of drug left in them; prepared chemotherapy IV bags; or syringes that are no longer needed—must be disposed of as bulk chemotherapy waste, which requires special handling to prevent environmental contamination.

For more detailed information, refer to the Web site for the American Society of Health-System Pharmacists (ASHP) for their publication *Guidelines on Handling Hazardous Drugs*.

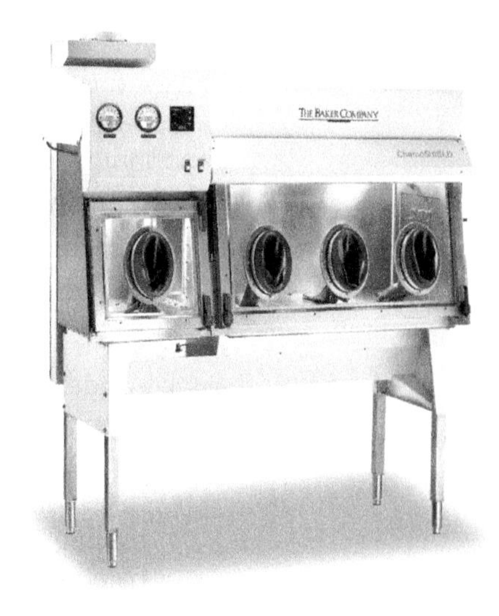

A Contained Aseptic Compounding Isolator (CACI) provides additional protection from hazardous drug exposure, for both the user and the environment, while ensuring a clean, aseptically prepared product.

Personal Protective Equipment

Personal protective equipment (PPE) should be used at all times when handling hazardous drugs, both oral and injectable. PPE protects the handler from being exposed to hazardous drugs or their residue (if left on the outside of vials or bottles). PPE also serves as product protection by keeping contaminants, such as lint or bacteria from the skin of the handler, away from the compound.

PPE includes:

- gloves that meet the American Society for Testing and Materials (ASTM) standard for resistance to chemotherapy drugs
- disposable, impermeable gowns with long sleeves, a closed front, and knit cuffs made of lint-free, polyethylene-coated polypropylene
- shoe covers
- hair cover
- respirator and safety goggles or glasses used during spill cleanup

Situations in which PPE should be used include:

- performing inventory control measures, such as unpacking a drug order
- assembling hazardous drugs for compounding
- compounding or cleaning up hazardous drugs, even when such takes place inside a BSC or a CACI with fixed gloves
- cleaning up spills inside or outside a BSC or a CACI

All PPE must be discarded as chemotherapy waste because it may be contaminated.

Aseptic and Negative Pressure Techniques

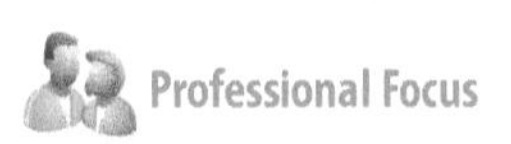

Professional Focus

When compounding hazardous drugs, you will first create a slight vacuum in the vial by pulling back on the plunger of the syringe to remove air from the vial. You can then exchange small amounts of diluent and air until all diluent is in the vial. Before removing the needle from the stopper, clear all drug from the needle and hub of the syringe by pulling back on the plunger while the needle is not submerged in the drug.

When compounding any IV preparation, it is very important to use proper **aseptic technique** to keep the product from being contaminated and harming the patient, the end user. In a laminar airflow workbench, to protect the product from contamination in a horizontal direction, the HEPA-filtered air blows across the work surface toward the technician.

When compounding hazardous preparations, however, care must also be taken to protect the technician and the environment. This protection is accomplished by using either a BSC or a CACI with a vertical airflow hood. The vertical airflow hood ensures that any potentially contaminated air exits the work chamber on the bottom and is first filtered through a HEPA filter before it is reintroduced to the work area or is exhausted outside. The vertical airflow makes it necessary to use a different technique in aseptic compounding to avoid blocking air coming from the top of the BSC or the CACI.

Attention must also be paid to the pressure in the vial when compounding hazardous drugs. **Positive pressure** (excess pressure inside a vial) may cause a drug to spray around the needle of the syringe when it is inserted into the vial, through the needle hole in the rubber stopper, or through a loose seal. A slight **negative pressure** (vacuum inside the vial) prevents such spraying or leaking. Too much negative pressure, however, could cause leakage from the needle when it is withdrawn from the vial. To create negative pressure in the vial, air is withdrawn from it. The size of the syringe is important. A syringe should never be filled to more than three-quarters of its capacity, in order to minimize the risk of the plunger separating from the barrel.

Handling Spills/Exposures

Pharmacy technicians working with hazardous drugs should be trained to clean up small **accidental spills** to reduce exposure to hazardous drugs. Four methods of possible accidental exposure to hazardous drugs are:

- inhalation
- ingestion (eating or drinking where hazardous drugs are stored or prepared; placing food on contaminated surfaces; touching food or mouth with contaminated hands)
- injection
- topical absorption (via skin and eyes)

Accidental spills, such as powder or liquid spillage from broken vials or leaking IV bags, can be sources of exposure in the pharmacy.

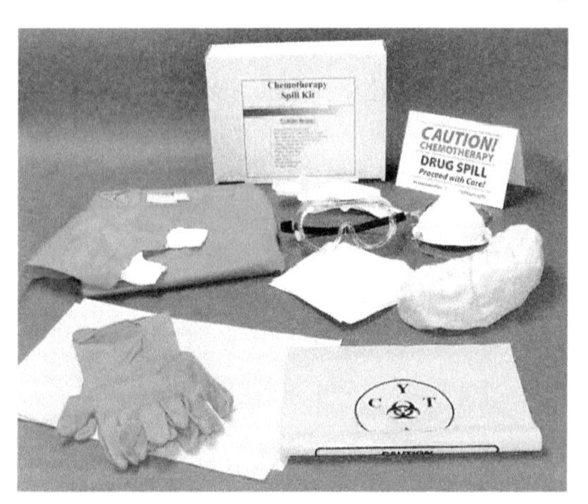

Chemotherapy spill kits should be kept in areas where chemotherapy drugs are prepared and administered. They should contain PPE such as gowns, gloves, goggles or safety glasses, and an N-95 disposable respirator; as well as disposable towels, absorbent pads, warning sign(s), and disposable bags.

Spill kits should be available in all areas where hazardous drugs are prepared, administered, or transported. All cleanup supplies must be placed in sealed plastic bags and disposed of as bulk chemotherapy waste. Large spills may need to be cleaned up by the hazardous materials (Hazmat) team.

The best source for information about hazardous drugs is the **Material Safety Data Sheet (MSDS).** MSDSs are available from manufacturers for all potentially hazardous drugs and chemical products. These sheets provide detailed information about the storage, handling, and cleanup of hazardous drug products. There are a variety of Internet resources for obtaining MSDSs for pharmaceutical products. Pharmacies handling hazardous drugs such as chemotherapy agents should keep a copy of the MSDS on file or have an established Internet link for each product they carry so that easy reference is possible when needed.

Contaminated clothing should be disposed of as bulk chemotherapy waste, and exposed skin should be thoroughly washed with soap and water. Every accidental exposure to hazardous drugs should be evaluated by a physician.

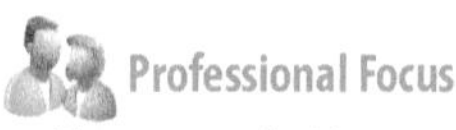

Professional Focus

Pharmacy technicians are often in charge of ordering and assembling equipment for spill kits, which should contain the items listed in the above photo. You may also be in charge of obtaining and filing MSDSs in the pharmacy.

Special Preparations

Many hazardous drugs require special handling during preparation or administration. Some medications are sensitive to light (e.g., cisplatin, doxorubicin) or need to be refrigerated (e.g., busulfan, dacarbazine) to extend their stability. Others break down plastic (e.g., etoposide, paclitaxel) or get absorbed by plastic (PVC or DEHP-containing) IV bags (e.g., carmustine), making it necessary to use special equipment such as non-PVC- or DEHP-free IV bags and tubing. Some drugs require filters in the infusion tubing (e.g., paclitaxel). Special care must be given to issues of compatibility and precipitation of drugs at certain concentrations and temperatures (e.g., etoposide, fluorouracil) as well as to special requirements in the choice of diluent for reconstitution and final dilution. Manufacturer and/or institutional guidelines must be strictly adhered to in preparing these products.

Oral product compounding is another area that requires special precautions. Pharmacy technicians need to be aware that the same rules for PPE that apply to IV product

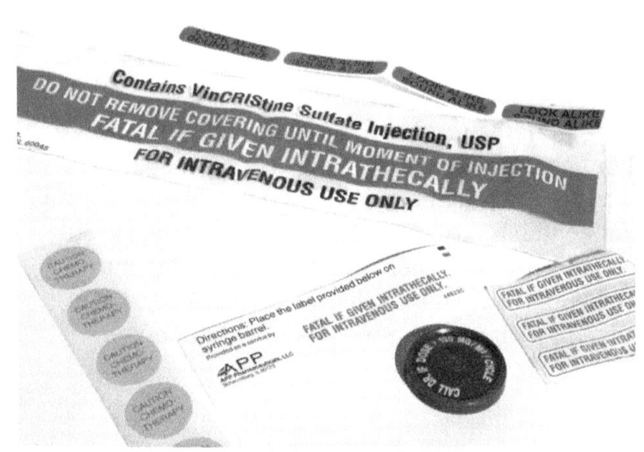

Vincristine and vinblastine can be fatal if given by the IT route. These medications come with an overwrap and a special warning label that *must* be used when dispensing these products to help prevent inadvertent IT administration.

compounding also apply to oral product compounding. Gloves, gowns, shoe covers, and respirators should be worn to protect individuals from exposure to hazardous drugs. Proper ventilation is also important. Compounding in a BSC or a CACI to prevent contaminating the environment is a good practice. Compounding includes activities such as breaking and crushing tablets or emptying capsules and mixing them with a base solution for administration in liquid form (e.g., for infants or patients with feeding tubes).

Special precautions need to be given to preparations of hazardous drugs administered **intrathecally (IT)**, via lumbar puncture into a special device called an Ommaya reservoir. IT administration delivers chemotherapy directly into the cerebrospinal fluid (CSF), the fluid that surrounds the brain and spinal cord. There are only a few drugs used for this type of injection, including methotrexate, cytarabine, and hydrocortisone. Because these drugs go directly into the CSF, caution must be taken to ensure that no preservatives are used in either the drug or diluent. Preservatives administered into the CSF can cause serious side effects, such as seizures and chemical irritation of the membranes that enclose the CSF. Filters are also used for the preparation of IT medications to eliminate any particulate matter. Fastidious use of aseptic technique is critical to minimize the risk of potential introduction of bacteria into the CSF. Special precautions are used so that the drugs intended for IV administration are not confused with drugs intended for IT administration. Such measures may include administering IT medications only in certain locations of the hospital or by specific, authorized personnel. Inadvertently giving vincristine or other medications by the IT route could be fatal to the patient.

Preventing Chemotherapy-Related Medication Errors

Pharmacy technicians play a vital role in preventing chemotherapy-related medication errors. They are responsible for drug inventory and medication storage. It is important to implement measures to prevent inadvertent drug and product mix-ups, especially in cases where the names sound or look similar or the packaging is similar. The acronym **SALAD** (i.e., **sound-alike, look-alike drugs**) is used. Care should be taken not to get these drugs confused accidentally. Examples of measures that prevent SALAD errors are:

- not storing SALADs next to each other
- drawing attention to the fact that there is another product with a similar name or appearance by applying sound-alike/look-alike stickers (e.g., for doxorubicin and liposomal doxorubicin [Doxil]).
- using colored and/or lidded storage bins
- noticing tall-man lettering on the labels (example: CISplatin vs. CARBOplatin, vinCRIStine vs. vinBLAStine) where differing parts of two similar words are emphasized in capital letters

Pharmacy technicians can help prevent multiple types of errors, including:

- errors in calculations: by double-checking every calculation and verifying that the correct concentration of the drug on hand was chosen
- errors in pharmacist order entry: by comparing the final product label to the original physician order for verification of drug, dose, administration schedule, route, and duration of therapy
- errors in dosing: by ensuring adherence to specific manufacturer-provided drug warnings (e.g., by questioning orders for cisplatin that exceed the maximum dose for an entire cycle as specified by the manufacturer on every vial as 100 mg/m^2)

- errors in administration route: by using a syringe overwrap (provided by the manufacturer) for vincristine and vinblastine to draw attention to the fact that giving these drugs by the IT route is lethal for the patient.

Overall, you should maintain a clean and organized work environment to avoid chemotherapy medication errors and unnecessary contamination. In a cluttered workplace, it is all too easy to accidentally mix the wrong base solution with the wrong drug, draw up the wrong dose, or inadvertently attach the wrong label to the finished product. Technicians need to ensure that there is no confusion about what is being mixed and which drug and concentration are being used. Ultimately, the pharmacist relies on the technician to complete compounding in a manner that results in a product that meets acceptable standards and is safe.

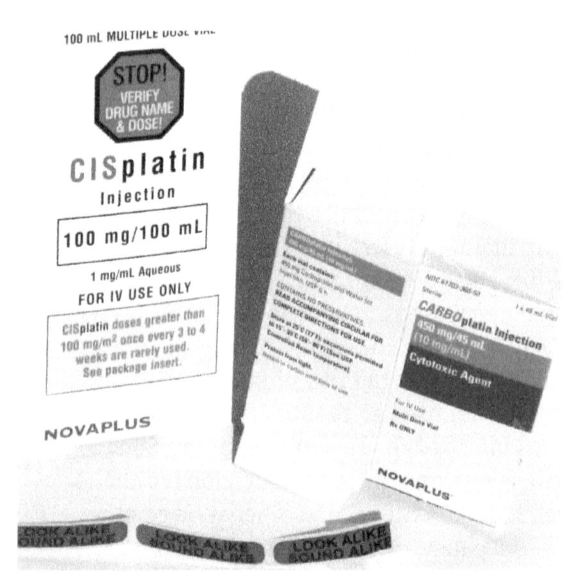

Cisplatin and carboplatin are look-alike, sound-alike drugs.

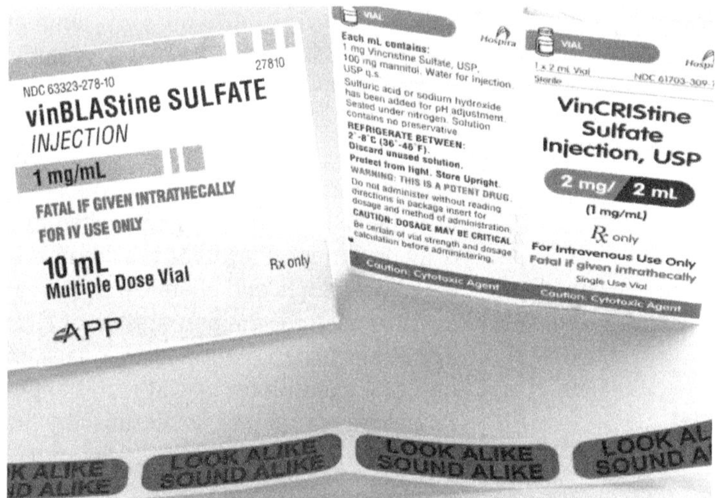

Tall-man lettering on the label of vinBLAStine and vinCRIStine is used to emphasize the difference in these similar drug names.

Chapter Summary

Cancer is a group of very complex and potentially fatal diseases. Treating cancer involves aggressive and rigorous therapy within multiple modalities, including surgery, radiation, and drug therapy. Chemotherapy drugs are a complicated group of medications with a narrow window between safe, therapeutic use and potential for great toxicity. Traditional cytotoxic agents are potent cancer-fighting drugs, but their spectrum of activity is not limited specifically to tumor cells. As a result, these drugs cause a lot of toxicities to normal tissue and put patients at risk for serious complications from treatment, including infection, organ failure, and death. Targeted drug therapies offer patients newer and smarter approaches to more selectively aim anticancer treatment specifically at tumor cells. Although targeted therapies are generally safer and better tolerated, these agents are not completely free of side effects and still pose a risk for serious side effects.

Chemotherapy agents have historically been administered to patients only in specialized inpatient or outpatient infusion settings. With the introduction of orally administered chemotherapy drugs, cancer treatment is expanding into community settings. This expansion increases the likelihood that technicians will handle these agents at some time in their careers. Because of potential harm resulting from personal, institutional, and environmental exposure to chemotherapy products, it is important that all pharmacy technicians have a basic understanding of these complex drugs and the unique issues associated with them.

Chapter Review

For the following sets of exercises, write the exercise heading, exercise numbers, and your answers on a separate sheet of paper. Your instructor may direct you to turn in the sheet of paper or discuss your answers as a class.

REVIEW THE BASICS

Circle a, b, c, d, or e as the correct answer to each multiple-choice question.

1. Heart failure is a serious toxicity of which drug?
   a. vincristine
   b. doxorubicin
   c. bleomycin
   d. etoposide
2. Which of the following best describes the treatment goal of palliative chemotherapy?
   a. chemotherapy given to cure a patient's disease
   b. chemotherapy given after surgery to eliminate residual disease
   c. chemotherapy given to decrease the size of a tumor to make it surgically removable
   d. chemotherapy given with the intention of decreasing symptoms
3. The acronym SALAD is used to describe which of the following?
   a. drug names that look alike and might be mistaken for each other
   b. drug names that sound alike and might be mistaken for each other
   c. toxic chemotherapy agents
   d. lettuce, cucumbers, and tomatoes mixed with balsamic vinaigrette
   e. both a and b
4. Which of the following drugs must *never* be administered by the IT route?
   a. methotrexate
   b. vincristine
   c. cytarabine
   d. hydrocortisone
5. Which of the following chemotherapy drugs does *not* cause bone marrow suppression as a common side effect?
   a. cyclophosphamide
   b. doxorubicin
   c. bleomycin
   d. topotecan
6. Which of the following scenarios requires preparation with proper PPE?
   a. preparation of hydroxyurea oral suspension for administration through a feeding tube
   b. cleanup of a chemotherapy spill in the BSC
   c. cleanup of a chemotherapy spill in a nursing unit
   d. reshelving deliveries of cytotoxic drugs
   e. all of the above
7. Which of the following is an example of an antimetabolite drug?
   a. cytarabine
   b. irinotecan
   c. paclitaxel
   d. vincristine
8. Which of the following chemotherapy agents comes in oral dosage forms?
   a. capecitabine
   b. cytarabine
   c. vincristine
   d. leuprolide
9. Which of the following best describes the rationale for giving sodium bicarbonate to patients receiving high-dose methotrexate?
   a. to help prevent mucositis
   b. to help prevent kidney damage
   c. to help prevent bone marrow suppression
   d. to help prevent diarrhea
10. Which of the following is appropriate in the preparation/handling of cytotoxic drugs?
    a. use of negative-pressure technique when withdrawing drug from vials
    b. preparation in a laminar airflow workbench
    c. use of a surgical mask to minimize drug inhalation
    d. filling syringes to full capacity to minimize waste

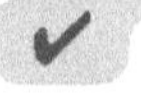

KNOW THE DRUGS

Match each brand name drug with its corresponding generic name and most common use. Your answers should follow this example format: Generic Name: 1. a; 2. b; 3. c; etc. Most Common Use: 1. h; 2. i; 3. j; etc.

Brand Name	Generic Name	Most Common Use
1. Xeloda	a. imatinib	h. brain tumors, melanoma
2. Sutent	b. erlotinib	i. breast cancer, immune system diseases
3. Sprycel	c. temozolomide	j. kidney cancer
4. Gleevec	d. cyclophosphamide	k. breast cancer, colon cancer
5. Tarceva	e. sunitinib	l. chronic myelogenous leukemia
6. Temodar	f. capecitabine	m. lung cancer
7. Cytoxan	g. dasatinib	

PUT IT TOGETHER

For each item, write down either true or false, or a single term to complete the sentence.

1. True or False: Cancer is the leading cause of death in the United States.
2. True or False: Pharmacy technicians who work in community practice settings will never encounter chemotherapy drugs.
3. ________________ is known as the tumor suppressor gene.
4. True or False: Traditional chemotherapy drugs exert their effects only on tumor cells.
5. ________________ is an anthracycline drug.
6. ________________ is a drug that "rescues" normal cells from methotrexate toxicities.
7. ________________ is the enzyme responsible for creating and repairing breaks in DNA during cell replication.
8. True or False: Some chemotherapy drugs are absorbed through the skin.

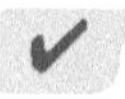

THINK IT THROUGH

Read and think through each numbered scenario carefully and then write several sentences in reply to the question(s) presented. Question 4 requires you to do some Internet research before completing your answer(s).

1. You are excited about your new job and responsibilities as a chemotherapy technician at a large cancer center. You are talking up your position to your friends over dinner. One of your friends stops you cold with, "I can't believe you are going to work with chemotherapy. You can get cancer just from handling those drugs. You should quit that job for a safer one." How would you respond?
2. You have a job in a community pharmacy. A customer comes in asking for something for his hands. His palms are very red and the skin is peeling. He says that the bottoms of his feet are even worse. You ask about any medications he is taking, and he says he is on Xeloda, for colon cancer. How should this patient be advised?
3. You are mixing chemotherapy in a large teaching hospital. The pharmacist hands you a profile and label for cisplatin 200 mg. When you read the order and the label, you realize that the order is written for cisplatin 200 mg/day IV infusion over 24 hours, daily for 4 days. This patient has a body surface area of 2 m^2. The cisplatin vial says that the maximum dose of cisplatin is 100 mg/m^2 *per cycle*. What should you do?

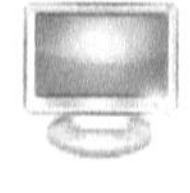

4. **On the Internet,** you can find many resources available to help look up standard chemotherapy regimens and dosing. Find a Web site by searching with the key term "chemoregimens" and review some of the commonly used cancer chemotherapy treatment regimens, based on the type of cancer being treated. Take extra time to familiarize yourself with the regimens for breast, prostate, and lung cancer, which are widely publicized and generate many questions. What are the treatment options? How might you use such Web sites as resources for yourself or pharmacy patients with questions about cancer treatment?

Appendices

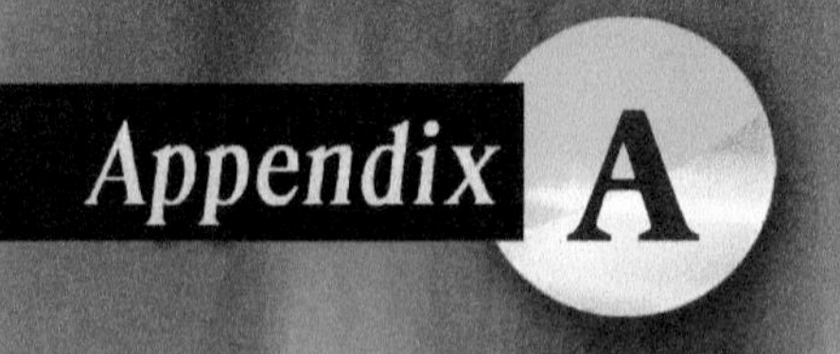

Appendix A The Pharmacists' Inventory of Learning Styles (PILS) Assessment

If you are interested in reading the full article on learning styles for pharmacy professionals, by Zubin Austin, from which this appendix information comes, check with your instructor or search the Web on your own using the following complete citation:

American Journal of Pharmaceutical Education 2004; 68 (2) Article 37. "Development and Validation of the Pharmacists' Inventory of Learning Styles (PILS)," by Zubin Austin, Associate Professor, PhD, MBA, MIS, BScPharm.

Think about a few recent situations where you had to learn something new to solve a problem. This could be any kind of situation: while you were taking a course at school, learning to use new software, or figuring out how to assemble a barbecue.

Now, circle the letter in the column that best characterizes what works best for you in situations like the one you've thought about.

When I'm trying to learn something new...	Usually	Some-times	Rarely	Hardly
1. I like to watch others before trying it for myself.	B	D	C	A
2. I like to consult a manual, textbook, or instruction guide first.	B	C	D	A
3. I like to work by myself, rather than with other people.	A	C	B	D
4. I like to take notes, or write things down as I'm going along.	B	C	D	A
5. I'm critical of myself if things don't work out as I hoped.	B	C	D	A
6. I usually compare myself to other people just so I know I'm keeping up.	B	D	C	A
7. I like to examine things closely instead of jumping right in.	B	D	C	A
8. I rise to the occasion if I'm under pressure.	C	A	B	D
9. I like to have plenty of time to think about something new before trying it.	D	B	C	A
10. I pay a lot of attention to the details.	B	C	A	D
11. I concentrate on improving the things I did wrong in the past.	C	A	D	B
12. I focus on reinforcing the things I got right in the past.	B	D	A	C
13. I like to please the person teaching me.	D	B	A	C
14. I trust my hunches.	D	C	A	B
15. In a group, I'm usually the first one to finish whatever we're doing.	A	C	D	B
16. I like to take charge of a situation.	C	A	B	D
17. I'm well organized.	B	A	C	D

Now, add up the number of times you circled each letter:

A = **B =** **C =** **D =**

Your DOMINANT learning style is the letter you circled most frequently. On this blank line, write the letter and its corresponding title from the following definitions:

____

Your SECONDARY learning style is the next most-frequently circled letter. On this blank line, write the letter and its corresponding title from the following definitions:

____

A = Enactor

You enjoy dealing directly with people, and have little time or patience for indirect or soft-sell jobs. You enjoy looking for, and exploiting, opportunities as they arrive, and have an entrepreneurial spirit. You learn best in a hands-on, unencumbered manner, not in a traditional lecture-style format. Though you don't take any particular pleasure in leading others, you do so because you sense you are best-suited for the job. You are confident, have strong opinions, and value efficiency. You are concerned about time, and like to see a job get done. Sometimes, however, your concern with efficiency means the quality of your work may suffer, and that you may not be paying as much attention to others' feelings and desires as you ought to.

B = Producer

You generally prefer working by yourself, at your own pace, and in your own time, or with a very small group of like-minded people. You tend to avoid situations where you are the center of attention, or you are constantly being watched—you prefer to be the one observing (and learning) from others. You have an ability to learn from your own—and other peoples'—mistakes. You place a high priority on getting things done properly, according to the rules, but at times, you can be your own worst critic. You value organization, and attentiveness to detail.

C = Director

You are focused, practical, and to the point. You usually find yourself in a leadership role, and enjoy this challenge. You have little time or patience for those who dither or are indecisive, or who spend too much time on impractical, theoretical matters. You are good at coming to quick, decisive conclusions, but recognize that at times your speed may result in less than perfect results. You would rather get a good job done on time, than get an excellent job delivered late. You like being in a high-performance, high-energy, fast-paced environment.

D = Creator

You enjoy out-of-the-box environments where time and resources are not particularly constrained. You have a flair for keeping others entertained and engaged, and sincerely believe this is the way to motivate others and get the best out of everyone. You are most concerned—sometimes too concerned—about how others perceive you, and you place a high priority on harmony. You find little difficulty dealing with complex, ambiguous, theoretical situations (provided there is not a lot of pressure to perform), but sometimes have a hard time dealing with the practical, day-to-day issues.

Your instructor may have you consider the five questions below and work in small groups based on your and your classmates' learning styles to discuss your answers.

Now, as a group of individuals with the same dominant learning style, think about the following questions and share your opinions:

1. What professional, social, or personal characteristics do you have in common?
2. What teaching and learning methods work best for you?
3. What teaching and learning methods do not work well for you?
4. Give some examples of the type of feedback that motivates you.
5. Give some examples of the type of feedback that discourages you.

Now, share your group's discussion with members of the other learning styles' groups.

Appendix B Look-Alike and Sound-Alike Drug Names

Although manufacturers have an obligation to review new trademarks for error potential before use, there are some things that prescribers, pharmacists, and pharmacy technicians can do to help prevent errors with products that have look- or sound-alike names. The following recommendations are designed to prevent dispensing errors and are based on recommendations from the Institute for Safe Medication Practices (ISMP). As new drugs come to market each year, the list of recognized look-alike, sound-alike drug names grows. For a complete and current listing of look-alike, sound-alike medications, please go to the ISMP Web site and search for that list.

- **Use electronic prescribing** to prevent confusion with handwritten drug names.
- **Encourage physicians to write prescriptions that clearly specify the dosage form, drug strength, and complete directions.** They should include the product's indication on all outpatient prescriptions and on inpatient *prn* orders. With name pairs known to be problematic, reduce the potential for confusion by writing prescriptions using both the brand and generic name. Listing both names on medication administration records and automated dispensing cabinet computer screens also may be helpful.
- **Whenever possible, determine the purpose of the medication** before dispensing or administering it. Many products with look-alike or sound-alike names are used for different purposes.
- **Accept verbal or telephone orders only when truly necessary.** Require staff to read back all orders, spell product names, and state their indication. Like medication names, numbers can sound alike, so staff should read the dosage back in numerals (e.g., "one five" for 15 mg) to ensure clear interpretation of dose.
- **When feasible, use magnifying lenses and copyholders under good lighting** to keep prescriptions and orders at eye level during transcription to improve the likelihood of proper interpretation of look-alike product names.
- **Change the appearance of look-alike product names** on computer screens, pharmacy and nursing unit shelf labels and bins (including automated dispensing cabinets), pharmacy product labels and medication administration records by highlighting—through boldface, color, and/or tall-man letters—the parts of the names that are different (e.g., hydr**OXY**zine, hydr**ALA**zine).
- **Install a computerized reminder** (also placed on automated dispensing cabinet screens) for the most serious confusing name pairs so that an alert is generated when entering prescriptions for either drug. If possible, make the reminder auditory as well as visual.
- **Affix "name alert" stickers** in areas where look-alike or sound-alike products are stored (available from pharmacy label manufacturers).
- **Store products with look-alike or sound-alike names in different locations.** Avoid storing both products in the fast-mover area. Use a shelf sticker to help locate the product that is moved.
- **Continue to employ an independent check in the dispensing process** (one person interprets and enters the prescription into the computer, and another reviews the printed label against the original prescription and the product).
- **Open the prescription bottle or the unit dose package in front of the patient** to confirm the expected product appearance and review the indication. Caution patients about error potential when taking products that have a look-alike or sound-alike counterpart. Take the time to fully investigate the situation if a patient states that he or she is taking an unknown medication.

- **Monitor reported errors caused by look-alike and sound-alike medication names**, and alert staff to mistakes.
- **Look for the possibility of name confusion when a new product is added to the formulary.** Have a few clinicians handwrite the product name and directions as they would appear in a typical order. Ask frontline nurses, pharmacists, technicians, unit secretaries, and physicians to view the samples of the written product name, as well as to pronounce it, to determine whether it looks or sounds like any other drug product or medical term. It may be helpful to have clinicians first look at the scripted product name to determine how they would interpret it before the actual product name is provided to them for pronunciation. Once the product name is known, clinicians may be less likely to see more familiar product names in the written samples. If the potential for confusion with other products is identified, then take steps to avoid errors as listed below.
- **Encourage reporting of errors and potentially hazardous conditions** with look-alike and sound-alike product names, and use the information to establish priorities for error reduction. Also maintain awareness of problematic product names and error prevention recommendations provided by the ISMP (and also listed on the quarterly *Action Agenda*), FDA, and USP.
- **Review periodically for the look-alike and sound-alike drug name pairs in use at your practice location**. Decide what actions might be warranted to prevent medication errors. Stay current with alerts from the ISMP, FDA, and USP in case new problematic name pairs emerge. Note that many sound-alike medications are indeed the same medication but in a different dosage form or drug delivery system (i.e., Metformin, Metformin XL).

Generic and Brand Name Drugs Index

*Page numbers with *f.* indicate figures; with *p.*, photographs, and with *t.*, tables.

A

D

R

S

T

Subject Index

*Page numbers with *f.* indicate figures; with *p.*, photographs, and with *t.*, tables.

B

D

I

N

Q

R

T